AF333888

GAIT DISORDERS OF AGING

FALLS AND THERAPEUTIC STRATEGIES

GAIT DISORDERS OF AGING

FALLS AND THERAPEUTIC STRATEGIES

Editors

Joseph C. Masdeu, M.D., Ph.D.
Professor and Chairman
Department of Neurology
New York Medical College
Munger Pavilion
Valhalla, New York

Lewis Sudarsky, M.D.
Assistant Professor
Department of Neurology
Harvard Medical School
Boston, Massachusetts

Leslie Wolfson, M.D.
Professor and Chairman
Department of Neurology
University of Connecticut
School of Medicine
Farmington, Connecticut

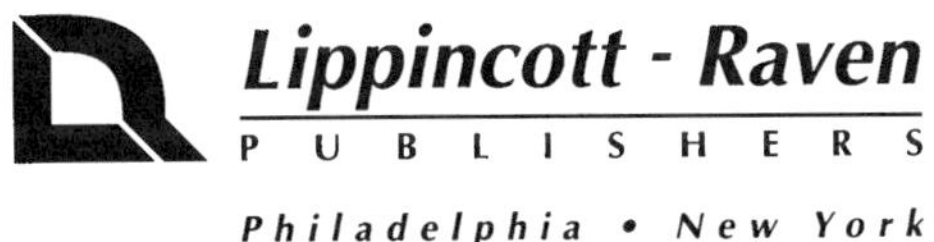

Acquisitions Editor: Nancy Megley
Development Editor: Mattie Bialer
Manufacturing Manager: Dennis Teston
Production Manager: Lawrence Bernstein
Production Editor: Janice Lochansky
Cover Designer: Ed Schultheis
Indexer: Lisa Mullenneaux
Compositor: Americomp
Printer: Maple Press

Printed in the United States of America

9 8 7 6 5 4 3 2 1

Library of Congress Cataloging-in-Publication Data
Gait disorders of aging : falls and therapeutic strategies / [edited
   by] Joseph C. Masdeu, Lewis Sudarsky, Leslie Wolfson.
      p.   cm.
   Includes bibliographical references and index.
   ISBN 0-316-54915-0
   1. Gait disorders in old age.   2. Falls (Accidents) in old age.   I. Masdeu, Joseph C.
II. Sudarsky, Lewis.   III. Wolfson, Leslie.   [DNLM: 1. Gait—in old age.   2. Movement
Disorders—in old age.   3. Accidental Falls—in old age.   4. Equilibrium—in old age.
5. Posture—in old age.   WE 103 G1437 1997]
RC376.5.G34   1997
618.97'683—dc21
DNLM/DLC
for Library of Congress   97-4217
                                                                                                    CIP

Contents

Contributors vii

Foreword xi

Preface xiii

1. Gait and Balance Impairment: An Overview 1
    Lewis Sudarsky, Joseph C. Masdeu, and Leslie Wolfson

2. Falls in the Elderly: Risk Factors and Prevention 13
    Michael C. Nevitt

3. Physiology of Balance, with Special Reference to the Healthy Elderly . . . 37
    Lewis M. Nashner

4. Neurophysiology of Locomotion: Recent Advances in the Study
    of Locomotion 55
    Shigemi Mori

5. Balance Decrements in Older Persons: Effects of Age and Disease 79
    Leslie Wolfson

6. Changes in Gait with Normal Aging 93
    Rodger J. Elble

7. Clinical and Research Methodology for the Study of Posture
    and Balance 107
    Marjorie H. Woollacott and Anne Shumway-Cook

8. Clinical and Research Methodology for the Study of Gait 123
    Rodger J. Elble

9. Toward a Nosology of Gait Disorders: Descriptive Classification 135
    C. David Marsden and Philip Thompson

10. Clinical Approach to Gait Disorders of Aging: An Overview 147
    Lewis Sudarsky

11. Foot and Ankle Disorders Affecting Gait and Balance 159
    Elly Trepman

12. Cervical Spondylotic Myelopathy 197
    Raj Murali and Joseph C. Masdeu

13. Gait Disorders in Parkinsonism and Other Movement Disorders 209
    Rajesh Pahwa and William C. Koller

14. Cerebrovascular Disorders 221
    Joseph C. Masdeu

15. A Clinical Approach to Symptomatic Hydrocephalus in the Elderly 245
   Neill R. Graff-Radford and John C. Godersky

16. Vestibular and Cerebellar Disorders of Equilibrium and Gait 261
   Hans Christoph Diener and John G. Nutt

17. Peripheral Neuropathy: Disorders of Proprioception 273
   Thomas D. Sabin

18. The Cautious Gait, Fear of Falling, and Psychogenic Gait Disorders ... 283
   Lewis Sudarsky and Rein Tideiksaar

19. Evaluating the Older Person Who Falls.......................... 297
   Mary B. King

20. Interventions to Reduce the Multifactorial Risks for Falling 309
   Laurence Z. Rubenstein and Karen R. Josephson

21. Physical Intervention for Elderly Patients with Gait Disorders 327
   Margaret Schenkman and Cheryl Riegger-Krugh

22. Improving Balance in Older Adults: Identifying the Significant
   Training Stimuli 355
   Robert H. Whipple

23. Resistance Training 381
   James O. Judge

24. Environmental Factors in the Prevention of Falls 395
   Rein Tideiksaar

Appendices

A. The Axial Mobility Exercise Program 415
   Margaret Schenkman

B. Performance-Oriented Environmental Mobility Screen 429
   Rein Tideiksaar

Index 433

Contributors

Hans Cristoph Diener, M.D.
Professor and Chairman
Department of Neurology
University of Essen
Essen FR6
Germany

Rodger J. Elble, M.D., Ph.D.
Professor and Chair
Department of Neurology and the Center for
*   Alzheimer Disease and Related Disorders*
Southern Illinois University School of Medicine
P.O. Box 19230
Springfield, Illinois 62794-9230

John C. Godersky, M.D.
Anchorage Neurosurgical Associates
2841 DeBarr Rd#34
Anchorage, Alaska 99508

Neill R. Graff-Radford, M.B.B.Ch,
M.R.C.P.
Professor and Chairman
Department of Neurology
Mayo Medical School
4500 San Pablo Road
Jacksonville, Florida 32224

Karen R. Josephson, M.P.H.
Senior Health Services Researcher
Geriatric Research Education Clinic Center
VA Medical Center
16111 Plummer Street
Sepulveda, California 91343

James O. Judge, M.D.
Assistant Professor of Medicine
University of Connecticut School of Medicine
Director of Geriatrics Associates
University of Connecticut Health Systems
Farmington, Connecticut 06030-5215

Mary B. King, M.D.
Assistant Professor
Department of Medicine
University of Connecticut School of Medicine
Farmington, Connecticut 06030; and
Hartford Hospital Geriatric Program
Hartford Hospital
Hartford, Connecticut 06106

William C. Koller, M.D., Ph.D.
Professor and Chairman
University of Kansas School of Medicine
3901 Rainbow Boulevard
Kansas City, Kansas 66103-7314

C. David Marsden, M.D., Ph.D.
Dean of the Institute of Neurology
Professor of Clinical Neurology
The National Hospital for Neurology and
*   Neurosurgery*
Queen Square
London, WC 1N 3BG
England

Joseph C. Masdeu, M.D., Ph.D.
Professor and Chairman
Department of Neurology
New York Medical College
Valhalla, New York 10595; and
Chairman of Neurology
Saint Vincents Medical Center
New York, New York 10011; and
Westchester County Medical Center
Valhalla, New York 10595; and
Adjunct Professor of Neurology
New York University School of Medicine
New York, New York 10016; and
Visiting Professor of Neurology
Albert Einstein College of Medicine
Bronx, New York 10461

Shigemi Mori, M.D., Ph.D.
Professor
Department of System Neurophysiology
National Institute for Physiological Sciences
Myodaigi-cho, Okazaki 444
Japan

Raj Murali, M.D.
Chairman
Department of Neurosurgery
St. Vincent's Hospital and Medical Center
153 West 11th Street
New York, New York 10011; and
Associate Professor of Clinical Neurosurgery
Department of Neurosurgery
New York Medical College
Valhalla, New York 10595

Lewis M. Nashner, Sc.D.
Adjunct Professor
Department of Physiology
Oregon Health Sciences University
Portland, Oregon 97015; and
Adjunct Senior Scientist
R.S. Dow Neurological
*   Sciences Institute*
Good Samaritan Hospital and Medical Center
Portland, Oregon 97015

Michael C. Nevitt, Ph.D., M.P.H.
Assistant Professor
Department of Clinical Epidemiology and
*   Biostatistics*
University of California
San Francisco, California 94105

Rajesh Pahwa, M.D.
Assistant Professor
Department of Neurology
University of Kansas Medical Center
Kansas City, Kansas 66160

Cheryl Riegger-Krugh, Sc.D., P.T.
Assistant Professor
Department of Rehabilitation Medicine
Physical Therapy Program
University of Colorado School of Medicine and
*   Health Sciences Center*
C244 4200 E. Ninth Avenue
Denver, Colorado 80262

Laurence Z. Rubenstein, M.D., M.P.H.
Professor
Department of Medicine
UCLA School of Medicine
Los Angeles, California 90024; and
Director
VA Medical Center
Geriatic Research Education and Clinical Center
16111 Plummer Street
Sepulveda, California 91343

Thomas D. Sabin, M.D.
Professor
Department of Neurology and Psychiatry
Boston University
Boston, Massachusetts 02118; and
Director of Neurology
Boston Medical Center
818 Harrison Avenue
Boston, Massachusetts 02118; and
Lecturer on Neurology
Harvard Medical School
Boston, Massachusetts 02115

Margaret Schenkman, Ph.D., P.T.
Associate Professor
Department of Physical Therapy
Duke University
Durham, North Carolina 27710; and
Senior Fellow Center on Aging
Duke University Medical Center
Durham, North Carolina 27710

Anne Shumway-Cook, Ph.D., P.T.
Clinical Assistant Professor
Department of Rehabilitation Medicine
University of Washington
Seattle, Washington 98195; and
Research Coordinator
Department of Physical Therapy
Northwest Hospital
Seattle, Washington 98133

Lewis Sudarsky, M.D.
Assistant Professor
Department of Neurology
Harvard Medical School
Boston, Massachusetts 02115; and
Assistant Chief
Neurology Service
VA Medical Center
West Roxbury, Massachusetts 02132; and
Associate Physician
Department of Neurology
Brigham and Womens Hospital
Boston, Massachusetts 02115

Rein Tideiksaar, Ph.D.
Director
Department of Geriatrics
Sierra Health Services, Inc.
Las Vegas, Nevada 89114

Philip Thompson
Assistant Professor
Department of Medicine
Royal Adelaide Hospital
Adelaide, South Australia 5000
Australia

Elly Trepman, M.D.
Co-director
Boston Foot and Ankle Center
New England Baptist Hospital
70 Parker Hill Avenue
Boston, Massachusetts 02120

Robert H. Whipple, M.A., P.T.
Assistant Professor
Department of Neurology
University of Connecticut Health Center
B.A.G.E.L.
Farmington, Connecticut 06030

Leslie Wolfson, M.D.
Professor and Chairman
Department of Neurology
University of Connecticut School of Medicine
263 Farmington Avenue
Farmington, Connecticut 06030; and
Chief
Department of Neurology
Hartford Hospital
Hartford, Connecticut 06106

Marjorie Hines Woollacott, Ph.D.
Professor
Department of Exercise and Movement Science
University of Oregon
1525 University Street
Eugene, Oregon 97403

Foreword

Currently, people in the geriatric age range constitute the most rapidly expanding segment of the population in the United States. In this age group, and particularly in those over age 85, neurologic disorders occur frequently. Neurodegenerative diseases are common, particularly Alzheimer's disease and Parkinson's disease. Other frequently encountered neurologic disorders in this group result from cerebrovascular diseases and the effects upon the nervous system of a variety of medical disorders, including cardiovascular disease, osteoporosis, the adverse effects of polypharmacy, trauma, and the difficulties resulting from decreasing vision and hearing.

Gait disorders are extremely common in the geriatric population and have many different etiologies. Although literature on this topic exists, there are few sources of comprehensive information. The present volume, edited by Drs. Masdeu, Sudarsky, and Wolfson, is a welcome contribution. The editors have brought together a group of clinicians who are familiar with the etiology, pathogenesis, clinical manifestations, and treatment of gait disorders. Many of the authors have participated in a special course in the American Academy of Neurology over an extended period. As with the special course, this book presents a multidisciplinary approach dealing with the systems important in coordinated gait, including the sensory pathways and motor components; the clinical and research tools available to evaluate gait and balance; the classification of gait disorders from physiological and descriptive perspectives; and an etiologic classification. The book includes substantial practical information about diagnostic and therapeutic interventions for the various disorders. This book will provide an excellent, up-to-date analysis of the types of gait disturbances that afflict the elderly. It is practically based and should be highly useful to all medical specialists dealing with gait disorders in the elderly, including neurologists, internists, geriatricians, physiatrists, nurses, and physical therapists.

Sid Gilman, M.D.
Professor and Chair
Department of Neurology
University of Michigan Medical Center

Preface

Unsteady gait leading to falls represents a major health problem for the geriatric segment of the population, the fastest expanding age group in the United States. In community surveys, gait abnormalities in people over 65 years of age have a higher prevalence than Alzheimer's disease. Falls from impaired equilibrium are the most common cause of unintentional injury in older people. They are also responsible for 1 in 5 days of restricted activity in the elderly, a higher proportion than for any other health condition. Despite the magnitude of the problem, comprehensive books dealing with this topic are scarce. For this reason, we decided to call on authorities on the different areas concerned with motor control and disorders of gait in older people to cull their knowledge and experience into a single, manageable text.

This book grew out of a course on gait disorders in the elderly at the American Academy of Neurology. Many of the contributors were participants in this course over a six-year period. While the editors are neurologists, we realize that the subject matter of this book requires a multidisciplinary treatment. Internists, geriatricians, neurologists, rehabilitation specialists, physiologists, and biomechanical engineers all deal with these problems from a different perspective. We have tried to craft a book that draws on all these disciplines to consider the problems of mobility in the elderly. We wanted to produce a book that would be useful to someone in clinical practice and also helpful to a researcher planning a clinical investigation. There is a detailed discussion of the basic physiology of postural control and locomotion, as well as a discussion of methodologic issues.

Therapeutic nihilism has often permeated the approach to gait disorders of aging. As a natural corollary of this attitude, professionals caring for older people with motility problems have lacked interest in understanding their causes and differential diagnosis. This book shows that an impaired gait and balance in an older person constitutes a syndrome that has a rich differential diagnosis and for which a treatable cause will be found in about one fourth of the cases, a proportion that compares favorably with the treatment of dementia in the elderly. Even in the case of individuals who still have unidentified causes of gait impairment, physical intervention programs can improve mobility, thereby facilitating activities of daily living and preventing falls.

JCM
LS
LIW

Acknowledgments

The editors wish to thank first the distinguished authors who contributed their expertise to *Gait Disorders of Aging*. We also gratefully acknowledge the contribution of our staff. Specially, we are thankful to the staff of the neurology departments at New York Medical College, St. Vincent's Medical Center, Westchester County Medical Center in New York, Harvard Medical School, West Roxbury V.A. Medical Center, Brigham and Women's Hospital in Boston, the University of Connecticut Medical School, and Hartford Hospital. We also thank our families and appreciate the support they have given us through the countless hours that we have dedicated to this endeavor.

JCM
LS
LIW

GAIT DISORDERS OF AGING

FALLS AND THERAPEUTIC STRATEGIES

1. Gait and Balance Impairment: An Overview

Lewis Sudarsky, Joseph C. Masdeu, and Leslie Wolfson

> In the summer of his seventh year in office, the 67 year old president looked the picture of health. His color was good; his clothes, impeccable as always, fit perfectly; his walk was firm and full of purpose.
>
> —David McCullough, *Truman*

Gait is a distinctive attribute of an individual, one that changes over the life span. Stage actors convey this instinctively; we marvel as they acquire the mannerisms of older characters. In his biography of Harry Truman, McCullough used a comment about gait to impart a physical and emotional vitality to his description of Truman. Indeed, preservation of thinking and walking are among the more distinctive features of successful aging.

This book considers some of the changes in gait and balance associated with aging and age-related disease. Special consideration is given to the problem of falls. Because of the substantial associated morbidity and mortality, there is a growing body of literature about the risk for falls and about prevention strategies.

HISTORICAL ASPECTS

Medical scholarship about gait disorders blossomed in the nineteenth century. Romberg, Gowers, and Charcot contributed to the description of locomotor ataxia in tabetic neurosyphilis. In his *Manual of Nervous Diseases* [1], Romberg describes the imbalance and staggering of a patient with tabes, who "walks with his legs apart; he leaves his heels as long as possible in contact with the ground and keeps his knees bent." Of another case, Romberg [1] writes, "If he is ordered to close his eyes while in the erect posture he at once commences to totter and swing from side to side." Gowers [2] adds the following description: "The patient sways about in the manner of one who has cerebellar disease . . . The early defect in coordination may be discovered by the patient when he walks in the dark or backwards, or, not uncommonly, when he shuts his eyes in the process of washing the face."

Cerebellar ataxia was recognized as distinct from sensory ataxia, principally by virtue of its persistence under visual control [3]. In Charcot's department at the Salpetriere, physical signs were developed to help differentiate cerebellar ataxia from staggering of spinal origin [4]. Friedreich [5] (in 1863) and Marie [6] (in 1892) addressed the problem of cerebellar degeneration in hereditary ataxia. The festinating gait of Parkinson's disease also was described in the nineteenth century [7], though little was known at that time about the contributions of the basal ganglia and cerebellum to the control of movement.

Literature describing the effects of the cerebrum on walking dates back to the turn of the century [8]. Astasia-abasia (discussed in Chapter 19) was described at approximately this time. In 1892, Bruns [9] reported four patients with ataxia and disequilibrium from frontal mass lesions. Inappropriate postural synergies were observed. Bruns' ataxia was attributed to a disorder of frontopontocerebellar connections. In 1901, Petren [10] described five patients with "trepident abasia." He observed start-hesitation, shuffling, and freezing—features typical of a frontal gait disorder. Petren speculated about a psychic element in the incapacity. In 1910, von Malaise [11] described the *marche à petits pas:* short steps, shuffling, and difficulty with initiation. He attributed the condition to multiple lacunar infarcts, a view that is surprisingly current. A concept of the frontal gait disorder as apraxia was advanced by Meyer and Barron and by Denny-Brown [12, 13].

Critchley [14] specifically addressed these various disorders of gait in his review of the neurology of old age. He discussed the progression from cautious gait to marche à petits pas and on to "senile paraplegia." He described a 98-year-old physician who lost his equilibrium and staggered, particularly if he looked up to see which way the wind was blowing. In an influential review of the senile disorders of gait in 1948, Critchley noted "a large group of cases where the gait in old people becomes considerably disordered, although the motor power of the legs is comparably well preserved" [15]. References to senile gait disorder persist in the literature today, though the term is vague and somewhat pejorative in nature. The disturbance of gait described above is nonspecific and by no means restricted to older people. As discussed in Chapter 18, this disturbance is not regarded as a necessary consequence of aging, nor is it a manifestation of senility. As senile gait is not a well-defined clinicopathological entity, the term probably should be abandoned.

SIGNIFICANCE, PREVALENCE, AND MORBIDITY

Gait disorders are common in older persons, although it is difficult to ascertain prevalence as no accepted definition exists. A functional definition of these disorders should include gait that is slow, unsteady, or biomechanically compromised so as to be ergonomically inefficient. In a study of 260 persons older than 60 living in Durham, North Carolina, 15% had some abnormality of gait as defined by standard neurological examination [16]. By age 80, one person in four will use assistive devices to help with ambulation [17]. In a recent survey of 467 older residents of East Boston, Massachusetts, shuffling or turn hesitation was noted in 14% of people age 65 to 74, 29% of those 75 to 84, and 49% of the oldest group, those 85 and older [18]. These data are particularly noteworthy, as this oldest group is the fastest-growing segment of the US population. Prevalence is somewhat higher in a population with more impairments, such as in an acute-care hospital or chronic nursing facility.

Balance difficulties also are common in an aging population, resulting in an increased risk of falls and fall-related injuries. Twenty to thirty percent of healthy older people living independently fall each year. Roughly 25% of these falls result in serious injury, and 5% result in a fracture [19]. Some 200,000 hip fractures occur each year in the United States [20]. Gait disorders contribute measurably to the risk of falls and fall-related injuries, as discussed in Chapters 2 and 20. Accidental injury is the sixth leading cause of death in people older than 65, with falls being the major cause of injury in this age group [21].

The statistics on falls and fall-related injuries understate the real impact of balance and gait impairment on an older population. Many older people voluntarily limit their activity because of concerns about mobility and fear of falling [22]. Because so many seniors live alone, poor ambulation may be a factor for some in electing nursing home placement. Loss of ambulation often is the marker of a downward spiral in health and functional status. Nonambulatory nursing home patients have an increased morbidity and mortality.

GAIT AND BALANCE DISORDERS OF AGING: A MULTIDISCIPLINARY APPROACH

Much is yet to be discovered if gait and balance disorders of aging are to be conquered. These disorders present a unique challenge, because the systems that mediate these important functions are among the most complex in the human body. These systems, discussed in Chapters 3 and 4, include sensory pathways, complex processing by the nervous system and, finally, motor components; their structure and function, in health and disease, fall within the realm of physiologists, biomechanical engineers, neurologists, and rehabilitation specialists. As part of these systems, muscles and joints play a key role in mobility. Indeed, aging-related mobility disorders often have been blamed on arthritis and other common musculoskeletal diseases prevalent in old age [22, 23]. Biomechanics, rheumatology, orthopedics and, particularly, rehabilitation medicine contribute important perspectives to the understanding of musculoskeletal disorders and their treatment. Geriatric medicine and epidemiology have pioneered the study of the impact of falls and mobility disorders on the health of this important and growing segment of the population [24]. To provide a balanced, useful view of the state of the art in this area, input from all the aforementioned disciplines is needed. This book contains contributions by a number of authors, from different disciplines, who have added to the emerging literature on gait and balance disorders of older people.

The advantages of a multidisciplinary approach to the problem of falls are evident when Chapters 19 and 20 are compared. In Chapter 19, Wolfson and King describe how a physician would approach someone who has sustained a fall. On the other hand, multidimensional assessment and treatment of falls is emphasized in Chapter 20. In that chapter, Rubinstein and Josephson acknowledge the research still needed to understand and treat falls. It is obvious that both approaches are needed. The former may be more helpful during evaluation; the latter might be used to plan and implement fall prevention programs and to design studies to better understand the causes of falls and how to remedy them.

BALANCE AND GAIT PHYSIOLOGY

Balance and gait are linked inextricably. To facilitate exposition, their discussions have been separated in Chapters 3 and 4, which address the physiology. Chapter 3 presents a systems approach to the physiology of balance that is very useful for the evaluation of patients with balance disorders and for the design of rehabilitation programs. Chapter 4 describes in detail the current knowledge of the complex circuitry underlying locomotor control. An understanding of these structures facilitates the correlation between patient's symptoms and lesion location(s) and eventually may help to clarify their etiology. Physiological and pharmacological research on the mechanisms of balance and gait rests on the body of knowledge summarized in Chapter 4.

Chapters 3 and 4 highlight the importance of adequate sensorimotor integration for balance and gait. Sensory information (particularly somatosensory, vestibular, and visual) is organized by the nervous system to generate the patterns of muscle contraction required for stance and gait [25]. Earlier approaches to the physiology of balance emphasized the contributions of specific sense organs and reflex responses. By contrast, a systems model considers mobility to be the product of an interaction among a network of component subsystems. By necessity, such a postural control network contains redundant capabilities. Impairment of a single component generally is not enough to cause mobility dysfunction. Likewise, a single lesion in an older person may not cause gait impairment. Typically gait-impaired elderly have sustained damage to several systems involved in mediating balance. An understanding of the underlying system physiology is paramount to design appropriate testing and treatment paradigms.

Based on work in experimental animals, a stepping generator was localized to the spinal cord. While spinal cats can walk on a treadmill, this capacity is regrettably lacking in humans with spinal cord injury. Stepping movements have been observed in humans who have lost supraspinal control; however, patients with spinal transection cannot stand or walk unsupported [26, 27].

Stepping movements of infants differ from the movements performed during gait and are inefficient in supporting the bipedal position [28]. Control centers higher than the spinal cord are critical for station and ambulation in humans. These control centers become integrated as pathway myelination proceeds in the young child. They include (1) the vestibular system, (2) the medullary locomotor region, (3) the pedunculopontine area, and (4) the basal ganglia circuits [29]. Several brain structures, particularly well-developed in humans, make up the basal ganglia loop. The dorsal medial frontal region projects to the putamen, which in turn projects to the globus pallidus. Modulated by the substantia nigra and subthalamic nucleus, the globus pallidus projects to the ventroantero-lateral thalamic nuclei, which in turn project to the dorsomedial frontal region. Axons from the medial frontal region, which project to the brainstem and spinal cord, play a major role in animal and human ambulation. These structures are important for gait and balance, as demonstrated by lesion anatomy in patients with deterioration of gait from stroke or other discrete disease.

AGE-RELATED CHANGES IN BALANCE AND GAIT

To define abnormality, first we need to know how normal, healthy elderly walk and maintain their balance. Chapters 5 and 6 describe the changes in mobility that accompany the last decades of life. Just as sensory systems and motor functions exhibit a modest but measurable decline with age, functional changes in gait and balance also are described in older people. The ability to control a narrow base of support is diminished, and stride is reduced. Conditions challenging balance are more likely to result in a fall. It is always difficult to establish whether any given change is the result of the aging process, with the connotation of irreversibility that this notion entails, or the result of diseases prevalent in older people. Chapters 5 and 6 address this problem, concluding that a large measure of the decline in mobility experienced with aging results not from the aging process itself but from disease. Some of the diseases responsible for mobility disorders are known, but they still account for only a minority of the disease burden found in mobility-impaired elderly.

BALANCE AND GAIT EVALUATION METHODOLOGY

Clinical and research tools to evaluate gait and balance with precision are described in Chapters 7 and 8. Chapter 16 describes testing procedures for the evaluation of patients with vestibulocerebellar impairment. These methods can be used to monitor the progress of a single patient and are essential for purposes of clinical investigation. Many tests are described in detail. All are referenced so that interested readers are able to access the original sources.

CLASSIFICATION AND ETIOLOGY OF GAIT DISORDERS

The classification of gait disorders is discussed in Chapters 9 and 10. Chapter 9 presents a physiological, descriptive approach to the problem, introducing the diversity of disorders of postural control and gait that confronts health care workers who see older patients. The pattern of impairment often leads the clinician to the identification of the relevant anatomy and, from there, the etiology of the problem. Sometimes this is not the case, however, and a phenomenological description is as far as the clinician can go. In these instances, clinical grouping can provide the groundwork for understanding the etiology of these disorders.

Chapter 10 contains an etiological classification for gait disorders. It provides an overview of the subjects discussed in detail in Chapters 11 through 18.

Mobility disorders of aging often are multifactorial. Identifying the causes and correcting the treatable disorders are key therapeutic principles in the approach to older people who have difficulty walking. Chapters 11 through 18 describe the most common etiologies of gait impairment and their treatment. The organization of this section follows a traditional outline. Motor disorders are considered first, from foot and ankle disorders to spinal cord disorders, and on to diseases affecting the brain, such as parkinsonism, vascular disease, and hydrocephalus. Disorders of balance and sensorimotor integration are discussed next, beginning with those involving the vestibular and cerebellar systems and proceeding to those of the peripheral proprioceptive pathways on which equilibrium depends. Finally, there is a review of psychogenic gait disorders and fear of falling, including the cautious gait.

To counteract the diagnostic and therapeutic nihilism that has permeated the field in the past, this section offers an important message: Most patients with gait disturbances can be assigned a diagnosis, and approximately one-fourth have a process that can be reversed by medication or surgery [20]. Many other patients will improve with physical therapy targeted at improving balance and strength. This outcome compares favorably with the yield in the management of dementia, another common problem of older people. Treatment approaches and their outcomes are discussed in detail in this section of the book, first as they relate to specific disorders, then as they relate to specific therapeutic modalities, including physical therapy, and to balance and resistance training.

Foot and Ankle Disorders

Musculoskeletal disorders affecting the foot and ankle are described in Chapter 11. Correction of some of these disorders can greatly improve mobility in older individuals. A delicate interplay of the bones, fat pads, muscles, and ligaments of the foot and ankle provide support for station and ambulation. Each component and its behavior during the gait cycle are described in detail. Foot or ankle diseases can affect gait by limiting joint motion or altering the normal patterns of weight bearing or as the result of muscle weakness. Weight shifting is a common strategy to prevent damage of a weakened structure, such as an inflamed joint. Then, however, weight is placed on other areas of the foot not normally as well suited to bear weight; these therefore may be easily damaged. Secondary changes may occur in adjacent joints and even at the hip if the foot condition is not identified and treated properly. Trauma, degenerative or rheumatoid arthritis or tendonitis, infection, congenital deformities, and tumors are some of the common conditions affecting the foot and ankle directly. Neurogenic disease, causing either a sensory loss that will predispose to repeated trauma or muscle weakness, may result secondarily in foot or ankle deformity and malfunction. Identification of the pathological process is done through a focused history and physical examination, occasionally supported by radiographic studies or magnetic resonance imaging. Each of the deformities affecting the ankle, the subtalar and transverse talar joints, the forefoot, or the toes has a specific treatment, sometimes surgical, often through the use of orthotic devices.

FALL PREVENTION

Impairment of balance and gait often leads to falls in older people. Once a fall has occurred, the clinician is left with two tasks: to address the effects of the fall and to prevent additional falls. Managing the effects of a fall is often a thankless task. The elderly person with a hip fracture from a fall may experience further deterioration of mobility. It is important to intervene when possible to avoid a recurrence. To this end, a careful evaluation of the patient and of the circumstances attending the fall is needed. The evaluation of someone who has fallen is described in detail in Chapter 19.

Fall prevention strategies are most effective if people at risk can be identified before they are injured. Strategies for fall prevention are discussed in Chapter 20. The perspective in Chapter 20, however, is different from that of Chapter 2, which reviews the epidemiology of falls. Chapter 20 examines the specific approaches that have been taken to reduce the multifactorial risks for falling and at the literature on intervention.

The multidimensional assessment explores medical, psychosocial, and functional aspects of the fall, thereby facilitating the development of a treatment plan. The specific components of fall assessment vary depending on the patient population being evaluated (e.g., community-living versus nursing home residents). The fall assessment includes a detailed inquiry into the circumstances of the fall, a physical examination, an evaluation of balance and gait, and an assessment of the subject's functional mobility and physical activity.

In cases in which the fall is due to an obvious acute problem, treatment may be relatively simple, direct, and effective (e.g., discontinuing medication that causes postural hypotension). However, patients with multiple risk factors often will require a combination of medical, rehabilitative, environmental, and behavioral intervention strategies (e.g., treating syncope, removing environmental hazards, prescribing a cane). Prevention strategies include interventions to reduce medical and environmental risk factors for falls, interventions to increase the subject's physical endurance and to enhance mobility, nursing interventions for institutionalized elderly and, finally, the use of assistive devices to decrease the risk of falling or to minimize the harmful effects of a fall. Although more data are needed to verify the usefulness of these different approaches, several studies show encouraging results in fall prevention with use of these strategies [30–32].

Physical Interventions to Treat Gait and Balance Disorders

Medical treatments for several of the causes of gait and balance disorders in older people are discussed in Chapters 10 through 18. Fortunately, drugs and surgery are not the only available means to improve mobility in the elderly. In many instances and for the majority of gait-impaired elderly, physical interventions partially restore lost mobility and may effectively reduce the risk of falling. Physical interventions are described and discussed critically in Chapters 21 through 24. This section is introduced by a chapter that describes the approach to physical intervention that may be taken in the treatment of an individual patient. Step by step, the clinician is guided through the nuances of the evaluation and treatment of an older patient with impaired mobility.

Balance Retraining

Not surprisingly, elderly who have poor balance tend to fall repeatedly [33]. Strategies designed to improve balance are reviewed in Chapter 22. To identify helpful training maneuvers or sets of exercises, the clinician needs to know the likely destabilizing situations that can occur during standing or walking. Some of these challenges are predictable, such as the displacement of the center of gravity with reaching or in the process of sitting on a chair. Others are unpredictable, such as tripping on a curb or missing a step while going downstairs. The complex sensorimotor system that mediates balance (discussed in Chapter 3) can normally negotiate these challenges. Abnormalities in any or, typically, several of the links of this system render some elderly prone to falls. The components of the balance system more critical for adequate standing and more amenable to correction are reviewed in Chapter 22.

Chapter 22 discusses the outcomes of the intervention studies on balance retraining in older people. Many of these interventions have focused too heavily on simple maneuvers that are for this reason easier to quantify but that may not address adequately the varied needs of different individuals. Programs that were successful at improving balance took a more intensive approach to training. Propulsive movements, in both the horizontal and vertical planes, and activities involving endurance and quick turns predominated in their exercise plans. Tasks combining multiple sensory and motor challenges under controlled conditions improved the participants' ability to respond to unexpected perturbations without falling. Examples of these tasks include walking backward on foam with eyes closed or tandem standing on foam with eyes closed while being pushed gently.

Other useful techniques are mental practice of balance and tai chi chuan, a movement technique that emphasizes directing attention to spatial intersegmental associations and to body orientation in space [34, 35].

Strength Training

Weight lifting is not a typical activity of nonagenarians. For this reason, the report that high-intensity resistance training can increase muscle strength and mobility in this age group was a discovery for many who work with older patients [36]. Chapter 23 reviews different types of resistance training, their effect on gait, and the theoretical justification for exploring this therapeutic modality. Older people walk more slowly because their steps are shorter. Hip extension and ankle plantar flexion are the most likely joint movements wherein muscle weakness could limit velocity. Unfortunately, to date, there have been no kinematic gait studies assessing directly whether weakness of these muscles does indeed limit velocity in older people. There is indirect evidence that muscle strength may be a determinant of velocity. Several cross-sectional studies have shown that older individuals with stronger ankle plantar flexion and knee extension walk more rapidly [36, 37].

Of even greater interest is the result of several interventional studies using resistance training and other training modalities to improve gait and balance in the elderly [36, 38]. They have shown that high levels of physical activity can maintain or increase strength gains achieved from resistance training. In addition, the performance gains are training specific. For instance, walking training improves walking more than resistance training does. Low levels of physical activity fail to accomplish these goals [39]. Gains with these interventions are more likely to be recorded in persons who have a very poor baseline gait than in community-living individuals with less-impaired gait [40]. However, physical activity does preserve independent function. Older persons with no complaints and with a clinically normal gait should perform enjoyable activities designed to preserve endurance and muscle strength. Walking programs probably are the most easily started and maintained and should be recommended to nearly all sedentary but able older persons. Those who have slow or impaired gait will experience increased muscle strength from resistance training. Resistance training alone, however, may have only a modest effect on gait velocity. Training that combines resistance and walking, either sequentially or simultaneously, seems to be most effective.

Correction of Environmental Hazards

The book concludes with a discussion of how to make the environment a safer place for older people with impaired gait and balance. This is appropriate because the environment has been implicated as a contributing factor in one-third to one-half of all falls occurring in the home and in institutional settings [41, 42]. Chapter 24 details a series of interventions to reduce environmental risks. Some interventions are meant to eliminate environmental conditions that interfere with mobility. This is accomplished by modifying or altering hazardous features of the existing physical environment. Hazards are discovered by a detailed review of the subject's living quarters, including circulation pathways, lighting, floor surfaces, stairs, beds, bathrooms, and storage areas. Another type of intervention strives to maintain safe mobility through use of appropriate ambulation devices and footwear. Yet another strategy attempts to reduce the risks associated with injurious falls (i.e., hip fractures; prolonged postfall lie times—the time spent on the ground after a fall before help arrives) by providing devices such as hip pads and personal emergency response systems. The management plan generally includes features of each approach. The recommended interventions will not yield any benefit if the individual at risk is not compliant. Compliance is enhanced when (1) the patient understands the reason for the environmental change, (2) that the modification improves mobility and is aesthetically appealing, and (3) that the modification is affordable and simple to implement [43].

Only recently have mobility disorders started to attract the attention they deserve. These disorders have a substantial impact on the lives of older persons. This book describes some of the initial efforts to come to terms with gait and balance problems of the elderly. Crucial issues regarding the normal physiology, disease mechanisms, therapeutic modalities, treatment efficacy, and cost require further research. It is hoped that this book will provide both practical information on the management of these common disorders and strategies and tools for future investigation.

REFERENCES

1. Romberg MH. *Manual of the Nervous System of Man (vol 2)*. Translated by EH Sieveking, Sydenham Society, London, 1853.
2. Gowers WR. *Diseases of the Nervous System*. Philadelphia: Blakiston Press, 1888. Pp 288–291.
3. Babinski JFF. Sur le role du cervalet dans les actes volitionnels necessitant une succession rapide des mouvements. *Rev Neurol* 1902;10:1013–1015.
4. Schiller F. Staggering gait in medical history. *Ann Neurol* 1995;37:127–135.
5. Friedreich N. Uber Ataxie mit Berucksichtigung der hereditaren Formen. *Virchows Arch* 1876;68:145–245.
6. Marie P. Sur l'heredo-ataxie cerebelleuse. *Semin Med Paris* 1892;239:331–337.
7. Parkinson J. *An Essay on the Shaking Palsy*. London: Sherwood, Neely, and Jones, 1817.
8. Nutt JG, Marsden CD, Thompson PD. Human walking and higher level gait disorders, particularly in the elderly. *Neurology* 1993;43:268–279.
9. Bruns L. Uber Sturugen des Gleichgewichtes bei Stirnhirntumoren. *Otsch Med Wochenschr* 1892;18:138–140.
10. Petren K. Uber den Zusammenhang zwischen anatomisch bedingter und functioneller Gangstorung im Greisenalter. *Arch Psychiatr Nerven* 1901;33:444–489.
11. von Malaise E. Studien uber wese grundlagen senile getstoringen. *Arch Psychiatr* 1910;46:902–1009.
12. Meyer JS, Barron DW. Apraxia of gait: A clinicophysiological study. *Brain* 1960;83:261–284.
13. Denny-Brown D. The nature of apraxia. *J Nerv Ment Dis* 1958;126:9–31.
14. Critchley M. The neurology of old age. *Lancet* 1931;1:1221–1230.

15. Critchley M. On senile disorders of gait, including the so-called "senile paraplegia." *Geriatrics* 1948;3:364–370.

16. Newman G, Dovenmuehle RH, Busse EW. Alterations in neurologic status with age. *J Am Geriatr Soc* 1960;8:915–917.

17. Lundgren-Lindquist B, Aniansson A, Rundgren A. Functional studies in 79 year olds (Part III). *Scand J. Rehabil Med* 1983;15:125–131.

18. Odenheimer G, et al. Comparison of neurological changes in "successfully aging" persons vs the total aging population. *Arch Neurol* 1994;51:573–580.

19. Tinetti ME, Speechley M, Ginter SF. Risk factors for falls among elderly persons living in the community, *N Engl J Med* 1988;319:1701–1707.

20. Sudarsky L. Geriatrics: Gait disorders in the elderly. *N Engl J Med* 1990;322:1441–1446.

21. Baker SP, Harvey AH. Fall injuries in the elderly. *Clin Geriatr Med* 1985;1:501–512.

22. Imms FJ, Edholm OG. Studies of gait and mobility in the elderly. *Age Ageing* 1981;10:147–156.

23. Aniansson A, Zetterberg C, Hedberg M, Henriksson K. Impaired muscle function with aging: A background factor in the incidence of fractures of the proximal end of the femur. *Clin Orthop* 1984;191:193–201.

24. Sheldon J. On the natural history of falls in old age. *Br Med J [Clin Res]* 1960;2:1685–1690.

25. Horak F, Shupert C, Mirka A. Components of postural dyscontrol in the elderly: A review. *Neurobiol Aging* 1989;10:727–738.

26. Dimitrijevic MR. Motor control in chronic spinal cord injury patients. *Scand J Rehabil Med Suppl* 1994;30:53–62.

27. Hanna J, Frank J. Automatic stepping in the pontomedullary stage of central herniation. *Neurology* 1995;45:985–986.

28. Forssberg H. Ontogeny of human locomotor control. I. Infant stepping, supported locomotion and transition to independent locomotion. *Exp Brain Res* 1985;57:480–493.

29. Garcia-Rill E. The pedunculopontine nucleus. *Prog Neurobiol* 1991;36:363–89.

30. Lauritzen J, Petersen M, Lund B. Effect of external hip protectors on hip fractures. *Lancet* 1993;341:11–13.

31. Rubenstein L, et al. The value of assessing falls in an elderly population: A randomized clinical trial. *Ann Intern Med* 1990;113:308–316.

32. Schmid N. Reducing patient falls: A research based comprehensive fall prevention program. *Mil Med* 1990;155:202–207.

33. Whipple R, et al. Altered sensory function and balance in older persons. *J Gerontol* 1993;48:71–76.

34. Fansler C, Poff C, Shepard K. Effects of mental practice on balance in elderly women. *Phys Ther* 1985;65:1332–1338.

35. Wolfson L, et al. Training balance and strength in the elderly to improve function. *Am Geriatr Soc* 1993;41:341–343.

36. Fiatarone M, et al. High-intensity strength training in nonagenarians, effects on skeletal muscle. *JAMA* 1990;263:3029–3034.

37. Bassey E, Bendal M, Pearson M. Muscle strength in the triceps surae and objectively measured customary walking activity in men and women over 65 years of age. *Clin Sci* 1988;74:85–89.

38. Brown M, Holloszy J. Effects of walking, jogging and cycling on strength, flexibility, speed and balance in 60- to 72-year olds. *Aging Clin Exp Res* 1993;5:427–434.

39. Brown M, Holloszy J. Effects of a low intensity exercise program on selected physical performance characteristics of 60- to 71-year olds. *Age Ageing* 1991;3:129–139.

40. Judge J, Underwood M, Gennosa T. Exercise to improve gait velocity in older persons. *Arch Phys Med Rehabil* 1993;74:400–406.

41. Kellogg International Work Group on the Prevention of Falls by the Elderly. The prevention of falls in later life. *Dan Med Bull* 1987;34:1–24.

42. Tinetti M, Speechley M. Prevention of falls among the elderly. *N Engl J Med* 1989; 320:1055–1059.

43. Tideiksaar R. Environment adaptations to preserve balance and prevent falls. *Top Geriatr Rehab* 1990;5:78–84.

2. Falls in the Elderly: Risk Factors and Prevention

Michael C. Nevitt

Recurrent falls are a marker of frailty, immobility, and acute and chronic health impairment in older persons. Falls, in turn, contribute to functional decline by causing injury, activity limitation, fear of falling, and loss of mobility and independence. Falls are the most frequent cause of unintentional injuries in the elderly. Fractures, the most common serious fall injury in the elderly, usually result from the combined effects of a fall and diminished bone strength.

A *fall* is defined as an unintentional event that results in a person's coming to rest on the ground or on another lower level [1]. Certain types of falls, such as those associated with loss of consciousness, an acute cerebrovascular event, overwhelming external force from motor vehicle accident, vigorous recreational activity, or violence, often are excluded from the definition of falls in older persons. The causes and risk factors for these falls may be different from the typical fall suffered by an older person and are, therefore, a separate distinct topic.

The etiology of falls in the elderly is multifactorial, often involving several intrinsic (host), behavioral, activity-related, and environmental factors. Epidemiological studies have identified several intrinsic risk factors for falls, which allow the identification of persons with an increased risk of falls and suggest potential preventive measures. Elderly individuals with multiple risk factors and, in particular, multiple physical impairments that affect balance and gait are at greatest risk; however, many apparently healthy older persons also fall.

Fall injuries typically result from the impact of the body on the floor or ground and the rapid transmission of forces to body tissues and organs. The potential for injury is a function of the magnitude and direction of the forces, the energy-absorbing characteristics of the impact surfaces, and the susceptibility of tissues and organs to damage. Factors affecting the risk of injury from a fall have received relatively little study but are a potential focus of prevention.

Prevention of falls and fall injuries must span the spectrum of ages and health characteristics within the older population and address the diverse causes of falls and their sequelae without unnecessarily compromising quality of life and independence. Information about the effectiveness of interventions to reduce falls and fall injuries is urgently needed to guide prevention efforts.

THE HEALTH BURDEN OF FALLS AND FALL-RELATED INJURIES IN OLDER PERSONS

Mortality

Unintentional injury is the sixth leading cause of death in the elderly, and falls are the single most common cause of unintentional injury deaths in persons aged 65 and older [2]. Approximately 70% of fall-related injury deaths occur in persons older than 65 (approximately 12% of the population) [3]. In 1986, the National Center for Health Statistics recorded 8,313 deaths from falls among elderly in the United States (Fig. 2-1). This number, derived from death certificates, almost certainly underestimates the number of deaths to which falls are a contributing factor [2, 4]. Falls account for one-third and one-fifth of all injury mortality in women and men, respectively [2]. The rate of fall-related deaths rises rapidly with age for whites aged 70 and older and less dramatically for non-whites aged 75 and older (see Fig. 2-1). By age 85, more than 50% of injury-related deaths in women and nearly 40% in men are due to falls [2]. Older men are more likely than older women to die from a fall. The highest mortality occurs in white men aged 85 and older (171 per 100,000), followed by white women aged 85 and older (127 per 100,000). This may reflect, in part, the much higher risk in older men of death after hip fracture [5].

The mortality rate from falls has declined in recent decades (Fig. 2-2), which may reflect, at least in part, general advances in trauma care and increased sur-

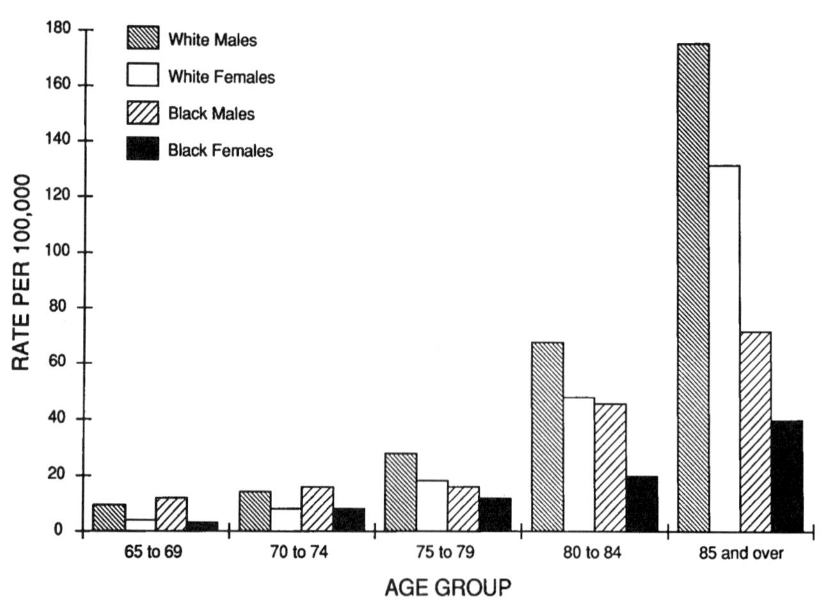

Figure 2-1. Death rates from falls per 100,000 persons by age, gender, and race: United States, 1986. (From MC Nevitt, Falls in Older Persons: Risk Factors and Prevention. In: RL Berg, JS Cassels, eds., *The Second Fifty Years: Promoting Health and Preventing Disability.* Washington, DC: National Academy Press, 1990.)

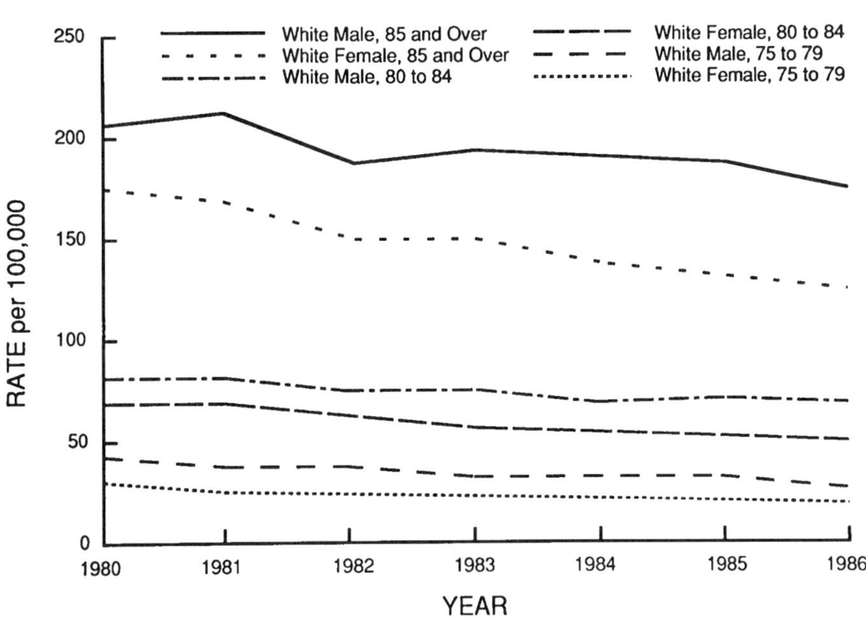

Figure 2-2. Death rates from falls per 100,000 persons by age, gender, race, and year: United States, 1986. (From MC Nevitt, Falls in Older Persons: Risk Factors and Prevention. In: RL Berg, JS Cassels, eds., *The Second Fifty Years: Promoting Health and Preventing Disability.* Washington, DC: National Academy Press, 1990.)

vival of patients with hip fractures in particular [6, 7]. Several studies suggest that falls in frail elderly, especially falls with a "long lie" (i.e., a long waiting time on the ground after a fall before help arrives), are associated with increased mortality, independent of injury severity [8–10] though this finding may be related to underlying medical conditions in persons who fall [11]. Rates of fall deaths may increase in the winter months, possibly due to an increase in outdoor environmental hazards [12], though this seasonal increase is uncertain [2]. Because a large proportion of fall-related deaths occur following a hip fracture, prevention of hip fractures in the elderly may significantly reduce mortality from unintentional injury.

Frequency of Falls

Several cross-sectional surveys of communities in the United States and other industrialized countries in recent years indicated that from one-fourth to one-third of persons aged 65 and older reported a fall in the previous year (Fig. 2-3) [13–16]. It should be noted that retrospective questions may underestimate the frequency of falls [17, 18]. However, several prospective population-based studies found a similar proportion of elderly falling each year [19–21]. From one-third to one-half of elderly persons who reported falling in the previous year fell two or more times [20–22].

Most studies find that the rate of falls is higher in women than in men [23] and

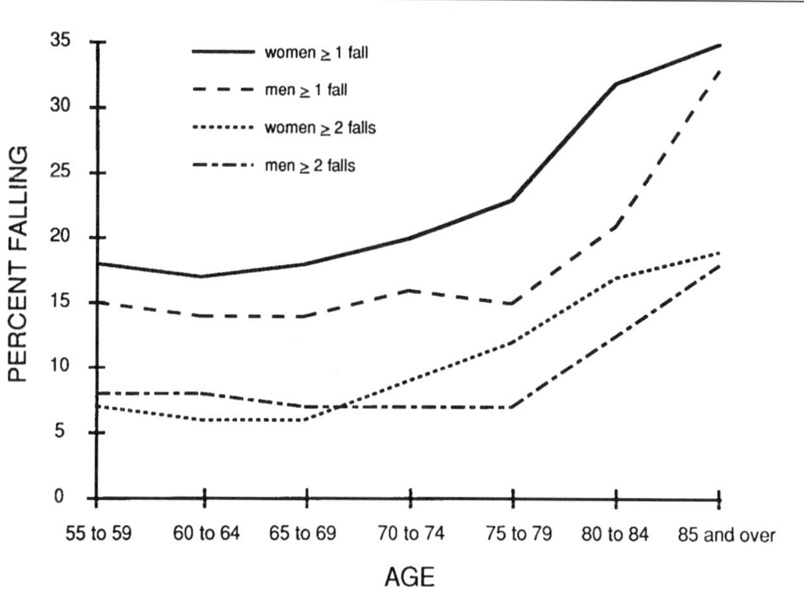

Figure 2-3. Percentage by age and gender of older individuals reporting falls in the previous 12 months in the United States. (From MC Nevitt, Falls in Older Persons: Risk Factors and Prevention. In RL Berg, JS Cassels, eds., *The Second Fifty Years: Promoting Health and Preventing Disability.* Washington DC: National Academy Press, 1990.)

increases with age, rising from about 30 to 50 falls per 100 person-years at ages 65 to 74 to about 60 to 90 falls per 100 person-years in those 75 and older [8, 20, 24]. The rate of falls is even higher in institutional settings, with an annual average published incidence of about 140 per 100 patient-years in nursing homes and 165 per 100 patient-years in hospitals [25, 26]. Rates in institutions vary substantially by organizational differences and level of care and by health characteristics of the patient population [26, 27]. For example, a study of nursing home residents with dementia reported a rate of 400 falls per 100 patient-years [28]. Falls in institutionalized populations may have more serious consequences; one in five fatal falls among persons aged 85 and older occurs in a nursing home [29].

Fall Injuries

Between 10% and 15% of falls in the elderly result in a serious injury [21, 25, 30]. Approximately 5–10% of falls in the elderly result in a fracture, 1–2% of falls cause a hip fracture, and approximately 5% of falls cause other serious injuries requiring medical care or causing disability [20, 21, 25, 31–33]. Most falls, however, do not cause sufficient injury to warrant medical attention. Between 30% and 50% of falls result in a variety of minor soft-tissue injuries, and the remainder cause no injury or only insignificant physical injury.

In a regional study in northeastern Ohio, the rate of emergency room treatment of fall-related injuries in persons aged 75 and older approached 80 per

Table 2-1. The percentage of fractures attributed to falls by older women who have recently suffered a fracture

Type of fracture	Percentage
Wrist	96
Proximal humerus	95
Elbow	95
Hip	92
Patella	89
Ankle	88
Foot or toes	82
Pelvis	80
Face	77
Hand or finger	68
Tibia or fibula	65
Rib	59
All nonspinal fractures	82
Vertebral fractures	<25

SOURCE: M Nevitt, SR Cummings. Falls and Fractures in Older Women. In: B Vellas et al, eds, *Falls, Balance and Gait Disorders in the Elderly.* Paris: Elsevier, 1992. Pp 69–80.

1,000 per year in women and 60 per 1,000 per year in men [34]. Another study in Dade County, Florida, found an exponential increase with age in the rate of fall injuries that were treated in acute-care settings. These rates were higher in women than in men at all ages [35]. The fall injury rate in women aged 75 and older was approximately 120 per 1,000 per year and in men of that age approximately 85 per 1,000 per year. More than 40% of those subjects with fall injuries were hospitalized, with an average length of stay of approximately 12 days.

Fractures account for the majority of all serious fall injuries [30, 33]. Nonspinal fractures in the elderly usually result from the combined effect of falls, osteoporosis, and other factors that increase susceptibility to injury [36, 37]. Each year in the United States, there are approximately 250,000 each of hip and wrist fractures in persons older than 65 [38]. Although precise national estimates are not available, there are one to two times as many fractures of other bones in the elderly as there are hip and wrist fractures combined [34, 39]. Falls are a factor in more than 85% of the most important osteoporotic fractures, such as those of the hip, wrist, pelvis, and humerus, but play a lesser role in distal extremity and rib fractures [31, 39] (Table 2-1) and infrequently are a factor in vertebral fracture.

Other serious injuries resulting from falls include hematoma, head injury with loss of consciousness, dislocation and other severe joint injury, severe laceration, sprain, and disabling soft-tissue injury [33, 35]. There are few data specifically relating to nonfracture fall-related injuries in the US population. Findings from regional studies indicate that injuries to the head comprise a substantial proportion of serious nonfracture injuries [35].

Disability

Approximately 25% of falls in the community result in an immediate activity limitation owing to injury or fear of falling [21, 30]. Falls are responsible for 1 in 5 of all days of restricted activity in the elderly, a higher proportion than for any other health condition [40]. Most of the 58.9 million days of restricted activity and 18.8 million bed-days among the elderly in 1986 from all forms of injury were due to falls [41].

Many falls also have a long-term impact. One study found that among persons who fell and were treated in an emergency room, 40% had continuing pain or disability 2 months later, and 16% had pain 7 months after the fall [42]. Persons who fall also have an increased risk of long-term decline in function [10, 11], in part due to coexisting medical conditions but also due to injury and fear of falling [43]. The devastating functional consequences of hip fractures are well-known; 20–30% of persons who lived in the community prior to hip fracture remain in long-term care 1 year after the injury [44]. The consequences of other fall injuries are less well-documented, but one study found that of elderly who lived at home and were then hospitalized for a fall injury other than hip fracture, nearly 40% died or were discharged to a nursing facility [35].

The psychological and functional consequences of falls can be significant, regardless of whether an injury occurs. Approximately 50% of community-living elderly who fall express fear of additional falls or injury [21, 30, 45]. Both the older person at risk and his or her family members and care givers experience anxiety about the older person's ability to avoid falls and injuries. This often leads to a reduction in the individual's activity, decreased mobility, social isolation, and loss of independence [1, 43, 45]. Between 10% and 25% of persons who fall say they restrict their activities due to fear of falling [21, 30]. After a fall, the inability to get up and a long lie may lead to serious physical complications, including pneumonia and hypothermia. Even in the absence of physical morbidity, a long lie may result in reduced self-confidence, feelings of helplessness, and loss of function [9, 30].

Costs

Meaningful estimates of the medical and other economic costs of falls in the elderly are difficult to make. One relatively recent study estimated that falls by elderly persons account for nearly 8% of the total lifetime economic cost of all unintentional injury in the United States [24]. Fractures that typically are the result of a fall constitute the major portion of the nearly $10 billion in annual costs of osteoporosis [46]. Approximately 90% of the estimated $5.2 billion in direct medical costs for osteoporosis in 1986 were attributable to hospital and nursing home care, and 66% of hospitalizations and 82% of nursing home care admissions for osteoporosis involved types of fractures that, among the elderly, usually were the result of falls [47]. In 1993, medical costs for elderly persons hospitalized for a fall averaged $10,000 to $12,000, approximately 50% more than for nonelderly adults hospitalized for a fall [48].

RISK FACTORS FOR FALLS AND FALL INJURIES

Risk factors are characteristics of individuals, behaviors, and environments that are associated with an increased likelihood of an adverse event or outcome, such as a fall. Even when etiological mechanisms are uncertain, identifying risk factors for falls is important for three reasons: (1) Understanding risk factors may help us to identify and understand the causes of falls; (2) risk factors can help to identify those at greatest risk who would benefit most from preventive measures; and (3) risk factors may be modifiable and suggest specific interventions to prevent falls in groups and in individuals, even those who do not have a history of falls. Though important, the study of risk factors for falls in the elderly presents many challenges.

Multifactorial Etiology

Falls in the elderly usually have a multifactorial etiology, resulting from the convergence of several intrinsic, pharmacological, environmental, behavioral, or activity-related factors [24, 25, 32, 49]. During normal movement and ambulation, the body's center of mass must be maintained dynamically over its base of support. Abnormal displacement of the center of mass beyond the base of support may result from a variety of causes, including sudden voluntary movements and environmental perturbations (e.g., tripping hazards) and from factors intrinsic to the individual, such as an abnormal gait, unreliable postural reflexes, unstable joints, and weak muscles. A fall may result when the body's postural control systems fail to detect a displacement and do not reposition the center of mass over the base of support in time to avoid a "loss of balance." This failure may be due to a variety of factors, including the abruptness, magnitude, and speed of the displacement, and intrinsic factors, such as the loss of sensory function essential to detecting movement of the body's center of mass, impaired ability of the central nervous system to organize and transmit a postural response, and an ineffective postural response due to neuromuscular abnormalities (e.g., muscle weakness) [49–51].

Many age-, disease-, and pharmacologically induced physiological changes can adversely affect postural control [51, 52]. Poor balance and falls often reflect the combined impact of several abnormalities, such as the combination of poor vision, loss of peripheral sensory function, and muscle weakness. In addition, activity-related and environmental factors, such as tasks that stress postural abilities and poor lighting, may interact with intrinsic (host) susceptibilities to precipitate a fall. Although activity-related and environmental factors are common contributors to falls in the elderly and could be the focus of widely applicable prevention strategies, their importance may differ between subgroups of elderly (e.g., healthy and frail elders) [53, 54]. Different types of falls, such as those due to external versus internal displacements, also may have different risk factors [55, 56]. Moreover, different falls experienced by one individual may involve unique combinations of causal factors. Thus, multiple risk factors may have to be identified and modified if efforts to prevent falls are to be effective [32].

Methodological Issues

Because risk factors for falls may differ between healthy and impaired or frail individuals [53, 54, 57], the selection of a study population may affect which combinations of risk factors are identified. Inconsistencies in fall risk factors across studies also may be due to other methodological differences. Most falls are not treated medically, so identification of falls can be problematic. Self-reporting of falls is susceptible to both over- and underreporting, and the accuracy of self-reporting may be affected by cognitive impairments and other subject characteristics [17, 18]. Different methods of fall surveillance, such as incident reports versus self-reporting or frequent versus infrequent self-reporting may yield different estimates of frequency and risk factors [58, 59]. However, for studies in the general population, there currently are no practical alternatives to self-reporting of nonmedically treated falls. Several attempts have been made to classify falls by their circumstances (e.g., intrinsic versus extrinsic perturbations) to increase the specificity of risk factor relationships and help to target preventive efforts [54–56, 60]. However, these classification systems differ considerably from one another, and there is no consensus on the best approach.

Some studies analyze fallers; others analyze fall rates per unit of time as the end point. In addition, there are several alternative statistical methods for analysis of fall rates. These different approaches to analysis of falls may identify different risk factors [58], in part because recurrent falls may be related more strongly to risk factors than are isolated falls [22, 61]. Other potential problems involve assessing exposure to such risk factors as medication use and symptoms, which can vary considerably over short periods, and measuring exposure to risk factors that are linked to a specific fall event, such as environmental and activity-related factors. Even with repeated measurement of time-varying risk factors, there may be difficulties in linking exposures with specific fall events and in making (and analyzing) comparable measurements in control subjects. Measurement of environmental hazards is especially challenging. No studies have quantified actual exposure to hazards (e.g., frequency of encounters); the usual approach simply is to note the presence of hazards in the homes of subjects. It is also difficult to standardize the definition and assessment of hazards [62].

Intrinsic Risk Factors

Characteristics of individuals that are associated with an increased susceptibility of falling have been identified in both prospective and retrospective studies comparing those who fall with those who have not fallen (Table 2-2). Extreme old age and the presence and severity of self-reported functional impairments and mobility limitations are strong indicators of an increased risk of falling (see Table 2-2). Data from the National Health Interview Survey's 1984 Supplement on Aging indicate that persons aged 75 to 84 who require help with activities of daily living are 14 times more likely, and those with limitations in walking, transfer, and balance activities are 10 times more likely to report having two or more falls in the previous 12 months than persons having no limitations [63]. The association of falls with frailty and functional disabilities in the elderly also is evident in the high rate of falls reported in nursing homes [25, 26, 28]. Thus, simple indicators of functional status can identify individuals or groups at high risk for falls.

The design of effective fall prevention measures, however, requires knowledge of more specific, modifiable risk factors. The search for modifiable intrinsic risk factors has focused largely on balance and gait impairments and their determinants, because these are recognized as central etiological factors in the occurrence of falls [52, 64].

Normal gait and postural stability depend on the proper functioning of sensory, neuromuscular, and musculoskeletal systems and the integrative processes of the central nervous system [51, 65]. Sensory function occupies an important place in many models of postural control [51, 52, 64]; limb tactile-proprioceptive sensation, vision, and vestibular input are critical for detecting movement of the body's center of gravity within its base of support. These sensory modalities may be compromised by age and disease [51, 65]. However, measures of visual and somatosensory impairment are not consistently associated with fall risk in epidemiological studies (see Table 2-2). Several studies have found that impaired visual functions, including acuity, contrast sensitivity, depth perception, and dark adaptation, increase the risk of falls, but other studies have not found an increased risk. Although vision impairment may play a direct role in poor balance [52, 66], its primary contribution to fall risk may be a reduced ability to negotiate environmental obstacles, especially under degraded visual conditions or in the presence of certain gait abnormalities, such as decreased step height [66]. Thus, these other conditions may have to be present before poor vision is associated with an elevated risk of falls. Similarly, measures of lower extremity somatosensory and proprioceptive impairment have been associated with fall risk in some studies but not in others. Clinical measures of these sensory modalities suitable for use in epidemiological studies may be too crude to detect functionally important differences. In addition, individual sensory organ system impairment may be less critical for balance than is the cumulative effect of multiple system deficits or the interactions between these deficits and sensory conditions, such as lighting. Other sensory deficits (e.g., mechanoreceptor and vestibular disorders), that may contribute to fall risk have received little epidemiological study, in part because they are difficult to measure.

Adequate skeletal muscle strength and joint range of motion, especially in the lower extremities, are essential to an effective response to postural perturbations and to the maintenance of postural control [64, 67]. Age-related slowing of pos-

Table 2-2. Intrinsic risk factors for falls

Type of risk factor	Measure (studies)	Strength of evidence*
Demographic	Age ≥ 80 yr [13, 14, 19, 21, 22, 27, 121]	Strong
	Female [11, 13, 14, 15, 22, 23, 76, 121]	Strong
General health and functioning	ADL, mobility impairment [11, 14, 21–23, 54, 57, 76, 78, 121–123]	Strong
	Low or high level of physical activity or exercise [19–22, 27, 54]	Moderate
	History of falls [19, 21, 22, 27, 57, 121, 123]	Strong
Gait, balance, physical performance	Clinical or activity-based tests of balance [21, 22, 56, 57, 60, 61, 70, 76, 78, 122–125]	Strong
	Laboratory tests of static balance (quiet standing) [19, 126, 127]	Weak
	Laboratory tests of balance with altered sensory or support conditions [56, 61, 128]	Moderate
	Slow gait speed, short step length [19, 22, 76, 129–131]	Strong
	Qualitative gait abnormalities [21, 22, 57, 78, 102, 123, 129, 131]	Moderate
	Poor physical performance (e.g., arise from chair, transfer, climb step) [19, 21, 22, 56, 57, 76, 102, 123]	Strong
Musculoskeletal and neuromuscular	Reduced knee, hip, or ankle strength [19, 21, 22, 61, 67, 70, 76, 78, 122, 123, 132]	Strong
	Reduced grip strength [13, 16, 19, 22, 132]	Strong
	Hip or knee pain or reduced range of motion [19, 22, 122]	Moderate
	Foot problems [13, 21, 22, 122]	Moderate
	Impaired knee or plantar reflexes [22, 78, 122]	Weak
	Slow reaction time [22, 61, 122]	Weak
Sensory	Impaired visual acuity [14, 19, 21, 22, 61, 76, 78]	Moderate
	Impaired contrast sensitivity or depth perception [22, 61]	Weak
	Visual perceptual error [19, 81, 128]	Weak
	Impaired lower extremity sensory function [21, 22, 61, 70, 76, 78, 123, 133]	Weak
Other neurological signs	Frontal cortex or release [78, 123]	Weak
	Cerebellar, pyramidal, extrapyramidal [22, 78]	Weak
Cognitive, psychological function	Cognitive impairment [14, 15, 19, 21, 22, 78, 123]	Strong
	Depression or anxiety [14, 21, 22, 27, 43, 123, 134]	Moderate
Medical conditions	Arthritis [13, 19, 21, 22, 70, 78, 123]	Moderate
	Stroke [15, 19, 22]	Moderate
	Parkinson's disease [19, 22, 57, 134]	Strong
	Dementia [70, 134, 135]	Moderate
	Incontinence [21, 22, 78, 121, 123]	Moderate
	Postural hypotension [14, 18, 19, 21, 22, 76, 123]	Weak
Medication use	Sedatives, hypnotics, anxiolytics [11, 13–16, 18, 19, 21, 22, 57, 123, 133, 134, 137]	Strong
	Antidepressants [13, 14, 22, 57, 76, 136]	Moderate
	Cardiovascular [13–15, 18–22, 123, 134, 136]	Weak
	Number of medications [13, 18, 19, 70, 123, 134]	Strong

ADL = activities of daily living

*Strong = associated with falls in most studies; moderate = associated with falls in several, but not all, studies; weak = associated with falls in just one or two studies, or generally conflicting and inconsistent findings across studies.

tural responses increases the muscular force required to mount an effective response to postural disturbances [50] but, at the same time, the strength of skeletal muscles involved in postural control and locomotion declines with age, disease, and inactivity [68, 69]. Weak muscles and unstable or painful joints also may be a source of postural disturbances during voluntary movement. Consistent with an important role in balance, most studies find that lower-extremity musculoskeletal and neuromuscular impairments increase the risk of falls (see Table 2-2). Leg and ankle muscle weakness and joint and foot problems generally are significant and consistent risk factors. Generalized muscle weakness, indicated by poor grip strengths, also is a major risk factor for falls.

Age-related slowing in the central neurological integration of sensory and motor systems, and disturbances in the organization of postural responses, may reduce the speed of postural reflexes and impair the effectiveness and reliability of postural control strategies [49–52]. Selective experimental alteration of sensory input in laboratory studies suggests that inability to compensate for sensory loss and to resolve conflict among sensory modalities increases with age and contributes to balance failure in the elderly [51, 52, 64]. Other age-related changes in higher-level neurological functioning, such as the slowing of choice reaction time, also has received attention in some models of postural control [50, 52]. Unfortunately, because they are difficult to measure, these central neurological processes have not been tested adequately in studies of risk factors for falls. A few studies have examined the association of falls with slowed reaction time, impaired reflexes, and a variety of nonspecific neurological signs, but the results generally have been inconclusive. The most appropriate measures of reaction time and other higher-level neurological processes for fall prediction remain uncertain.

Indirect support for the role of abnormal higher-level neurological function in postural instability comes from several studies finding that impaired cognitive function, depression, and fall-related anxiety are associated with an increased risk of falls (see Table 2-2). Cognitive impairment may increase the risk of falls due to direct effects on postural control as well as through compromised judgment, visuospatial disorientation, and related behavioral changes (e.g., wandering) [70, 71]. Affective disorders, such as anxiety or depression, also may have direct effects on postural control [72] and may decrease attention to environmental hazards.

Simple, clinical tests of gait, functional balance, and physical function based on observed performance of standardized tasks are strong predictors of falls in many studies (see Table 2-2). This may be because these measures (1) summarize the combined impact of sensory, neurological, and musculoskeletal abnormalities on postural stability; and (2) assess dynamic postural stability in response to the challenges presented by daily tasks (e.g., walking and transfer maneuvers) in which falls commonly occur [73, 74]. For example, the ability to stand from a chair without the use of arms, a simple test which assesses leg strength, range of motion, and balance during a common daily task [75], is a strong indicator of fall risk [19, 22, 76].

Laboratory measures of static balance, such as postural sway and center of pressure displacement during quiet stance, on the other hand, are not associated as strongly or consistently with fall risk. These measures also do not show substantial declines with age [52] and may be relatively poor indicators of dynamic postural stability during the range of tasks typical of daily life. In contrast, laboratory measures of balance during stressed or altered sensory and support conditions show more marked declines with age, may more closely approximate challenges to balance in daily life, and may be better predictors of fall risk than are static measures [49, 64, 73]. One study [56] found that sway during two-legged stance with eyes closed was as good or better a predictor of falls than task-specific clinical measures. The authors speculated that the activity-specific tests only assessed risk associated with situations similar to the limited range of tasks simulated, whereas sway during altered sensory conditions seemed applicable to a wider variety of balance challenges. Additional research is needed to compare clinical and laboratory tests of balance and the relative usefulness of each type of measure for fall prediction.

Psychotropic, diuretic, antihypertensive, and antiparkinsonian medications, especially if used in improper doses, may contribute to falls in the elderly by decreasing alertness, depressing psychomotor function, or causing weakness, fatigue, dizziness, or postural hypotension [77]. These adverse physiological effects may be exacerbated by altered drug metabolism in elderly individuals. There is good evidence that use of hypnotic-anxiolytic drugs, particularly benzodiazepines (see Table 2), increase the risk of falls, though not all studies support this [22, 57, 76, 78]. The role of diuretic, antihypertensive, and other medications linked to orthostatic hypotension in increasing the risk of falls is uncertain and needs further investigation [77]. As shown in Table 2-2, several studies have found an association of falls with the number of medications being taken. This could reflect synergistic effects among drugs but also could be due to the poorer health of individuals taking multiple medications.

A number of medical conditions, including arthritis (especially with lower-extremity involvement), dementia, stroke, Parkinson's disease, and cataracts were associated with the risk of falls in one or more studies. These conditions may have direct adverse effects on postural control or may affect balance indirectly as a result of physical deconditioning. Although most studies have not found an association of falls with chronic cardiovascular conditions, including postural hypotension, their role as risk factors remains uncertain.

Some studies have evaluated persons who fall clinically in order to determine a "cause" of the fall [26, 76, 78]. Among the most common causes to which falls are attributed are muscle weakness, generalized weakness, dizziness and vertigo, gait and balance disorders, confusion, drug-induced postural hypotension, visual impairment, specific neurological disorders (including parkinsonism and stroke), and arthritis. Although these findings are largely consistent with those of risk-factor studies, results from the two types of analysis may conflict even within a single study. For example, in a study of ambulatory nursing home residents, Lipsitz et al. [76] did not find an association of recurrent falls with cardiovascular medications, orthostatic dizziness, or orthostatic hypotension. However, in assessing likely causes of individual falls, they determined that drug-induced hypotension was a factor in more than 10% of falls. Differences in the approach to defining causes (e.g., making diagnoses versus assessing functional impairments) and in the assignment of falls to causes makes comparison among these attribution studies difficult. In addition, these studies often lack controlled comparisons; the clinical findings to which falls are attributed in older persons also may be common in persons who do not fall.

Environmental, Activity-Related, and Behavioral Risk Factors

Environmental, activity-related, and behavioral factors may be important in the etiology of falls in the elderly and present a promising focus for preventive measures. A useful model for understanding the role of these factors in fall risk posits that risk is increased when the postural demands of an activity or task stress or exceed the postural competence of the individual. Factors that influence the equilibrium between task demands and individual competence, such as the environmental and behavioral context of the task, can increase or decrease the risk of falls [79]. This model has several implications for understanding falls and for prevention. First, it suggests that the importance of activity-related, behavioral, and environmental factors will vary depending on the health and mobility level of subgroups of the population. For example, postural maneuvers and environmental obstacles that are easily negotiated under most conditions by a healthy person can become serious threats to mobility and safety in those with gait or balance impairments or in those suffering from fatigue, anxiety, or stress. Second, fall risk may be reduced by behavioral and environmental modifications that improve the balance between task demands and the physiological limits of postural competence.

Conventional wisdom holds that in frail and physically dependent elders and in those with severe balance and mobility problems falls typically occur during routine ambulation and transfer tasks required for basic mobility, usually without an obvious environmental hazard and, most frequently, within familiar environments such as the bedside or bathroom. This characterization is supported by recent studies of the circumstances of falls [26, 53, 54, 76, 80], underscoring the importance of interventions to improve postural competence and basic mobility skills in frail and physically dependent elders.

Lipsitz et al. [76] analyzed the causes of falls in frail, ambulatory nursing home residents and concluded that environmental hazards rarely were implicated as primary causes of falls and that when hazards contributed to a fall, there was usually an underlying pathological condition that reduced the individual's ability to compensate for the hazardous situation. Overt hazards may be relatively uncommon in well-designed long-term care and structured living environments. However, another study of nursing home residents [80] implicated environmental factors in one-half of the nearly 300 falls examined. Long-term care environments may vary a great deal in the presence of more overt hazards. However, it is also possible that the latter study identified more subtle environmental characteristics as potential hazards (e.g. slippery bedspreads and floor finishes, improper bed heights, absence of handrails). Subtle features like lighting and visual and spatial design also may have direct effects on postural stability [50, 66, 81]. Although familiarity with a particular environment may reduce the risk per exposure [32], circumstances that suddenly precipitate a fall in these familiar contexts are poorly understood. Clearly, there is need for a better understanding of environmental and behavioral factors that affect the ability of frail and impaired individuals to cope with challenges to balance during basic transfer and mobility maneuvers.

In contrast to falls in frail and impaired elderly, in healthy and mobile elders, falls are believed to be less common and more frequently to involve overt environmental hazards, including risk-taking activities such as climbing ladders, hurrying, or running [1]. Falls in this population are more likely to occur away from home [1]. Exposure to fall risks is spread over a wider range of physical environments and activities for individuals with good mobility. Studies of the circumstances of falls tend to support this conventional wisdom [21, 22, 24, 53, 54]. For example, Speechley et al. [54] found that falls in a group of vigorous elders were about one-third as common as in a group of frail elders and were more likely to involve an environmental hazard or a large displacement of the center of gravity from the base of support.

Environmental hazards faced by ambulatory, community-living elderly include poor stairway design and disrepair, inadequate lighting, clutter, slippery floors, unsecured mats and rugs, and lack of nonskid surfaces in bathtubs, among many others. Environmental factors are implicated by self-report as contributing to one-third to one-half of falls in community-dwelling subjects [1, 21, 25, 26, 30], but only a few studies have compared exposure to environmental hazards in those who fall and those in a control group. Although exposure to environmental hazards was not associated with an increase in risk of falls among all subjects in two studies [22, 21], Northridge [53] reanalyzed data from one of these studies and found that the presence of home hazards predicted falls in a subgroup of healthy and active subjects but not in a subgroup of frail individuals. In addition, Studenski et al. [57] studied mobile older men who had balance or gait abnormalities and found that increased home hazards and a decreased regard and concern for personal safety predicted a greater risk of falls.

These studies support the idea that fall risk factor modification needs to be tailored to the functional status and mobility level of the individual [54]. By extension, as an individual ages and the level of function declines, new risk factors for falls emerge, and new interventions become appropriate for that person. Behavioral, cognitive, and psychosocial factors that enhance an individual's adaptation to the dynamic and changing relationship between physical capabilities and environmental and task demands are a potentially productive focus for fall prevention [79, 82–84].

Individuals who have lost a measure of postural competence but remain active and mobile, take personal risks, and are exposed to hazardous environments may have an especially high risk of falling [57]. O'Laughlin et al. [20] found that moderately active elderly living in the community had a decreased risk of falls; however, those who were very active had an increased risk. High activity levels also have been associated with the risk of wrist fractures [85] and serious fall injuries

[33]. Fortunately for these individuals, there are many applicable interventions for building postural competence and of reducing behavioral and environmental risk. Changes in activities to reduce fall risk sometimes are appropriate; however, a balance always must be struck between reduction in risk and maintenance of mobility, quality of life, and independence. Although severe curtailment of activities might decrease falls in the short term by reducing exposure, over the long-term reduced self-confidence and physical deconditioning serves only to increase the risk of falls and functional decline [43].

Risk Factors for Injurious Falls

If risk factors for injurious falls are different from risk factors for falls in general, the finding might have important implications for the design and targeting of interventions to prevent morbidity from falls. However, risk factors for injurious falls and determinants of whether a fall causes serious injury have received relatively little study. Most of the work in this area has investigated determinants of whether a fall results in a fracture, one of the most common and serious fall injuries.

On average, a fall from a standing height has approximately 400 to 500 joules of potential energy, an order of magnitude greater than that required to fracture almost any bone of an elderly woman and enough to cause a variety of other serious injuries [86]. A fall directly onto the greater trochanter generates femoral impact forces that are 30–50% greater than the average needed to fracture the proximal femur of an older woman [87]. Yet, only approximately 15% of falls in older persons cause serious injuries requiring medical care or causing disability; approximately 5–10% cause fractures; and only 1–2% result in hip fractures [20, 25, 30, 31, 33].

For injuries resulting from mechanical energy, such as a fall, the forces generated on impact, the resistance of the body through inertial forces, the elastic capacity of tissue, and the viscous tolerance of organs play an important role in the risk of injury [88]. Because of declines in the strength and resiliency of muscle, bone, and other tissues, older persons have an increased risk of injury compared to a younger person subjected to similar impact forces. Bone mineral density is highly correlated with bone strength [86]; after age 50, bone density declines approximately 1% per year, on average, at key sites such as the proximal femur [89]. Differences within the older population in the strength of bone, muscle, and skin and other tissue may explain, in part, why some falls result in serious injury and others do not. For example, the risk of most fractures increases with decreasing bone density, independent of age in the elderly population in general [90] and in those who fall [37].

Most elderly women, however, have a low bone density (at least 2 SD below the mean for normal young women) [91] which puts them at increased risk for fractures. Yet, even in women with low bone density, most falls do not result in a fracture. The mechanics of falls also may play an important role in determining the risk of fracture. Whereas much attention has been given to factors affecting the strength of bone and to ways to preserve or increase it, little attention has been paid to the mechanics of falls. This is due in part to the lack of simple non-invasive methods for measuring forces generated in falls, the tremendous diversity of circumstances and human characteristics that affect these forces, and the difficulty of observing falls.

Several hypotheses have been proposed for how the mechanics of falls affect the risk of fractures, particularly hip fractures [36, 86, 92]. For a fall to result in a fracture of a particular bone, the fall must be oriented in such a way that there is impact on the bone. The fall must have enough energy (a product of the velocity and mass of the falling body) to fracture the bone. The energy of the fall that is transmitted to the bone can be reduced by protective responses, such as putting out an arm to break the fall. The amount and rate of energy transmitted to the bone also can be reduced by the ability of skin, fat, and muscle overlying the bone, and impact surfaces (such as carpeting) to absorb and distribute the mechanical energy. The bone will fracture if the residual energy transmitted to it exceeds its strength when applied in that particular direction.

Evidence from several case-control studies of persons who fall provides support for these hypotheses [37, 93, 94]. These studies found that individuals who suffered a hip fracture as a result of a fall were 20 to 30 times more likely to have fallen on the hip and 3 to 5 times more likely to have fallen sideways than were controls who fell without a fracture. An increased potential energy of the fall [93, 94] and greater stature of the faller [37] (which increases the potential energy) also increased the risk of hip fracture. Women who landed on an outstretched hand or who broke the momentum of the fall by grabbing or hitting an object had approximately one-third the risk of fracture, whereas those who landed on hard surfaces (tile, concrete) had approximately a threefold higher risk of hip fracture [37]. Greater arm extensor strength reduced the risk of hip fracture. When an individual landed on or near the hip, decreased bone density at the hip greatly increased the risk of hip fracture [37].

Obesity confers protection against hip fracture, but whether this is due primarily to the higher bone mass of obese persons or is partly attributable to their having more padding is uncertain. A greater body mass index was associated with a reduced risk of fracture, even after adjusting for hip bone density in one of the case-control studies [93] but not in another [37]. Whether the amount of soft-tissue padding over the trochanter influences the risk of hip fracture is unclear from these studies as this was not measured directly. However, a recent controlled trial conducted in a Danish nursing home demonstrated that wearing protective pads over the hips greatly reduced the risk of hip fractures [95].

There has been little research about the role of the mechanics of falls in other types of fracture. Most wrist fractures involve a fall onto an outstretched hand. One of the case-control studies mentioned earlier included women who had a wrist fracture from a fall. Orientation of the fall and site of impact were the most important factors in whether an individual fractured a wrist or a hip [37]. Thus, the orientation of the fall and the site of impact are important factors in determining the type of fracture that will result from a fall.

The overall risk of any fracture with each fall remains fairly constant with increasing age, but the risk of hip fracture per fall increases substantially with advancing age [31]. Changes in the mechanics of falls with age may account, in part, for the increasing risk of hip fracture per fall. These changes may include an increasing likelihood with age of an unprotected fall onto the greater trochanter, a weakening of protective arm responses, and loss with age of energy-absorbing soft tissue over the trochanter. Bone loss in the proximal femur also continues into very old age [89].

There are few studies examining whether risk factors for injurious falls are different from risk factors for either noninjurious falls or all falls. In one study [20], risk factors for falls that result in any injury, including minor ones, were similar to risk factors for all falls. However, in other studies, risk factors for more severe injury falls were different from those for noninjurious falls [33] and from those causing minor injury [30]. Nevertheless, some risk factors for falls also are associated with the risk of hip and other fractures. These include a history of past falls, impaired vision, disabling stroke, neuromuscular and balance impairments, cognitive impairment, and use of long-half-life sedatives, especially benzodiazepines [31, 85, 96–101].

In general, risk factors associated with both the likelihood of falling and impaired protective responses when a fall occurs (e.g., muscle weakness and other neuromuscular abnormalities) may be the best predictors of injurious falls and the most promising targets of interventions to reduce serious morbidity from falls. In addition, interventions that attenuate the force of impact of the fall, such as the application of protective padding over the hip or the use of energy-absorbent floor coverings in places where elderly reside, may decrease the risk of hip fracture.

Conclusion: Implications for Prevention

Individuals who fall, especially those who fall repeatedly, tend to have greater functional and mobility limitations, to have more neurological conditions, to be taking more medications, and to have more neuromuscular, balance, and gait impairments than do elderly persons who do not fall. Several studies find that an individual's risk of falls can be predicted from a few simple measures of these intrinsic risk factors and that an individual's risk increases with the number of risk factors present [21, 22, 61, 76, 102], which underscores the multifactorial etiology of falls and suggests that those at increased risk can be identified. Though several determinants of balance, such as sensory impairments, have not demonstrated consistent associations with falls in risk factor studies, in some cases this may reflect a lack of functionally relevant and practical measures of these parameters. In addition, identification of thresholds below which certain deficits (e.g., strength) increase risk may further enhance prediction of falls and identification of those at risk [103]. Environmental, behavioral, and activity-related factors probably also play an important role as risk factors for falls, but these require further investigation.

Current prospects for the prevention of falls are promising, but uncertainties remain. Many of the known risk factors for poor balance and falls can be modified by remedial therapy and other interventions (see Chaps. 20 and 24). Approaches to improving balance, gait, and strength in the elderly are discussed in detail in Chapters 21, 22, and 23.

The health benefits of exercise are supported by a substantial body of evidence [104, 105]. Exercise might prevent falls and injury by strengthening muscles and increasing endurance; maintaining and improving posture, joint motion, and postural competence; enhancing cardiopulmonary function; and improving alertness. An increasing number of studies show that endurance training in the elderly results in modest increases in aerobic capacity, whereas strength training results in substantial increases in muscle strength and muscle mass; these beneficial effects continue at very old ages, in extremes of frailty, and in those with chronic conditions [68, 103, 106]. In addition, weight-bearing exercise [107] and resistance training [108] may preserve bone strength, although this is controversial [109].

The type, level, intensity, and duration of exercise needed to achieve a reduction in falls and fall injuries are uncertain [104]. Aerobic training and low-level exercises, such as walking, may have insufficient effects on muscle strength, balance, and other risk factors for falls. High-intensity resistance training may be required to achieve the levels of improvement in muscle strength required to prevent falls [68]. Inadequate nutrition also may contribute to muscle weakness and should be considered a target for intervention [68].

Balance and gait abnormalities may be ameliorated through focused exercise and rehabilitative therapies, including strength training targeted to lower-extremity muscle groups, habituation exercises for vestibular problems, motor coordination and proprioception exercises to improve postural control, and gait training [84, 110, 111]. Strength training and other forms of exercise may have beneficial effects on balance and gait [103], particularly when combined with postural exercises designed to improve balance [52, 111, 112]. However, several well-done trials have failed to prove a beneficial effect of exercise and strength training on balance [113, 114].

More than 70% of persons 65 and older living in the community currently have at least one prescribed medication [115], and the percentage is even higher among nursing home residents [116]. However, there is evidence that polypharmacy can be reduced through medication review [117]. Conservative guidelines for use of psychotropic medications to prevent falls should be tested [77].

Environmental modifications focusing on removal of hazards (e.g., sidewalks and stairways in disrepair, poor lighting, slippery surfaces in bathrooms, unstable footwear) and improved functioning (e.g., grab bars, better positioning of handrails, improved design of furniture) are feasible in both clinical and community-based interventions [82, 118]. Because falls tend to occur where people spend the most time, a home-oriented environmental modification strategy may be effective. Many checklists are available to help identify fall hazards in the home [1, 119]. Attention to the interaction of specific physical disabilities and environmental factors may help prioritize remediation of the many potential problems that may be found.

It has not been established convincingly that efforts to modify risk factors reduce the risk of falling. Multifactorial interventions combining exercise and education about modifying fall risk factors have been tested in two randomized trials; one found no effect on falls [83] the other found a 15% reduction in the risk of falling but no effect on medically treated falls [82] and included minor home safety modifications. These trials used low-intensity exercises in an unscreened population, and the interventions were not targeted specifically to the risk factors present in individuals. In a group of nursing home residents with recent falls, Rubenstein et al. [118] randomized them to conventional care versus an intensive geriatric medical evaluation, treatment, and remediation of probable causes of the fall and risk factors. In the intervention group, nearly three treatment recommendations per subject were made to the primary care physician, approximately two-thirds of which were implemented. The intervention reduced hospitalization, but there was only a small (9%) nonsignificant reduction in falls. The subjects in this study had a very high risk of falls (two-thirds fell during 2 years of follow-up), and the efforts to modify risk factors were not standardized.

To be successful, it is likely that fall prevention interventions will have to identify populations with an increased risk of falls, to include standardized interventions for multiple risk factors, and to tailor the interventions to the presence of these risk factors in individuals [120]. Intervention components will need to address the strength, balance, and gait impairments that contribute to functional and mobility problems during routine tasks and should include interventions of sufficient focus and intensity, such as resistance and strength training and stimulation of postural responses, to effect an improvement in these impairments. Behavioral, environmental, and medication modifications should be included in multiple risk-factor interventions. However, it is important that study designs allow comparison of the efficacy of different intervention components, either through factorial designs or by testing specific components separately. Finally, whenever feasible, study end points should include serious fall injuries, physical function, and mobility, for it is the effect of falls on these outcomes that makes falls a major public health concern.

REFERENCES

1. Kellogg International Work Group on the Prevention of Falls by the Elderly. The prevention of falls in later life. *Dan Med Bull* 1987;34(4):1–24.
2. Sattin RW. Falls among older persons: A public health perspective. *Annu Rev Public Health* 1992;13:489–508.
3. National Safety Council. *Accident facts.* Chicago: National Safety Council, 1987.
4. Fife D. Injuries and deaths among elderly persons. *Am J Epidemiol* 1987;126(5):936–941.
5. Fisher ES, et al. Hip fracture incidence and mortality in New England. *Epidemiology* 1991;2:116–122.
6. Riggs JE. Mortality from accidental falls among the elderly in the United States, 1962–1988: Demonstrating the impact of improved trauma management. *J Trauma* 1993;35(2):212–219.
7. Rodriguez JG, Sattin RW, Waxweiler RJ. Incidence of hip fractures, United States, 1970–1983. *Am J Prev Med* 1989;5(3):175–181.
8. Campbell AJ, et al. Circumstances and consequences of falls experienced by a community population 70 years and over during a prospective study. *Age Ageing* 1990;19:136–141.

9.   Tinetti ME, Liu WL, Claus EB. Predictors and prognosis of inability to get up after falls among elderly persons. *JAMA* 1993;269(1):65–70.

10.   Wolinsky FD, Johnson RJ, Fitzgerald JF. Falling, health status, and the use of health services—A prospective study. *Med Care* 1992;30(7):587–597.

11.   Dunn JE, Rudberg MA, Furner SE, Cassel CK. Mortality, disability, and falls in older persons: The role of underlying disease and disability. *Am J Public Health* 1992;82(3):395–400.

12.   Hemenway D, Colditz GA. The effect of climate on fractures and deaths due to falls among white women. *Accid Anal Prev* 1990;22(1):59–65.

13.   Blake AJ, et al. Falls by elderly people at home: Prevalence and associated factors. *Age Ageing* 1988; 17:365–372.

14.   Campbell A, et al. Falls in old age: A study of frequency and related clinical factors. *Age Ageing* 1981;10:264–170.

15.   Prudham D, Evans J. Factors associated with falls in the elderly: A community study. *Age Ageing* 1981;10:141–146.

16.   Wickham C, Cooper C, Margetts BM, Barker DJP. Muscle strength, activity, housing and the risk of falls in elderly people. *Age Ageing* 1989;18:47–51.

17.   Cummings SR, Nevitt MC, Kidd S. Forgetting falls: The limited accuracy of recall of falls in the elderly. *J Am Geriatr Soc* 1988;36:613–616.

18.   Nevitt MC. Ascertainment and Description of Falls. In: Weindruch R, Ory M, eds. *Frailty Reconsidered: Reducing Frailty and Fall-Related Injuries in the Elderly.* Springfield, IL: Thomas, 1991. Pp 476–495.

19.   Campbell A, Borrie MJ, Spears GF. Risk factors for falls in a community-based prospective study of people 70 years and older. *J Gerontol* 1989;44(4):112–117.

20.   O'Laughlin JL, Robitaille Y, Boivin J, Suissa S. Incidence of and risk factors for falls and injurious falls among the community-dwelling elderly. *Am J Epidemiol* 1993;137(3):342–354.

21.   Tinetti ME, Speechley M, Ginter SF. Risk factors for falls among elderly persons living in the community. *N Engl J Med* 1988;319(26):1701–1707.

22.   Nevitt MC, Cummings SR, Kidd S, Black D. Risk factors for recurrent nonsyncopal falls: A prospective study. *JAMA* 1989;261(18):2663–2668.

23.   Campbell AJ, Spears GF, Borrie MJ. Examination by logistic regression modelling of the variables which increase the relative risk of elderly women falling compared to elderly men. *J Clin Epidemiol* 1990;43(12):1415–1420.

24.   Runge JW. The cost of injury. *Emerg Med Clin North Am* 1993;11(1):241–253.

25.   Rubenstein LZ, et al. Falls and instability in the elderly. *J Am Geriatr Soc* 1988;36(3):266–278.

26.   Rubenstein LZ, Josephson KR. Causes and Prevention of Falls in Elderly People. In: Vellas B, et al., eds. *Falls, Balance and Gait Disorders in the Elderly.* Paris: Elsevier, 1992. Pp 21–38.

27.   Myers AH, et al. Risk factors associated with falls and injuries among elderly institutionalized persons. *Am J Epidemiol* 1991;133(11):1179–1190.

28.   van Dijk PT. Meulenberg OG, van de Sande HJ, Habbema JD. Falls in dementia patients. *Gerontologist* 1993;33(2):200–204.

29.   Baker S, O'Neill B, Karpf RS. *The injury fact book.* Cambridge, MA: Lexington Books, 1984.

30.   Nevitt MC, Cummings SR, Hudes ES. Risk factors for injurious falls: A prospective study. *J Gerontol Med Sci* 1991;46(5):M164–170.

31.   Nevitt M, Cummings. SR. Falls and Fractures in Older Women. In: Vellas B, et al., eds. *Falls, Balance and Gait Disorders in the Elderly.* Paris: Elsevier, 1992. Pp 69–80.

32.   Tinetti ME, Speechley M. Prevention of falls among the elderly. *N Engl J Med* 1989; 302(16):1055–1059.

33.   Tinetti ME, Claus E, Liu WL. Risk Factors for Fall-Related Injuries Among Community Elderly: Methodological Issues. In: Vellas B, et al., eds. *Falls, Balance and Gait Disorders in the Elderly.* Paris: Elsevier, 1992. Pp 7–19.

34.   Fife D, Barancik JI, Chatterjee MS. Northeastern Ohio trauma study II: Injury rates by age, sex and cause. *Am J Public Health* 1984;74(5):473–478.

35.   Sattin RW, et al. The incidence of fall injury events among the elderly in a defined population. *Am J Epidemiol* 1990;131(6):1028–1037.

36. Cummings SR, Nevitt MC. A hypothesis: The causes of hip fractures. *J Gerontol* 1989; 44(4):M107–111.

37. Nevitt MC, Cummings SR. Type of fall and risk of hip and wrist fractures: The Study of osteoporotic fractures. *J Am Geriatr Soc* 1993;41(11):1226–1234.

38. Melton L. Osteoporosis. In: Berg, RL, Cassells JS, eds. *The Second Fifty Years: Promoting Health and Preventing Disability*. Washington, DC: National Academy Press, 1990. Pp 76–100.

39. Griffin MR, Ray WA, Fought RL, Melton LJ. Black-white differences in fracture rates. *Am J Epidemiol* 1992;136(11):1378–1385.

40. Kosorok MR, et al. Restricted activity days among older adults. *Am J Public Health* 1992; 82(9):1263–1267.

41. National Center for Health Statistics. Current estimates from the National Health Interview Survey, United States, 1986. *Vital and Health Statistics, Series 10(164)*. Washington, DC: US Government Printing Office, 1987. Pp 16–52.

42. Grisso JA, et al. The impact of falls in an inner-city elderly African-American population. *J Am Geriatr Soc* 1992;40(7):673–678.

43. Tinetti ME, Mendes de Leon CF, Doucette JT, Baker DI. Fear of falling and fall-related efficacy in relationship to functioning among community-living elders. *J Gerontol* 1994; 49(3):M140–M147.

44. Ray WA, Griffin MR, Baugh DK. Mortality following hip fracture before and after implementation of the prospective payment system. *Arch Intern Med* 1990;150:2109–2114.

45. Vellas B, et al. Prospective study of restriction of activity in old people after falls. *Age Ageing* 1987;16:189–193.

46. Peck WA, et al. Research directions in osteoporosis. *Am J Med* 1988;84:275–282.

47. Phillips S, Fox N, Jacobs J, Wright WE. The direct medical costs of osteoporosis for American women aged 45 and older, 1986. *Bone* 1988;9:271–279.

48. Covington DL, Maxwell JG, Clancy TV. Hospital resources used to treat the injured elderly at North Carolina Trauma Centers. *J Am Geriatr Soc* 1993;41:847–852.

49. Wolfson L, et al. The Effects of Age, Disease and Gender on the Balance of Healthy Elderly. In: Vellas B, et al., eds. *Falls, Balance and Gait Disorders in the Elderly*. Paris: Elsevier, 1992. Pp 129–135.

50. Stelmach CE, Worringham CJ. Sensorimotor deficits related to postural stability: Implications for falling in the elderly. *Clin Geriatr Med* 1985;1(3):679–694.

51. Woolacott MH. Age-related changes in posture and movement. *J Gerontol* 1993;48(S):55–60.

52. Alexander NB. Postural control in older adults. *J Am Geriatr Soc* 1994;42(1):93–108.

53. Northridge ME, Nevitt MC, Kelsey JL, Link B. Home hazards and falls in the elderly: The role of health and functional status. *Am J Public Health* 1995; 85(4):509–515.

54. Speechly M, Tinetti M. Falls and injuries in frail and vigorous community elderly persons. *J Am Geriatr Soc* 1991;39:46–52.

55. Northridge ME, Nevitt MC, Kelsey JL. Nonsyncopal falls in the elderly in relation to home hazards. *Osteoporos Int* 1996;4:249–255.

56. Topper AK, Holliday PJ. Are activity-based assessments of balance and gait in the elderly predictive of risk of falling and/or type of fall? *J Am Geriatr Soc* 1993;41(5):480–487.

57. Studenski S, et al. Predicting falls: The role of mobility and nonphysical factors. *J Am Geriatr Soc* 1994;42:297–302.

58. Cumming RG, Kelsey JL, Nevitt MC. Methodologic issues in the study of frequent and recurrent health problems, falls in the elderly. *Ann Epidemiol* 1990;1(1):49–56.

59. Kanten DN, et al. Falls: An examination of three reporting methods in nursing homes. *J Am Geriatr Soc* 1993;41:662–666.

60. Lach HW, et al. Falls in the elderly: Reliability of a classification system. *J Am Geriatr Soc* 1991;39:197–202.

61. Lord SR, Clark RD, Webster IW. Physiological factors associated with falls in an elderly population. *J Am Geriatr Soc* 1991;39:1194–1200.

62. Rodriguez JG, Sattin RW, DeVito CA, Wingo PA. Developing an Environmental Hazards Assessment Instrument for Falls Among the Elderly. In: Weindruch R, Ory M, eds. *Frailty Re-*

considered: Reducing Frailty and Fall-Related Injuries in the Elderly. Springfield, IL: Thomas, 1991. Pp 263–276.

63. Harris T, Kovar MG. National statistics on the functional status of older persons. In: Weindruch R, Ory M, eds. *Frailty Reconsidered: Reducing Frailty and Fall-Related Injuries in the Elderly.* Springfield, IL: Thomas, 1991. Pp 15–28.

64. Whipple R, et al. Altered sensory function and balance in older persons. *J Gerontol* 1993; 48(S):71–76.

65. Wolfson LI, Whipple R, Amerman P. Gait and balance in the elderly: Two functional capacities that link sensory and motor ability to falls. *Clin Geriatr Med* 1985;1(3):649–660.

66. Owen DH. Maintain posture and avoid tripping. *Clin Geriatr Med* 1985;1(3):581–600.

67. Studenski S, Duncan PW, Chandler J. Postural responses and effector factors in persons with unexplained falls: Results and methodologic issues. *J Am Geriatr Soc* 1991;39:229–234.

68. Fiatarone MA, Evans WJ. The etiology and reversibility of muscle dysfunction in the aged. *J Gerontol* 1993;48(S):77–83.

69. Grimby G, Saltin B. Mini-review: The aging muscle. *Clin Physiol* 1983;3:209–218.

70. Buchner DM, Larson EB. Falls and fractures in patients with Alzheimer's type dementia. *JAMA* 1987;257(11):1492–1495.

71. Mossey JM. Social and psychologic factors related to falls among the elderly. *Clin Geriatr Med* 1985;1(3):541–554.

72. Maki BE, Holliday PJ, Topper AK. Fear of falling and postural performance in the elderly. *J Gerontol* 1991;46(4):M123–31.

73. Horak FB. Effects of Neurological Disorders on Postural Movement Strategies in the Elderly. In: Vellas B, et al., eds. *Falls, Balance and Gait Disorders in the Elderly.* Paris: Elsevier, 1992. Pp 137–151.

74. Tinetti ME. Performance-oriented assessment of mobility problems in the elderly. *J Am Geriatr Soc* 1986;34(2):119–126.

75. Alexander NB, Schultz AB, Warwick DN. Rising from a chair: Effects of age and functional ability on performance biomechanics. *J Gerontol Med Sci* 1991;46(3):M91–98.

76. Lipsitz LA, Jonsson PV, Kelley MM, Koestner JS. Causes and correlates of recurrent falls in ambulatory frail elderly. *J Gerontol Med Sci* 1991;46(4):M114–122.

77. Ray WA, Griffin MR. Prescribed Medications, Falling, and Fall-Related Injuries. In: Weindruch R, Ory M, eds. *Frailty Reconsidered: Reducing Frailty and Fall-Related Injuries in the Elderly.* Springfield, IL: Thomas 1991. Pp 76–89.

78. Robbins AS, et al. Predictors of falls among elderly people: Results of two population-based studies. *Arch Intern Med* 1989;194:1628–1633.

79. Hogue CC. A Person-Environment Model for Understanding Fall Risk. In: Weindruch R, Ory M, eds. *Frailty Reconsidered: Reducing Frailty and Fall-Related Injuries in the Elderly.* Springfield, IL: Thomas 1991. Pp 96–105.

80. Fleming BE, Pendergast DR. Physical condition, activity pattern, and environment as factor in falls by adult care facility residents. *Arch Phys Med Rehabil* 1993;74:627–630.

81. Tobis JS, et al. Visual perception dominance of fallers among community-dwelling older adults. *J Am Geriatr Soc* 1985;33(5):330–333.

82. Hornbrook MC, et al. Preventing falls among community-dwelling older persons: Results from a randomized trial. *Gerontologist* 1994;34(1):16–23.

83. Reinsch S, MacRae P, Lachenbruch PA, Tobis JS. Attempts to prevent falls and injury: A prospective community study. *Gerontologist* 1992;32(4):450–456.

84. Tobis JS, Reinsch S. Postural instability in the elderly: Contributing factors and suggestions for rehabilitation. *Crit Rev Phys Rehabil Med* 1989;1(2):59–65.

85. Kelsey J, et al. Risk factors for fractures of the distal forearm and proximal humerus. *Am J Epidemiol* 1992;135(5):477–489.

86. Hayes WC, Piazza SJ, Zysset PK. Biomechanics of fracture risk prediction of the hip and spine by quantitative computed tomography. *Radiol Clin North Am* 1991;29(1).

87. Courtney AC, Wachtel EF, Myers ER, Hayes WC. Effects of loading rate on strength of the proximal femur. *Calcif Tissue Int* 1994;55:53–58.

88. Committee on Trauma Research, Commission on Life Sciences, National Research Council, and the Institute of Medicine. *Injury in America.* Washington, DC: National Academy Press, 1985.

89. Steiger P, et al. Age-related decrements in bone mineral density in women over 65. *J Bone Miner Res* 1992;7(6):625–632.

90. Seeley D, et al. Which fractures are associated with low appendicular bone mass in elderly women? *Ann Intern Med* 1991;115(1):837–842.

91. Melton L, et al. How many women have osteoporosis? *J Bone Miner Res* 1992;7(9):1005–1010.

92. Melton LJ III, Riggs BL. Risk factors for injury after a fall. *Clin Geriatr Med* 1985; 1(3): 525–530.

93. Greenspan SL, et al. Fall severity and bone mineral density as risk factors for hip fracture in ambulatory elderly. *JAMA* 1994;271(2):128–133.

94. Hayes W, et al. Impact near the hip dominates fracture risk in elderly nursing home residents who fall. *Calcif Tissue Int* 1993;52:192–198.

95. Lauritzen J, Petersen M, Lund B. Effect of external hip protectors on hip fractures. *Lancet* 1993;341:11–13.

96. Cumming RG, Klineberg J. Fall frequency and characteristics and the risk of hip fractures. *J Am Geriatr Soc* 1994;42(7):774–778.

97. Felson DT, et al. Impaired vision and hip fracture: The Framingham Study. *J Am Geriatr Soc* 1989;37:495–500.

98. Grisso JA, et al. Risk factors for falls as a cause of hip fracture in women. *N Engl J Med* 1991;324:1326–1331.

99. Nguyen T, et al. Prediction of osteoporotic fractures by postural instability and bone density. *BMJ* 1993;307:1111–1115.

100. Porter RW, Miller CG, Grainger D, Palmer SB. Prediction of hip fracture in elderly women: A prospective study. *BMJ* 1990;301:638–641.

101. Ray WA, Griffin MR, Downey W. Benzodiazepines of long and short elimination half-life and risk of hip fracture. *JAMA* 1989;262:3303–3307.

102. Clark RD, Lord SR, Webster IW. Clinical parameters associated with falls in an elderly population. *Gerontology* 1993;39:117–123.

103. Buchner DM. Effects of physical activity on health status in older adults II: Intervention studies. *Annu Rev Public Health* 1992;13:469–488.

104. Harris SS, Caspersen CJ, DeFriese GH, Estes H Jr. Physical activity counseling for healthy adults as a primary preventive intervention in the clinical setting. *JAMA* 1989;261 (24):3590–3598.

105. US Preventive Services Task Force. Recommendations for physical exercise in primary prevention. *JAMA* 1989;261(24):3588–3589.

106. Fiatarone MA, et al. High-intensity strength training in nonagenarians, effects on skeletal muscle. *JAMA* 1990;263(22):3029–3034.

107. Krall EA, Dawson-Hughes B. Walking is related to bone density and rates of bone loss. *Am J Med* 1994;96:22–26.

108. Pruitt LA, Jackson RD, Bartels RL, Lehnhard HJ. Weight-training effects on bone mineral density in early postmenopausal women. *J Bone Miner Res* 1992;7(2):179–185.

109. Gutin B, Kasper M. Can vigorous exercise play a role in osteoporosis prevention? *Osteoporosis Int* 1992;2:55–69.

110. Shumway-Cook A, Horak FB. Vestibular rehabilitation: An exercise approach to managing symptoms of vestibular dysfunction. *Semin Hearing* 1989;10(2):196–209.

111. Judge JO, Underwood M, Gennosa T. Exercise to improve gait velocity in older persons. *Arch Phys Med Rehabil* 1993;74(4):400–406.

112. Judge JO, Lindsey C, Underwood M, Winsemius D. Balance improvements in older women: Effects of exercise training. *Phys Ther* 1993;73(4):254–262.

113. Crilly RG, et al. Effect of exercise on postural sway in the elderly. *Gerontology* 1989;35:137–143.

114. Lichtenstein MJ. Exercise and balance in aged women: A pilot controlled clinical trait. *Arch Phys Med Rehabil* 1989;70:138–143.

115. Havlik RJ, et al. Health statistics on older persons, United States, 1986. (DHHS pub. no. [PHS] 87-1409.) Hyattsville, MD: National Center for Health Statistics, 1987.

116. Beers M, et al. Psychoactive medication use in intermediate-care facility residents. *JAMA* 1988;260:3016–3020.

117. Gurwitz JH, Soumerai SB, Avorn J. Improving medication prescribing and utilization in the nursing home. *J Am Geriatr Soc* 1990;38:542–552.

118. Rubenstein LZ, et al. The value of assessing falls in an elderly population—a randomized clinical trial. *Ann Intern Med* 1990;113(4):308–316.

119. Tideiksaar R. Preventing falls: Home hazard checklists to help older patients protect themselves. *Geriatrics* 1986;41(5):26–28.

120. Tinetti ME, et al. Yale ficsit: Risk factor abatement strategy for fall prevention. *J Am Geriatr Soc* 1993;41:315–320.

121. Teno K, Kiel DP, Mor V. Multiple stumbles: A risk factor for falls in community-dwelling elderly. A prospective study. *J Am Geriatr Soc* 1990;38:1321–1325.

122. Gabell A, Simons MA, Nayak USL. Falls in the healthy elderly: Predisposing causes. *Ergonomics* 1985;28(7):965–975.

123. Tinetti ME, Williams FT, Mayewski R. A fall risk index for elderly patients based on number of chronic disabilities. *Am J Med* 1986;80:429–434.

124. Duncan PW, Studenski S, Chandler J, Prescott B. Functional reach: Predictive validity in a sample of elderly male veterans. *J Gerontol* 1992;47(3):M93–98.

125. Wolfson LI, Whipple R, Amerman P. Stressing the postural response: A quantitative method for resting balance. *J Am Geriatr Soc* 1986;34:845–850.

126. Fernie G, et al. The relationship of postural sway in standing to the incidence of falls in geriatric subjects. *Age Ageing* 1981;11:11–16.

127. Overstall P, et al. Falls in the elderly related to postural imbalance. *Br Med J* 1977;(1):261–264.

128. Ring C, Nayak USL, Isaacs B. Balance function in elderly people who have and who have not fallen. *Arch Phys Med Rehabil* 1988;69:261–264.

129. Guimaraes RM, Isaacs B. Characteristics of the gait in old people who fall. *Int Rehabil Med* 1980;2:177–180.

130. Imms F, Edholm O. Studies of gait and mobility in the elderly. *Age Ageing* 1981;10:147–156.

131. Wolfson L, Whipple R, Amerman P, Tobin JN. Gait assessment in the elderly: A gait abnormality rating scale and its relation to falls. *J Gerontol* 1990;45(1):M12–19.

132. Whipple RH, Wolfson LI, Amerman PM. The relationship of knee and ankle weakness to falls in nursing home residents: An isokinetic study. *J Am Geriatr Soc* 1987;35:13–20.

133. Sorock GS, Shimkin EE. Benzodiazepine sedatives and the risk of falling in a community-dwelling elderly cohort. *Arch Intern Med* 1988;148:2441–2444.

134. Granek, E, et al. Medications and diagnoses in relation to falls in a long-term care facility. *J Am Geriatr Soc* 1987;35:503–511.

135. Morris JC, Rubin EH, Morris EJ, Mandel SA. Senile dementia of the Alzheimer's type: An important risk factor for serious falls. *J Gerontol* 1987;42:412–417.

136. Cumming RG, et al. Medications and multiple falls in elderly people: The St Louis OASIS study. *Age Ageing* 1991;20(6):455–461.

3. Physiology of Balance, with Special Reference to the Healthy Elderly

Lewis M. Nashner

CHRONIC BALANCE AND MOBILITY DISORDERS

A Major Medical Problem

Balance and mobility disorders are the single largest cause of chronic disability in individuals aged 60 or older, according to a British study [1]. A probable cause for the prevalence of balance and mobility problems among the elderly is the relatively high percentage of cases that are not resolved by medical intervention [2]. Clinical resolution by traditional medical means is frustrated by the fact that balance and mobility impairments in the elderly frequently cannot be attributed to specific localized diseases [3].

Need for Multidisciplinary Management

This chapter presents a systems model of balance and mobility control. According to this model, balance and mobility functions are maintained by cooperative interactions among the biomechanical, musculoskeletal, sensory, and central nervous system components. As an individual's age advances, the potential for one or a combination of these components to suffer impairment increases. When impairment is limited to a single component, the impact on overall function frequently is masked by the compensatory actions of the other healthy components. In contrast, the cumulative impact on overall function may exceed a simple sum of the individual effects when multiple components are impaired. In these cases, the additional cumulative impairment is due to the loss of compensatory interactions among the impaired components.

The systems model suggests why traditional treatment approaches that focus on single localized disease process frequently are ineffective in reducing the disabilities of elderly persons with chronic balance and mobility disorders. The systems model of balance and mobility suggests that an alternative multidisciplinary management approach focused on the treatable functional impairments and their interactions can prove more beneficial in reducing chronic disability [3–5].

BIOMECHANICS OF POSTURE AND MOVEMENT

Definition of Balance

A standing person is inherently unstable and will fall in the absence of active balance controls, because the body's center of gravity (COG) is located well above a relatively small base of support. As long as the COG is maintained over the base of support, a person can both resist the destabilizing influence of gravity and actively move the COG to perform activities, such as rising from a chair, reaching, turning, and walking [6–8]. Once the COG deviates beyond the perimeter of the base of support, however, a rapid step, stumble, or external support is required to prevent a fall.

Base of Support

The base of support during standing is the area contained within the perimeter of the area of contact between the support surface and the feet. The base of support is nearly square when the feet are placed comfortably apart on a flat surface. A diagonal stance produces a parallelogram shaped base of support extending forward on one side and backward on the other. Tandem stance substantially extends the length of the support base but produces a very narrow width.

When the support surface is shorter than the feet are long or when surface irregularities limit areas of contact between the feet and the surface, the base of support is reduced. Standing perpendicular to the longitudinal axis of a narrow beam, for example, substantially reduces the length of the support base but does not affect the width.

Limits of Stability

The family of COG sway angles that place the COG at the outer perimeter of the base of support form a two-dimensional quantity termed the *limits of stability* (LOS) [7,9]. In normal adults standing on a flat, firm surface with feet spaced comfortably apart, the theoretical LOS perimeter forms an ellipse similar to that shown in Fig. 3-1. The anteroposterior (AP) dimension of the ellipse is approximately 12.5 degrees from the backwardmost to the forwardmost points on the perimeter [10–12]. Both the height of the COG above the surface and foot length affect the AP limits of stability. Because subject height and foot length co-vary, the AP limits are similar for people of various heights [13]. The lateral dimension of the LOS depends on the person's height relative to the spacing of the feet. For a typical spacing, the lateral dimension is approximately 16 degrees.

Factors influencing an individual's actual LOS are similar when standing in place, walking, and sitting without trunk support as shown in Fig. 3-2. During in-place standing, the COG moves randomly within an LOS perimeter determined by the base of support and the placement of the feet. During sitting without trunk support, the height of the COG above the support surface is less, and the base area is larger. Therefore, the LOS perimeter is larger in sitting than in quiet standing. During walking, a new LOS is established with each step. During progression of the step, the COG moves from the rear boundary of the LOS to the front.

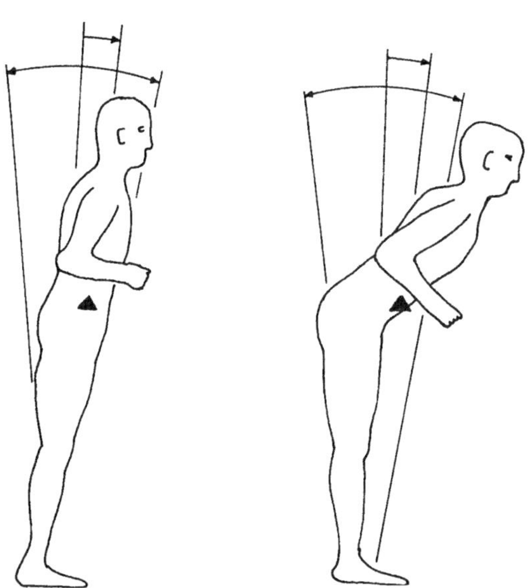

Figure 3-1. Center of gravity (COG) sway angle in relation to the limits of stability cone. The figure on the left is moving about the ankles, the figure on the right is moving about the hips. COG sway angles of the two figures are the same. Filled diamonds show the body COG positions. (From LM Nashner, Computerized Dynamic Posturography. In: GP Jacobson, CW Newman, JM Kartush, eds. *Handbook of Balance Function Testing.* Chicago: Mosby–Year Book, 1993. Pp 280–307.)

Postural Movement Strategies

To maintain balance and perform purposeful activities while standing and walking, a person must be able to actively control the movements of the COG relative to the base of support. Because there are three joints located between the support base and the COG in the lower abdomen, a wide variety of ankle, knee, and hip joint movement patterns can (in theory) be used to move the COG. Functionally effective patterns of ankle, knee, and hip joint movements are constrained to a relatively few patterns generally referred to as *movement strategies* (Fig. 3-3). The number of effective movement strategies is limited by the height of the body in relation to its relatively small base of support. The stepping strategy is the only effective way to prevent a fall once the COG has deviated beyond the LOS perimeter. The step establishes a new base of support beneath the COG.

Two movement strategies are used to move the COG to positions within the LOS perimeter without the feet either losing contact with or changing position on the surface. Rotating the body as an approximately rigid mass about the ankle joints is commonly referred to as the *ankle strategy* [11,14]. The ankle strategy moves the body COG by generating ankle torque against the support surface and counteracting knee and hip torques to stabilize these proximal joints. A rapid

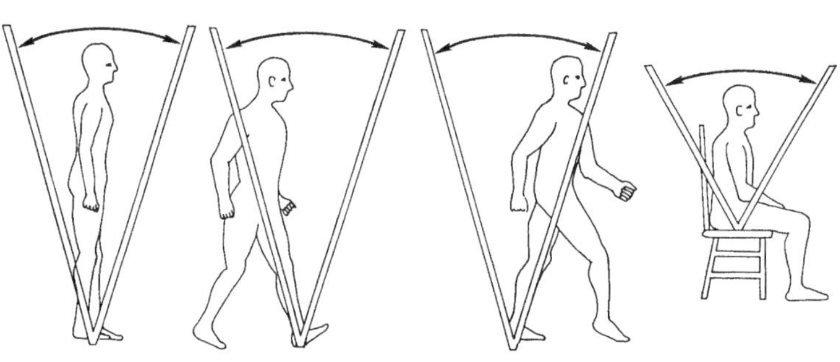

Figure 3-2. Limits of stability boundaries during standing, walking, and sitting. (From LM Nashner, Computerized Dynamic Posturography. In: GP Jacobson, CW Newman, JM Kartush, eds. *Handbook of Balance Function Testing*. Chicago: Mosby–Year Book, 1993. Pp 280–307.)

movement of the trunk about the hip joints accompanied by smaller opposing rotation about the ankles is commonly referred to as the *hip strategy*. The hip strategy relies on the inertia of the rapidly moving trunk to generate a horizontal shear force against the support surface to move the COG.

There is no single appropriate movement strategy for balancing under all conditions. The relative effectiveness of ankle, hip, and stepping strategies depends on the configuration of the base of support, the COG alignment in relation to the LOS perimeter, and the speed of the desired COG movement [11, 13, 15]. Because the ankle strategy relies on the exertion of ankle torque against the support surface, it is most effective when the COG movements are slow and well within the LOS perimeter and when the support base is sufficiently firm and

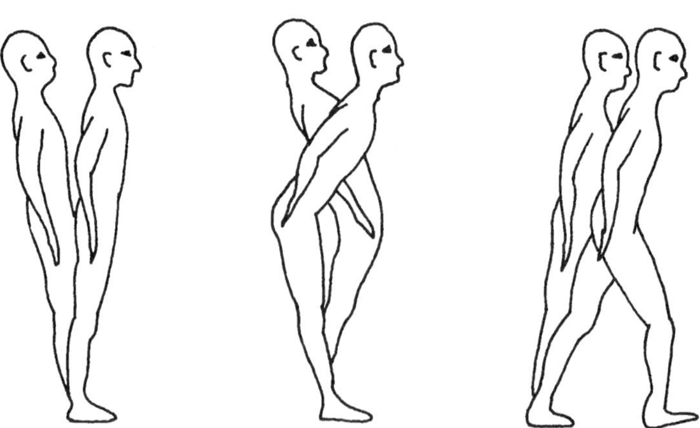

Figure 3-3. Functional properties of the ankle, hip, and stepping strategies for moving the center of gravity relative to the base of support. (From LM Nashner, Computerized Dynamic Posturography. In: GP Jacobson, CW Newman, JM Kartush, eds. *Handbook of Balance Function Testing*. Chicago: Mosby–Year Book, 1993. Pp 280–307.)

broad to support the exertion of torque. When these constraints are met, ankle torques do not cause the toes or heels to lift off the support surface.

For rapid COG movements and movements near the LOS perimeter; hip movements are effective when ankle movements are not. However, because the hip strategy relies on transient inertial forces generated by rapid trunk motions rather than ankle torques, hip movements can displace the COG only short distances, and they cannot be used to maintain the COG in an off-center position.

When conditions are intermediate between those favoring use of an ankle or hip strategy and when subjects are adapting to a new surface condition, combinations of ankle and hip movements commonly are observed. In response to changes in conditions, transitions from one strategy to another occur progressively over a series of responses rather than instantaneously. The reader can experience the biomechanical constraints on ankle and hip movements by swaying with increasing speed back and forth about the ankles. As body speed and ankle torques increase, a limit is reached when the toes or heels lift from the surface and no further increases are possible. Use of the hip strategy is experienced by shifting one's posture while standing on tip toes or with the feet placed laterally heel to toe.

PHYSIOLOGY OF POSTURAL MOVEMENT CONTROL

Three Movement Systems

The three systems for organizing the activation levels of muscles are reviewed in Table 3-1. The myotatic stretch reflex is the first mechanism to respond to external perturbations. The major role of this mechanism is believed to be the regulation of muscle contractile forces. Automatic postural movements are the earliest functionally effective responses helping to regain stability following an external challenge to a standing individual's balance [16–18]. In contrast to reflex

Table 3-1. Roles of the three movement systems

Property	Movement System		
	Reflex	Automatic	Voluntary
Mediating pathways	Spinal cord	Brain stem and subcortical	Brainstem and cortical
Mode of activation	External stimulus	External stimulus	Self-generated or stimulus
Response properties	Localized to point of stimulus and highly stereotyped	Coordinated among leg and trunk muscles, and stereotyped but adaptable	Limitless variety
Role in posture control	Regulate muscle forces	Coordinate movements across joints	Generate purposeful behaviors
Onset times	Fixed at 35–40 msec	Fixed at 85–95 msec	Varies with difficulty; 150+ msec

and automatic movements, voluntary postural movements can be either self-initiated or initiated in response to an external stimulus. The variety of voluntary movement patterns possible is almost limitless.

Automatic Postural Movements

Automatic postural movements resemble reflex responses in some respects and voluntary movements in others. Like reflexes, automatic movements are triggered by abrupt, unexpected external stimuli, occur at fixed latencies, and are relatively stereotyped. Like voluntary postural movements, automatic responses involve the coordinated actions of many leg and trunk muscles. Also, automatic response amplitudes and patterns are strongly influenced by the individual's most recent performance experiences and by the external task conditions under which they are executed.

When an automatic postural movement is initiated by an abrupt external stimulus, the onset of muscular electromyelography activity occurs within 90 to 100 msec, and the resulting patterns of activation among leg and lower trunk muscles are directionally specific and relatively stereotyped, as shown in Fig. 3-4. The onset of active force as measured by a force plate is delayed an additional 20 to 40 msec beyond the electromyography, owing to the delay between electrical activation and force generation of muscle [20].

The neural pathways mediating automatic postural movements have not been identified, although the 90 to 100-msec electromyography latencies suggest sufficient time for participation of brainstem and cortical structures [21, 22]. Additional evidence for brainstem and cortical involvement is provided by clinical observations of delayed long-latency (automatic) responses in patient populations with brain and spinal cord lesions [23].

Local somatosensory input from the feet and proprioceptive input from the ankle joint muscles are sufficient to trigger an automatic postural response [24] and to determine the direction of the resulting movement [14, 17, 18]. A backward movement is triggered by forward displacement of the body COG (e.g., when the support surface moves backward or when the subject pulls backward on a rigid object). A forward movement follows a backward COG displacement caused by forward movement of the surface or by pushes against a rigid object.

Although there is a relationship between the amplitude of the triggering somatosensory stimulus and the automatic movement [24], visual input, vestibular input, and the recent experiences of the individual also strongly influence the response amplitudes [25–27]. The pattern of leg and lower trunk muscle contractions depends on the movement strategy that in turn is determined by the configuration of the support surface and the recent performance experience of the individual.

The importance of somatosensory, visual, and vestibular inputs in modulating the amplitudes of automatic postural responses has been illustrated in studies of patients with known neurological diseases. Peripheral neuropathy and multiple sclerosis, for example, not only delay automatic response latencies but also impair the ability to modulate response amplitudes in relation to stimulus size

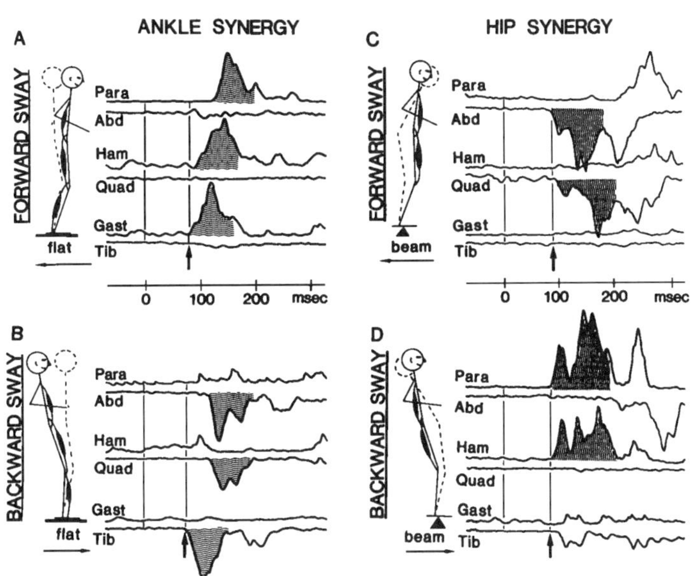

Figure 3-4. Patterns of ankle, thigh, and lower trunk muscle electromyography (EMG) responses during executions of movements organized into ankle (*A, B*) and hip (*C, D*) strategies. EMG signals full-wave rectified and low-pass filtered. Traces show averages of five trials. Traces of antagonist muscles acting about the same joint are grouped. The trace of the functional extensor muscle is displaced upward by increased activation. The functional flexor trace is displaced downward during activation. Para = paraspinal; Abd = abdominal; Ham = hamstrings; Quad = quadriceps; Gast = gastrocnemius; Tib = tibialis anterior. (From JV Begbie, Some Problems of Postural Sway. In: AVS de Reuck, J Knight, eds. CIBA Foundation Symposium on Myotatic, Kinesthetic and Vestibular Mechanisms. London: Churchill, 1967. Pp 80–92.)

[28–30]. In contrast, automatic responses are inappropriately small but not delayed in patients with bilateral peripheral vestibular deficits [27].

Coordination of Automatic Postural Responses

The movement strategy with which a subject responds to an external perturbation is set in advance, depending on the person's recent performance experience, not on an unconscious or conscious decision made at the time of the stimulus [14, 15]. Individuals well-practiced at standing on a firm support surface can use relatively pure ankle strategies. Similarly, subjects well-practiced at standing on a narrow beam may use relatively pure hip strategies. During initial practice trials following changes in support surface conditions, in contrast, more complex movements combining the two pure strategies are observed.

Clinical studies demonstrate the importance of sensory information and central mechanisms in selection of functionally appropriate movement strategies. Patients with profound bilateral vestibular deficits (absence of responses under high-frequency rotary chair testing) persist in using ankle strategies under conditions in which hip movements are functionally more effective, despite their apparent ability to voluntarily produce hip movement patterns [31]. Theory suggests that vestibular inputs may be critical to proper coordination of trunk and head movements associated with the hip strategy. For reasons not fully understood, individual patients with partial peripheral or central vestibular system lesions may persist in the use of either ankle or hip movements, even when the other strategy is more efficient. Normal subjects deprived of somatosensory inputs from the feet by bilateral ischemia preferentially use hip movements when ankle strategies are more effective [23]. Finally, parkinsonian patients persist in using ineffective combinations of ankle and hip strategies and show inflexibility in modifying patterns in response to changes in surface conditions [32].

Research studies have demonstrated no single characteristic change in movement strategies in elderly populations. The prevalence in elderly populations of many of the diseases just mentioned suggests that no single deficit will be found. Depending on the combination of subtle biomechanical, sensory, and neurological deficits, an elderly individual may display a number of different forms of inappropriate strategies.

Voluntary Postural Movements

Unlike the relatively fixed latencies of automatic responses, voluntary response latencies vary with the complexity of, and the person's attention to the task, ranging from a minimum of approximately 150 msec for leg muscles to much longer times [33]. In further contrast to automatic responses, persons performing complex voluntary movements as rapidly as possible frequently make execution errors, such as responding in the inappropriate direction.

A person's voluntary actions either may alter balance directly or may involve the arms, trunk, and head in ways that have an indirect effect. One example of a direct voluntary change is a weight shift from one leg to the other prior to initiating a step or changing the placement of the feet on the surface.

Another is a forward shifting of the COG from over the buttocks to over the feet during initiation of the sit-to-stand maneuver. Actions having the largest indirect effects on balance are those during which forces are exerted against external objects. When a freely standing person pulls open a heavy door or lifts a heavy object, for example, the forces exerted against the external objects generate equal and opposite forces on the COG. Voluntary actions not involving external objects (e.g., raising an arm) have small but nevertheless significant effects on a person's stability.

Research has shown that voluntary actions with the potential for disturbing balance are delayed actively so that an anticipatory postural response can establish a stable base of support. When a freely standing person pulls on an object, for example, an automatic postural movement is initiated in leg muscles in advance of the activation of the arm muscles, and the direction and amplitude of the anticipatory action are scaled to the expected direction and size of the external load [33–35]. Coordination of voluntary and postural components depends on the requirements for postural stability. When the need for active stabilization is removed by providing trunk support during the standing arm pull, the stabilizing postural responses in the leg muscle are abolished, and voluntary activation of arm muscles is initiated more quickly.

PHYSIOLOGY OF SENSORY POSTURAL CONTROL

Senses Involved in Postural Control

Sensing the position of the COG relative to the base of support requires a combination of visual, vestibular, and somatosensory (tactile, deep-pressure, joint receptor, and muscle proprioceptor) inputs. Use of the three balance senses is reviewed in Table 3-2. Three senses are required because no single sense can measure directly the COG position relative to gravity and the base of support. Vision measures the orientation of the eyes and head in relation to surrounding objects. The somatosensory input provides information on the orientation of body parts relative to one another and to the support surface. The vestibular input does not provide orientation information in relation to external objects. Rather, it measures gravitational, linear, and angular accelerations of the head in relation to inertial space.

There is no single combination of the three senses providing accurate COG information under all performance conditions. This is because one or more of the senses may provide information that is misleading or inaccurate for purposes of balance control. For example, when a person stands next to a large bus that suddenly begins to move forward, momentary disorientation or unsteadiness may result. A fraction of a second is required for the brain to determine whether the resulting visual stimulus indicates backward sway or forward movement of the bus. Similarly, a downward tilting support surface may be confused with a backward swaying of the body.

During sensory conflict situations, the brain must quickly select the sensory inputs providing accurate orientation information and must ignore the other

Table 3-2. Use of the senses for balance

Sense	Reference	Conditions favoring use	Conditions disrupting use
Somatosensory	Support surface	Fixed support surface	Irregular or moving support
Visual	Surrounding objects	Fixed visible surrounds and irregular or moving support	Moving surrounds or darkness
Vestibular	Gravity and inertial space	Irregular or moving support and moving surrounds or darkness	Unusual motion environments

misleading ones. Failure to ignore conflicting sensory inputs can lead to instability or surface and surround motion illusions. The process of selecting and combining appropriate sensory information has been termed *sensory organization.*

Somatosensory Input

Under fixed support surface conditions, somatosensory input derived from the contact forces and motions between the feet and the support surface dominates the control of balance [36–40]. When a person stands on a firm, level surface, the extent of COG sway is very small relative to the LOS. Closing the eyes to eliminate vision or moving the visual surround to disrupt it causes little if any functionally significant increase in COG sway, although some studies have reported very slight but statistically significant increases. The strength of the somatosensory input allows a well-compensated patient with a bilateral vestibular loss to maintain sway well within the LOS with the eyes closed [41–44].

Visual Input

Vision plays a significant role in balance when the support surface is unstable [45–49]. For example, when toes-up and toes-down tilting of the surface in direct relation to the anteroposterior sway disrupts somatosensory input useful for balance, COG sway is significantly less with eyes open than with eyes closed [41–43]. The stabilizing effect of vision also is illustrated by comparing eyes-open and eyes-closed sway while a person stands on a compliant foam rubber pad.

Vision influences COG alignment. When a person is exposed to a constant linear or rotational movement of the visual field, for example, the alignment of the COG over the base of support shifts in the direction of the visual field's motion [50, 51].

Vestibular Input

When functionally useful somatosensory and visual inputs are available under fixed support and visual surround conditions, the vestibular input plays a lesser role in direct control of the COG position [43, 44, 52]. This is probably because the somatosensory and visual inputs are more sensitive to body sway than is the vestibular system [53]. The primary role of vestibular input under these conditions is to enable independent and precise control of head and eye movements. Precise head and eye control is critical in the execution of many complex daily life motor activities, such as running and either kicking or catching a moving ball.

Vestibular input, however, is critical for balance under sensory conflict conditions and when somatosensory and visual inputs are unavailable [54, 55]. The patient with a profound bilateral vestibular loss, for example, is unsteady standing in darkness on a compliant or irregular surface. Because input from the healthy vestibular system is seldom if ever misleading (the exception being unusual motion environments), the vestibular input plays a critical role when conflicting visual or somatosensory information requires a person to identify and quickly ignore a misleading input [42, 54]. This is probably why patients with vestibular system deficits frequently complain of problems with vision and report dizziness, unsteadiness, and unusual sensory illusions when exposed to conflicting visual and support surface environments.

Isolating the Sensory Inputs to Balance

Isolating deficits in sensory organization can be difficult, because redundant information from one sense can mask a problem in another sense under normal performance conditions. To overcome this limitation, the sensory organization test comprising six different conditions has been devised to isolate and assess the functional effectiveness of visual, vestibular, and somatosensory inputs to balance. This test also is designed to assess an individual's ability to select the input(s) providing the most appropriate functional orientation information under a variety of conditions.

In the computed version of the test, the six conditions shown in Fig. 3-5 consists of all combinations of normal (fixed), eyes-closed, and "sway-referenced" visual and support surface sensory conditions [43, 56]. Sway-referencing involves the tilting of the support surface and the visual surround about an axis colinear

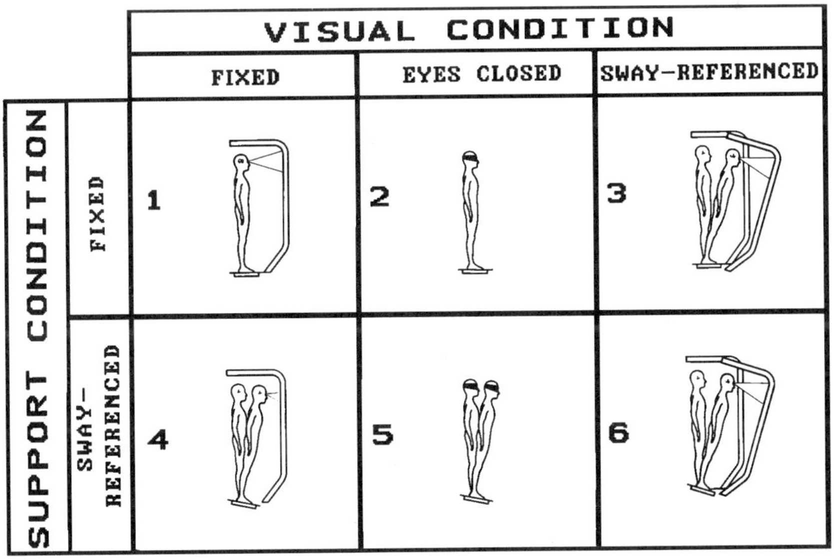

		VISUAL CONDITION		
		FIXED	EYES CLOSED	SWAY-REFERENCED
SUPPORT CONDITION	FIXED	1	2	3
	SWAY-REFERENCED	4	5	6

Figure 3-5. The six sensory organization test conditions.

with the ankle joints, thereby directly following the patient's COG sway in the AP direction [43]. In the clinical version of the sensory organization test, the six conditions and order of presentation are similar [57]. In place of the sway-referenced surface condition, however, the subject stands on a thick foam rubber pad.

The dominance of the somatosensory input to balance is demonstrated by the high degree of postural stability of normal subjects under the first three conditions, during which time the support surface is fixed [58–61]. Under fixed surface conditions, increases in sway with eye closure and sway-referenced motions of the visual surround are measurable but not functionally significant in normal subjects.

When somatosensory information useful for balancing is virtually eliminated under the last three test conditions (see Fig. 3-5), functionally significant influences of vestibular and visual inputs are evident. Under condition 5, both somatosensory and visual inputs are absent, and subjects must rely principally on the vestibular input. Under this condition, sway is increased substantially, although it is still well within the LOS in normal individuals. When useful visual as well as vestibular inputs are available in condition 4, sway still is functionally significant but only approximately one-half as great as under condition 5. When visual inputs are available but not functionally useful under condition 6, sway is approximately the same as under condition 5, indicating that the conflicting visual information is largely ignored by normal subjects.

Sensory Balance Control Under Changing Conditions

Certain adaptive changes in balance responses occur progressively over 3 to 10 trials following changes in task conditions. For example, the first of a sequence of (unexpected) toes-up rotations of the support surface is more destabilizing than are the subsequent (expected) rotations [16, 58]. An interpretation consistent with this observation is that the normally useful somatosensory input is unexpectedly disturbed by the first toes-up surface rotation. Following a short period of exposure to this altered condition, the magnitude of automatic responses triggered by the disturbed input is reduced in favor of higher-level responses mediated by the more useful visual and vestibular inputs.

Exposure to conditions in which both the support surface and the visual surround are rotating in relation to the individual's COG sway will result in larger increases in sway during the first trial as compared to the third trials of a sequence [58, 61]. Simultaneous surface and surround movements create a challenging sensory conflict condition in which neither the visual nor the somatosensory inputs are functionally useful, and the individual must suppress these and rely principally on the vestibular input.

Sensory Organization Patterns with Known Diseases

A number of abnormal sensory organization patterns are seen in patients with sensory balance deficits. Patients who perform within normal limits under conditions 1 through 4 but are repeatedly unstable under conditions 5 and 6 are not making effective use of the vestibular input (see Fig. 3-5). This pattern occurs in patients with substantial bilateral peripheral vestibular loss but also may appear in patients with uncompensated unilateral peripheral vestibular deficits, central vestibular system lesions, and lesions of such brain centers as the cerebellum [23, 43, 44, 62–67].

In patients with an abnormal preference for vision, stability under the sway-referenced visual condition is poorer than is the equivalent eyes-closed condition. This pattern occurs most frequently in patients with posttraumatic balance system deficits and in some elderly with unsteadiness [41, 58]. The site or sites of lesions responsible for posttraumatic balance system deficits are unknown.

Other patient groups with more severe sensory balance deficits rely on a single sensory input for balance. Those dependent on the somatosensory input alone are destabilized under conditions 4 through 6 of the sensory organization test (see Fig. 3-5) [68, 69]. Finally, an occasional patient may be dependent on the visual input to balance and is destabilized under all combinations of eyes-closed or sway-referenced visual conditions (conditions 2, 3, 5, and 6 in Fig. 3-5) [29]. The literature indicates that patients dependent on a single sensory input are substantially more impaired in daily life functions, have more extensive central nervous system disorders, and are less likely to have positive treatment outcomes [70, 71].

INTEGRATION OF BALANCE AND STEPPING FUNCTIONS DURING WALKING

Biomechanics of Balance During Walking

The biomechanical principles of balance during walking and in-place standing are similar. Rather than the fixed LOS of standing, a new LOS perimeter is established with the placement of each new step [72, 73]. As the step progresses, the COG moves forward from the posterior LOS perimeter in a smooth trajectory. As the COG approaches the anterior LOS perimeter, a succeeding step establishes a new LOS boundary before balance is lost, and the entire process is repeated.

Coordination of Stepping and Balance Movements

Although relatively little is known about the coordination of stepping and balance during walking, a few kinematic and EMG studies suggest that the mechanisms of balance control are similar during the two activities. EMG postural responses triggered by external perturbations during walking (resembling those seen during standing) were superimposed on the background stepping activities of the support phase leg [73]. A kinematic study of COG control during gait indicated that coarse balance control is achieved by foot placement, whereas fine control is provided by the ankle musculature of the weight-bearing leg [74].

CONCLUSIONS: IMPLICATIONS FOR CLINICAL MANAGEMENT OF ELDERLY BALANCE AND MOBILITY DISORDERS

The traditional approach to patients with balance and mobility disorders has been to identify the site of the lesion responsible for the patient's symptoms and then to focus drug or surgical treatments where appropriate to arrest or reduce the effects of the underlying disease process. Though the "localized" treatment model has worked well for managing disorders in the acute phases, a growing body of evidence suggests that it is substantially less effective for managing chronic problems, such as those affecting balance and mobility in the elderly [75]. Recent controlled intervention management programs for elderly and other patients with chronic balance and mobility disorders have been undertaken based on the "cumulative effect" systems model of impairment [71, 76]. Retrospective reviews of results are finding that, in contrast to acute intervention programs, the functional performance information is the most useful in treatment planning and outcome prediction [77]. Most importantly, these management programs now are demonstrating improved outcomes in the form of reduced numbers of falls and decreased dizziness symptoms [71, 76].

REFERENCES

1. Squires A, Livesley B. The future of physiotherapy with older people: Demographic, epidemiological and political influences. *Physiotherapy* 1993;79:851–857.
2. Fife TD, Baloh RW. Disequilibrium of unknown cause in older people. *Ann. Neurol* 1993; 34:694–702.
3. Duncan PW, et al. How do physiological components of balance affect mobility in elderly men? *Arch Phys Med Rehabil* 1993;74:1343–1349.
4. Horak FB, Shupert CL, Mirka A. Components of postural dyscontrol in the elderly: A review. *Neurobiol Aging* 1989;10:727–738.
5. Tinetti ME, Ginter SF. Identifying mobility dysfunctions in elderly patients. *JAMA* 1988; 259:1190–1193.
6. Gurfinkel VS, Osevets M. Dynamics of the vertical posture in man. *Biophysics* 1972;17:496–506.
7. Koozekanni SH, Stockwell CW, McGhee RB, Firoozmand F. On the role of dynamic models in quantitative posturography. *IEEE Trans Biomed Eng* 1980;27:605–609.
8. Nashner LM. Analysis of Stance Posture in Humans. In: Towe AL, Luschei ES, eds. *Handbook of Behavioral Neurobiology* (vol 5). New York: Plenum, 1981. Pp 527–565.
9. McCollum G, Leen TK. Form and exploration of mechanical stability limits in erect stance. *J Motor Behav* 1989;21:225–244.
10. Blaszcyk JW, Lowe DL, Hansen PD. Ranges of postural stability and their changes in the elderly. *Gait Posture* 1994;2:11–17.
11. Nashner LM, McCollum G. The organization of human postural movements: A formal basis and experimental synthesis. *Behav Brain Sci* 1985;8:135–172.
12. Schieppati M, et al. The limits of equilibrium in young and elderly normal subjects and in parkinsonians. *Electroenceph Clin Neurophysiol* 1994;93:286–298.
13. Duncan PW, Weiner DK, Chandler J, Studenski S. Functional reach: A new clinical measure of balance. *J Gerontol* 1990;45:M192–197.

14. Horak FB, Nashner LM. Central programming of postural movements: Adaptation to altered support surface configurations. *J Neurophysiol* 1986;55:1369–1381.

15. McCollum G, Horak FB, Nashner LM. Parsimony in Neural Calculations for Postural Movements. In: Bloedel J, Dichgans J, Precht W, eds. *Cerebellar Functions.* Berlin: Springer-Verlag, 1984. Pp 52–66.

16. Nashner LM. Adapting reflexes controlling the human posture. *Exp Brain Res* 1976;26:59–72.

17. Nashner LM. Fixed patterns of rapid postural responses among leg muscles during stance. *Exp Brain Res* 1977;150:403–407.

18. Nashner LM, Woollacott M, Tuma G. Organization of rapid responses to postural and locomotor-like perturbations of standing man. *Exp Brain Res* 1979;36:463–476.

19. Bawa P, Stein RB. Frequency response of human soleus muscle. *J Neurophysiol* 1976;39: 788–793.

20. Marsden CD, Merton PA, Morton HB. Latency measurements compatible with a cortical pathway for the stretch reflex in man. *J Physiol (Lond)* 1973;230:58–59.

21. Melvill-Jones G, Watt DGD. Observations on the control of stepping and hopping movements in man. *J Physiol (Lond)* 1971;219:709–727.

22. Diener HC, Ackermann H, Dichgans J, Guschlbauer B. Medium- and long-latency responses to displacements of the ankle joint in patients with spinal and central lesions. *Electroenceph Clin Neurophysiol* 1985;60:407–416.

23. Horak FB, Nashner LM, Diener HC. Postural strategies associated with somatosensory and vestibular loss. *Exp Brain Res* 1990;82:167–177.

24. Diener HC, Horak FB, Nashner LM. Influence of stimulus parameters on human postural responses. *J Neurophysiol* 1988;59:1888–1895.

25. Wolfson LI, Whipple R, Amerman P, Kleinberg A. Stressing the postural response: A quantitative method of testing balance. *J Am Geriatr Soc* 1986;34:845–850.

26. Nashner LM, Berthoz A. Visual contribution to rapid motor responses during posture control. *Brain Res* 1978;150:403–407.

27. Allum JHJ, Honegger F, Schicks H. The influence of a bilateral vestibular deficit on postural synergies. *J Vestib Res* 1994;4:49–70.

28. Inglis JT, Horak FB, Shupert CL, Rycewicz C. The importance of somatosensory information in triggering and scaling automatic postural responses in humans. *Exp Brain Res* 1994;101: 159–164.

29. Nelson SR, DiFabio RP, Anderson JH. Vestibular and sensory interaction deficits assessed by dynamic platform posturography in patients with multiple sclerosis. *Ann Otol Rhinol* 1995; 104:62–68.

30. Jackson RT, Epstein CM, De l'Amme WR. Abnormalities in posturography and estimations of visual vertical and horizontal in multiple sclerosis. *Am J Otol* 1995;16:88–93.

31. Shupert CL, Horak FB, Black FO. Hip sway associated with vestibulopathy. *J Vestib Res* 1994:231–234.

32. Horak FB, Nutt JG, Nashner LM. Postural inflexibility in parkinsonian subjects. *J Neurol Sci* 1994;111:46–58.

33. Nashner LM, Cordo PG. Relation of automatic postural responses and reaction-time voluntary movements of human leg muscles. *Exp Brain Res* 1981;43:395–405.

34. Belen'kii VY, Gurfinkel VS, Pal'tsev YI. On the elements of voluntary movement control. *Biophysics* 1967;12:135–141.

35. Cordo PJ, Nashner LM. Properties of postural adjustments associated with rapid arm movements. *J Neurophysiol* 1982;47:287–302.

36. Stelmach GE, Populin L, Muller F. Postural muscle onset and voluntary movement in the elderly. *Neurosci Lett* 1990;117:188–193.

37. Diener HC, Dichgans J. On the role of vestibular, visual, and somatosensory information for dynamic postural control in humans. *Brain Res* 1988;76:253–262.

38. Diener HC, Dichgans J, Guschlbauer B, Mau H. The significance of proprioception on postural stabilization as assessed by ischemia. *Exp Brain Res* 1989;296:103–109.

39. Dietz V, Horstmann GA, Berger W. Significance of proprioceptive mechanisms in the regulation of stance. *Prog Brain Res* 1989;80:419–423.

40. Gurfinkel VS, Lipshits MI, Mori S, Popov KE. The state of the stretch reflex during quiet standing in man. *Prog Brain Res* 1976;44:473–490.

41. Black FO, Nashner LM. Vestibulospinal control differs in patients with reduced versus distorted vestibular function. *Acta Otolaryngol (Stockh)* 1984;406:110–114.

42. Black FO, Nashner LM. Postural Control in Four Classes of Vestibular Abnormalities. In: Igarashi M, Black FO, eds. *Vestibular and Visual Control of Posture and Locomotor Equilibrium.* Basel: Karger, 1985. Pp 271–281.

43. Nashner LM, Black FO, Wall C. Adaptation to altered support and visual conditions during stance: Patients with vestibular deficits. *J Neurosci* 1982;2:536–544.

44. Shupert CL, Black FO, Horak FB, Nashner LM. Coordination of Head and Body in Response to Support Surface Translations in Normals and Patients with Bilaterally Reduced Vestibular Function. In: Amblard B, Berthoz A, Clarac F, eds. *Posture and Gait: Development, Adaptation and Modulation.* New York: Elsevier, 1988. Pp 281–289.

45. Begbie JV. Some Problems of Postural Sway. In: de Reuck AVS, Knight J, eds. *CIBA Foundation Symposium on Myotatic, Kinesthetic and Vestibular Mechanisms.* London: Churchill, 1967. Pp 80–92.

46. Diener HC, Dichgans J, Guschlbauer B, Bauer M. Role of visual and static vestibular influences on dynamic posture control. *Hum Neurobiol* 1986;5:105–113.

47. Lee DN, Lishman JR. Visual proprioceptive control of stance. *J Hum Move Stud* 1975;1:87–95.

48. Paulus WM, Straube A, Brandt Th. Visual stabilization of posture: Physiological stimulus characteristics and clinical aspects. *Brain* 1984;107:1143–1163.

49. Paulus W, Straube A, Brandt Th. Visual postural performance after loss of somatosensory and vestibular function. *J Neurol Neurosurg Psychiat* 1987;50:1542–1545.

50. Brandt Th, Paulus W, Straube A. Vision and Posture. In: Bles W, Brandt Th, eds. *Disorders of Posture and Gait.* New York: Elsevier, 1986. Pp 157–175.

51. Lestienne F, Soechting J, Berthoz A. Postural readjustments induced by linear motion of visual scenes. *Exp Brain Res* 1977;28:363–384.

52. Bles W, de Jong JMBV, de Wit G. Somatosensory compensation for loss of labyrinthine function. *Acta Otolaryngol (Stockh)* 1984;97:213–221.

53. Nashner LM, Shupert CL, Horak FB, Black FO. Organization of Posture controls: An analysis of sensory and mechanical constraints. *Prog Brain Res* 1989;80:411–418.

54. Allum JHJ, Honegger F, Pfaltz CR. The role of stretch and vestibulo-spinal reflexes in the generation of human equilibrating reactions. *Prog Brain Res* 1989;80:399–409.

55. Bles W, de Jong JMBV. Uni- and Bilateral Loss of Vestibular Function. In: Bles W; Brandt Th, eds. *Disorders of Posture and Gait.* New York: Elsevier, 1986. Pp 127–139.

56. Fregly AR. Vestibular Ataxia and its Measurement in Man. In: Kornhuber HH, ed. *Handbook of Sensory Physiology* (vol 6; no. 2). Berlin: Springer-Verlag, 1974. Pp 321–360.

57. Shumway-Cook A, Horak FB. Assessing the influence of sensory interaction on balance: Suggestion from the field. *Phys Ther* 1986;66:1548–1550.

58. Wolfson L, et al. A dynamic posturography study of balance in healthy elderly. *Neurology* 1992;42:2069–2075.

59. Jackson RT, Epstein CM. Effect of head extension on equilibrium in normal subjects. *Ann Otol Rhinol Laryngol* 1991;100:63–67.

60. Peterka RJ, Black FO. Age-related changes in human posture control: Sensory organization tests. *J Vestib Res* 1990;1:73–85.

61. Nashner LM. Computerized Dynamic Posturography. In: Jacobson GP, Newman CW, Kartush JM, eds. *Handbook of Balance Function Testing.* Chicago: Mosby–Year Book, 1993. Pp 280–307.

62. Black FO, Wall III C, Nashner LM. Effect of visual and support surface references upon postural control in vestibular deficit subjects. *Acta Otolaryngol Scand* 1983; 95:199–210.

63. Mirka A, Black FO. Clinical Application of Dynamic Posturography for Evaluating Sensory In-

tegration and Vestibular Dysfunction. In: Arenberg IK, Smith DB, eds. *Neurologic Clinics: Diagnostic Neurology.* Philadelphia: Saunders, 1990. Pp 351–359.

64. Black FO, Shupert C, Peterka RJ, Nashner LM. Effects of unilateral loss of vestibular function on the vestibulo-ocular reflex and posture control. *Ann Otol Rhinol Laryngol* 1989;98:884–889.

65. Fetter M, Diener HC, Dichgans J. Recovery of postural control after an acute unilateral vestibular lesion in humans. *J Vestib Res* 1991;1:373–383.

66. Goebel JA, Paige GD. Dynamic posturography and caloric test results in patients with and without vertigo. *Otolaryngol Head Neck Surg* 1989;100:553–558.

67. Nashner LM, Shumway-Cook A, Marin O. Stance posture control in selected groups of children with cerebral palsy: Deficits in sensory organization and muscular coordination. *Exp Brain Res* 1983;197:393–409.

68. Hamid MA, Hughs GB, Kinny SE. Specificity and sensitivity of dynamic posturography: A retrospective analysis. *Acta Otolaryngol (Stockh)* 1991;481(Suppl):596–600.

69. Nashner LM, Peters, JF. Dynamic Posturography in the Diagnosis and Management of Dizziness and Balance Disorders. In: Arenburg IK, Smith DB, eds. *Neurologic Clinics: Diagnostic Neurotology.* Philadelphia: Saunders, 1990. Pp 331–349.

70. Jacobson GP, Newman CW, Hunter L, Balzer GK. Balance function test correlates of the dizziness handicap inventory. *J Am Acad Audiol* 1991;2:253–260.

71. Shepard NT, Telian SA. Programmatic vestibular rehabilitation. *Otolaryngol Head Neck Surg* 1995;112:173–182.

72. Nashner LM. The Organization of Human Postural Movements During Standing and Walking. In: Grillner S, et al., eds. *Neurobiology of Posture and Locomotion.* London: Macmillan; 1986. Pp 637–648.

73. Nashner LM, Forssberg H. Phase-dependent organization of postural adjustments associated with arm movements while walking. *J Neurophysiol* 1986;55:538–548.

74. Yuancheng J, Winter DA, Ishac MG, Gilchrist L. Trajectory of the body COG and COP during initiation and termination of gait. *Gait Posture* 1993;1:9–22.

75. Hoenig H, et al. Geriatric rehabilitation: What do physicians know about it and how should they use it? *Geriatr Soc* 1994;42:341–347.

76. Tinetti ME, et al. A multifactorial intervention to reduce the risk of falling among elderly people living in the community. *N Engl J Med* 1994;331:821–827.

77. Shepard NT, Telian SA, Smith-Wheelock M, Raj A. Vestibular and balance rehabilitation therapy. *Ann Otol Rhinol Laryngol* 1994;102:198–205.

4. Neurophysiology of Locomotion: Recent Advances in the Study of Locomotion

Shigemi Mori

In 1941, Sherrington wrote, "The dog not only walks but also it walks to greet its master. In a word, the component from the roof-brain alters the characteristics of the motor act from one of generality of purpose to one of narrowed and specific purpose fitting a specific occasion" [1]. Recent studies have shown that information routed through both the cerebrocerebellar and spinocerebellar pathways plays a crucial role in changing locomotor behavior, by modifying signals descending from the motor cortex and the brain stem [2–4]. During locomotion, an animal controls, without interruption, its speed and direction, deals with unexpected perturbations, circumvents obstacles, and anticipates necessary conditions [5]. Although there is a standard posture of the body during locomotion, systematic modifications occur to meet both internal and external requirements. These modifications necessitate a flexible neural control structure for posture and locomotion. Animals solve this problem by using a combination of neural mechanisms related to *reflex-dependent adaptation* and *context-dependent adaptation* [4, 6].

This chapter considers four major aspects of the supraspinal control of locomotion: (1) contribution of dorsolateral and ventromedial descending systems to the control of locomotor movements, (2) central programs related to the control of locomotor movements and to integration of posture and locomotor movements, (3) adaptation of locomotor movements to suit environmental needs and purpose, and (4) requirements for satisfactory execution of bipedal locomotion in humans.

CONTRIBUTION OF CORTICOSPINAL AND SUBCORTICOSPINAL PATHWAYS TO THE CONTROL OF LOCOMOTION IN MONKEYS

The general control of locomotion is presumably accomplished by varying the level of cortical drive to posture and locomotor-related centers in the diencephalon, mesencephalon, and the pontomedullary reticular formation [2]. Global changes, such as stopping, starting, and changing speed or direction, are produced in this fashion. Descending pathways from the brain stem to the spinal

This study was supported by a Grant-in-aid for Scientific Research (H06404087), the Ministry of Education, Science, Sports, and Culture of Japan.

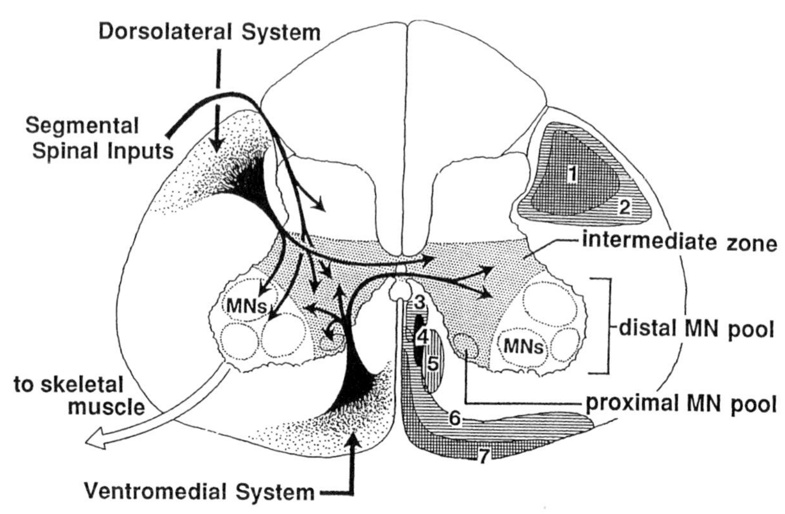

Figure 4-1. Convergence of supraspinal and spinal inputs to interneurons and motoneurons (*MNs*). The intermediate zone includes Rexed's laminae V, VI, and VII. 1 = corticospinal tract (lateral); 2 = rubrospinal tract; 3 = corticospinal tract (medial); 4 = interstitiospinal tract; 5 = tectospinal tract; 6 = reticulospinal tract; 7 = vestibulospinal tract.

cord constitute the main route by which the higher nervous system governs the spinal mechanisms related to locomotion. Before discussing specific studies on locomotion in monkeys, the pertinent anatomy will be briefly reviewed. Descending afferents to the spinal gray matter are summarized schematically in Fig. 4-1.

Trajectory and Terminal Distribution of the Descending Pathways

The corticospinal fibers descend into the dorsolateral funiculus of the spinal cord and terminate bilaterally in the internuncial zone of the spinal gray matter, especially contralaterally in its dorsolateral parts. In addition, corticospinal fibers terminate on motoneurons, primarily in the lateral motoneuronal cell group. In the cervical and lumbosacral enlargements of the spinal cord, the lateral motoneuronal cell group of the ventral horn innervates the limb muscles, whereas the medial group innervates axial musculature. The subcortical pathways to the spinal cord are grouped into the ventromedial system and dorsolateral system, based on their terminal distribution [7]. The fibers of the ventromedial system occupy a ventral and medial position in the lower brain stem and descend in the spinal cord in the ventral, the ventrolateral, and the medial parts of the lateral funiculi. These fibers are derived primarily from the vestibular nuclei, the interstitial nucleus of Cajal, the tectum, and the medial pontine and medullary reticular formation. They terminate preferentially in the ventral and medial parts of the intermediate zone, where long propriospinal neurons are located. The fibers of the dorsolateral system occupy a lateral position in the lower brain stem and descend contralaterally into the lateral funiculus of the spinal cord. The majority of these fibers are derived from the pars magnocellularis of the red nucleus and terminate preferentially in the dorsal and lateral parts of the intermediate zone of the spinal gray matter, where short propriospinal neurons are located.

One of the major differences between the ventromedial and dorsolateral systems is that the descending fibers of the ventromedial system give off numerous axon collaterals along their trajectory through the spinal cord. Some of these fibers also make monosynaptic connections with motoneurons innervating axial and proximal limb muscles [7, 8]. The trajectory of reticulospinal fibers descending from the pontine reticular formation have been traced [9], and it was found that a single reticulospinal fiber gives off axon collaterals at each segmental level of the cervical and thoracic cord as it descends. Each axon collateral further gives off a number of terminal and preterminal fibers. Many of these axon collaterals terminate in the gray matter ipsilateral to the location of the stem axons, but some of them innervated both ipsilateral and contralateral gray matter. Terminal fibers are found around small to large-size neurons in Rexed's laminae VII and VIII, where propriospinal neurons and premotor interneurons are located. By reconstructing branching patterns of axon collaterals, each axon collateral is found to innervate spinal neurons located in a disc-like spinal segment with a width less than 1 mm. These results support a view of the spinal cord and lower brain stem (medulla oblongata and pons) as a functional unit [7].

The Effects of Chronic Ablation of Pyramidal Tracts and Dorsolateral and Ventromedial Systems

Lawrence and Kuypers [10] surgically interrupted the pyramidal tracts of adult rhesus monkeys between the caudal border of pons and the rostral tip of the inferior olives, bilaterally. In examining the recovered animals, Lawrence and Kuypers studied their ability to orient themselves to targets, sit, stand, walk, run, and climb, and the finger movements used for picking up food. In animals with lesions strictly limited to the pyramidal tracts, there was an immediate ability to sit with the head up and to stand, walk, run, and climb. When they ran across the floor, movements of the forelimbs and hindlimbs were well coordinated. When the pyramidal lesions extended into the ventral reticular formation, righting was delayed, and the hand and trunk were always flexed, though the animals were still able to progress.

Lawrence and Kuypers [11] further interrupted selectively the ventromedial and dorsolateral systems at various levels in monkeys that had recovered from a prior pyramidotomy. In these animals, interruption of the respective brain stem pathways produced contrasting disturbances of motility. Interruption of the dorsolateral pathways produced an impairment of independent distal extremity and hand movements and impaired capacity to flex the extended limb. Total limb movements and combined movements of the body and limbs were relatively unaffected. They sat unsupported in their cages and could stand, walk, run, and climb. Initially, some were mildly unsteady in standing and walking, but this condition cleared within 1 week. In contrast, interruption of the ventromedial pathways resulted in a flexion bias of trunk and limbs and a severe impairment of axial and of proximal extremity movements. Animals with lesions in the medulla oblongata could not right up for 40 days. When they finally could sit and walk, they were unsteady and walked with a narrow-based gait and abduction of the limbs. They had serious difficulties in staying on course and avoiding obstacles. Independent distal extremity movements, however, were relatively unaffected. They could pick up pieces of food with their hands, even in the early postoperative phase.

These observations led Lawrence and Kuypers [11] to conclude that the ventromedial pathways function as the basic system by which the brain exerts control over movement. This control is concerned especially with maintenance of erect posture, integrated movements of body and limbs, and directing the course of progression. The dorsolateral systems superimpose on that control the capacity for the independent use of the extremity, particularly the hand. The corticospinal connections mediate a control similar to that of the brain stem system but, in addition, provide the capacity for further fractionation of movements as exemplified by individual finger movements. Drew et al. [12] confirmed the importance of the ventromedial system, particularly the reticulospinal tract, for the integrated control of posture and locomotion in cats. Eidelberg et al. [13] demonstrated that monkeys with incomplete spinal transection could regain the capacity for stepping and walking, provided that at least one ventral quadrant was preserved.

CORTICAL AND SUBCORTICAL SYSTEMS FOR THE CONTROL OF LOCOMOTION IN CATS

The cat with transection of the brain stem has mechanisms for the "automatic" control of posture and locomotion, but an intact nervous system is required for "volitional" control [2, 4, 14]. This volitional control is exercised through some of the same mechanisms already in place for automatic control. It is postulated that the main objective of this supraspinal control network is to automatize movement rather than keeping it at a fully conscious level.

Compartmental Models for the Study of Posture and Locomotion

Before considering higher nervous control of posture and locomotion in detail, it is instructive to compare the results obtained by lesion experiments with findings from recordings in awake, behaving animals. In the lesion studies, a part of the central nervous system is ablated, the brain stem is transected, and a particular nucleus is lesioned. Representative compartmental models, which have been employed by a number of scientists during past decades, are illustrated in Fig. 4-2. They include the whole-brain cat or the cat with intact central nervous system, the

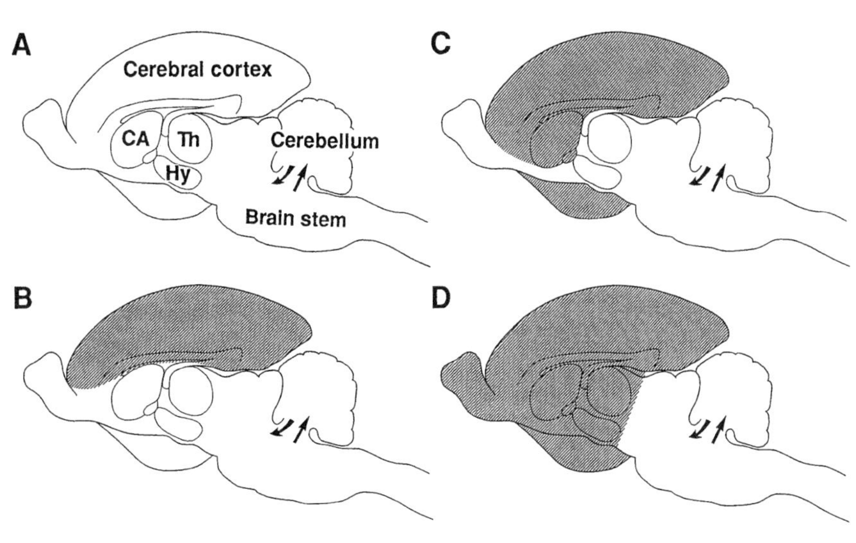

Figure 4-2. Representative compartmental models. *A.* Intact whole-brain cat. *B.* Decorticate (striate) cat. *C.* Thalamic cat (diencephalic cat). *D.* Decerebrate cat. CA = caudate nucleus; Th = thalamus; Hy = hypothalamus.

decorticate or striate cat, the thalamic cat, the decerebrate cat, and the decerebellate cat. In the decorticate cat, basal ganglia are in functional connection with the brain stem and the cerebellum, whereas in the thalamic cat, only the thalamus and the hypothalamus are in connection with the brain stem and the cerebellum [6]. Major features of postural and locomotor changes observed in each compartmental model follow. (All the behavioral observations were made after the recovery of the animals from the ablations.)

Decorticate Cat (Striate Cat)

Loss of the cortex does not impair the locomotion process but disturbs the context in which these movements are performed. In general, decorticate cats tend to be hyperactive as well as hyperreactive. Schaltenbrandt and Cobb [15] observed the behavior of chronically decorticate cats as early as 1930:

> Decorticate cats are able to walk; they have normal muscle tone; they are able to perform isolated movements of the extremities. They keep a normal body temperature, and have a normal rhythm of wakening and sleeping. They show signs of different emotional states such as satisfaction and anger. They react to sounds; but they appear to be completely 'idiotic,' if such a word may be applied to the animals. They do not recognize particular sounds and do not recognize objects by vision, though pupillary reflexes are intact.

These results demonstrate that the decorticate cat, in which the cerebrocerebellar connections are interrupted and the highest level of motor center is the basal ganglia, is capable of activating both the brain stem and spinal locomotor automatisms with an adequate degree of postural control.

Armstrong et al. [16–18] recorded the activity of neurons in the forelimb area of the motor cortex and in the cerebellar nuclei of the intact cat during steady walking on a moving belt. In the cortex, they recorded both pyramidal tract neurons (PTNs) and nonpyramidal tract neurons (non-PTNs). During locomotion, no fewer than 80% of units discharged rhythmically. Population activity in interpositus neurons with elbow-related receptive fields was almost precisely opposite in phase to that in PTNs recorded via electrodes from which elbow flexion was evoked by electrical stimulation. These investigators also studied discharge patterns of cortical neurons during locomotion on a flat boardway and on two horizontal ladders, one with wide flat rungs and another with similarly spaced, narrow, round rungs. The population output of these neurons was phased similarly during all three tasks, but activity was slightly greater for the flat-runged ladder, and a substantial increase was evident for the round-runged ladder. Armstrong [2] suggested that the cerebral motor cortex participates in the production of some of the more specific changes, such as step-by-step adaptive changes in the movements that are needed to fit the movements to particular behavioral context, in addition to the production of general or global changes.

Acaudate Cat

The basal ganglia, thalamus, and hypothalamus are located between the lesion of decortication and decerebration. Somewhere in these structures are neuronal circuits that activate spinal locomotor automatisms and modify them to meet environmental conditions. Visual and proprioceptive information is integrated by the basal ganglia in conjunction with the motor cortex, providing the animal with a capacity for reflex adjustment of locomotion [19]. Villablanca et al. [20, 21] studied the behavior of chronic acaudate cats in which the caudate nuclei were ablated bilaterally. Acaudate cats exhibit a "compulsory approach syndrome." This syndrome is expressed by a tendency to approach, follow, and stick to the investigator or moving objects presented to the cat. Although this syndrome is elicited by external stimuli, the subsequent walking is highly stimulus-bound. Any obstacle or impending danger arrests the movement. Visual stimuli are the most effective in eliciting this behavior, but the cats also are markedly attracted to auditory and tactile cues. The caudate nucleus is an input nucleus of the basal ganglia, which receives afferents from sensory cortex via the cortico-striatal pathway.

Thalamic (Diencephalic) Cat

The thalamic cat exhibits "obstinate progression" [22]. The main feature is a pervasive tendency of the animal to walk incessantly in a totally nondirected, blind manner. An attempt to stop the cat only enhances the strength of its progression. The tendency to follow or attend to the environmental stimuli is absent. The other striking behavioral feature of the chronic thalamic cat is its increased irritability in response to minor environmental changes. Because obstinate progression differs from compulsory approach syndrome in its transient nature, Garcia-Rill [19] suggested that it may be a nonspecific consequence of the removal of inhibitory telencephalic influences. Removal of the cortex and basal ganglia activates or disinhibits locomotor centers, such as the subthalamic locomotor region (SLR) in the lateral hypothalamic area and the mesencephalic locomotor region (MLR) [23–25]. The MLR corresponds to the caudal portion of the nucleus cuneiformis and includes a part of the pedunculopontine nucleus in the posterior midbrain (Fig. 4-3). Based on the observations in the cats with bilateral SLR lesion, Shik and Orlovsky [14] suggested that the SLR is responsible only for the initiation of locomotion as a part of goal-directed behavior— searching, hunting, defending, and so on—in the behavioral and emotional life of the animal. In intact cats, searching-like locomotor movements are evoked by stimulating the lateral hypothalamic area [26].

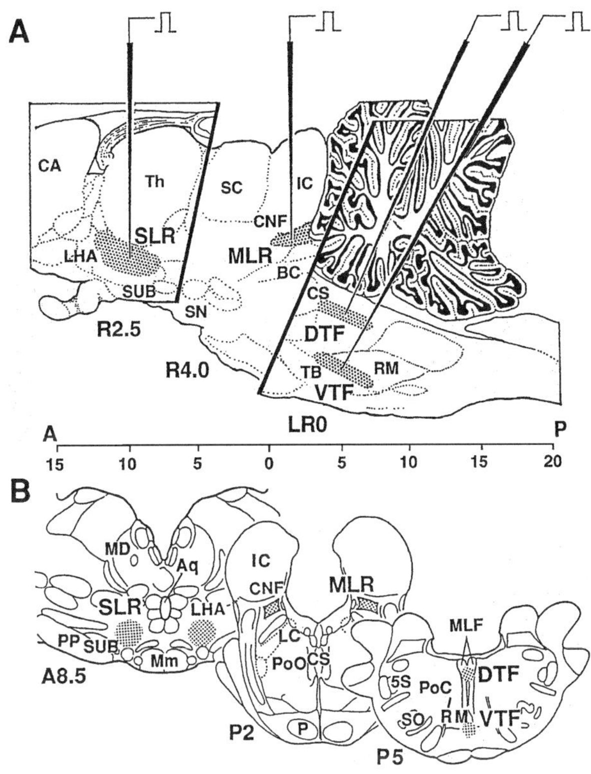

Figure 4-3. Location of the subthalamic locomotor region (SLR), mesencephalic locomotor region (MLR), dorsal tegmental field (DTF), and ventral tegmental field (VTF) areas on the parasagittal planes along R2.5, R4.0 and LR0 (*A*) and frontal planes at A8.5, P2, and P5 (*B*) of the brain stem. The horizontal axis under the parasagittal planes in *A* represents the rostrocaudal Horsley-Clarke coordinates. 5S = spinal trigeminal nucleus; BC = brachium conjunctivum; CNF = cuneiform nucleus; CS = nucleus centralis superior; IC = inferior colliculus; LC = nucleus locus coeruleus; MLF = medial longitudinal fasciculus; Mm = mammillary body; NRPc = nucleus reticularis pontis caudalis; NRPo = nucleus reticularis pontis oralis; P = pyramidal tract; RM = nucleus raphe magnus; SUB = subthalamic nucleus; SC = superior colliculus; SO = superior olive; SN: substantia nigra; TB = trapezoid body.

Decerebrate Cat

Rigidity is one of the most important features of decerebration, and the extent of its development depends on the level of brain stem transection. Decerebrate cats have either precollicular-postmammillary or precollicular-premammillary lesions, and most of them maintain a standing posture with or without the aid of external support [14]. Such a reflexively standing posture was noted by Sherrington in 1906 [27]. A striking difference between the precollicular-premammillary and precollicular-postmammillary decerebrate cats is that the former cats often walk on a moving treadmill without external stimuli. The precollicular-postmammillary decerebrate cat has been called a *locomotor preparation*; it exhibits locomotion only with the electrical or chemical stimulation of the MLR [25]. Within a narrow region of the upper brain stem bounded by the two transection levels, there must be a population of cells with tonic inhibitory effects on the MLR. The substantia nigra (SN) is one such neuronal structure.

Garcia-Rill et al. [28] focally injected putative neurotransmitters and their agonists and antagonists into the MLR and substantia nigra (SN) and studied the effects on locomotor movements. In the locomotor preparation, MLR injections of the gamma-aminobutyric acid (GABA) antagonists bicuculine and picrotoxin evoked locomotion, whereas application of muscimol or GABA blocked both the chemically and electrically evoked locomotion. In the precollicular-premammillary decerebrate cat, SN injections of GABA antagonists blocked spontaneous locomotion, whereas injections of GABA and muscimol restored walking. Because the only known afferent to SN within the wedge of tissue remaining after the premammillary (compared to postmammillary) transection is the subthalamic nucleus, Garcia-Rill et al. suggest that subthalamic projections to SN inhibit the GABAergic SN projections to the MLR, effectively releasing (disinhibiting) locomotion in the premammillary transected cat, resulting in spontaneous locomotion. The subthalamic influence on SN may be removed by a postmammillary transection, leaving the SN free to inhibit the MLR. Locomotion then must be induced by electrical activation of the MLR or blockade of its GABAergic afferents from SN postsynaptically by injections of GABA antagonist. These studies reveal some of the basal ganglia mechanisms for the control of locomotor movements.

Decerebellate Cat

Broadly speaking, both postural and locomotor control can be regarded as a form of motor synergy [29]. The cerebellum selects only essential parts of the detailed information about the current state of the synergies and the environment [30]. The cerebellum is informed constantly of the activity of the spinal locomotor automatism by way of the spinocerebellar tract. The dorsal spinocerebellar tract transmits detailed information about the operation of the peripheral motor apparatus, such as the phase and strength of contraction of single muscles, the joint angles, and the time at which the hind limb touches the ground. The ventral spinocerebellar tract and the spinoreticulocerebellar pathways convey information about the activity of the spinal rhythm generatory mechanisms. The cerebellum also is informed of the cerebral activity via the cerebrocerebellar pathways arising from the pericruciate cortex. In addition, posture and locomotor-related information, processed at the level of the cerebellum, is fed back to the cerebral cortex by way of the cerebellocerebral pathway, such as the interpositothalamocortical projection [18].

The cells of origin of the descending tracts from the brain stem, such as the vestibulospinal, reticulospinal, and rubrospinal tracts, are under the control of the cerebellum. The spinocerebellar loop, which comprises the spinal cord, spinocerebellar pathways, the cerebellum, and the descending tracts from the brain stem, serves as *the locomotor phase control system* [30]. Each of these descending tracts carries both tonic (unpatterned) and phasic (patterned) signals to the spinal cord. These signals eventually regulate the movements of the forelimbs and hindlimbs by exciting and inhibiting the activity of spinal interneurons and motoneurons. Accordingly, removal of the cerebellum results in profound locomotor disturbances in otherwise intact animals. The deficits add up to a "drunken" gait, and they include abnormally variable coupling between the step cycles in the different limbs, which leads to frequent loss of equilibrium, and also abnormal variation in the speed and range of movement at different joints in the individual limbs, which leads to unevenness in stride length [14, 31].

Postural and Locomotor Changes in Acutely Decerebrate Cats

There are four principal locomotor centers in the cat, neuronal areas from which postural changes and locomotor movements can be expressed by stimulation. These areas are (1) the SLR in the lateral hypothalamic area, (2) the MLR, (3) the dorsal tegmental field (DTF), and (4) the ventral tegmental field (VTF) in the caudal pons (see Fig. 4-3). Homologous regions exist in the macaque monkey and quite likely in humans as well [13, 32]. When Shik et al. [25] first evoked locomotion by stimulating the MLR, the results were dramatic. The decerebrate cat, which was immobile before stimulation, suddenly came to life, stood up, and began to walk on the treadmill. With increases in the speed of a moving belt and increases in the stimulus intensity delivered to the MLR, the locomotor pattern could be changed from a slow walk to a fast walk, and then to a trot, and even from a trot to a gallop (Fig. 4-4). In decerebrate macaque monkeys, Eidelberg et al. [13] evoked similar locomotor movements by stimulating the posterior subthalamic region and the vicinity of the cuneiform nucleus.

Stimulation of the MLR in this fashion overcomes tonic inhibitory influences on the region, which in turn activates a spinal stepping generator, or central pattern generator (CPG) [5]. The decerebrate preparation affords good access to neural locomotor mechanisms and has been studied extensively. Shik and Orlovsky [14] view the basic locomotor automatism exhibited by the decerebrate cat in terms of two principal tasks: interlimb coordination and maintenance of equilibrium. Later evidence suggests that stimulation of the MLR activates si-

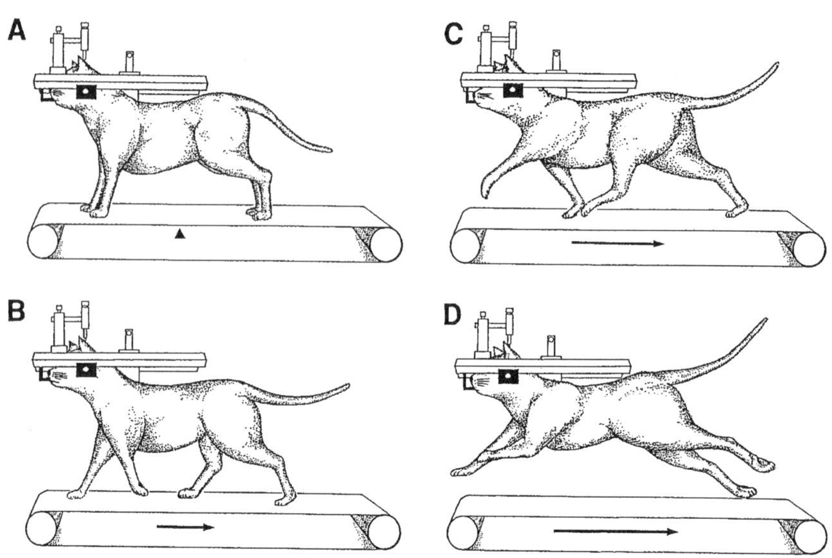

Figure 4-4. Schematic illustrations of postural and locomotor movements. (*A*) Reflexively standing posture, (*B*) slow walk, (*C*) trot, and (*D*) gallop. The head and the first three thoracic vertebrae of the cat are fixed to the stereotaxic instrument, and the length of the arrows represents the speed of the moving treadmill.

multaneously three major subsystems for control of locomotion: the locomotor rhythm-releasing or activating system, the postural tonus or power control system, and the locomotor phase control system [4, 33].

The Locomotor Rhythm-Releasing or Activating System

The locomotor rhythm-releasing or generating system has two components: the pontomedullary locomotor region and the reticulospinal pathway originating from the ventromedial part of brain stem reticular formation. The pontomedullary locomotor region extends ventrocaudally throughout the lateral tegmentum of the brain stem from the MLR to the cervical spinal cord. Stimulation of any site within this strip generally is capable of eliciting locomotion of the subject on a moving belt [34]. The pontine locomotor region consists primarily of descending axons from the cells located in the MLR, whereas the medullary locomotor region contains a column of reticular cells medially and a tract of their axons laterally [35]. Stimulation of the MLR and the pontine locomotor region is relayed to the spinal cord by way of this column of reticular neurons. The spinal cord then is switched into a locomotor state by the activation of the CPGs located at the cervical and lumbar segments and the propriospinal polysynaptic pathway connecting these segments.

Orlovsky [36] demonstrated the presence of monosynaptic excitatory connections between the MLR and the medioventral reticulospinal neurons in the pons and the medulla and suggested that the MLR-reticulospinal system is used for initiation of locomotion. Reticulospinal cells in this area are rhythmically active during MLR-evoked locomotor movements [37]. They receive convergent inputs from the SLR, the MLR, and other brain regions involved in the initiation of locomotion and provide a descending "command" pathway for the activation of the CPG. In fact, stimulation of the VTF area (including the medioventral part of the caudal pons) can produce hindlimb or quadrupedal locomotion or facilitate locomotion produced by MLR stimulation [38]. Jordan [39] proposed that the cells of origin of the descending message are localized within the magnocellular and gigantocellular tegmental fields of the pons and medulla. The reticulospinal fibers originating from these areas terminate on interneurons in laminae V, VI, and VII of the lumbar spinal cord (see Fig. 4-1).

In chronically prepared unrestrained cats walking on a treadmill, Drew et al. [12] examined the temporal relationship between the activity of reticulospinal cells and forelimb and hindlimb muscles. The goal of the study was to determine the relationship between cell activity and aspects of the locomotor cycles and to demonstrate the correlation with specific muscle groups. These cells were recorded from the medial regions of the gigantocellular, magnocellular, and lateral tegmental fields. The discharge of many of these cells was frequency-modulated during locomotion. Roughly one-third of these units fired in direct relation to electromyographic (EMG) activity in flexor or extensor muscles of the limbs. Correlations were found with muscles lying both ipsilaterally and contralaterally to the site of the recordings. Drew et al. [12] were able to divide the reticulospinal cells into three groups: EMG-related cells, locomotor-related cells, and unrelated cells. They suggest that the medullary reticulospinal neurons are involved in the control of individual muscles and in postural adjustments that would require simultaneous activation of muscles in different limbs or in the neck and limbs.

The Postural Tonus-Regulating or Power Control System

The decerebrate preparation is capable of maintaining a standing posture due to decerebrate rigidity, with or without the aid of external support. During stance, the EMG activity of the hindlimb muscles and the force exerted by each of the hindlimbs are considered to represent the degree of postural muscle tone developed in the hindlimbs [4, 40]. Specific areas in the caudal pons have been identified for the regulation of postural muscle tone in cats [33] and in rats [41]. Stimulation of the DTF area decreases, whereas that of VTF areas increases, the tone of the hindlimb muscles. With DTF stimulation, the reflexively standing cat is unable to maintain a standing posture without external support, but with the VTF-induced increase in the level of postural muscle tone, it regains the standing posture. Anatomically, the DTF area for postural tone corresponds to the caudal portion of the nucleus centralis superior in which there are only a few cell bodies, so the DTF stimulation probably results in an activation of passing fibers. The VTF area corresponds to the rostral portion of the nucleus raphe magnus and the adjacent medioventral tegmentum.

How are the MLR-induced locomotor movements in the decerebrate cat modified by changing the level of postural muscle tone? In an attempt to answer this question, MLR stimulation was combined with the DTF and the VTF stimulations, respectively [4]. MLR-elicited controlled locomotion was suppressed completely with a DTF-induced decrease in the level of postural muscle tone. With a VTF-induced increase in the level of postural muscle tone, hindlimb stepping was converted to coordinated four-legged locomotion. Stimulation of the VTF area alone also evokes spastic locomotor movements, with a substantial increase in extensor muscle tone of the hindlimbs. Because postural control is manifested through the adjustment tone in postural muscles, these results clearly indicate that an increase in the level of postural muscle tone and an activation of the spinal stepping generator are not independent phenomena [42]. The results also demonstrate that postural muscle tone or a power control system is one of the subsystems involved in locomotor control.

Some fibers that descend from the pontine reticular formation terminate on the reticulospinal cells in the medullary reticular formation [9]. These reticuloreticular fibers together with those connecting the left and the right pontine reticular formation pass through the DTF area. Takakusaki et al. [43] demonstrated that MLR-induced rhythmical oscillation of the hindlimb extensor motoneurons is terminated with DTF-induced membrane hyperpolarization. A study by the author also has shown that DTF stimulation activates orthodromically those reticulospinal cells in the nucleus reticularis gigantocellularis. They, in turn, exert postsynaptic inhibitory effects on extensor and flexor hindlimb motoneurons by way of inhibitory interneurons. These inhibitory interneurons also could exert inhibitory effects on rhythmically discharging premotor interneurons of the locomotor-related CPG, terminating MLR-evoked locomotor movements [38].

The Locomotor Phase Control System

Purkinje cells are the output neurons of the cerebellar cortex. They exert tonic inhibitory effects on the neurons of the cerebellar nuclei (e.g., the fastigial and interpositus nuclei) and of the lateral vestibular (Deiters') nucleus. Orlovsky [44] recorded Purkinje cell simple-spike activity from the hindlimb projection zone of the cerebellum. Although closely neighboring cells tend to discharge with similar patterns during locomotion, there is nevertheless a very wide range of patterns among cells sampled from within restricted regions of the anterior lobe. During locomotion, the discharge of most Purkinje cells is modulated in the rhythm of stepping. Usually, the Purkinje cells discharge in bursts separated by periods of silence. The discharge frequency within the bursts reached 100–150 spikes per second and sometimes up to 200–250 spikes per second. The overall activity of the entire population of Purkinje cells is maximal at the beginning of the stance phase. The population of cells in the fastigial nucleus is maximally active in the swing phase of the ipsilateral hindlimb. The overall activity of the population of cells in the interpositus nucleus is maximal at the beginning of the swing phase and minimum in the stance phase of the ipsilateral hindlimb.

Most reticulospinal, vestibulospinal, and rubrospinal neurons exhibit weak background activity before initiation of locomotion, but during locomotion most of these neurons exhibit rhythmical bursting discharges [45]. In general, the discharge frequency of the neurons increased in a certain phase of the step cycle but decreased in other phases. The phases of maximal activity differ in different neurons. Rubrospinal neurons exert excitatory effects on flexor motoneurons, innervating contralateral hindlimb muscles. These neurons are maximally active in the swing phase. Reticulospinal cells exert excitatory and inhibitory effects mainly on flexor and extensor motoneurons of the ipsilateral hindlimbs, respectively. They were maximally active in the flexor or swing phase of locomotion. Vestibulospinal cells exert excitatory effects on extensor alpha-motoneurons of the ipsilateral hindlimb. They are maximally active at the beginning of the extensor or stance phase of locomotion [31]. In decerebrate cats, the phases of maximal activity of the descending pathways coincided mainly with the phases of activity of those muscles on which the same pathways exerted excitatory effects.

Rhythmical modulation of rubrospinal, reticulospinal, and vestibulospinal neurons is mostly abolished after cerebellar ablation. Orlovsky and Shik [31] conclude that the rhythmic signals reaching the cerebellum via the spinocerebellar pathways modulate activity of cerebellar neurons, whose output, in turn, rhythmically entrains the activity of cells of origin of the descending brain-stem pathways. After cerebellectomy, background activity of the vestibulospinal neurons increases considerably, whereas the activity of the rubrospinal and reticulospinal neurons diminishes. Shik and Orlovsky [14] suggest that uncoupling of the descending pathways results in abnormal relations between flexor and extensor muscle tone, yielding locomotor ataxia observed after cerebellar ablation. All these results indicate that the spinocerebellospinal closed circuit serves as the locomotor phase control system [42]. It is noteworthy that cells in the pontomedullary reticular formation influence not only the rhythm but also the power and phase of ongoing locomotor movements, reinforcing the importance of the ventromedial system for locomotor control in both cats and monkeys [7, 12].

Changes in Gait Pattern: Modifiability of the Descending Systems

At the appropriate moment, the cat changes its locomotor pattern from a slow walk to a fast walk and then even to a gallop. In an attempt to understand this critical event, changes in the discharge property of the vestibulospinal neurons were analyzed in relation to systematically changing patterns of induced locomotor movements [46]. With transition of locomotion from a slow walk to a fast walk, those vestibulospinal neurons, which exhibit single bursting discharges in the extensor phase of the ipsilateral hindlimb, start to exhibit double bursting discharges in a single step cycle. Each bursting discharge is observed in phase with the stance phase of the left or the right hindlimb. With these changes, previously silent vestibulospinal neurons start to discharge tonically, with a gradual increase in the discharge frequency, and some of them even start to discharge rhythmically. With modification of the discharge properties, single vestibulospinal neurons become capable of controlling the movements of not only the ipsilateral but also the contralateral hindlimb. During a gallop in which the left and the right hindlimb moved more or less in phase, each of the double bursting discharges of the single vestibulospinal neurons fuse, increasing dramatically their average firing frequency.

Changes in the locomotor patterns were evoked by increasing both the stimulus intensity delivered to the MLR and the speed of the moving treadmill. Thus, it is conceivable that an increase in the tonic excitatory output from the MLR to Deiters' nucleus and a change in the rhythmical feedback signals related to the movements of the hindlimb influence the systematic modifications of the discharge property of the vestibulospinal neurons. The recruitment of vestibulospinal neurons, regardless of whether they are tonically or phasically active, along with an increase in the discharge frequency and modulation depth of individual neurons, would contribute to an increase in power or postural muscle tone. Enhanced tone in postural muscles is required not only for shifting a locomotor pattern from a slow walk to a trot and then to a gallop but also for adequately setting the accompanying posture.

All these results demonstrated that Deiters' nucleus itself flexibly changes the magnitude of populational activity of vestibulospinal neurons, depending on the internal and external demands, and contributes to the simultaneous control of rhythm, power, and the phase of required locomotor movements [29]. Conversely, the reverse shifting of the locomotor patterns from a gallop to a trot, and even from a fast walk to a slow walk and then to the quiet standing posture, can be established by a sequential derecruitment of the vestibulospinal neurons and by systematic decrease in the modulation depth of their bursting discharges. It is highly possible that descending signals carried by the reticulospinal and rubrospinal pathways also are modified sequentially in this manner with transition from locomotor movements to a standing posture.

Postural and Locomotor Changes in a Cat with an Intact Central Nervous System

Stimulation of the SLR, the MLR, the DTF, and the VTF areas in intact animals also evokes stimulus site–specific behavioral changes [26]. Postural and locomotor changes for each of the four stimulus sites are illustrated in Fig. 4-5. Although mechanical features of the stimulus-induced postural and locomotor movements are essentially similar among decerebrate and intact cats for each of the stimulus sites, a cat with an intact central nervous system always shows "behavioral" arousal reactions, such as alerting and orienting reactions. These arousal reactions are not observed in the decerebrate locomotor preparation, although other categories of arousal reactions, such as pupil dilatation and cardiovascular and respiratory changes, have been reported to occur during treadmill-induced locomotor movements [14]. The induced behavioral changes are accompanied by electroencephalographic arousal reactions. These results support a proposition that the reticular formation is one of the major sources for generalized motor drive [4, 47]. The stimulation delivered to each of the four posture-related and locomotor-related areas in the brain stem invariably activates ascending fibers coursing through the reticular formation to the sensori-

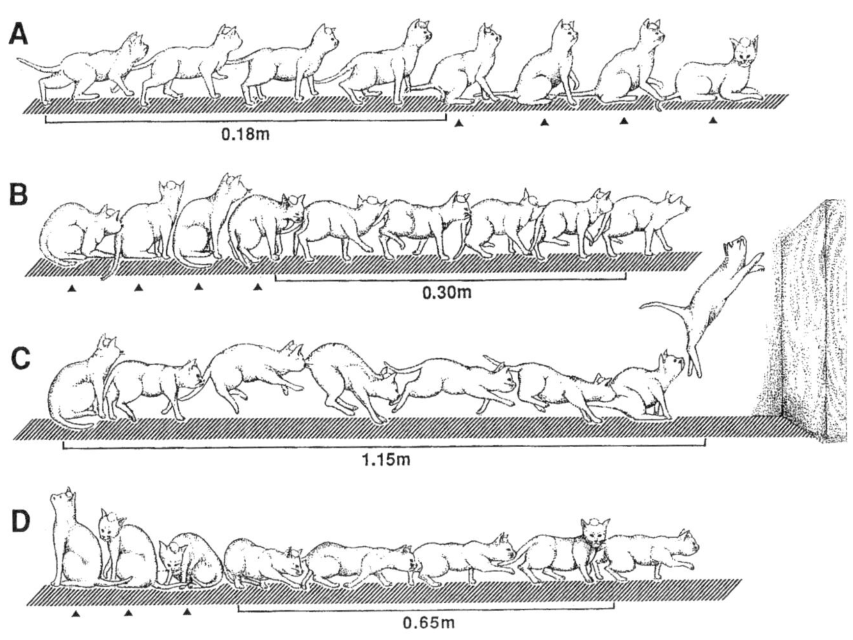

Figure 4-5. Behavioral changes evoked by stimulating four neural areas in the brain stem of a cat with an intact central nervous system. The sketches show postural and loco-motor changes evoked by stimulating the (*A*) DTF area, (*B*) VTF area, (*C*) MLR, and (*D*) SLR. Behavioral changes were analyzed by recording them on a video-recording system (Sony 208V). They were sketched sequentially at regular intervals of 0.2 sec from the rep-resentative frames of the videotape. The stimuli were delivered at the beginning of each series of sketches from the left to the right. Sketches indicated with closed triangles indi-cate that the cat changed its posture without changing its position on the floor. The lines under each series indicate the distance the animal moved. (Redrawn from S Mori, K Takakusaki. Integration of Posture and Locomotion. In: B Amblard, A Bertohoz, F Clarac, eds. *Posture and Gait*. Amsterdam: Exerpta Medica, 1988. Pp 341–354.)

motor cortex. The ascending fibers may include those belonging to the reticular activating system [26].

Stimulus Site–Specific Postural and Locomotor Changes

Within 1 second from the beginning of DTF stimulation, the cat ceases to walk but maintains a standing posture. With continuation of the stimulation, it squats without changing its position and then lies on the floor. DTF stimulation results in a sequential transition to a final lying posture. VTF stimulatioin evokes a se-ries of postural changes almost opposite to those induced by DTF stimulation. Within a few seconds from the beginning of VTF stimulation, the cat changes from a lying to a squatting position or to a standing position and then starts to walk during continuation of the stimulation. Induced locomotion is charac-terized by an enhanced swing phase and an enhanced stance phase without a preferred direction. However, a forelimb-hindlimb diagonal pattern is well maintained. After cessation of the stimulation, locomotion usually stops, and the cat remains standing.

Following MLR stimulation, intact cats invariably exhibit fast walking and then running movements. With the beginning of MLR stimulation, the cat often retraces its steps before initiation of locomotion, but the transition from a prestimulus posture, such as a squatting posture, to a running movement is very fast. The induced running movement is propulsive in nature, and the cat runs straight forward, avoiding collisions with walls or other obstacles. Furthermore, MLR-induced locomotor movements do not necessarily require continuous stimulation, in contrast to DTF- and VTF-induced postural and locomotor changes. Observation of the cat on MLR stimulation gives the impression of an animal trying to avoid noxious stimuli. When the SLR in the lateral hypothalamic area is stimulated, the cats exhibits searching-like locomotor behavior. In the sketches in Fig. 4-5, the cat is in a squatting position initially. A few seconds after the beginning of SLR stimulation, the cat starts to walk slowly, extending its head forward and looking around repeatedly. The cat tends to walk with a stoop and stealthy steps along the corners of the rooms. On termination of SLR stimulation, the cat ceases to walk and assumes a squatting or crouching posture. Locomotion was evoked only during lateral hypothalamic stimulation, and it was indistinguishable from spontaneous locomotion. With DTF stimulation, the cat shifts its center of gravity backward, a reaction specifically related to suppression of postural support. With this, the cat is forced to adopt a squatting posture.

It should be mentioned that the more rostral was the stimulus level (such as the SLR), the more natural were the evoked postural and locomotor changes. Bernstein [48] assumed the presence of some higher motor centers and the motor hierarchy. Each level of command relies on interaction with those above and below. According to Bernstein's view, for realization of movement, the higher motor centers have only to select and, possibly, tune the motor synergies, with resultant reduction in the number of degrees of freedom of the motor apparatus. The aforementioned observations indicate that the postural and locomotor synergies are structured in a hierarchy within the rostrocaudal axis of the brain stem and that the command routing through the brain stem relies on interactions with the SLR, the MLR, the DTF, and the VTF areas, and possibly on those within the pontomedullary reticular formation, forming a central program for locomotor control. In order to understand the neuronal mechanisms underlying such interactions and the central program, attempts have been made to selectively activate a group of cells in the pontine reticular formation.

Pontine-Induced Modification of Locomotor Movements

In acute decerebrate cats, focal microinjection of carbachol (a long-acting cholinomimetic chemical agent resistant to acethylcholinesterases) and serotonin (5-HT) into the medial pontine reticular formation (mPRF) results in suppression and augmentation of postural muscle tone, respectively [49]. MLR-induced locomotion is suppressed with carbachol-induced postural suppression, whereas it is restored and even enhanced with 5-HT–induced postural augmentation. Corresponding to carbachol- and 5-HT–induced postural suppression and augmentation, activities of fast-conducting reticulospinal cells in the nucleus reticularis gigantocellularis increase along with membrane hyperpolarization of hindlimb motoneurons and decrease along with membrane depolarization. Based on these findings, an attempt was made to study the behavioral changes possibly evoked by intrapontine injections of bethanechol in freely walking cats [50]. Bethanechol (a short-acting cholinergic agent) was injected into the mPRF by an injecting cannula inserted through a previously implanted guide tube. Bethanechol injections into the mPRF in freely moving, awake cats result in a reproducible modification of posture and locomotion. The animals were conditioned to walk around the room in which observations were made, with presentation of food as a reward. When they approached the food plates, the animals adopted a postural synergy adequate for feeding. They extended and flexed their hindlimbs and forelimbs, respectively, along with slight ventroflexion of their heads. Approximately 5 to 10 minutes after bethanechol injections, the cats showed the following reproducible behavioral changes: Once they began to walk, they walked continuously for a period without showing any deficit. However, once they stopped at the food plate and prepared a postural synergy adequate for feeding, postural muscle tone started to decrease, and the cats became unable to maintain a standing posture, even falling asleep. With auditory stimuli, the cats immediately became alert and began to walk again. Their locomotor behavior was the same as that observed before bethanechol injection, and it was difficult to detect any sign of postural suppression. By repeating a similar procedure and simply interrupting the ongoing locomotion of the animals, it was possible to reproduce intermittently these two extreme behavioral changes. One hour after bethanechol injection, the animals reverted to a normal pattern of behavior. These results suggest that intrapontine injection of bethanechol disturbs the cat's automatic and volitional control of motor performance. Both the ascending pathways to the cerebral cortex and the descending pathways to the medullary reticular formation and the spinal cord originate from the mPRF [7–9]. Because integration of locomotor drive signals and locomotor-related feedback signals could occur at the level of the pontomedullary reticular formation, it is conceivable that dissociation of these two different signals has taken place at the level of the mPRF via bethanechol injection, resulting in the disturbance of locomotor behaviors. The results also support the proposition that one of the sources of "drive signals" related to the activation of volitional control system is in the mPRF [4].

CONTEXT-DEPENDENT AND REFLEX-DEPENDENT ADAPTATION

In awake and behaving animals, the neural control of locomotion must be flexible and adaptive. The motor cortex receives somatosensory, visual, and vestibular inputs, integrating representation of posture and movements of the body through extrapersonal space. This integrated input may be considered to be the basis for an internal and external reference system for formulating locomotor movements [6]. The flow of locomotor control is illustrated in diagrammatic

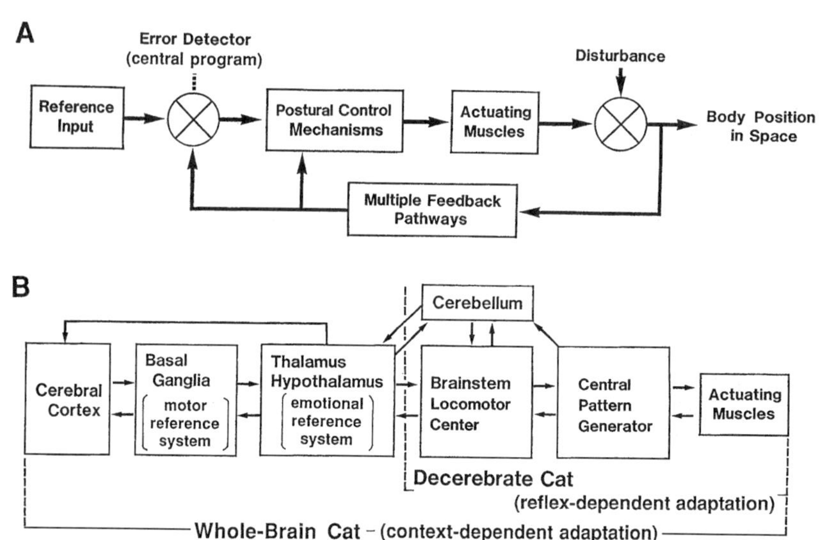

Figure 4-6. Block diagrams of postural and locomotor control systems. *A*. A block diagram of the postural control system. *B*. A block diagram of the locomotor control system. The level of brain-stem transection is indicated by a vertical broken line between the thalamus (hypothalamus) and the brain stem. Note that adjacent upper and lower structures are mutually and functionally connected.

form in Fig. 4-6A. Reference input arising from the sensorimotor cortex is fed into the error detector or higher-order central program and is compared with the multiple feedback signals. The summed outputs become so-called locomotor drive signals. They are fed forward into the postural and locomotor control mechanisms existing in the basal ganglia, diencephalon, brain stem, cerebellum, and spinal cord. These events result in an activation of postural muscles and locomotor synergies. Disturbances applied to the executive locomotor apparatus can be detected by a number of interoceptive and exteroceptive receptors, and the detected signals are fed back, not only to the cerebellum but also to the sensorimotor cortex. The locomotor-related signals flow recurrently through the loop in Figure 4-6A, and the final body position of the animal in space will be corrected constantly in relation to the reference input.

From a functional point of view, the reference system can be divided tentatively into a motor reference system and an emotional reference system (see Fig. 4-6B). It is assumed that by daily experience, training, and learning processes, the reference input is transcribed by not only the basal ganglia but also by a number of posture- and locomotor-related areas in the central nervous system. In the absence of the motor cortex (e.g., in a decorticate cat), the motor reference system in the basal ganglia becomes the highest motor center. With such transcription, the decorticate cat now becomes capable of executing locomotor behaviors, to a certain degree without reference input from the motor cortex. The emotional reference system is inherently stored in the thalamus and in the hypothalamus [47]. Thus, the thalamic cat exhibits, with removal of inhibitory inputs from the motor cortex and basal ganglia, general hyperactivity and hyperreactivity. These are manifested in the form of obstinate progression, which probably is the result of tonic activation of the basic locomotor automatism by the emotional reference system. By using the reference input, the cat with an intact central nervous system exhibits a variety of locomotor behaviors, adapting itself to the context. This type of adaptation can be context-dependent adaptation, and the information routed through the cerebrocerebellar and cerebellocerebral pathways play an essential role for its execution.

Studies of locomotion no longer are limited to the understanding of reflex-dependent adaptation in the decerebrate cat but can now encompass an understanding of context-dependent adaptation in the essentially intact cats. Wetzel et al. [51] made a very important observation in this regard. They cinematographically compared treadmill and overground locomotion and revealed considerable flexibility in the neural control program for locomotion. They suggested that segmental afferent input, visual and other suprasegmental inputs, and motivational variables probably all contribute to the separation of treadmill and overground timing profiles of limb movements. It appears that reflex-dependent adaptation is established by automatic interactions of neuronal subsystems in the brain stem and in the cerebellum with the environment. Context-dependent adaptation is established by the purposive or higher-order interactions of the cerebrocerebellar neuronal subsystems with the environment (see Fig. 4-6B). It appears also that "behavioral arousal" plays a crucial and additional role for purposive interactions.

NEUROPHYSIOLOGY OF BIPEDAL LOCOMOTION

Bipedal locomotion in humans and quadrupedal locomotion in animals need to satisfy the following four requirements: (1) antigravity support of the body, (2) stepping movements, (3) an adequate degree of equilibrium and, when these have been provided, (4) a means of propulsion [32]. For satisfactory execution of bipedal locomotion, all four requirements must be coordinated simultaneously and continuously. The support of the body against gravity is a general requirement for nearly all motor activities related to the external environment. In a vertical, standing, symmetrical rest position, the center of gravity of the body is situated at the forward edge of the second sacral vertebra. Because the human body in walking progresses on a narrow base, it is always in a posture of unstable equilibrium. It then must be controlled in such a way that its center of gravity always remains within the vertical projections of the narrow alternating bases [52]. The forward movement of the center of gravity provides propulsion. The force providing the propulsion is that produced by the weight of the body sliding down an incline with forward movements. The forward tilting of the body is also part of the necessary and adequate stimulus to evoke stepping and therefore serves a double purpose: If an individual leans forward beyond a certain degree he or she must either make a step forward or fall. This step forward is a defensive reaction, but it also ensures that stepping continues as long as propulsion is applied.

Primitive stepping is present in the newborn baby, but it cannot support the body against gravity because of immature development of postural muscle tone [53]. In the spinal human, there is no effective stepping movement [54] nor is there in spinal monkeys [13]. These results suggest that spinal circuits producing locomotor activity may be present in the adult human spinal cord but that they are not sufficient to generate locomotor activity by themselves. Martin [32] suggested that the most important coordinating mechanism or "center" for stepping is situated in the midbrain in humans. Inhibition and excitation of postural muscles related to locomotor activity most likely are due to the direct action of command signals descending from the midbrain on alpha-motoneurons. Command signals subsequently "switch on" a stereotyped repertoire of events, the function of a central program for locomotor control. The central program thus requires (at least to a certain degree) supraspinal and peripheral modulating inputs to sustain fine-tuning of the step cycle. Under normal environmental conditions, both supraspinal programs and the inherent passive and active (contractile) properties of muscle are adequate to control the dynamic performance of stepping, with sufficient stability and without further compensation by reflex activity [55]. As already demonstrated in the animal experiments, a variety of afferents are required to modulate supraspinal structures related to the central program for locomotor control (e.g., cerebellum, sensorimotor cortex) [2, 3].

It is useful to distinguish afferent pathways (which carry information into the nervous system that does not enter consciousness but may influence movement) from sensory pathways (which contribute to conscious perception). Balance is mediated largely by the specialized receptors of the vestibular apparatus, whereas the position and movement of the limbs are mediated by muscle afferent fibers. The spinocerebellar tracts provide information about the position of the body in space and about the position of the body segments relative to one another. Proprioception is the sense of balance, position, and movement of the limbs. The proprioceptive information from the limbs is used in two ways. First, it mediates reflex responses through a local circuit in the spinal cord. Some of these data, which are relayed to the cerebellum, modulate unconsciously the actions of spinal reflexes and the central program contributing to the "automatic" or reflex-dependent adaptation of locomotor movements (as is well demonstrated in the studies in decerebrate cats) [3, 31]. Second, proprioceptive information projects to the cerebral cortex, where it is used for the perception of limb position and, possibly, even for the voluntary control of posture during locomotion.

Two parallel ascending systems for somatic sensation are important clinically: the dorsal column–medial lemniscal system and the anterolateral system. These systems relay afferent information to the somatic sensory cortex for three purposes: perception, arousal, and motor control. The dorsal column–medial lemniscal system mediates tactile sensation, including vibration sense, joint position, and proprioception from the contralateral side of the body. The parallel anterolateral system (including spinothalamic, spinoreticular, and spinotectal tracts) carry information, chiefly about pain and temperature, and also some tactile information. The information relayed by the dorsal column–medial lemniscal system and the anterolateral system will be used for context-dependent adaptation of locomotor movements. Postural reactions (including the voluntary adjustments) are dependent on afferent impulses from (1) proprioception, (2) labyrinthine function, (3) vision, and (4) contact.

According to Martin [32], a normal individual blindfolded and walking on a smooth pavement shortens the step by approximately 5%. On uneven ground, this shortening of the step is more pronounced. Subjects devoid of labyrinthine function show very little disturbance in ordinary walking. Such individuals feel unsteady in an open space and cannot come down stairs without holding on to the banister, so that at all times they are dependent to some extent on vision. When blindfolded, they remain able to make normal stepping movements and do not fall or festinate forward or backward, indicating that such individuals are dependent for their postural reactions on proprioception alone. Martin [32] also emphasized the importance of proprioception in the automatic control aspects in bipedal human locomotion. Lipschitz and Block [56] reported a particular case in which a young man lost all sense of position below his face and ears, all other functions of his spinal cord being normal. His greatest difficulty was in starting to walk and in propelling himself forward. If he lost his balance, he showed no reactions to protect his equilibrium. When standing and walking, he was entirely dependent on vision and fell down if he closed his eyes [56]. Just recently, Ishii et al. [57] studied the human brain function associated with bipedal gait, using injection of 18F-fluorodeoxyglucose and positron emission tomography. Although the study was preliminary, these investigators found a marked activation of cerebellar vermis and occipital cortices bilaterally with treadmill walk in all subjects.

SUMMARY AND CONCLUSIONS

More than 80 years have passed since the pioneer studies by Sherrington [27] and Graham-Brown [58, 59] regarding postural control and locomotion. In 1914, Graham-Brown described the phenomenon of decerebrate reflex standing and stepping and proposed the existence of a "central rhythm generator" relating to locomotion. The "half-center model" was the basis for the concept of central pattern generator (CPG) or spinal stepping generator [5, 14]. Shik et al. [25] identified neural centers or networks active in control of locomotion. Engberg and Lundberg [60] provided evidence that the limb movements associated with locomotion are programmed centrally. The contribution of dorsolateral and ventromedial descending systems to the integration of posture and locomotion was studied in monkeys by Lawrence and Kuypers [10, 11]. We have provided evidence indicating that an activation of setting mechanisms in the level of postural muscle tone and that of the "spinal stepping generator" are not separate phenomena [33, 38], emphasizing the necessity of postural and locomotor integration for the satisfactory expression of locomotor movements. The results obtained from the cat experiments have been used for the better understanding of locomotor movements in monkeys and bipedal human locomotion.

It is our current understanding that postural and locomotor control systems do not reside clustered in particular sites; instead, they are formed by subprograms that are distributed within the central nervous system [61]. Postural and locomotor control systems share their subprograms at several levels in the central nervous system, especially in the brain stem and spinal cord. The neuronal circuitry related to each of the subprograms is connected functionally and is refined in parallel with the acquisition and execution of locomotor movements. Afferent impulses from various sources play a crucial role in the task. In 1979, Brookhart [62] explicitly stated that "we must devise ways to determine whether parts of the system function with the whole in the same way they do in isolation. Learning how a system subcomponent behaves in a carefully defined and constrained set of circumstances gives us no guarantee that our subcomponent will behave according to the same rules if the circumstances were changed." Further studies aimed at elucidating context-dependent adaptation in the overground locomotion of both quadrupeds and bipeds will allow us to understand the higher nervous control that alters the character of the locomotor act from one of generality of purpose to one of narrowed and specific purpose fitting a specific occasion.

References

1. Sherrington CD. *Man on His Nature*. London: Macmillan, 1941.
2. Armstrong DM. Supraspinal contributions to the initiation and control of locomotion in the cat. *Prog Neurobiol* 1986;26:273–361.
3. Arshavsky YuI, Gelfand IM, Orlovsky GN. *Cerebellum and Rhythmical Movements*. Berlin: Springer-Verlag, 1986.
4. Mori S. Integration of posture and locomotion in acute decerebrate cats in awake, freely moving cats. *Prog Neurobiol* 1987;28:161–195.
5. Grillner S. Locomotion in vertebrates: Central mechanisms and reflex interactions. *Physiol Rev* 1975;55:247–304.
6. Mori S, Takakusaki K. Integration of Posture and Locomotion. In: Amblard B, Bertohoz A, Clarac F, eds. *Posture and Gait*. Amsterdam: Excerpta Medica, 1988. Pp 341–354.
7. Kuypers HGJM. Anatomy of the Descending Pathways. In: Brookhart JM, Mountcastle VB, eds. *Handbook of Physiology* (vol 2): *The Nervous System*. Bethesda, MD: American Physiological Society, 1981. Pp 597–666.
8. Brodal A. *Neurological Anatomy in Relation to Clinical Medicine* (3rd ed). Oxford: Oxford University Press, 1981.
9. Matsuyama K, et al. Termination mode and branching patterns of reticuloreticular and reticulospinal fibers of the nucleus reticularis pontis oralis in the cat: An anterograde PHA-L tracing study. *Neurosci Res* 1993;17:9–21.
10. Lawrence DG, Kuypers HGJM. The functional organization of the motor system in the monkey: I. The effects of bilateral pyramidal lesions. *Brain* 1968;91:1–14.
11. Lawrence DG, Kuypers HGJM. The functional organization of the motor system in the monkey: II. The effects of lesions of the descending brain stem pathways. *Brain* 1968;91:15–36.

12. Drew T, Dubuc R, Rossignol S. The discharge patterns of reticulospinal and other reticular neurons in chronic unrestrained cats walking on a treadmill. *J Neurophysiol* 1986;55:375–401.

13. Eiderberg E, Walden JG, Nguyen H. Locomotor control in macaque monkeys. *Brain* 1981;104:647–663.

14. Shik ML, Orlovsky GN. Neurophysiology of locomotor automatism. *Physiol Rev* 1976;55:465–501.

15. Schaltenbrandt G, Cobb S. Clinical and anatomical studies on two cats without neocortex. *Brain* 1930;53:449–488.

16. Armstrong DM, Drew T. Discharges of pyramidal tract and other motor cortical neurones during locomotion in the cat. *J Physiol* 1984;346:471–495.

17. Armstrong DM, Drew T. Locomotor-related neuronal discharges in cat motor cortex compared with peripheral receptive fields and evoked movements. *J Physiol* 1984;346:497–515.

18. Armstrong DM, Edgley SA. Discharges of nuclues interpositus neurones during locomotion in the cat. *J Physiol* 1984;351:411–432.

19. Garcia-Rill E. The basal ganglia and the locomotor regions. *Brain Res Rev* 1986;11:47–63.

20. Villablanca JR, Marcus RJ. Sleep-wakefulness, EEG and behavioral studies of chronic cats without neocortex and striatum: The 'diencephalic' cat. *Arch Ital Biol* 1972;110:348–382.

21. Villablanca JR, Olmstead CE. The striatum: A fine tuner of the brain. *Acta Neurobiol Exp* 1982;42:227–229.

22. Villablanca JR, Marcus RJ, Olmstead CE. Effects of caudate nuclei or frontal cortical ablations in cats: II. Sleep-wakefulness, EEG and motor activity. *Exp Neurol* 1976;53:31–50.

23. Hinsey JC, Ranson SW, McNattin RF. The role of the hypothalamus and mesencephalon in locomotion. *Arch Neurol Psychiatr* 1930;23:1–43.

24. Waller WH. Progression movements elicited by subthalamic stimulation. *J Neurophysiol* 1940;3:300–307.

25. Shik ML, Severin FV, Orlovsky GN. Control of walking and running by means of electrical stimulation of the mid-brain. *Biophysics* 1966;11:756–765.

26. Mori S, et al. Site-specific postural and locomotor changes evoked in awake, freely moving intact cats by stimulating the brainstem. *Brain Res* 1989;505:66–74.

27. Sherrington CS. *The Integrative Action of the Nervous System.* New Haven: Yale University Press, 1906.

28. Garcis-Rill E, Skinner RD, Fitzgerald JA. Chemical activation of the mesencephalic locomotor region. *Brain Res* 1985;330:43–54.

29. Mori S, et al. Neuronal constituents of postural and locomotor control systems and their interactions in cats. *Brain Dev* 1992;14(suppl):S109–120.

30. Arshavsky YuI, Gelfand IM, Orlovsky GN. The cerebellum and control of rhythmical movements. *Trends Neurosci* 1983;6:417–422.

31. Orlovsky GN, Shik ML. Control of locomotion: A neurophysiological analysis of the cat locomotor system. *Int Rev Physiol Neurophysiol* 1976;2:282–317.

32. Martin JP. *The Basal Ganglia and Posture.* London: Pitman Medical, 1967.

33. Mori S, et al. Setting and resetting of level of postural muscle tone in decerebrate cat by stimulation of brain stem. *J Neuroiphysiol* 1983;48:737–748.

34. Mori S, Yagodnitsyn AS, Shik ML. Role of pontine tegmentum for locomotor control in mesencephalic cat. *J Neurophysiol* 1977;40:284–295.

35. Selionov VA, Shik ML. Medullary locomotor strip and column in the cat. *Neuroscience* 1984;13:1267–1278.

36. Orlovsky GN. Connexions of the reticulo-spinal neurons with the "locomotor regions" of the brain stem. *Biophysics* 1970;15:178–186.

37. Shimamura M, Kogure I. Discharge patterns of reticulospinal neurons corresponding with quadrupedal leg movements in thalamic cats. *Brain Res* 1983;230:27–34.

38. Mori S, et al. Controlled locomotion in the mesencephalic cat: Distribution of facilitatory and inhibitory regions within pontine tegmentum. *J Neurophysiol* 1978;41:1580–1591.

39. Jordan LM. Brainstem and Spinal Cord Mechanisms for the Initiation of Locomotion. In: Shi-

mamura M, Grillner S, Edgerton VR, eds. *Neurobiological Basis of Human Locomotion.* Tokyo: Japan Scientific Societies Press, 1991. Pp 3–20.

40. Mori S. Contribution of postural muscle tone to full expression of posture and locomotor movements: Multifaceted analyses of its setting brainstem-spinal cord mechanisms in the cat. *Jpn J Physiol* 1989;39:785–809.

41. Iwahara T, Wall PT, Garcia-Rill E, Skinner RD. Stimulation-induced setting of postural muscle tone in the decerebrate rat. *Brain Res* 1991;557:331–335.

42. Mori S, Kawahara K, Sakamoto T. Supraspinal Aspects of Locomotion in the Mesencephalic Cat. In: Roberts A, Roberts BL, eds. *Neural Origin of Rhythmic Movements.* Cambridge: Cambridge University Press, 1983. Pp 445–468.

43. Takakusaki K, Ohta Y, Mori S. Membrane Potential Oscillations of Hindlimb Alpha-Motoneurons Associated with Alternating Hindlimb Loading in Reflexively Standing Cats. In: Shimamura M, Grillner S, Edgerton VR, eds. *Neurological Basis of Human Locomotion.* Tokyo: Japan Scientific Societies Press, 1991. Pp 159–166.

44. Orlovsky GN. Work of the Purkinje cells during locomotion. *Biophysics* 1972;17:935–941.

45. Orlovsky GN. The effect of different descending systems on flexor and extensor activity during locomotion. *Brain Res* 1972;40:359–371.

46. Mori S, Matsuyama K, Takakusaki K, Kanaya T. The behavior of lateral vestibular neurons during walk, trot and gallop in acute decerebrate cats. *Prog Brain Res* 1988;76:211–220.

47. Roberts WW. Hypothalamic Mechanism for Motivational and Species Typical Behavior. In: Walen RE, ed. *The Neural Control of Behavior.* New York: Academic, 1970. Pp 175–210.

48. Bernstein N. *The Coordination and Regulation of Movements.* Oxford: Pergamon, 1967.

49. Takakusaki K, Kohyama J, Matsuyama K, Mori S. Synaptic mechanisms acting on lumbar motoneurons during postural augmentation induced by serotonin injection into the rostral pontine reticular formation in decerebrate cats. *Exp Brain Res* 1993;93:471–482.

50. Mori S, Sakamoto T, Takakusaki K. Interaction of Posture and Locomotion in Cats: Its Automatic and Volitional Control Aspects. In: Shimamura M, Grillner S, Edgerton VR, eds. *Neurobiological Basis of Human Locomotion.* Tokyo: Japan Scientific Societies Press, 1991. Pp 21–32.

51. Wetzel MC, Atwater AE, Wait JV, Stuart DG. Neural Implications of different profiles between treadmill and overground locomotion timings in cats. *J Neurophysiol* 1975;38:492–501.

52. Carlsoo S. *How Man Moves: Kinesiological Methods and Studies.* London: Heinemann, 1972.

53. Kuhn RA. Functional capacity of the isolated human spinal cord. *Brain* 1950;73:1–51.

54. Forssberg H, Hirschfeld H, Stokes VP. Development of Human Locomotor Mechanisms. In: Shimamura M, Grillner, S, Edgerton, VR, eds. *Neurobiological Basis of Human Locomotion.* Tokyo: Japan Scientific Societies Press, 1991. Pp 259–274.

55. Herman H, Cook T, Cozzens B, Freedman W. Control of Postural Reactions in Man: The initiation of gait. In: Stein RB, Pearson, KG, Smith, RS, Redford, IB, eds. *Control of Posture and Locomotion.* New York: Plenum, 1973. Pp 363–388.

56. Lipschitz R, Block J. Stab wounds of the spinal cord, *Lancet* 1962;2:169–172, 1962.

57. Ishii K, et al. Brain function in bipedal gait studied with PET. *Abstr Soc Neurosci* 1993;19:145.

58. Graham-Brown T. The intrinsic factors in the act of progression in the mammal. *Proc R Soc Lond [B]Biol Sci* 1911;84:308–319.

59. Graham-Brown T. On the fundamental activity of the nervous centers. *J Physiol* 1914;48:1846.

60. Engberg I, Lundberg A. An electromyographic analysis of muscular activity in the hindlimb of the cat during unrestrained locomotion. *Acta Physiol Scand* 1969;75:614–630.

61. Mori S. Motor Control in Relation to Postural and Locomotor Control. *Electrophysiological Kinesiology.* In: Pedotti A, ed. Amsterdam: IOS Press, 1993. Pp 1–8.

62. Brookhart JM. Convergence on an Understanding of Motor Control. In: Talbott RE, Humphrey DR, eds. *Posture and Locomotion.* New York: Raven, 1979. Pp 295–304.

5. Balance Decrements in Older Persons: Effects of Age and Disease

Leslie Wolfson

Biological functions decline with age. This decrease varies for different functions, as was shown in a recent longitudinal study of cognition that demonstrated a consistent although variable decrease in markers of primary mental abilities as well as the constructs of these abilities [1]. The major problem in defining age-dependent changes is the role of age-related diseases in producing the decrements. Thus, diseases that have not manifested themselves overtly (i.e., subclinical) may affect these functions, giving the appearance of age-associated change. Nevertheless, data from well-screened subjects consistently demonstrate the decrements in almost all areas studied. This chapter examines the changes that have been observed with increasing age, both in balance and in its component neuromuscular functions. Finally, mobility, functional capacity, and the justification for balance training in older persons are discussed in terms of these changes.

AGE-ASSOCIATED CHANGES IN UNDERLYING NEUROMUSCULAR FUNCTION

Sensory Function

Vision Is Fundamental for Balance

Visual input is important for automatic balance responses that allow for the reflexlike response to uneven floors or other hazards commonly encountered (see Chapter 3). In addition, the ability to perceive normal surface conditions (e.g., a curb or step edge) and hazards (e.g., a wet floor) under a wide variety of lighting conditions helps to frame the voluntary responses that allow us to avoid falls.

Common age-related changes in visual function include presbyopia (due to decreasing lens accommodation) and cataracts. Other visual changes include diminished visual acuity due to macular degeneration [2] and decreased response to spatial frequency, contrast, stereopsis, and diminished adaptation to dark and glare [3–4]. Age-related diseases involving the visual system are common and include glaucoma and macular degeneration.

Pain and Thermal Sensitivity

Pain and thermal sensitivity decrease with age, although consistent decrements are not demonstrable on neurological examination [6–10]. Similarly, psychophysiological measurement has demonstrated decrements in tactile sensitivity

[11], two-point discrimination [12], joint position sense, and stereognosis [11] with increasing age, although a quantitative neurological examination did not demonstrate a significant decrement in tactile perception and two-point discrimination [13, 14]. Clinical studies are consistent with these modest decrements, as less than one-third of older patients have abnormalities of these sensory modalities [6–10].

By contrast, vibratory sensitivity demonstrates a major decrement with age. There is a two- to tenfold increase in the vibratory threshold of older persons [13–15]. Diminished vibratory function is present in two-thirds of older persons evaluated in six previously reported clinical studies [6–10]. These changes in vibratory sensation are more prominent in the lower than in the upper extremities [7]. The prominence of the vibratory changes and the lack of comparable changes in any other modalities are not consistent with the presence of a generalized sensory neuropathy in older persons. Nerve conduction velocities and action potential amplitudes decrease gradually, and F-wave latencies increase from the third to the eighth decades but not to the extent that brings them close to the neuropathic range [16]. Thus, though changes in sensory function are associated with age, they are unlikely to be the result of a functionally significant sensory neuropathy. Conceivably, age-related changes in receptor function could account for the modest sensory decrements observed, particularly those reported in vibratory sensation. The likelihood is, therefore, that for most older persons, change in lower-extremity sensory function is not the primary causative factor in balance decrements.

Hearing and Vestibular Functions

Age-related changes in hearing start in young adult life but do not become significant until after age 65 [17, 18]. Speech and loudness discrimination are particularly affected, with high frequencies commonly involved. As a result, older persons have particular difficulty understanding speech in rooms with a high ambient noise level [19]. For most older persons, hearing aids provide a measure of relief. The role of hearing in postural responses as well as in avoiding falls appears to be relatively minor.

By contrast (see Chapter 3), vestibular function is an essential part of the postural response. A substantial literature details the effects of vestibular dysfunction on balance. Vestibular dysfunction often produces impaired balance in younger persons. A critical question has been whether this is a factor in the balance changes reported in older persons. No direct evidence addresses this question, although a reduction in the number of hair cells in the maculae and cristae may be the anatomical substrate for diminished vestibular function [20]. In contrast to the anatomical changes, vestibular evaluation using oculocaloric and vestibulo-ocular testing demonstrates minor decrements with age [21, 22]. A recent study demonstrated no caloric response changes with age and only modest changes during rotational testing. The authors suggest that adaptive mechanisms within the central nervous system (CNS) are important in maintaining the vestibulo-ocular response [21]. The importance of vestibular function in age-related balance changes remains unclear, although there are no data to suggest that it is a major factor.

In the presence of inaccurate tactile-proprioceptive input, the sway of older persons increases to a greater extent than that of younger persons. Platform posturography demonstrates a significant decrement in balance performance with absent or blocked visual and tactile-proprioceptive input. It is unlikely that this is primarily the result of diminished vestibular input, as balance performance on difficult motor tasks decreases to a comparable extent, suggesting higher-order organizational or biomechanical dysfunction [23].

Motor Function

Muscle mass declines between 0.5% and 1.0% annually in men and women (respectively) aged 60 or older [24, 25]. Cross-sectional studies have demonstrated a 20–40% decrease in strength from the third to the eighth decades [26–28]. These declines in strength are greater than the loss of muscle mass [29, 30]. Quantitative neurological assessment has demonstrated decreased coordination and hand dexterity, with diminished ability to perform simulated activities of daily living (e.g., buttoning a shirt or cutting a steak) [13, 14].

Changes in reaction time as a result of age have been well studied. The studies indicate that reaction times decrease from childhood to young adulthood, prolong slowly until the sixth decade, and increase more rapidly thereafter. Afferent and efferent transmission of reaction-time tasks consume a modest portion of the time required for these tasks and change only nominally with increasing age. Even though they represent only a minor portion of reaction time, the time required for transduction of the stimulus into a nerve impulse and the time required for the nerve impulse to activate muscles have been reported to demonstrate moderate changes with increasing age. By far, the largest part of the response time is consumed by sensorimotor processing (i.e., definition of the sensory input and choice of the motor response). The time required for sensorimotor processing is influenced by the number of choices and complexity of those choices. Thus, the time required for choice reaction-time tasks increases more than that of simple reaction-time tasks with increasing age. Similarly, more complicated tasks result in greater increments in the processing time required in older subjects. Thus, sensorimotor processing represents the largest portion of reaction time and the part most influenced by age [31]. An important element of balance requires sensorimotor processing with the choice of an effective motor response.

Sensorimotor Processing

Visual, vestibular, and tactile-proprioceptive input provide the internal representation of an individual's position, motion, and surroundings in external space. As with other motor functions, the balance response is modifiable and influenced by prior experience (e.g., learning) and perceptual set, among other factors. This is likely to occur at a time and locus proximate to the synthesis of the sensory input, so that what is produced is an integrated postural response appropriate to current conditions and that uses an individual's prior experience. The association of gait and balance dysfunction with frontal lobe and, to a lesser extent, thalamic lesions suggests that these are important sites for this integration, although the anatomical site(s) of sensorimotor processing have not been determined definitely. Although controversy exists, morphological changes within the nervous system are well-documented with age. Postmortem study of the frontal cortex (precentral gyrus) from 80- to 90-year-old subjects suggests a decrement of approximately 40% of neurons, with a loss of dendrites and dendritic spines by comparison with young adults [32]. The role of morphology in balance changes is unclear. In addition to the morphological changes, significant neurochemical changes are reported in the motor system. Most notable is the 50% decrease in the dopamine content of the human neostriatum in 80-year-olds that is associated with changes in concentration of subtypes of the dopamine receptor [32, 33]. The role of changes within the dopamine system in age-related motor changes is unclear. Dopamine replacement does not improve performance of motor tasks in nonparkinsonian subjects [34].

Measures of Sway During Standing and with Blocked or Inaccurate Visual Input

During normal standing, the sway amplitude of subjects 70 and older (average age = 76 ± 5 years) relatively free of neurological disease known to compromise balance was only 3% lower (difference not significant) than a group of controls (average age = 35 ± 12 years) [23]. The sway velocity of subjects 75 and older who were comparably screened was considerably greater than that of young controls [35]. Other studies have demonstrated small differences in the spontaneous sway of older persons, suggesting that even during normal standing, small differences exist between the balance of older and younger persons [36, 37]. Differences of sway amplitude are greater when the subjects close their eyes or are presented with inaccurate visual input [23, 38]. Sway velocity also becomes accentuated with eyes closed, although the differences are still modest [35]. Sensory information is overlapping via tactile-proprioceptive, vestibular, and visual inputs. Thus, even if visual input is blocked, sway during quiet standing increases only modestly in older persons.

Measures of Sway with Inaccurate Tactile-proprioceptive Input and Blocked or Inaccurate Visual Input

When the tilt of the support surface is programmed to follow that of the subject, thus providing inaccurate tactile-proprioceptive input, the sway amplitude of older persons increases only modestly over that of the eyes-closed condition [23, 38]. When, in addition to visual input, tactile-proprioceptive input is blocked, the balance performance of older persons deteriorates markedly by comparison with younger subjects. Under these conditions, 30% to 50% of older persons demonstrate a loss of balance on their initial exposure to testing (Fig. 5-1) [23,

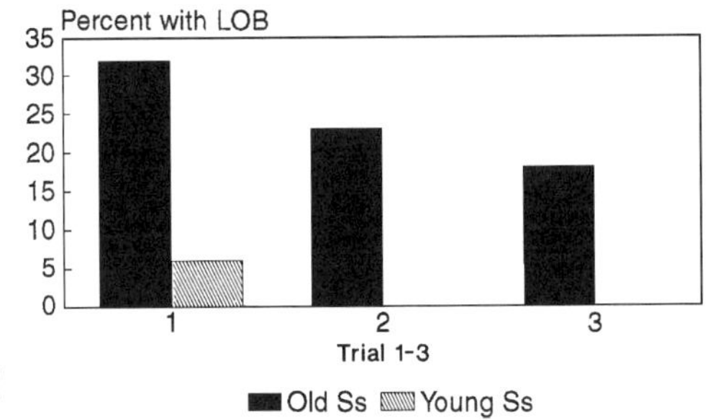
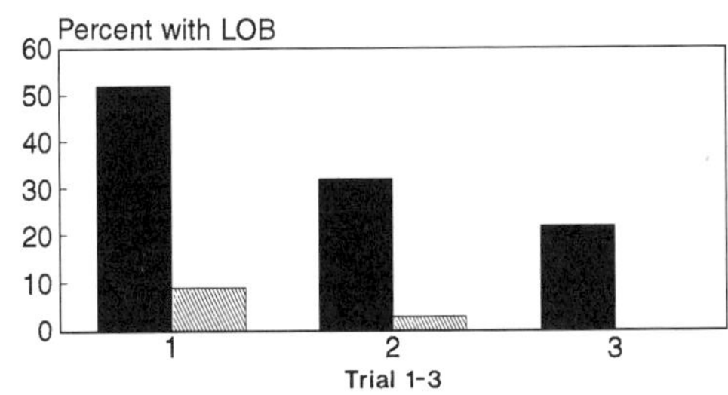

Figure 5-1. The percentage of old compared to young subjects (*Ss*) with loss of balance (*LoB*) during conditions that limit or distort visual and tactile-proprioceptive input. *A*. Eyes closed, sway-referenced surface. *B*. Sway-referenced vision and surface. Significant differences in the performance of older subjects compared to younger persons were present in each trial of both conditions (p <.005, Fisher exact test). Performance improved comparably with repetitive trials for both groups. (From L Wolfson et al. A dynamic posturography study of balance in healthy elderly. *Neurology* 1992; 42:2069–2075.)

38]. This suggests that in older persons, the processing of sensory information into an effective postural response may require redundant sensory information. Comparable data in older persons has been reported during balance perturbations with peripheral vision blocked [39]. The data suggest that under conditions that restrict sensory input from two modalities, the balancing ability of older persons is limited.

Response to Perturbations

Fast

Daily activities require postural adjustments as one encounters the hazards that surround all individuals at home and work. The ability to make corrective postural responses (termed *long-loop reflexes*) can be evaluated by moveable force platforms that can present destabilizing surface movements. Balance differences between old and young, which are minimal during unperturbed stance, become prominent with movement of the support surface. In older subjects, movement-induced sway amplitude, sway velocity, and the occurrence of loss of balance are significantly poorer than in younger persons [23, 35, 38]. Furthermore, with increasing difficulty of the test conditions (e.g., larger, higher acceleration movement), older persons demonstrate larger performance decrements in comparison to young persons (Fig. 5-2) [23, 35].

Slow

Large, rapid surface movements activate long-loop reflexes, whereas small, slow movements induce the higher level sensory integration facets of postural con-

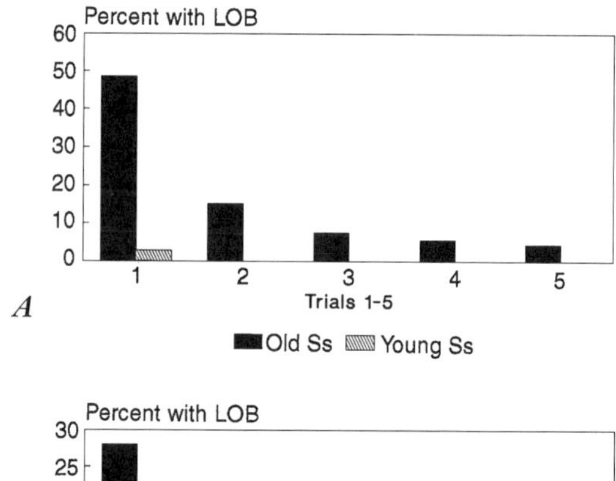

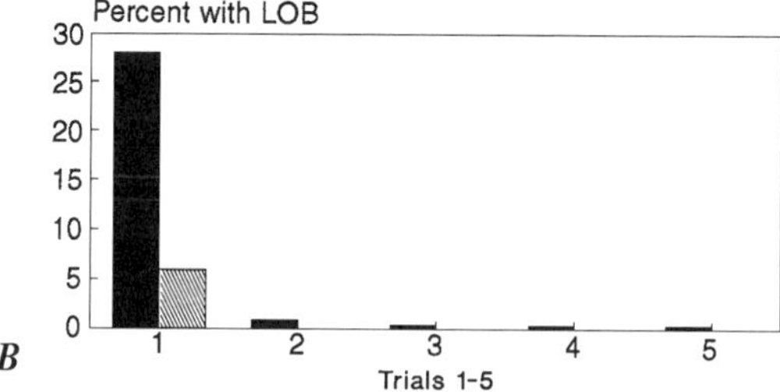

Figure 5-2. The percentage of old compared to young subjects (*Ss*) with loss of balance (*LoB*) during challenging motor tasks, (i.e., toes-up [*A*] and toes-down [*B*] rotations of the platform). Significant differences in the performance of older subjects compared to younger persons were present for trials one and two of the toes-up rotations and the first trial of the toes-down rotations ($p < .05$, Fisher exact test). Performance improved with repetitive trials for both toes-up and toes-down rotations. (From L Wolfson et al. A dynamic posturography study of balance in healthy elderly. *Neurology* 1992; 42:2069–2075.)

trol. Surprisingly, older persons demonstrate greater decrements in response to small, slow movements, with slower response time and increased sway amplitude. In addition, improvement of performance (adaptation) with repetitive long-loop trials during serial small, slow movements is not observed in older persons but is present in young persons. Older persons seem to demonstrate poorer balance when posture is controlled by a higher level sensorimotor integration mechanism [40]. In addition, during voluntary movement, older persons demonstrate slower, less reactive postural responses [41].

Adaptation and Learning

The presentation of repetitive motor tasks produces an improvement in performance called *adaptation*, which is an important element of balance function [23]. Thus, although the balance of older persons initially is poor, with limited sensory input, repetitive trials lead to a major improvement in performance (see Fig. 5-1). Similarly, the performance on difficult motor tasks (e.g., platform tilts) is enhanced at all ages with serial presentation (see Fig. 5-2). Adaptation implies that the nervous system can monitor performance and has the flexibility to improve execution of the balance response with repetition. Moreover, short-term learning of adaptive postural responses supports the potential of training that would expose older persons to balance stimuli that would develop adaptation. This potential for long-term improvement has been shown in a study demonstrating meaningful improvements of balance at the end of a 3-month intervention and following the completion of a 6-month maintenance period (see Chapter 22).

Muscle Activation

Following platform movement, the muscle response latency of older persons is the same as that of younger persons [39] or is increased modestly [23, 42]. Older persons demonstrated greater activation of antagonist muscles and used muscle sequences not observed in young persons (e.g., use of hips) [39, 42]. Older persons also have poorer integration between postural reflexes and voluntary movement, with slower stabilizing responses to postural disturbances during voluntary sway. In addition, there was less integration of the bilateral activation required in postural responses [41]. Therefore, the choice, sequence, and timing of muscle activity is, at least in part, responsible for the changes in balance observed in older persons.

Limits of Stability

To maintain bipedal stance, body weight must be maintained within a stability zone on each foot so that the center of body mass is directly above this zone. When turns, transfers, reaching, or destabilizing forces cause body mass to leave this zone (i.e., exceed the limit of stability), a motor response (i.e., balance response) or step(s) must occur to restore vertical alignment. A gauge of the limit of stability in the anteroposterior (AP) plane is the functional base of support (FBOS), which requires a force platform to determine the portion of foot length used to support body mass during maximal sustained backward and forward lean. FBOS was 0.60 ± 0.07 in subjects younger than 60 and 0.42 ± 0.12 for those 60 and older. FBOS was relatively constant until age 60, after which it declines 16% per decade (Fig. 5-3) [43]. Functional reach, the difference between arm length and maximal forward reach, is determined in part by the anterior limit of stability and can be assessed with a yardstick. Functional reach decreases approximately 25% from adulthood to age 70 or older [44].

Decreases in strength and range of motion are likely to be major factors in diminished FBOS. This is particularly true for the posterior portion of the FBOS. Normally the tibialis anterior develops far less strength than does the gastrocnemius, providing little functional reserve of power. Thus, if tibialis strength is diminished (age- or disease-associated), weakness may become a factor in controlling backward lean as well as in checking posteriorly directed perturbations.

Narrowed Base of Support

As the base of support is narrowed both in the AP and mediolateral planes, maintaining stance becomes more difficult. Single-stance, which represents a special condition of a narrowed base of support, is a difficult balancing task for older persons. In part because of simplicity of its measurement (measurement is fast and requires no specialized equipment), it has been used widely as a balance measure. The ability to maintain single-stance for 30 seconds (eyes open) changes little from the third to the sixth decade and then decreases to 22 seconds in the

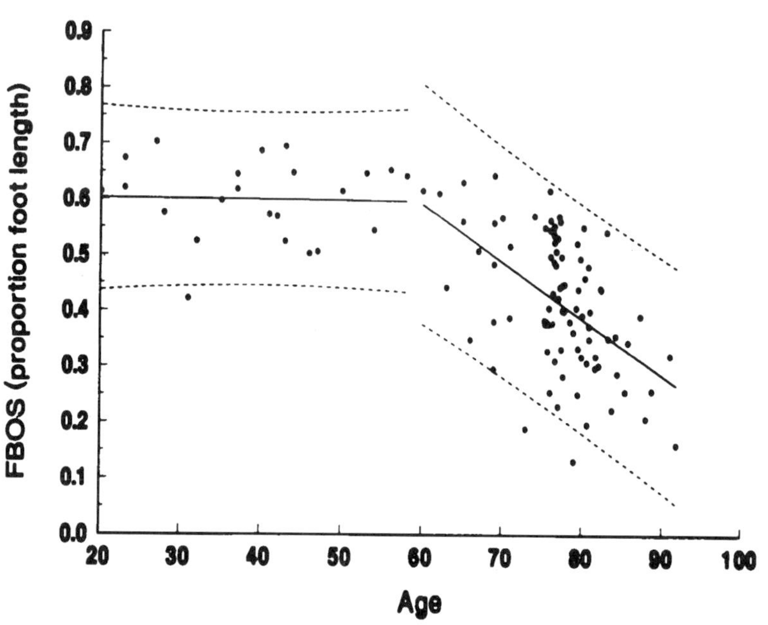

Figure 5-3. Functional base of support (*FBos*) plotted against age. A two-phase function was observed with separate regression lines for subjects 20–59 years old and for subjects 60–91 years old. The 95% confidence intervals are denoted by the dashed lines. (From MB King, JO Judge, L Wolfson. Functional base of support decreases with age. *J Gerontol Med Sci* 1994; 48:M258–263.)

seventh decade and to 14 seconds in the eighth decade (Fig. 5-4). Single-stance time (eyes closed) decreases modestly in the fifth and sixth decades and then drops rapidly to 4 seconds in the seventh and eighth decades (see Fig. 5-4) [45]. Concurrently, length of the sway path during single-stance almost doubles in subjects from the third through the seventh decades, also indicating the compromise of single-stance ability with increasing age [46]. Though single-stance describes the balance changes in healthy older persons, it is above the capacity for individuals with significant elements of motor dysfunction and becomes increasingly difficult for persons older than 80. For these individuals, tandem-stance becomes a test of increasing value. A recently described test, suitable for the frail and for individuals older than 80, uses the narrowest base a subject can maintain (i.e., parallel, semitandem, tandem, and single) as a measure of performance [47].

Gender and Age

During quiet standing and mild balance stresses and when support surface and visual input were manipulated separately, the balance of older women was comparable to that of their male counterparts. When both vision and support surface inputs were compromised and during challenging stresses (e.g., platform tilts),

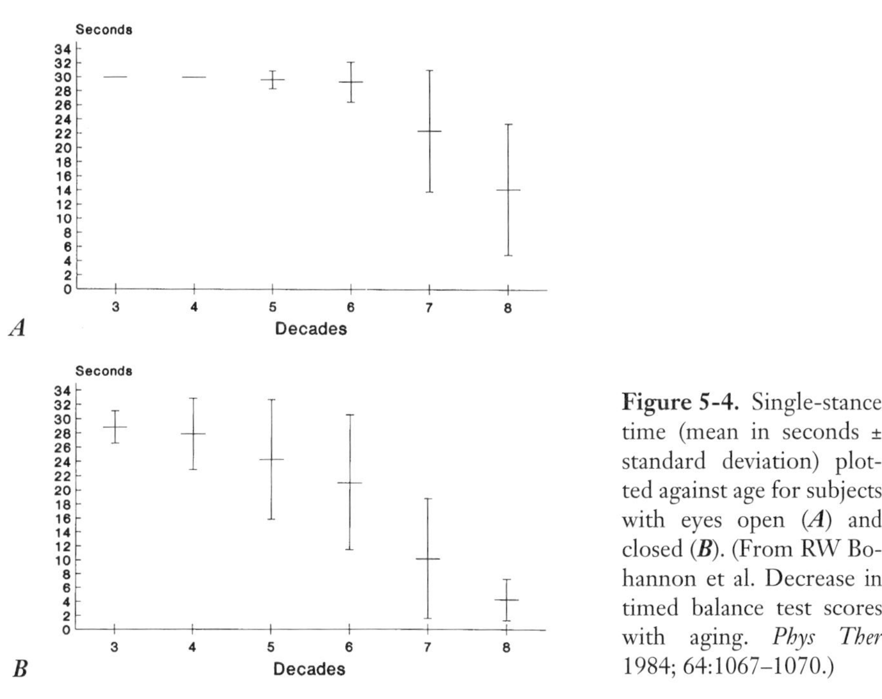

Figure 5-4. Single-stance time (mean in seconds ± standard deviation) plotted against age for subjects with eyes open (*A*) and closed (*B*). (From RW Bohannon et al. Decrease in timed balance test scores with aging. *Phys Ther* 1984; 64:1067–1070.)

the balance of older women was significantly poorer than that of men (Fig. 5-5). Women demonstrated adaptation during repetitive testing, although this was less evident for backward destabilization [48]. There are minimal data to support a CNS cause for this gender difference, so that biomechanical origins (e.g., dorsiflexion strength or ankle mobility) seem more likely.

FUNCTIONAL AND THERAPEUTIC IMPLICATIONS OF BALANCE DECREMENTS

What is the functional significance of the balance changes that have been presented? Older persons demonstrate a restricted limit of sway and diminished ability to control a narrowed base of support (i.e., single-stance). Therefore, even in relatively routine activity, they may approach their limit of stable stance, are closer to using postural responses, and may require a more vigorous response to restore a secure posture. The data also suggest that the balance of older persons differs most from that of younger individuals under challenging conditions (e.g., single modality sensory input or platform tilt) that produce both increased sway and the occurrence of loss of balance. Thus, effectiveness of the postural response is diminished in a group in which it will be increasingly used. Moreover, postural response is compromised most in those challenging conditions that elicit falls. It is likely, therefore, that even these relatively modest age-related changes are a significant factor in the increased incidence of falls in older per-

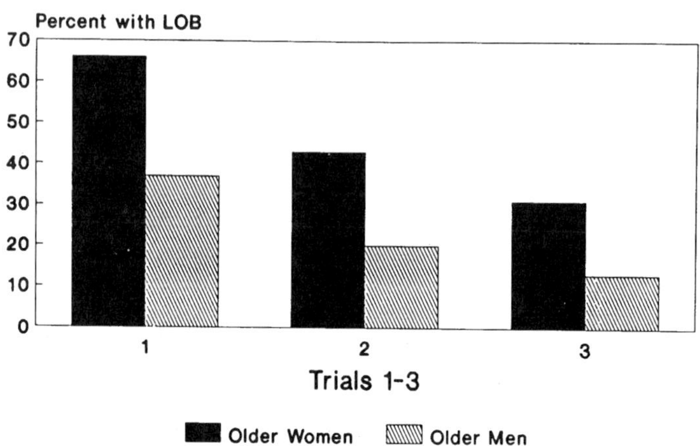

Figure 5-5. The percentage of older men compared to older women with loss of balance *LoB*) during a condition (sway-referenced vision and surface) distorting visual and tactile-proprioceptive input. Significant differences were present between older women and men for all three trials ($p < .05$, Fisher exact test), although both genders improved comparably during repetitive testing. (From L Wolfson et al. Gender differences in the balance of healthy elderly as demonstrated by dynamic posturography. *J Gerontol Med Sci* 1994; 49:M160–167.)

sons. This also may explain the increased incidence of falls in older women, as gender differences in balance become prominent under challenging conditions.

Under most circumstances, however, the balance of older persons functions effectively. In older persons screened for diseases known to impair balance, we observed that the response of older persons to difficult balance challenges (e.g., single modality sensory input or platform tilt) demonstrated modest decrements in subjects 80 and older by comparison with those from aged 70 to 74 and 75 to 79 years (Table 5-1) [23]. These data suggest that dysfunctional balance associated with impaired mobility and multiple falls may be less a result of age than an effect of age-related disease. Our experience in frail nursing home residents with recurrent falls supports these data. These patients had severely compromised balance, gait, and strength in contrast with nonfalling controls also enrolled in this study [49–51]. The differences are even greater when the balance and gait of frail nursing home residents are compared with the 80-year-old and older patients screened for disease known to impair balance. These findings reinforce the importance of the superimposed effects of age-associated disease in producing functionally meaningful balance impairment [49–51].

We propose that age-related balance decrements may be significantly improved by interventions that use exposure to postural stresses to train balance. It is likely that this training can augment the choice, sequence, and timing of muscle activation that may be responsible for age-related balance decrements.

Disease-related balance decrements are treated most effectively by efforts directed at the underlying pathophysiology (e.g., L-DOPA for Parkinson's disease). Moreover, as noted earlier, the disease-related decrements often are of such

Table 5-1. Percentage of elderly subjects with loss of balance (LOB) by age group during difficult test conditions

| | | Percentage of subjects with LOB | | |
		70–74 yr (N = 114)	75–79 yr (N = 75)	≥ 80 yr (N = 45)
Test	Trial			
Absent vision, sway-	1	31	33	33
referenced, support	2	18	24	32
	3	18	19	16
Sway-referenced;	1	46	60	53
vision, and support	2	24	39	42
	3	17	23	34
Toes-up rotation	1	43	49	64
	2	15	9	27
	3	8	7	9
Toes-down rotation	1	26	32	27
	2	1	0	2
	3	0	0	2

(See Fig. 3-5 on page 47 for more details on the test conditions.)

magnitude that training cannot be expected to make significant inroads. There are, however, a significant number of older individuals with a mild or moderate multifactorial compromise of balance for which training should be effective. This is discussed in Chapter 22.

The definition of age-related balance changes leads to the conclusion that despite the decrements described, the balance of older persons is remarkably flexible and effective under most conditions. Changes in balance are similar to the effects of age on other important CNS functions (e.g., cognition). Furthermore, it suggests that the term *senile* is no more appropriate in describing gait and balance than in describing cognition. Most importantly, knowledge of age-related balance change is the foundation for understanding the superimposed effects of disease and the feasibility of intervention.

REFERENCES

1. Schaie KW. The course of adult intellectual development. *Am Psychol* 1994;49:304–313.
2. Wright BE, Henkind P. Aging Changes and the Eye. In: Katzman R, Terry R, eds. *The Neurology of Aging* Philadelphia: Davis, 1983.
3. Sekuler R, Hutman LP, Owsley CJ. Human aging and spatial vision. *Science* 1980;209: 1255–1256.
4. Carter JH. The Effects of Aging on Selected Visual Functions: Color Vision, Glare Sensitivity, Field of Vision, and Accommodation. In: Sekuler R, Kline D, Dismukes K, eds. *Aging and Human Visual Function*. New York: Alan R. Liss, 1982. Pp 121–130.
5. Pitts DG. The Effects of Aging on Selected Visual Functions: Dark Adaptation, Visual Acuity, Stereopsis, and Brightness Contrast. In: Sekuler R, Kline D, Dismukes K, eds. *Aging and Human Visual Function*. New York: Alan R. Liss, 1982. Pp 131–159.
6. Howell TH. *Old Age—Some Practical Points in Geriatrics*, 3rd ed. London: HK Lewis, 1975. Pp 38–47.

7. Klawans HL, Tufo HM, Ostfeld AM. Neurologic examination in an elderly population. *Dis Nerv Syst* 1971;32:274–279.

8. Prakash C, Stern G. Neurological signs in the elderly. *Age Ageing* 1973;2:24–27.

9. Kokmen E, Bossemeyer RW, Barney J, Williams WJ. Neurological manifestations of aging. *J Gerontol* 1977;32:411–419.

10. Carter AB. The Neurologic Aspects of Aging. In: Rossman I, ed. *Clinical Geriatrics*, 2nd ed. Philadelphia: Lippincott, 1979. Pp 292–316.

11. Welford AT. Sensory Perceptual and Motor Processes in Older Adults. In: Birren JE, Swane RB, eds. *Handbook of Mental Health and Aging.* Englewood Cliffs, NJ: Prentice-Hall, 1980. P 192.

12. Skinner HB, Barrack RL, Cook SD. Age-related decline in proprioception. *Clin Orthop* 1984;184:208–211.

13. Potvin AR, et al. Quantitative Evaluation of Normal Age-Related Changes in Neurologic Function. In: Pirozzolo FJ, Maletta GJ, eds. *Advances in Neurogerontology* (vol 2). New York: Praeger, 1980.

14. Potvin, AR, et al. Human neurologic function and the aging process. *J Am Geriatr Soc* 1980; 28:1–9.

15. Perret E, Reglis F. Age and the perceptual threshold for vibratory stimuli. *Eur Neurol* 1970; 4:65–76.

16. Dorfman LJ, Bosley TM. Age-related changes in peripheral and central conduction in man. *Neurology* 1979;29:38–44.

17. Bentzen O. Disorder of Hearing in the Elderly. In: Hinchcliffe R, *Hearing and Balance in the Elderly.* London: Churchill Livingstone, 1983. Pp 123–144.

18. Moller MB. Changes in Hearing Measures with Increasing Age. In: Hinchcliffe R, ed. *Hearing and Balance in the Elderly.* London: Churchill Livingstone, 1983. Pp 97–122.

19. Schow RL, Christensen JM, Hutchinson JM, Nerbonne MA. Communication disorders of the aged. Baltimore: University Park Press, 1978.

20. Rosenhall U. Degenerative patterns in the aging human vestibular neuroepithelia. *Acta Otolaryngol* 1973;76:208–220.

21. Peterka RJ, Black FO, Schoenfoff MB, Age-related changes in human vestibulo-ocular reflexes: Sinusoidal rotation and caloric tests. *J Vestib Res* 1994;1:49–59.

22. Bruner A, Norris TW. Age-related changes in caloric nystagmus. *Acta Otolaryngol Suppl* (Stockh), 1971;282:1–24.

23. Wolfson L, et al. A dynamic posturography study of balance in healthy elderly. *Neurology* 1992;42:2069–2075.

24. Aloia JF, et al. Relationship of menopause to skeletal and muscle mass. *Am J Clin Nutr* 1991;53:1378–1383.

25. Flynn MA, et al. Total body potassium in aging humans: A longitudinal study. *Am J Clin Nutr* 1989;50:713–717.

26. Larsson L. Aging in Mammalian Skeletal Muscles. In: Mortimer JA, Pirazzolo FJ, Maletta GJ, eds. *The Aging Motor System.* New York: Praeger, 1982. Pp 60–96.

27. Murray PM, et al. Age-related changes in knee muscle strength in normal women. *J Gerontol* 1985;40:275–280.

28. Stalberg E, et al. The quadriceps femoris muscle in 20- to 70-year-old subjects: Relationship between knee extension torque, electrophysiologic parameters and muscle fiber characteristics. *Muscle Nerve* 1989;12:382–389.

29. Frontera WR, et al. A cross-sectional study of muscle strength and mass in 45- to 78-yr-old men and women. *J Appl Physiol* 1991;71(2):644–650.

30. Kallman DA, Plato CC, Tobin JD. The role of muscle loss in the age-related decline of grip strength: Cross-sectional and longitudinal perspectives. *J Gerontol* 1990;45(3):M82.

31. Welford AT. Reaction time, speed of performance and age. *Ann NY Acad Sci* 1988; 515:1–17.

32. Katzman R, Terry R. Normal Aging of the Nervous System. In: Katzman R, Rowe J, eds. *Principles of Geriatric Neurology.* Philadelphia: Davis, 1992.

33. Morgan DG, Finch CE. Dopaminergic changes in the basal ganglia: A generalized phenomenon of aging mammals. *Ann NY Acad Sci* 1988;515:145–159.

34. LeWitt PA. Neuropharmacologic intervention with motor system aging. *Ann NY Acad Sci* 1988;515:376–381.

35. Baloh RW, Fife TD, Zwerling L. Comparison of static and dynamic posturography in young and older normal people. *J Am Geriatr Soc* 1994;42:405–412.

36. Maki BE, Holliday PJ, Fernie GR. Aging and postural control, a comparison of spontaneous and induced-sway balance tests. *J Am Geriatr Soc* 1990;38:1–9.

37. Ring C, Nayak SL, Isaacs B. The effect of visual deprivation and proprioceptive change on postural sway in healthy adults. *J Am Geriatr Soc* 1989;37:745–749.

38. Schultz A, Alexander NB, Gu MJ, Boismier T. Postural control in young and elderly adults when stance is challenged: Clinical versus laboratory measurements. *Ann Otol Rhinol Laryngol* 1993;102:508–517.

39. Manchester D, Woollacott M, Zederbauer-Hylton N, Marin O. Visual, vestibular and somatosensory contributions to balance control in the older adult. *J Gerontol* 1989;44(4):118–127.

40. Stelmach GE, Teasdale N, DiFabio RP, Phillips J. Age-related decline in postural control mechanisms. *Int J Aging Hum Dev* 1989;29:205–223.

41. Stelmach GE, Phillips J, DiFabio RP, Teasdale N. Age, functional postural reflexes, and voluntary sway. *J Gerontol* 1989;44:B100–106.

42. Woollacott MH, Shumway-Cook, A, Nashner LM. Aging and posture control: Changes in sensory organization and muscle coordination. *Int J Aging Hum Dev* 1986;23:97–114.

43. King MB, Judge JO, Wolfson L. Functional base of support decreases with age. *J Gerontol Med Sci* 1994;48:M258–263.

44. Duncan PW, Weiner DK, Chandler J, Studenski S. Functional reach: A new clinical measure of balance. *J Gerontol Med Sci* 1990;45:M192–197.

45. Bohannon RW, et al. Decrease in timed balance test scores with aging. *Phys Ther* 1984;64:1067–1070.

46. Ekdahl C, Jarnlo GB, Anderson SI. Standing balance in healthy subjects. *Scand J Rehabil Med* 1989;21:187–195.

47. Fornoff JE, et al. A cross-sectional validation study of the FICSIT common database static balance measure. *Gerontologist* 1993;335:173.

48. Wolfson L, et al. Gender differences in the balance of healthy elderly as demonstrated by dynamic posturography. *J Gerontol Med Sci* 1994;49:M160–167.

49. Wolfson LI, Whipple R, Amerman P, Kleinberg A. Stressing the postural response: A quantitative method for testing balance. *J Am Geriatr Soc* 1986;34:845–850.

50. Whipple R, Wolfson LI, Amerman P. The relationship of knee and ankle weakness to falls in nursing home residents: An isokinetic study. *J Am Geriatr Soc* 1987;35:13–20.

51. Wolfson L, Whipple R, Amerman P, Tobin J. Gait assessment in the elderly: A case-control study of abnormalities and their relation to falls. *J Gerontol Med Sci* 1990;45:M12–19.

6. Changes in Gait with Normal Aging

Rodger J. Elble

The definition of normal aging is unclear because the unavoidable consequences of aging are defined poorly. Most age-associated changes in posture and locomotion are attributable to one or more diseases. However, age-associated changes can be so mild and nonspecific that the presence of disease is uncertain. Such changes are reviewed in this chapter.

GAIT INITIATION

Normal locomotion requires the integrated control of limb movement and posture. Gait initiation is an elegant example of this important concept [1–8]. In gait initiation, one lower extremity is destined to leave the ground (swing leg) while the other provides support. Brisk gait initiation begins with relaxation of the triceps surae, which are tonically active during quiet stance. Relaxation of the triceps surae is followed almost immediately by a synergistic contraction of the ventral muscles of the lower extremities and torso. Contraction of the ventral muscles produces a sagittal moment of force that propels the body about the ankles, into forward motion. A posterior displacement of the center of pressure beneath the feet underlies this sagittal moment (Figs. 6-1, 6-2). A coronal moment of force is produced by swing hip abduction and a few degrees of flexion in the support hip and knee. Both events begin nearly simultaneously with the activation of the ventral muscles, and they displace the center of pressure laterally toward the swing foot (see Figs. 6-1, 6-2), creating a coronal moment of force that propels the body toward the support foot. Thus, gait initiation is achieved with purposeful postural shifts that culminate in a forward step. A steady-state velocity of gait is achieved in less than two steps [9].

Coronal postural shifts from one support limb to the next continue throughout steady-state walking [10]. The integration of postural control with movement is necessary in all aspects of locomotion, including turning and stopping. Diseases such as Parkinson's disease, multiple cerebral infarcts, normal-pressure hydrocephalus, progressive supranuclear palsy, and cervical myelopathy affect postural control and limb movement. Patients with these disorders may move relatively well while seated or recumbent, because they are not faced with the added postural demands of bipedal stance and locomotion.

This work was supported by grants P30 AG08014 and RO1 AG10837 from the National Institute on Aging.

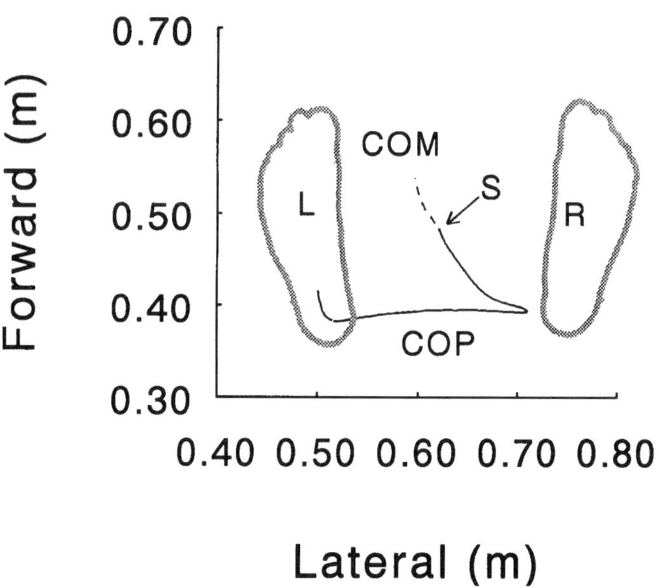

Figure 6-1. An overhead view of the paths of the resultant center of pressure (COP) of the feet and the total-body center of mass (COM, *broken line*) during the brisk initiation of gait. The COP and COM are superimposed during quiet stance (S) and are located 3–8 cm anterior to the angles. Gait initiation begins with a posterolateral movement of the COP toward the right swing foot (R). The COM begins moving in the opposite direction after a delay of approximately 0.45 sec. By this time, the COP has begun moving toward the left support foot (L). Total elapsed time is 0.7 sec.

My colleagues and I [5] found that six normal people aged 64 to 82 (mean, 74 years) initiated gait in nearly the same manner as six younger people aged 22 to 47 (mean, 28 years). The older people generated smaller ankle moments of force during the initial contraction of their ventral muscles, possibly due to weaker muscles in the older people or to a desire to limit forward acceleration, thereby reducing the potential of postural instability. Additional study is needed to fully understand the effects of aging on gait initiation and similar transitional tasks in locomotion.

Sitting and Standing

The ability to rise from a chair is a critical aspect of normal mobility. The total body center of mass of an average adult seated in a typical chair is approximately 33 cm behind the ankles [11]. In preparation for standing, the knees are flexed to bring the feet closer to the chair, thereby reducing the distance that the center of mass must move anteriorly. This important preparation for standing frequently is omitted by patients with Parkinson's disease and other neurological disturbances of gait. Standing from a chair then proceeds with bilateral hip flexion, ankle dorsiflexion, and anterior rotation of the trunk and pelvis, which propel

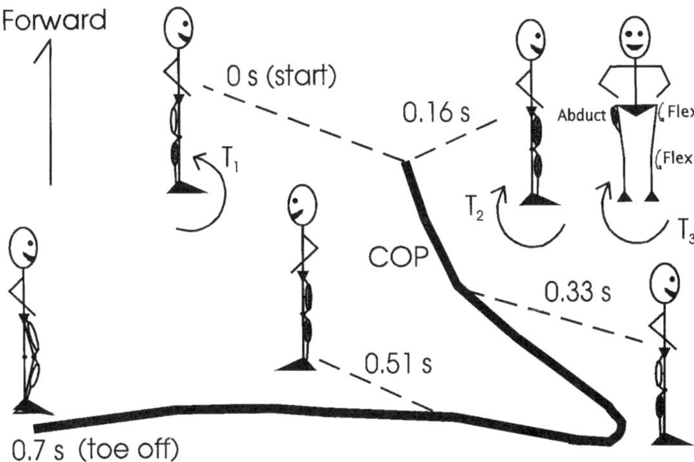

Figure 6-2. The resultant center of pressure (COP) beneath the feet during gait initiation with the right foot, as in Figure 6-1. Cartoon stick figures are shown to illustrate the critical patterns and approximate times of muscle activation and joint rotations that underlie this COP trajectory. Prior to the start of gait initiation, the COP and center of mass are located a few centimeters anterior to the angles. Therefore, the center of mass produces a forward moment of force (torque) about the ankles, which is balanced by the torque T_1 produced by tonic ankle plantar flexion. This plantar flexing ankle torque suddenly changes to a dorsiflexing torque T_2 when the ventral muscles are activated and the dorsal muscles are silenced at the onset of gait initiation (time = 0.16 sec). Ankle dorsiflexion propels the body into forward motion. Abduction at the swing hip and a few degrees of flexion in the support hip and knee create a coronal torque T_3 that propels the body toward the support limb.

the center of mass over the feet [12–14]. The associated pattern of muscle activation in the lower extremities is similar to the ventral muscle activation that occurs in gait initiation [4]. Finally, extensor moments of force at the hips and knees and plantarflexor moments at the ankles are developed and propel the body into an erect stance.

The kinematic and dynamic events that occur when rising from a chair are reversed when sitting [12]. The base of support provided by the feet first is located as closely as possible to the ultimate base of support provided by the chair, thus minimizing the required posterior displacement of the center of mass. Sitting proceeds with flexion of the knees and hips, anterior rotation of the trunk and pelvis, and plantarflexion of the ankles. These events propel the center of mass downward and backward toward the chair. Last, extensor moments of force are produced at the hips and knees to decelerate the center of mass as the body is seated.

The transition from sitting to standing or vice versa is a period of postural instability that is conducive to falls [11]. These locomotor tasks, like gait initiation, are impaired by disturbances of postural control or movement. Reduced range of motion in the hips, pelvis, knees, and spine is common in older people and will impede the initial shift of the total body center of mass over the feet when standing and over the chair when sitting. Similarly, weakness in the hips and knees may reduce the attainable moments of force to such a level that use of the upper extremities and possibly additional assistance are needed to accelerate and decelerate the body in the appropriate directions.

WALKING

Walking is a cyclical movement. The gait cycle is defined arbitrarily as the time between successive heel-floor contacts with the same foot (Fig. 6-3). The time from right heel-floor contact to left toe-off is the first of two periods (phases) of double-limb support, each lasting approximately 10% of the gait cycle. The first double-limb support phase is followed by the left swing phase, which is simultaneous with and equal to the right single-limb support phase. The time from left heel-floor contact to right toe-off is the second double-limb support phase and is followed by the right swing phase and left single-limb support phase. Stride length and cadence (steps per minute) generally are regarded as the independent variables of walking. Stride and cadence determine the velocity of walking $\left(\dfrac{\text{stride length} \times \text{cadence}}{2} \right)$ and the magnitudes of many other kinematic variables of

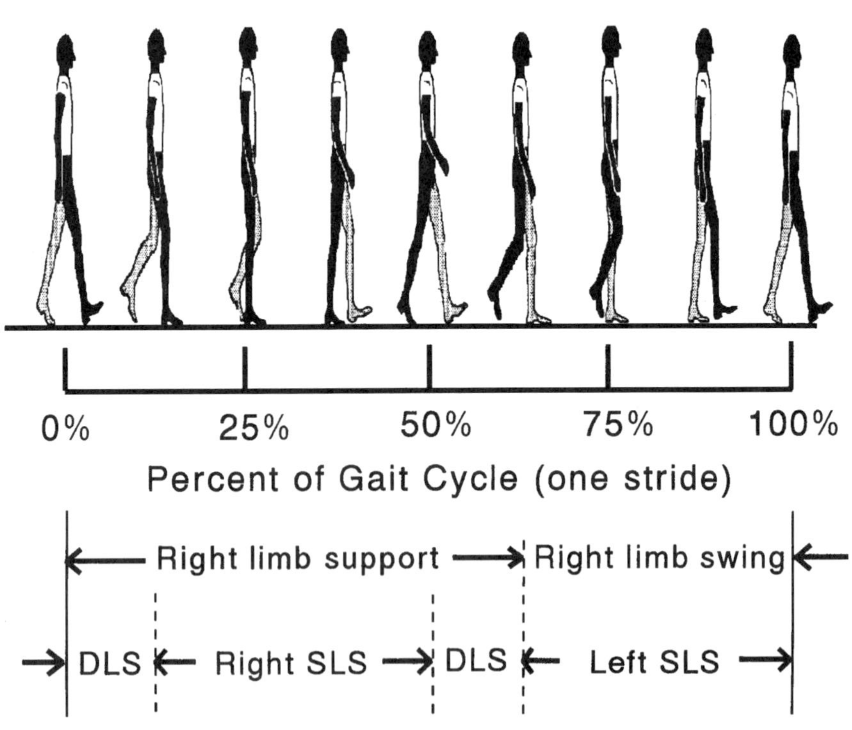

Figure 6-3. The gait cycle extends from the time of heel-floor contact to the time of next heel-floor contact with the same (right) foot. DLS = double-limb support; SLS = single-limb support.

gait, such as arm swing, lower-extremity joint rotations, and time in double-limb support [15–20].

Many studies have examined quantitatively the kinematics of walking in older people, with the principal goal of defining those changes that can be attributed to normal aging [21–29]. Most quantitative studies have found that healthy older people walk more slowly than do young adults. In addition, older people exhibit a shorter stride, which necessitates a faster cadence for a given speed of walking [21–26, 28, 30]. We [31] used computer infrared stroboscopic photometry to quantify the kinematic profiles of fast and natural walking in 20 young adults (mean age, 30.0 ± 6.1 years) and 19 older adults (mean age 76 ± 6 years) who had no history of falling, fear of falling, or abnormal neurological signs other than reduced vibratory sensation in the feet and absent ankle reflexes. The average natural and fast velocities of walking in the older people were, respectively, 20% and 17% less than in the young. These differences in gait velocity were produced by comparable differences in stride length. Cadence did not differ between the young and old for fast or natural walking.

Kinematic data from our studies [31, 32] are summarized in Table 6-1. Velocity (meters per second), cadence (steps per minute), percentage of stride in double-limb support, stride length (meter), maximum vertical toe displacement (meter; occurs at initial heel-floor contact) minimum vertical toe displacement (meter; occurs in midswing phase), maximum vertical wrist displacement (a measure of arm swing in meters), and maximum and minimum hip and knee flexion (degrees; rotation = maximum − minimum flexion) were measured in the sagittal plane, and step width (i.e., base; distance in meters between the heel markers at successive heel-floor contacts) was measured in the coronal plane. Although the healthy young and older volunteers differed in several respects, analysis of covariance revealed that these differences were attributable statistically to the reduced strides of the elderly. Cadence, height, and age did not contribute. This dependence of kinematic variables on stride was similar to that reported by Kirtley et al. [16] and explains why stride and gait velocity are useful, albeit nonspecific, measures of clinical performance and disability [33–35].

Many older adults exhibit a slightly increased toe-floor clearance during the swing phase of walking (see Table 6-1). This change is possibly a compensatory adaptation to a greater risk of falling. An increased foot clearance and reduced cadence also are observed during stair descent with reduced vision and possibly with normal aging [36]. When approaching obstacles on a floor, older adults reduce their gait velocity and clear the object with a slower, shorter step. Foot clearance over the obstacle is normal, but the shortened step occasionally causes the older adult to step on the obstacle rather than over it [37]. This strategy of negotiating obstacles reduces the risk of catching a toe and tripping but increases the risk of less hazardous heel or sole contact with the obstacle.

The effects of reduced stride and velocity on the other characteristics of gait must be considered when assessing an older person's pattern of walking. Increased time spent in double-limb support, reduced arm swing, reduced rotation of the hips, knees, and ankles, and a more flat-footed foot-floor contact and liftoff occur whenever stride is reduced [15–20]. A reduction in stride could be

Table 6-1. Kinematics of natural walking exhibited by young and older healthy adults and by neurological patients with a symmetrical disturbance of gait

Variable	Young adults (N = 20)	Older adults (N = 19)	Patients (N = 10)
Age	30.0 (6.1)[a]	76 (6)[b]	79 (4)
Velocity (m/sec)	1.18 (0.15)	0.96 (0.15)[b]	0.338 (0.16)[c]
Stride length (m)	1.32 (0.12)	1.08 (0.11)[b]	0.49 (0.17)[c]
Cadence (steps/min)	107 (7.3)	106 (10)	80 (18)[c]
Step width (m)	0.109 (0.041)	0.11 (0.03)	0.14 (0.04)[c]
Double-limb stance (%)	23.8 (4.09)	26.0 (3.9)	47.0 (7.5)[c]
Minimum vertical toe-floor clearance (m)	0.014 (0.004)	0.015 (0.006)	0.013 (0.010)[c]
Vertical toe displacement at initial heel-floor contact (m)	0.069 (0.009)	0.055 (0.008)[b]	0.025 (0.01)[c]
Vertical wrist displacement during arm swing (m)	0.081 (0.018)	0.068 (0.03)[b]	0.036 (0.01)[c]
Minimum hip flexion (degrees)	−4.21 (7.79)	−2.9 (6.5)	7.7 (12.0)[c]
Maximum hip flexion (degrees)	31.2 (6.28)	30.0 (6.4)	27.7 (7.6)
Hip rotation (degrees)	35.4 (4.88)	32.9 (4.3)	20.8 (7.7)[c]
Minimum knee flexion (degrees)	−0.50 (2.93)	2.2 (5.3)[b]	8.7 (9.3)[c]
Maximum knee flexion (degrees)	61.2 (4.38)	56.3 (5.0)[b]	43.9 (10.5)[c]
Knee rotation (degrees)	61.7 (4.19)	54.1 (4.5)[b]	30.8 (17.0)[c]

[a] Mean (SD).
[b] Different from young adults at $p < .05$ (two-tailed Student's t test).
[c] Different from normal older adults at $p < .05$.
NOTE: All kinematic measures except step width were taken in the sagittal plane.
SOURCE: Data from RJ Elble, SS Thomas, C Higgins, J Colliver. Stride-dependent changes in gait of older people. *J Neurol* 1991;238:1–5; RJ Elble, C Higgins, L Hughes. The syndrome of senile gait. *J Neurol* 1991;239:71–75.

precautionary or compensatory in a neurologically normal person confronted with a threatening environment or afflicted with a systemic disease. Consider, for example, a person who is negotiating a room full of hazardous obstacles or who has poor cardiopulmonary function. Reduced stride also is common in patients with musculoskeletal and neurological diseases.

We quantified the kinematic features of gait in 10 elderly patients with vascular dementia, shunt-responsive normal-pressure hydrocephalus, dementia of Alzheimer type, levodopa-resistant parkinsonism, or sensorimotor polyneuropathy [32]. These patients exhibited greatly reduced arm swing (vertical wrist displacement), increased time in double-limb support, reduced lower-extremity joint rotations, and a more flat-footed foot-floor contact at the end of single-limb swing (see Table 6-1), but analysis of covariance revealed that these changes in gait were attributable statistically to the patients' shortened strides. Stride-dependent changes in gait provide no clue to the underlying diagnosis and often dominate the patterns of walking in mildly to moderately impaired patients with bilateral subdural hematomas [38], Binswanger disease [39], normal-pressure hydrocephalus [40–47], Parkinson's disease [48, 49], and high cervical myelopathy [50].

AGE-ASSOCIATED CAUSES OF IMPAIRED LOCOMOTION

Critchley [51] warned that "an abnormal gait in the aged is frequently the result of disease outside the nervous system." The musculoskeletal, circulatory, and respiratory systems play an important role in determining stride length and gait velocity, because the need to minimize energy expenditure largely dictates the cadence-stride relationship exhibited at a particular velocity of walking [25, 52–58]. Furthermore, reduced stride and velocity can result from such nonneurologic causes as increased stiffness or reduced muscular power at the hips and knees. People with stiff joints are likely to minimize energy expenditure by taking shorter, more frequent steps to accomplish a particular velocity and distance of walking. People with reduced skeletal muscle power or with reduced cardiopulmonary reserve [59] must walk at a reduced velocity (i.e., stride and cadence). These nonneurologic reductions in stride cause increased time in double-limb support, reduced arm swing, and reduced lower-extremity joint rotations.

Increased musculoskeletal stiffness in the limbs, spine, and pelvis make sitting, standing turning, and rolling over very difficult [60, 61]. Maintenance of joint flexibility and range of motion, therefore, are critical to normal balance and mobility. The importance of good spinal and pelvic flexibility in balance and ambulation is experienced when one imitates the stooped posture of many older people (i.e., lumbothoracic kyphosis with posterior pelvic tilt; Fig 6-4). Attempts to walk, sit, stand, turn, and adjust to postural disturbances (e.g., a nudge to the chest) become exceedingly difficult while maintaining this posture.

Age-related degeneration in monoaminergic pathways frequently is proposed as a mechanism of gait senescence. Age-related loss of nigrostriatal dopaminergic input occurs at an estimated rate of 8% per decade of life but would not cause parkinsonism in most people before the tenth decade of life [62–64]. An average 20% cell loss in the locus ceruleus occurs by age 85 [65] but is not likely to have an appreciable effect on locomotion [66]. Age-related cell loss in the cholinergic pedunculopontine nucleus and adjacent noncholinergic neurons has not been demonstrated, but loss of these neurons probably plays a significant role in the gait disturbances of Parkinson's disease and progressive supranuclear palsy [67–71]. This region of the brain stem plays an important role in the supraspinal control of locomotion [72–75]. Cell loss in the neocortex and cerebellum occurs with aging [76, 77] and could contribute to locomotor impairment in the elderly [78, 79]. Age-related atrophy of Purkinje cells, superior vermian atrophy, and possibly other changes in cerebellar anatomy and physiology [80–82] probably reduce the locomotor capacity of older people.

Type II (fast-twitch) muscle fiber atrophy and muscle weakness are well-

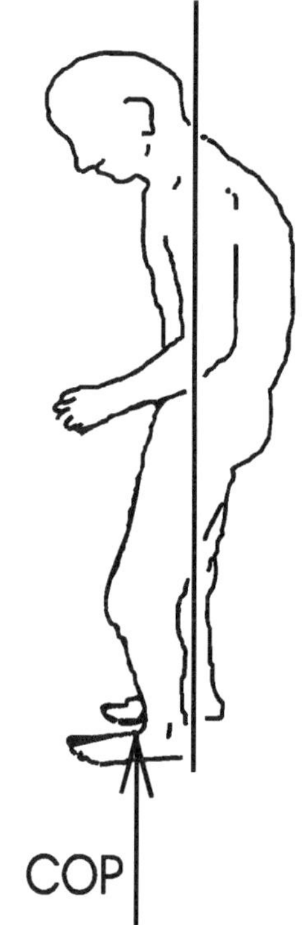

Figure 6-4. The normal location of the center of pressure (COP, *arrow*) and center of mass during quiet stance may be displaced posteriorly (*vertical line*) by thoracolumbar kyphosis and posterior pelvic tilt. This posture promotes backward falls and greatly restricts the purposeful postural shifts required in locomotion.

documented accompaniments of aging [83–86]. Type II muscle fiber atrophy is a nonspecific phenomenon caused by reduced activity, toxins, systemic metabolic disturbances, and endocrine disorders. This form of muscle atrophy is seen more frequently in older patients who fall [83, 87] and is reversed by exercise, which improves ambulation [88].

Multiple sensory deficits or conflicts are common in older people and are particularly destabilizing [89]. Vision, somatosensation, and vestibular feedback are used continuously in the control of posture and movement. Mild disturbances in any two of these modalities can combine synergistically to produce significant functional impairment. Loss of vibration sensation is common in the feet of older people [90, 91] and is attributable in many older people both to a loss of cutaneous sensory receptors and to arthritic joint disease [92, 93]. Mild somatosensory loss in the lower extremities could be symptomatic in a person with concomitant visual or vestibular dysfunction.

An age-related decline in vestibular hair cells and nerve cells in Scarpa's ganglion is particularly prominent after age 60 [94], and Fife and Baloh [95] found impaired peripheral vestibular function in 7 of 26 patients with cryptogenic disequilibrium. Age-related visual impairment is common, and its neurological impact can be complex. The treatment of refractive errors with bifocals, trifocals, and lens implants can distort peripheral vision sufficiently to cause sensory conflicts and disequilibrium. Older people have more difficulty adapting to such conflicts, particularly when other central or peripheral neurological deficits exist. Macular degeneration, cataracts, and other forms of ocular disease force an elderly person to depend more on somatosensory and vestibular functions, which also may be impaired. Finally, the central integration of visual input with other somatosensory and vestibular information is slower in older people [96], and older people tend to have reduced visual perception of motion, perhaps due to impairment of peripheral vision and the magnocellular visual pathway [97].

CONCLUSIONS

Putative age-related changes in neurological and musculoskeletal function are reviewed in this chapter while evading the uncertain definition of *normal*. Some abnormalities of posture and movement probably are inevitable at some advanced age, but this age is not defined. Abnormalities of locomotion frequently are attributed to old age when the underlying disease is obscure. However, older people and their physicians are becoming increasingly aware that advanced age usually is an incorrect or incomplete explanation.

The locomotor capacity of most older people is reduced by a combination of age-associated systemic, musculoskeletal, and neurological factors, but the extent to which these factors are attributable to normal aging is unclear. The speed, range, and functional flexibility of locomotion are reduced in ostensibly healthy older people. Many older people ambulate normally when conditions are ideal but perform inadequately in tasks requiring great speed, strength, or agility. Such tasks include the rescue responses that are necessary to prevent or cushion a fall.

The importance of postural control in all aspects of locomotion cannot be overstated. Gait initiation, walking, turning, sitting, and other locomotor tasks require carefully formulated postural changes integrated with limb motion. Consequently, musculoskeletal limitations and sensory impairments can have a surprising impact on the locomotor function of older people, who are likely to have reduced compensatory reserve within the CNS.

Older people walk more slowly due to a modest reduction in stride. Arm swing, lower-extremity rotations, and time in double-limb support are changed in proportion to the reduction in stride. Similar but greater nonspecific, stride-dependent changes in gait are the principal features of many mild to moderate neurological gait disturbances. Consequently, pathological gait disturbances can be mistaken as extremes of normal aging.

REFERENCES

1. Brenière Y, Do MC, Sanchez J. A biomechanical study of the gait initiation process. *J Biophys et Méd Nucl* 1981;5:197–205.
2. Carlsöö S. The initiation of walking. *Acta Anat* (Basel) 1966;65:1–9.

3. Cook T, Cozzens B. Human Solutions for Locomotion. III. The Initiation of Gait. In: Herman RM, Grillner S, Stein PSG, Stuart DG, eds. *Neural Control of Locomotion.* New York: Plenum, 1976. Pp 65–76.

4. Crenna P, Friggo C. A motor programme for the initiation of forward-oriented movements in humans. *J Physiol (Lond)* 1991;437:635–653.

5. Elble RJ, Moody C, Leffler K, Sinha R. The initiation of normal walking. *Mov Disord* 1994;9:139–146.

6. Herman R, Cook T, Cozzens B, Freedman W. Control of Postural Reactions in Man: The Initiation of Gait. In: Stein RB, Pearson KG, Smith RS, Redford JB, eds. *Control of Posture and Locomotion.* New York: Plenum Press, 1973. Pp 363–388.

7. Mann RA, Hagy JL, White V, Liddel D. The initiation of gait. *J Bone Joint Surg* 1979;61:232–239.

8. Nissan M, Whittle MW. The initiation of gait in normal subjects: A preliminary study. *J Biomed Eng* 1990;12:165–171.

9. Brenière Y, Do MC. When and how does steady state gait movement induced from upright posture begin? *J Biomech* 1986;19:1035–1040.

10. MacKinnon CD, Winter DA. Control of whole body balance in the frontal plane during human walking. *J Biomech* 1993;26:633–644.

11. Schultz AB, Alexander NB, Ashton-Miller JA. Biomechanical analyses of rising from a chair. *J Biomech* 1992;25:1383–1391.

12. Kralj A, Jaeger RJ, Munih M. Analysis of standing up and sitting down in humans: Definitions and normative data presentation. *J Biomech* 1990;23:1123–1138.

13. Millington PJ, Myklebust BM, Shambes GM. Biomechanical analysis of the sit-to-stand motion in elderly persons. *Arch Phys Med Rehabil* 1992;73:609–617.

14. Pai Y-C, Rogers MW. Speed variation and resultant joint torques during sit-to-stand. *Arch Phys Med Rehabil* 1991;72:881–885.

15. Hirokawa S. Normal gait characteristics under temporal and distance constraints. *J Biomed Eng* 1989;11:449–456.

16. Kirtley C, Whittle MW, Jefferson RJ. Influence of walking speed on gait parameters. *J Biomed Eng* 1985;7:282–288.

17. Larrson L-E, et al. The phases of the stride and their interaction in human gait. *Scand J Rehabil Med* 1980;12:107–112.

18. Murray MP, Clarkson BH. The vertical pathways of the foot during level walking: I. Range of variability in normal men. *J Am Phys Ther Assoc* 1966;46:585–589.

19. Murray MP, Kory RC, Clarkson BH, Sepic SB. A comparison of free and fast speed walking patterns of normal men. *Am J Phys Med* 1966;45:8–24.

20. Murray MP, Sepic SB, Barnard EJ. Patterns of sagittal rotation of the upper limbs in walking. *J Am Phys Ther Assoc* 1967;47:272–284.

21. Blanke DJ, Hageman PA. Comparison of gait of young men and elderly men. *Phys Ther* 1989;69:144–148.

22. Finley FR, Cody KA, Finizie RV. Locomotion patterns in elderly women. *Phys Med Rehabil* 1969;50:140–146.

23. Hageman PA, Blanke DJ. Comparison of gait of young women and elderly women. *Phys Ther* 1986;66:1382–1387.

24. Imms FJ, Edholm OG. The assessment of gait and mobility in the elderly. *Age Ageing,* 1979;8(suppl):261–267.

25. Inman VT, Ralston HJ, Todd F. *Human Walking.* Baltimore: Williams & Wilkins, 1981.

26. Jansen EC, Vittas D, Hellberg S, Hansen J. Normal gait of young and old men and women: Ground reaction force measurement on a treadmill. *Acta Orthop Scand* 1982;53:193–196.

27. Larish DD, Martin PE, Mungiole M. Characteristic patterns of gait in the healthy old. *Ann NY Acad Sci* 1988;515:18–31.

28. Murray MP, Kory RC, Clarkson BH. Walking patterns in healthy old men. *J Gerontol* 1969;24:169–178.

29. Imms FJ, Edholm OG. Studies of gait and mobility in the elderly. *Age Ageing* 1981;10:147–156.
30. Lundgren-Lindquist B, Aniansson A, Rundgren Å. Functional studies in 79-year-olds. III. Walking performance and climbing capacity. *Scand J Rehabil Med* 1983;15:125–131.
31. Elble RJ, Thomas SS, Higgins C, Colliver J. Stride-dependent changes in gait of older people. *J Neurol* 1991;238:1–5.
32. Elble RJ, Higgins C, Hughes L. The syndrome of senile gait. *J Neurol* 1991;239:71–75.
33. Nakamura R, Handa T, Watanabe S, Morohashi I. Walking cycle after stroke. *Tohoku J Exp Med* 1988; 154:241–244.
34. Smidt GL. Gait Assessment and Training in Clinical Practice. In: Smidt GL, ed. *Gait in Rehabilitation*. New York: Churchill Livingstone, 1990. Pp 301–315.
35. Wade DT, et al. Walking after stroke: Measurement and recovery over the first 3 months. *Scand J Rehabil Med* 1987;19:25–30.
36. Simoneau GG, et al. The influence of visual factors on fall-related kinematic variables during stair descent by older women. *J Gerontol* 1991;46:M188–195.
37. Chen H-C, Ashton-Miller JA, Alexander NB, Schultz AB. Stepping over obstacles: Gait patterns of healthy young and old adults. *J Gerontol* 1991;46:M196–203.
38. Goto I, Kuroiwa Y, Kitamura K. The triad of neurological manifestations in bilateral chronic subdural hematoma and normal pressure hydrocephalus. *J Neurosurg Sci* 1986;30:123–128.
39. Thompson PD, Marsden CD. Gait disorder of subcortical arteriosclerotic encephalopathy: Binswanger's disease. *Mov Disord* 1987;2:1–8.
40. Adams RD, et al. Symptomatic occult hydrocephalus with "normal" cerebrospinal fluid pressure. *N Engl J Med* 1965;273:117–126.
41. Black PMcL. Idiopathic normal-pressure hydrocephalus: Results of shunting in 62 patients. *J Neurosurg* 1980;52:371–377.
42. Fisher CM. The clinical picture of occult hydrocephalus. *Clin Neurosurg* 1977; 24:270–284.
43. McHugh PR. Occult hydrocephalus. *Q J Med* 1964;33:297–308.
44. Messert B, Wannamaker BB. Reappraisal of the adult occult hydrocephalus syndrome. *Neurology* 1974;24:224–231.
45. Sorensen PS, Jansen EC, Gjerris F. Motor disturbances in normal-pressure hydrocephalus. *Arch Neurol* 1986;43:34–38.
46. Sudarsky L, Simon S. Gait disorder in late-life hydrocephalus. *Arch Neurol* 1987;44:263–267.
47. Woollacott MH, Inglin B, Manchester D. Response preparation and posture control: Neuromuscular changes in the older adult. *Ann NY Acad Sci* 1988;515:42–55.
48. Knutsson E. An analysis of parkinsonian gait. *Brain* 1972;95:475–486.
49. Murray MP, Sepic SB, Gardner GM, Downs WJ. Walking patterns of men with parkinsonism. *Am J Phys Med* 1978;57:278–294.
50. Murray PK. Cervical spondylotic myelopathy: A cause of gait disturbance and urinary incontinence in older persons. *J Am Geriatr Soc* 1984;32:324–330.
51. Critchley M. The neurology of old age. *Lancet* 1931;1:1221–1230.
52. Alexander RMcN. Optimization and gaits in the locomotion of vertebrates. *Physiol Rev* 1989;69:1199–1227.
53. Cavagna GA, Franzetti P. The determinants of the step frequency in walking in humans. *J Physiol (Lond)* 1986;373:235–242.
54. Cavagna GA, Thys H, Zamboni A. The sources of external work in level walking and running. *J Physiol (Lond)* 1976;262:639–657.
55. Heglund NC, Taylor CR. Speed, stride frequency and energy cost per stride: How do they change with body size and gait? *J Exp Biol* 1988;138:301–318.
56. Nilsson J, Thorstensson A. Adaptability in frequency and amplitude of leg movements during human locomotion at different speeds. *Acta Physiol Scand* 1987;129:107–114.
57. Ralston HJ. Energy-speed relation and optimal speed during level walking. *Int Z Angew Physiol* 1958;17:277–283.

58. Zarrugh MY, Todd FN, Ralston HJ. Optimization of energy expenditure during level walking. *Eur J Appl Physiol* 1974;33:293–306.

59. Buskirk ER, Hodgson JL. Age and aerobic power: The rate of change in men and women. *FASEB* 1987;46:1824–1829.

60. Schenkman M, Butler RB. A model for multisystem evaluation treatment of individuals with Parkinson's disease. *Phys Ther* 1989;69:932–943.

61. Schenkman M, et al. Management of individuals with Parkinson's disease: Rationale and case studies. *Phys Ther* 1989;69:944–955.

62. De Keyser J, Ebinger G, Vauquelin G. Age-related changes in the human nigrostriatal dopaminergic system. *Ann Neurol* 1990;27:157–161.

63. McGeer PL, Itagaki S, Akiyama H, McGeer EG. Comparison of Neuronal Loss in Parkinson's Disease and Aging. In: Calne DB, et al., eds. *Parkinsonism and Aging.* New York: Raven, 1989. Pp 25–34.

64. Scherman D, et al. Striatal dopamine deficiency in Parkinson's disease: Role of aging. *Ann Neurol* 1989;26:551–557.

65. Marcyniuk B, Mann DMA, Yates PO. The topography of nerve cell loss from the locus caeruleus in elderly persons. *Neurobiol Aging* 1989;10:5–9.

66. Fishman RHB, Feigenbaum JJ, Yanai J, Klawans HL. The relative importance of dopamine and norepinephrine in mediating locomotor activity. *Prog Neurobiol* 1983;20:55–88.

67. Hirsch EC, Graybiel AM, Duyckaerts C, Javoy-Agid F. Neuronal loss in the pedunculopontine tegmental nucleus in Parkinson disease and in progressive supranuclear palsy. *Proc Natl Acad Sci USA* 1987;84:5976–5980.

68. Jellinger K. Neuropathological substrates of Alzheimer's disease and Parkinson's disease. *J Neural Transm* 1987;24:109–129.

69. Jellinger K. The pedunculopontine nucleus in Parkinson's disease, progressive supranuclear palsy and Alzheimer's disease. *J Neurol Neurosurg Psychiatr* 1988;51:540–543.

70. Rye DB, Lee HJ, Saper CB, Wainer BH. Medullary and spinal efferents of the pedunculopontine tegmental nucleus and adjacent mesopontine tegmentum in the rat. *J Comp Neurol* 1988;269:315–341.

71. Rye DB, Saper CB, Lee HJ, Wainer BH. Pedunculopontine tegmental nucleus of the rat: Cytoarchitecture, cytochemistry, and some extrapyramidal connections of the mesopontine tegmentum. *J Comp Neurol* 1987;259:483–528.

72. Armstrong DM. The supraspinal control of mammalian locomotion. *J Physiol (Lond)* 1988;405:1–37.

73. Austin MC, Kalivas PW. Dopaminergic involvement in locomotion elicited from the ventral pallidum/substantia innominata. *Brain Res* 1991;542:123–131.

74. Mori, S. Integration of posture and locomotion in acute decerebrate cats and in awake, freely moving cats. *Prog Neurobiol* 1987;28:161–195.

75. Mori S, et al. Site-specific postural and locomotor changes evoked in awake, freely moving intact cats by stimulating the brainstem. *Brain Res* 1989;505:66–74.

76. Coleman PD, Flood DG. Neuron numbers and dendritic extent in normal aging and Alzheimer's disease. *Neurobiol Aging* 1987;8:521–545.

77. Flood DG, Coleman PD. Neuron numbers and sizes in aging brain: Comparisons of human, monkey, and rodent data. *Neurobiol Aging* 1988;9:453–463.

78. Scheibel AB. Falls, motor dysfunction, and correlative neurohistologic changes in the elderly. *Clin Geriatr Med* 1985;1:671–676.

79. Scheibel ME, Tomiyasu U, Scheibel AB. The aging human Betz cell. *Exp Neurol* 1977;56:598–609.

80. Raz N., Torres IJ, Spencer WD, White K, Acker JD. Age-related regional differences in cerebellar vermis observed in vivo. *Arch Neurol* 1992;149:412–416.

81. Rogers J. The neurobiology of cerebellar senescence. *Ann NY Acad Sci* 1988;515:251–268.

82. Torvik A, Torp S, Lindboe CF. Atrophy of the cerebellar vermis in ageing: A morphometric and histologic study. *J Neurol Sci* 1986;76:283–294.

83. Aniansson A, Zetterberg C, Hedberg M, Henriksson KG. Impaired muscle function with aging: A background factor in the incidence of fractures of the proximal end of the femur. *Clin Orthop* 1984;191:193–201.

84. Bassey EJ, Bendall MJ, Pearson M. Muscle strength in the triceps surae and objectively measured customary walking activity in men and women over 65 years of age. *Clin Sci* 1988;74:85–89.

85. Larsson L, Grimby G, Karlsson J. Muscle strength and speed of movement in relation to age and muscle morphology. *J Appl Physiol* 1979;46:451–456.

86. Vandervoort AA, McComas AJ. Contractile changes in opposing muscles of the human ankle with aging. *J Appl Physiol* 1986;61:361–367.

87. Whipple RH, Wolfson LI, Amerman PM. The relationship of knee and ankle weakness to falls in nursing home residents: An isokinetic study. *J Am Geriatr Soc* 1987;35:13–20.

88. Fiatarone MA, et al. High-intensity strength training in nonagenarians: Effects on skeletal muscle. *JAMA* 1990;263:3029–3034.

89. Wolfson L, et al. A dynamic posturography study of balance in healthy elderly. *Neurology* 1992;42:2069–2075.

90. Newman G, Dovenmuehle RH, Busse EW. Alterations in neurologic status with age. *J Am Geriatr Soc* 1960;8:915–917.

91. Prakash C, Stern G. Neurological signs in the elderly. *Age Ageing* 1973;2:24–27.

92. Bolton CF, Winkelmann RK, Dyke PJ. A quantitative study of Meissner's corpuscles in man. *Neurology* 1966;16:1–9.

93. Newman HW, Corbin KB. Quantitative determination of vibratory sensibility. *Proc Soc Exp Biol* 1936;35:273–276.

94. Richter E. Quantitative study of human Scarpa's ganglion and vestibular sensory epithelia. *Acta Otolaryngol* 1980;90:199–208.

95. Fife TD, Baloh RW. Disequilibrium of unknown cause in older people. *Ann Neurol* 1993;34:694–702.

96. Teasdale N, Stelmach GE, Breunig A, Meeuwsen HJ. Age differences in visual sensory integration. *Exp Brain Res* 1991;85:691–696.

97. Gilmore GC, Wenk HE, Naylor LA, Stuve TA. Motion perception and aging. *Psychol Aging* 1992;7:654–660.

7. Clinical and Research Methodology for the Study of Posture and Balance

Marjorie H. Woollacott and Anne Shumway-Cook

It has been shown repeatedly that falls are a cause of accidental injury and death in older adults [1]. One major factor that contributes to the high incidence of falls in the elderly is decreased balance control leading to instability during stance and gait. The contribution of poor balance to falls has led to a growing emphasis within the health care system on assessment and treatment of balance as one approach to fall prevention in the older adult.

This chapter focuses on the assessment of balance in the elderly from both a research and a clinical perspective. Traditional global methods of measuring balance in the elderly are described and their limitations discussed.

TRADITIONAL APPROACHES TO ASSESSING BALANCE

Classically, the assessment and treatment of balance function in older adults has been centered around global measures of balance abilities (e.g., the measurement of total body sway) or the measurement of postural reflex function [2].

Early research by Sheldon [3] in exploring balance changes in older adults surveyed the degree to which subjects in groups aged 6 through 80 swayed during quiet stance. Sheldon used a very simple instrument for measuring global body sway that he could take into institutional settings. He devised a triangular metal frame with U-shaped pads that fit over the shoulders of the subject. He placed a pencil at the apex of the triangle, and the pencil marked a subject's sway on graph paper, which was placed directly below the pencil. Using this technique to measure global body sway, he observed that subjects at both ends of the age spectrum (6–14 yr and 50–80 yr) had greater difficulty in minimizing sway during quiet stance than those in the midrange of the age spectrum.

Fernie et al. [4] examined sway amplitude and velocity in institutionalized elderly and found that sway velocity was significantly greater for those who fell one or more times in a year than for those who had not fallen. Thus, sway velocity was correlated with frequency of balance loss. More recently, *stabilometry*, or the use of force plates, also has been used as a measure of balance during quiet stance [5]. Subjects stand quietly on a force plate, and the excursion of the center of pressure is calculated and used to infer the degree of stability. The center of pressure is the location of the net force on the support surface.

However, a number of methodological issues have been raised regarding the validity of center-of-pressure measures as a gauge of stability. One problem is that changing the relationship of body segments can alter the center of pressure without affecting stability of the subject [6]. In addition, such measures have not always been shown to correlate well with postural instability in daily life [5]. For example, many patients with severe neurological deficits, such as Parkinson's disease or severe loss of vestibular function, show normal sway in quiet stance [7, 8]. This suggests that a single measure, such as sway, is not always a valid measure of stability.

Other traditional approaches to assessing balance function in older adults typically evaluate function by using a reflex model of motor control [9]. For example, clinical assessment traditionally has included the evaluation of such reflexes as tendon reflexes, righting and equilibrium reflexes, and vestibulo-ocular reflexes. This type of evaluation was based on a theoretical framework that hypothesizes that reflexes are the basic elements of motor control [10, 11].

Conclusions about aging that have come from this perspective tend to view many of the problems associated with neural function in the elderly as resulting from a release of primitive reflexes. For example, Paulus and Gottlieb [2] noted a reappearance of primitive reflexes in aging patients with pathology, which they viewed as a "release" of lower levels of nervous system function.

Traditional approaches to assessment often were based on the assumption that one could find a single cause of falls for a given individual (e.g., vertigo, sensory neuropathy, or postural hypotension). More recent research has taken a broader approach to determining the cause of falls in older adults. Current definitions of posture and balance reflect a "systems theory" of motor control (as reviewed in Chap. 3). This view has led to an increasing number of new approaches to assessing posture and balance control in older adults.

CURRENT RESEARCH METHODS FOR STUDY OF BALANCE CONTROL

Balance, or stability, is defined as the ability to maintain the center of body mass within stability limits largely determined by the base of support. *Stability limits* are boundaries of an area of space in which the body can maintain its position without changing the base of support. Stability limits are not fixed boundaries but change according to the task, the individual's biomechanics, and aspects of the environment.

Postural orientation is defined as the ability to maintain an appropriate relationship between the various body segments and between the body and the environment for a task [12]. For most functional tasks, we maintain a vertical orientation of the body.

Current views of the physiological basis for balance suggests it is not simply the result of reflexes organized hierarchically within the nervous system. Rather, stability and orientation result from a complex interaction of sensory, motor, and cognitive systems typically referred to collectively as the *postural control system* [13–15].

Motor processes, including both musculoskeletal and neuromuscular components, are essential to the generation and coordination of forces for controlling the body's position in space. Sensory aspects involve processing visual, vestibular, and somatosensory inputs reporting the body's position relative to gravity and the environment. Higher-level (cognitive) processes are essential for adaptive and anticipatory aspects of postural control.

Motor Components

Researchers have explored the different types of movement strategies that people use to control balance under several different contexts.

Reactive Balance Control

When simply sitting or standing, we are swaying constantly and receiving information about that sway from the visual, somatosensory, and vestibular systems. When the center of mass moves toward our perceived stability limits, a postural response is activated to control sway. This type of balance control has been referred to as *static balance control*, because it is used while standing quietly.

Reactive balance control also can be more dynamic. For example, if an older adult is standing on a bus and the bus begins to move forward, the adult will sway backward. A reactive balance response will be required to regain stability.

Research methods to explore underlying patterns of muscle coordination related to reactive balance control have relied largely on moving platforms to perturb balance in a standing subject. An example of a moving platform used to study stance postural control is shown in Fig. 7-1. A variety of surface perturbations are used to study reactive balance control, including anterior and posterior translations that cause the subject to sway in the opposite direction of platform motion, surface rotations that stretch the distal ankle muscles without producing associated sway, and vertical displacements of the platform [16].

To study the adaptation of movement strategies, subjects often are asked to stand on one foot, across narrow beams, or on compliant surfaces [17].

Surface electromyography is used to record the onset, latency, amplitude, and duration of muscle activation patterns in response to surface perturbations. Motion analysis systems are used to quantify the kinematics of body movements associated with recovery of balance, whereas force plates measure ground reaction forces [16–18].

Using moving platform methodology, researchers have identified at least three different types of reactive postural response strategies used to recover balance in response to a forward or backward perturbation: an ankle strategy, a hip strategy, and a stepping strategy (see Fig. 3-3 on page 40).

An ankle strategy typically is used to compensate for small amounts of sway. In response to backward sway, the normal muscle response synergy that underlies this strategy is the activation of tibialis anterior, then quadriceps, followed by abdominal muscles at latencies of approximately 100, 120, and 140 msec, respec-

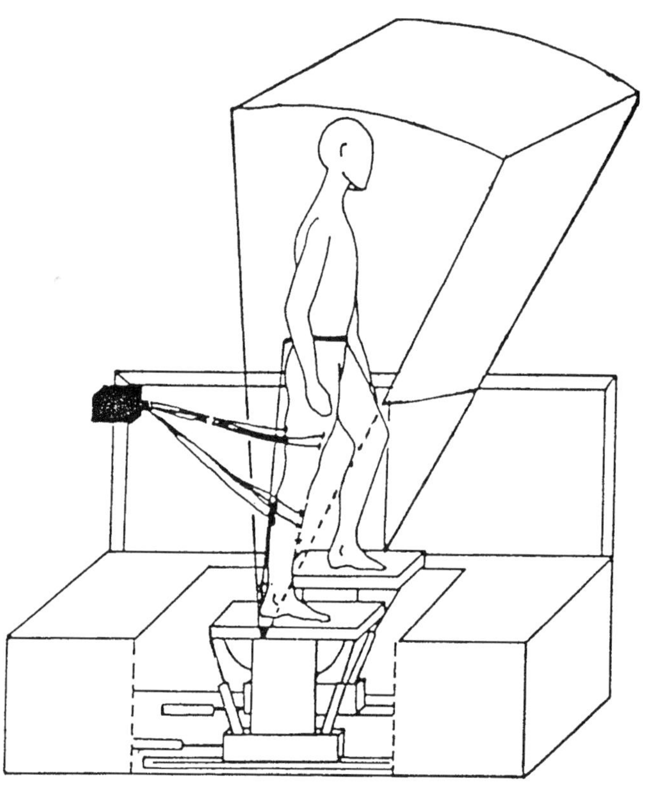

Figure 7-1. Schematic drawing of a moving platform with a moving visual surround used to examine sensory and motor aspects of stance postural control. (Adapted from M. Woollacott, A. Shumway-Cook, L. Nashner. Aging and posture control: changes in sensory organization and muscular coordination. *Int. J. Aging Hum. Dev.* 1986; 22:332.)

tively. Similarly, in response to forward sway, gastrocnemius, hamstrings, and trunk extensors are activated at similar latencies. Note that these latencies are too long to be monosynaptic spinal reflexes. Rather, they are longer loop responses that are more adaptable to changes in task conditions [15, 16].

A hip strategy typically is used to compensate for larger amounts of sway or faster perturbations to balance, which still are within the limits of stability. The hip strategy also is used when standing on a small support surface wherein the generation of torque around the ankle is more difficult. In this case, when the support surface is moved backward, the subject bends forward at the hip, activating the abdominal and quadriceps muscles (the hip synergy) [17].

A stepping strategy is used in response to perturbations that cause a subject to sway beyond stability limits. In this case, a step must be taken to regain balance.

Proactive Balance Control

Normal balance control requires more than the ability to respond to an external perturbation. Humans also typically activate balance adjustments before voluntary movements to minimize potential disruptions to balance that the movement may cause. For example, when reaching forward to take a large bowl out of the cupboard, an older adult will need to activate postural muscles in the legs in an anticipatory manner before reaching, so as to compensate in advance for the shift in the center of mass caused by the voluntary movement.

A number of approaches are used by researchers to study proactive (or anticipatory) balance control. Subjects are asked to maintain stance balance while performing a lifting or pushing task with the upper extremities. Another approach to studying proactive balance control has examined the adaptation of gait patterns to both expected and unexpected obstacles. The same technology described earlier (i.e., electromyography, kinematics) is used to quantify muscle response patterns, body motions, and forces associated with proactive balance control.

It has been shown that the same muscle response synergies activated in reactive postural control are used in proactive postural control [19]. Most functional activities require both reactive and proactive balance control (e.g., walking on uneven surfaces while carrying a heavy object).

Sensory Components

Balance requires more than the ability to generate and apply forces for controlling the body's position in space. To know when to apply restoring forces, the nervous system must have an accurate picture of where the body is in space and whether it is stationary or in motion. Balance control requires the ability to adapt the use of vision, somatosensory, and vestibular inputs according to the task and environment. This allows the preservation of balance in situations in which one sense is unavailable or inaccurate for orientation [20].

Researchers have explored how sensory information from visual, somatosensory, and vestibular systems is organized to enable the body to maintain a vertical orientation. Using a moving platform with a moving visual surround (see Fig. 7-1), Nashner et al. [16, 18, 21] developed an approach to investigating how the CNS organizes multiple sensory inputs for postural control.

In Nashner's protocol, body sway is measured while the subject stands quietly for 20 seconds under six different conditions that alter the availability and accuracy of visual and somatosensory inputs for postural orientation. This practice is referred to as a *Sensory Organization Test* (see Fig. 3-5 on page 47). Differences in the amount of body sway in the different conditions are used to determine a subject's ability to organize and select appropriate sensory information for postural control.

Research on normal balance control suggests that multiple sensory inputs are organized into *sensory strategies* for postural control based on a hierarchical ordering of sensory frames of reference, ensuring that the most appropriate sense is selected for both the environment and the task [22].

ASSESSING BALANCE IN THE CLINIC

The clinical assessment of balance from a systems perspective evaluates both functional performance and the subsystem contributing to balance. The systems approach has a number of advantages for the assessment and treatment of balance dysfunction. First, it aids clinicians in assessing and documenting a patient's overall level of function related to balance. Second, it allows clinicians to determine the extent to which deterioration in specific neural and musculoskeletal components contributes to loss of balance (stability) and mobility in older adults [23].

Functional Balance Tests

A number of clinical tools currently are used for assessing functional balance skills in older adults. Many of these tests have been developed as quick screening tests to identify older adults at risk for falls.

Get-Up-and-Go Test and Timed Get-Up-and-Go Test
The *Get-up-and-Go* test is a quick screening tool for detecting balance problems in the elderly. As part of this screening tool subjects are required to stand up from a chair, walk 3 meters, turn around, and return. Performance is judged subjectively and is graded using the following scale:

1 = normal
2 = very slightly abnormal
3 = mildly abnormal
4 = moderately abnormal
5 = severely abnormal

The test has been shown to be both reliable and consistent. It has been shown that older adults who scored 3 or higher on this test had an increased risk for falls [24].

More recently, a timing component has been added to the test, and the modified test is known as the *Timed Get-Up-and-Go test*. It has been shown that neurologically normal adults who are independent in balance and movement skills can finish the test in fewer than 10 seconds, whereas patients independent in basic transfers can finish the test in fewer than 20 seconds. Patients who required more than 30 seconds to finish the test were dependent in most activities of daily living and mobility skills. This test thus correlates well with a patient's functional capacity as measured by the Barthel Index [25].

Functional Reach Test
Another simple test developed as a fast screening aid for detecting balance problems in older adults is *The Functional Reach Test*. In this test, an older adult is asked to stand with feet shoulder-width apart and with an arm raised to 90 degrees to the front. Without moving the feet, the person is asked to reach as far forward as possible while still maintaining stability. The distance that can be reached is determined and compared to established norms as presented in Table 7-1. This test also is reliable and highly predictive of falls in the elderly [26].

Table 7-1. Functional reach test norms (Inches)

Age (yr)	Men	Women
20–40	16.7 + 1.9	14.6 + 2.2
41–69	14.9 + 2.2	13.8 + 2.2
70–87	13.2 + 1.6	10.5 + 3.5

NOTE: The goal is the clinical measure of balance, which is defined as the maximal distance of reach forward beyond arm's length, with a fixed base of support during stance.
SOURCE: P Duncan, et al. Functional reach: A new clinical measure of balance. *J Gerontol* 1990; 45:192–195.

Tinetti's Balance and Mobility Scale

The *Tinetti Balance and Mobility Scale* also was developed to screen for balance and mobility skills in older adults and to determine the risk for falls [22, 27–29]. The balance portion of Tinetti's scale rates performance on 11 different tasks and grades each item 0, 1, or 2 (Table 7-2). This scale often is used with the Tinetti Gait evaluation, and a total score then is used to predict the risk for falls.

Mobility Skills Protocol

The *Mobility Skills Protocol*, a tool for measuring functional performance on tasks that depend on posture and balance control, was developed at the Fall Prevention Center at Duke University. The test consists of 12 different items scored on a scale of 0 to 2. It has been tested for reliability and also shows good validity in predicting the probability of falls in the elderly [30].

Limitations of Functional Tests

Functional tests of balance control have certain limitations. For example, most tests of this type do not assess functional tasks within changing contexts and thus may miss problems in individuals who can carry out a task in one environmental context but not in another. For example, if a test examines an older adult only under normal lighting conditions in a clinic, it may not identify the person who has difficulty walking in dim lighting or on uneven surfaces.

These tests also focus on quantitative assessment and indicate the extent to which an older adult can perform a task; however, they seldom measure how a patient performs a task. This may be important in determining the quality of a person's movements. In addition, these measures do not specifically indicate dysfunction in neuronal or musculoskeletal subsystems that may be the cause of performance decline.

Evaluating the Subsystems of Balance Control

A comprehensive assessment of balance control in the older adult also requires evaluating the efficacy of sensory, motor, and cognitive systems contributing to

Table 7-2. Tinetti's balance and mobility assessment

Balance tests

Initial instructions: Subject is seated in a hard, armless chair. The following maneuvers are tested.

1. **Sitting balance**
   Leans or slides in chair = 0
   Steady, safe = 1

2. **Arises**
   Unable without help = 0
   Able, uses arms to help = 1
   Able without using arms = 2

3. **Attempts to rise**
   Unable without help = 0
   Able, requires >1 attempt = 1
   Able to rise, 1 attempt = 2

4. **Immediate standing balance (first 5 seconds)**
   Unsteady (staggers, moves feet, trunk sway) = 0
   Steady but uses walker or other support = 1
   Steady without walker or other support = 2

5. **Standing balance**
   Unsteady = 0
   Steady but wide stance (medial heels >4 in. apart) and uses cane or other support = 1
   Narrow stance without support = 2

6. **Nudged (subject at maximum position with feet as close together as possible, examiner pushes lightly on subject's sternum with palm of hand 3 times)**
   Begins to fall = 0
   Staggers, grabs, catches self = 1
   Steady = 2

7. **Eyes closed (at maximum position no. 6)**
   Unsteady = 0
   Steady = 1

8. **Turning 360 degrees**
   Unsteady (grabs, staggers) = 0
   Discontinuous steps = 1
   Continuous = 2

9. **Sitting down**
   Unsafe (misjudged distance, falls into chair) = 0
   Uses arms or not a smooth motion = 1
   Safe, smooth motion = 2

Balance score: _________________ /16

Gait tests

Initial instructions: Subject stands with the examiner, walks down hallway or across room, first at usual pace, then back at rapid but safe pace (usual walking aids)

10. **Initiation of gait (immediately after told to "go")**
    Any hesitancy or multiple attempts to start = 0
    No hesitancy = 1

Table 7-2. (continued)

11. Step length and height
    a. Right swing foot
        Does not pass left stance foot with step = 0
        Passes left stance foot = 1
        Right foot does not clear floor completely with step = 0
        Right foot completely clears floor = 1
    b. Left swing foot
        Does not pass right stance foot with step = 0
        Passes right stance foot = 1
        Left foot does not clear floor completely with step = 0
        Left foot completely clears floor = 1

12. Step symmetry
    Right and left step length not equal (estimate) = 0
    Right and left step appear equal = 1

13. Step continuity
    Stopping or discontinuity between steps = 0
    Steps appear continuous = 1

14. Path (estimated in relation to floor tiles, 12-in. diameter; observe excursion of 1 foot over approximately 10 ft of the course)
    Marked deviation = 0
    Mild to moderate deviation or uses walking aid = 1
    Straight without walking aid = 2

15. Trunk
    Marked sway or uses walking aid = 0
    No sway but flexion of knees or back pain or spreads arms out while walking = 1
    No sway, no flexion, no use of arms, and no use of walking aid = 2

16. Walking time
    Heel apart = 0
    Heels almost touching while walking = 1

Gait score: _______________ /12 _______________

Balance and gait score: _______________ /28 _______________

SOURCE: M Tinetti, Performance-oriented assessment of mobility problems in elderly patients. *J Am Geriatr Soc* 1986;34:119–126.

postural control. Both clinical and research methods have been developed to assess specific sensory and motor aspects of postural control.

Motor Aspects of Postural Control

An assessment of motor aspects of postural control examines both musculoskeletal and neural components. Evaluation of musculoskeletal function includes measures of range of motion, strength, body alignment, pain, and muscle tonus. Evaluation of musculoskeletal constraints is important because they may limit the ways in which older adults are able to move to maintain or regain balance. An older adult with restricted ankle motion or reduced strength in the ankle muscles may be unable to use an ankle strategy for controlling upright posture. In contrast, an older adult with musculoskeletal limitations at the hips may find use of the hip strategy difficult.

Evaluation of body alignment also is important, because alignment of the body segments over the base of support contributes to the effort required to support the body against gravity. Assessment may be performed with a plumb line in conjunction with a grid to quantify changes in alignment. The width of an older adult's standing base of support also may be determined by using a tape to measure the distance between the medial malleoli.

Other ways to measure placement of the center of mass during standing include static force plates to measure the center of pressure or two standard scales to determine weight discrepancy between left and right.

Assessment of neuromuscular constraints includes the examination of strategies used to control balance when standing. In assessment of movement strategies, the key point is to determine the flexibility of the patient in adapting the strategy to different sensory and movement contexts.

Strategies used for the control of self-initiated movements of the center of mass may be evaluated by asking older adults voluntarily to shift their weight forward, backward, and side to side and observing the type of movement coordination they employ to maintain balance. For example, when asked to sway forward without taking a step, an older adult may (1) sway forward primarily at the ankle joint, using an ankle strategy to control center of mass motion; or (2) sway primarily at the hips, which decreases forward displacement of the center of mass.

Varied protocols are available for the evaluation of strategies used to recover balance in response to an external perturbation, or push [17, 31, 32]. For example, a clinician may hold the older adult at the hips and displace him or her slightly forward, backward, and side to side. The normal adult responds to a small perturbation backward or forward by using sway principally about the ankles. One can carefully observe the ankle joints to determine if the tibialis anterior muscles are active in both legs. Absence of knee and hip motion during these compensatory ankle movements indicates that the appropriate proximal muscle synergists have been activated in addition to the tibialis anterior muscles.

More significant displacements by a clinician usually cause greater amounts of hip and trunk movement as the subject attempts to maintain the center of mass within the base of support. If the clinician makes a displacement large enough to move the center of body mass outside the base of support, a normal subject will take a step.

Part of the Tinetti Balance Test is *The Nudge Test*, which evaluates the ability of an older adult to regain stability when gently pushed backward [27]. The clinician gently pushes on the person's sternum, displacing the subject in the backward direction, three times. Scoring of the response is

2, if steady
1, if there is a stagger but the subject regains balance
0, if the subject begins to fall.

In the clinic, the most frequently used method to evaluate balance coordination problems is by subjective analysis of movement patterns (e.g., extreme flexion of the knees or trunk or asymmetrical movements of the body). However, electromyography or motion analysis is required to determine whether there are specific timing or amplitude errors in the activation of synergistic muscles used in balance control.

One also may evaluate an older adult's skill in anticipating possibly destabilizing voluntary movements by making anticipatory postural adjustments. For example, one may ask an older adult to lift a heavy object quickly. Normally, a small amount of backward sway precedes the lift, indicating the activation of anticipatory postural responses in the legs. If the subject does not make these adjustments, it shows forward instability.

Sensory Aspects of Postural Control

Assessment of the sensory systems contributing to balance control includes (1) evaluation of the individual visual, somatosensory, and vestibular systems that contribute to balance function; and (2) the patient's ability to adapt sensory strategies to changing contexts. Assessing sensory adaptation will allow a clinician to determine if an older adult is most dependent on one of these senses for sway orientation information. For example, some adults are visually dominant, whereas others are proprioceptively dominant. It is important also to determine the ability of a person to switch to the use of an alternative sense in situations of intersensory conflict.

To determine the ability of patients to use different sensory strategies, a patient is asked to balance under conditions wherein one or more of the sensory inputs contributing to balance is inappropriate or reduced, thus requiring the appropriate selection of specific sensory inputs for use in balance function (e.g., standing on foam or in poor lighting).

One method for clinical assessment of the ability of patients to adapt to changing sensory contexts is *The Clinical Test for Sensory Interaction in Balance* (CTSIB) [13, 20]. A clinician uses a 24×24–in. piece of medium-density Temper foam in conjunction with a modified Japanese lantern (vertical stripes are placed inside) that has been cut down the back and attached to a head band. This method, based on a protocol developed by Nashner [21], asks the subject to balance for 30 seconds under six different sensory conditions as illustrated in Fig. 7-2. Sensory conditions are altered by either eliminating or altering the accuracy of visual or surface orientation inputs (standing on a normal surface or a foam surface or with eyes open, closed, or with vision stabilized by wearing the lantern). The subject is tested with feet together and hands on the hips.

Neurologically intact young adults are able to maintain balance for 30 seconds under all six conditions with minimal amounts of body sway. In conditions 5 and 6, normal adults sway on the average 40% more than they do in condition 1.

Results from a number of research studies using the CTSIB suggest the following scoring criteria [4]: A single fall, regardless of the condition, is not

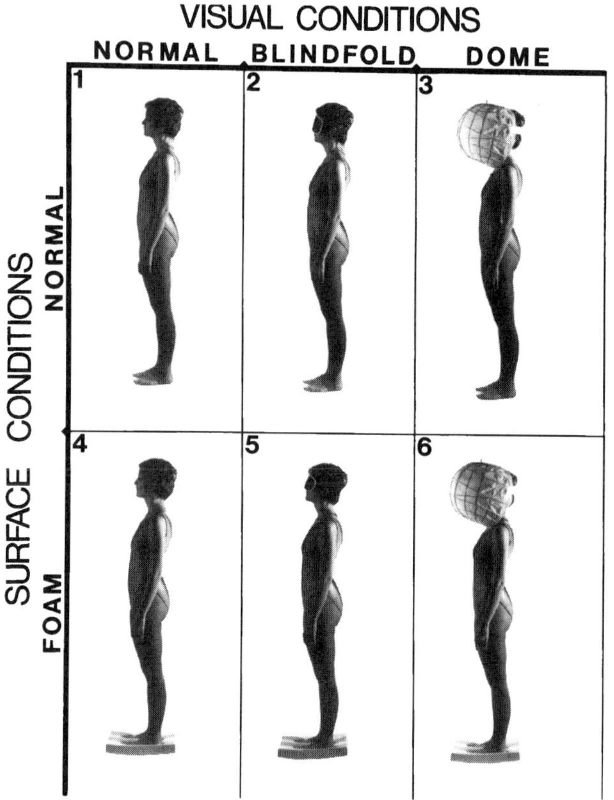

Figure 7-2. The six sensory conditions used as part of the clinical test for sensory interaction in balance, a test of postural orientation under altered sensory conditions. (From A Shumway-Cook, F Horak. Assessing the influence of sensory interaction on balance. *Phys Ther* 1986; 10:1548. Reprinted with permission of the American Physical Therapy Association.)

considered abnormal; however, two or more falls are indicative of difficulties in adapting sensory information for postural control.

Patients who show increased amounts of sway or fall under conditions 2, 3, and 6 are considered to be visually dependent (i.e., highly dependent on vision for postural control). Patients who have problems under conditions 4, 5, and 6 are considered to be surface-dependent (i.e., rely for postural control primarily on somatosensory information from the feet in contact with the surface).

In interpreting increased sway on a compliant surface, it must be noted that whereas we suppose that the primary effect of standing on a foam surface relates to altering the availability of incoming sensory information for postural orientation, there are additional effector factors that potentially affect performance in this condition. Standing on foam changes the dynamics of force production with respect to the surface and may be a significant factor in performance under this condition. There has been no research examining the dynamics of standing on foam; thus, clinicians should be careful in interpreting results of the use of the foam condition.

Patients who sway more, or fall, under conditions 5 and 6 of the CTSIB demonstrate a vestibular loss pattern, suggesting an inability to select vestibular inputs for postural control in the absence of useful visual and somatosensory cues. Finally, patients who lose balance under conditions 3, 4, 5, and 6 are said to have a *sensory selection problem*, defined as an inability to effectively adapt sensory information for postural control [12].

SUMMARY

The prevention and rehabilitation of balance decline in an older adult requires (1) developing appropriate clinical and research methodology for measuring balance function in older adults, and (2) developing effective training programs for both reducing balance decline in the elderly and ameliorating balance dysfunction. This chapter has reviewed several approaches to the assessment of balance in the elderly from both a research and a clinical perspective.

Early approaches to the assessment of balance function in an older adult often assumed that balance could be represented by a single measure such as sway, measured by a static force plate. In addition, it often was assumed that one could find a single cause of falls for a given individual (e.g., vertigo, sensory neuropathy, or postural hypotension).

More recent research has taken a broader approach to determining the cause of falls in older adults. First, clinicians have begun to be aware of the complex interactions between intrinsic factors related to the individual and extrinsic environmental factors that contribute to falls in the elderly.

A new method for the assessment of balance function uses a systems approach to quantify performance on functional tests of balance and to study the relative contribution of specific neural and musculoskeletal variables to normal postural control. This approach aids clinicians in determining the extent to which deterioration in the function of specific subsystems contributes to loss of balance (stability) and mobility in the older adult.

Recent experiments have aimed at determining if older adults could improve their balance, using a balance training protocol focused on the ability to adapt the use of sensory inputs to different environmental contexts. (Approaches to balance retraining are described in Chapter 22.) The results of such studies suggest that older adults given a sensory training program in balance control are able to significantly improve sway, and this training effect transfers to other balance conditions as well [33, 34].

REFERENCES

1. Ochs AL, Newberry J, Lenhardt ML, Harkins SW. Neural and Vestibular Aging Associated with Falls. In: Birreny J, Schaie KW, eds. *Handbook of Psychology of Aging*. New York: Van Nostrand Reinhold, 1985.

2.   Paulus G, Gottlieb G. Developmental reflexes: The reappearance of foetal and neonatal reflexes in aged patients. Brain 1968;91:37–52.

3.   Sheldon JH. The effect of age on the control of sway. *Gerontol Clin* 1963;5:129–138.

4.   Fernie GR, Gryfe CI, Holliday PJ, Llewellyn A. Relationship of postural sway in standing to incidence of falls in geriatric subjects. *Age Ageing* 1982;11:11–16.

5.   Horak FB. Effects of Neurological Disorders on Postural Movement Strategies in the Elderly. In: Vellas B, et al., eds. *Falls, Balance and Gait Disorders in the Elderly.* Amsterdam: Elsevier, 1992.

6.   Keshner E. Postural Abnormalities in Vestibular Disorders. In: Herdman S, ed. *Vestibular Rehabilitation.* Philadelphia: FA Davis, 1994.

7.   Black FO, Shupert C, Horak FB, Nashner L. Abnormal Postural Control Associated with Peripheral Vestibular Disorders. In: Pompeiano, Allum J, eds. *Vestibulospinal Control of Posture and Locomotion.* Amsterdam: Elsevier, 1988.

8.   Horak FB, Mirka A, Shupert C. Vestibular Dyscontrol in Aging Adults. In: Woollacott M, Shumway-Cook A, eds. *Posture and Gait Across the Lifespan.* Columbia, SC: University of South Carolina Press, 1989.

9.   Woollacott M, Shumway-Cook A. Changes in posture control across the life span—A systems approach. *Phys Ther* 1990;70:799–807.

10.   Sherrington, C. *The Integrative Action of the Nervous System,* 2nd ed. New Haven, CT: Yale University Press, 1947.

11.   Milani-Comparetti A, Gidoni EA. Pattern analysis of motor development and its disorders. *Dev Med Child Neurol* 1967;9:625–630.

12.   Shumway-Cook A, Horak FB. *Balance Rehabilitation in the Neurologic Patient: Course Syllabus.* Seattle: Neuroscience Education and Research Associates, 1993.

13.   Horak FB. Clinical measurement of postural control in adults. *Phys Ther* 1987;12:1881–1885.

14.   Shumway-Cook A, Horak FB. Rehabilitation strategies for patients with vestibular deficits. *Neurol Clin* 1990;2:441–457.

15.   Shumway-Cook A, Woollacott M. *Motor Control: Theory and Practical Applications.* Baltimore: Williams & Wilkins, 1995.

16.   Nashner L, Woollacott, MH. The Organization of Rapid Postural Adjustments of Standing Humans: An Experimental-Conceptual Model. In: Talbott RE, Humphrey DR, eds. *Posture and Movement.* New York: Raven, 1979.

17.   Horak FB, Nashner L. Central programming of postural movements: Adaptation to altered support surface configurations. *J Neurophysiol* 1986;55:1369–1381.

18.   Nashner L, McCollum G. The organization of human postural movements: A formal basis and experimental synthesis. *Behav Brain Sci* 1985;9:135–172.

19.   Cordo P, Nashner L. Properties of postural adjustments associated with rapid arm movements. *J Neurophys* 1982;47:287–302.

20.   Shumway-Cook A, Horak FB. Assessing the influence of sensory interaction on balance. *Phys Ther* 1986;66:1548–1550.

21.   Nashner LM. Adaptation of human movement to altered environments. *Trends Neurosci* 1982;5:358–361.

22.   Woollacott MH, Shumway-Cook A, Nashner LM. Aging and posture control: Changes in sensory organization and muscular coordination. *Int J Aging Hum Dev* 1986;23:97–114.

23.   Bernstein N. *Coordination and Regulation of Movements.* New York: Pergamon, 1967.

24.   Mathias S, Nayak USL, Isaacs B. Balance in elderly patients: The "Get-up-and-go test." *Arch Phys Med Rehabil* 1986;67:387-389.

25.   Mahoney RI, Barthel DW. Functional evaluation: The Barthel Index. *Maryland Med J* 1965;14:61–65.

26.   Duncan P, et al. Functional reach: A new clinical measure of balance. *J Gerontol* 1990; 45:192–195.

27.   Tinetti ME. Performance-oriented assessment of mobility problems in elderly patients. *J Am Geriatr Soc* 1986;34:119–126.

28. Tinetti ME, Ginter SF. Identifying mobility dysfunctions in elderly patients: Standard neuro-muscular examination or direct assessment? *JAMA* 1988;259:1190–1193.

29. Speechley M, Tinetti M. Assessment of risk and prevention of falls among elderly persons: Role of the physiotherapist. *Physiother Can* 1990;2:75–79.

30. Duncan P. Balance Dysfunction and Motor Control Theory: Implications for Neurologic and Geriatric Rehabilitation. Washington Physical Therapy Association, Annual Meeting, 1993.

31. Carr JH, Shepherd RB. *Motor Relearning Programme for Stroke.* Rockville, MD: Aspen Publications, 1983.

32. Bobath B. *Adult Hemipleaia: Evaluation and Treatment.* London: Heinemann, 1978.

33. Hu M, Woollacott M. A Training Program to Improve Standing Balance Under Different Sensory Conditions. In: Woollacott M, Horak F, eds. *Posture and Gait: Control Mechanisms.* Eugene, OR: University of Oregon Books, 1992.

34. Hu MH, Woollacott M. Multisensory training of standing balance in older adults: I. Postural stability and one-leg stance balance. *J Gerontol* 1994;49:M52–M61.

8. Clinical and Research Methodology for the Study of Gait

Rodger J. Elble

The title of this chapter is misleading because it implies that clinical and research methodologies are distinct when, in fact, a sharp distinction is not possible. Granted, there are clinical measures that are too crude to be of much utility in research, and some laboratory methods are too time consuming and expensive to be clinically useful. However, future technological advancements undoubtedly will make sophisticated motion analysis systems more amenable to routine clinical applications. The intent of this chapter is to provide an overview of clinical and laboratory methods of gait analysis from a clinician's perspective, with emphasis on the strengths and limitations of each method. The methodology in this review is discussed in order of increasing technological sophistication. The strengths and limitations are emphasized without strictly categorizing a method as clinical or experimental.

QUALITATIVE (ORDINAL) AND SIMPLE TIMED MEASURES

Posture, balance, and rhythmic body movement are highly integrated components of normal locomotion. All three components and their integration must be assessed in a comprehensive study of gait. The biomechanical and neurophysiological complexities of walking become painfully obvious when a clinician or therapist is confronted with the task of assessing an abnormal gait.

Assessments of muscle strength, stretch reflexes, somatosensory function, and extremity movement usually are crucial to making a correct clinical diagnosis, but they provide little indication of a patient's ability to walk [1]. One or more severe deficits in these measures may be found in patients who are still ambulatory, and it is common to see little or no abnormality in these measures in an elderly patient with a markedly impaired gait. This is particularly true of the gait disorders caused by normal-pressure hydrocephalus, chronic subdural hematomas, Binswanger's disease, and high cervical myelopathies. Patients with such disorders may move their lower extremities surprisingly well when supine or sitting, only to appear frozen to the floor when they attempt to stand and walk [2]. Similarly, the ability to stand unaided with eyes either open or closed is common in patients who fall frequently and require assistance in walking. Such observations

This work was supported by grants P30 AG08014 and RO1 AG10837 from the National Institute on Aging.

123

suggest that impaired integration of posture, balance, and movement is the crucial deficit in many patients, and they illustrate the need for a comprehensive performance-oriented (i.e., functional) assessment of locomotion.

Clinical assessments of mobility typically include measures of a patient's ability to walk short distances, turn, get in and out of bed, and sit and rise from a toilet or chair. Tests of balance include tandem walking, the Romberg test, and the response to a sternal push. Ordinal scales of performance are used to quantify these tests. These measures of gait and balance are contained in the clinically valid and reliable functional assessment protocol of Tinetti et al. [3], which is summarized in Table 7-2, page 114. A total mobility score on the Tinetti protocol (gait plus balance) of less than 19 (maximum, 28) is a strong predictor of falling. The ability to predict falling is enhanced further by documenting the presence of dementia, depression, need for a walking aid, polypharmacy, history of falling, orthostatic hypotension, poor endurance, reduced lower-extremity strength or coordination, flexed posture, restricted neck mobility, poor hearing, and poor vision [8].

Protocols like Tinetti's are time-consuming and must be administered by trained personnel. Consequently, clinicians continue to seek simpler quantitative measures of mobility for screening patients for impaired mobility. In the *Get-up-and-go test* of Mathias et al. [4] (see Chapter 7), patients are evaluated with five-point ordinal scales as they rise from an arm chair, walk 3 meters, turn, and return to the chair. The imprecision of the ordinal scales led Podsiadlo and Richardson [5] simply to measure the time necessary to complete the *Get-up-and-go task*. This measure of mobility is reliable and valid. Patients who perform this task in less than 20 seconds usually are independently mobile, whereas those who require more than 30 seconds generally are immobile or mobile only with assistance.

Stride length, cadence, and gait velocity are measured easily and inexpensively with a stop watch and 10-meter walkway. Stride length and cadence may be viewed as the two independent variables of walking. These variables, in combination, determine gait velocity and influence most other gait variables [6, 7]. Measurements of gait velocity, cadence, and stride length therefore have considerable utility in the quantitative assessment of mobility [8–12]. Strong correlations typically are found between gait velocity and performance on ordinal rating scales such as the *Get-up-and-go test* of Mathias et al. [4]. Although measures of gait velocity, cadence, and stride are useful indices of performance, specific aspects of a patient's disability must be defined in terms of other dependent variables of gait, such as joint rotations, ground reaction forces, and electromyography (EMG). These measurements usually are performed in modern motion analysis laboratories.

VIDEO RECORDING

Standard video equipment is invaluable in the assessment of complex motor behaviors such as walking. The old adage "a picture is worth a thousand words" certainly is apropos to gait analysis. It is difficult to grasp and record the complexities of a gait disturbance in their entirety without the aid of a video recording. A patient's performance of clinical protocols can be videotaped for subsequent checking of the accuracy of scoring, testing of inter-rater reliability, and performing of post hoc analyses. Video recording is popular among specialists in movement disorders but is still an underused clinical tool.

The limitations of videotaping stem mainly from the methods of data analysis. Standard video recordings are evaluated with the same ordinal scales and limited quantitative measures (gait velocity, stride, and cadence) used in other clinical examinations. Trained observers are needed for adequate inter-rater reliability [12, 13]. Detailed quantitative motion analysis requires high-speed, high-resolution video equipment and a digital computer. This equipment is found in most research motion analysis laboratories and is becoming increasingly prevalent in the clinical setting.

MOTION ANALYSIS LABORATORIES

In studies of balance and walking, the body is modeled as a series of linked rigid segments. The lack of rigidity in various segments is ignored in most studies. Gait is an integrated pattern of movement. The motion of one segment generally affects the motion of many others through biomechanical interactions and neurological integration. For example, knee rotation affects hip rotation and visa versa.

A burgeoning technology is available for the laboratory analysis of gait, and the complexity of locomotion seems, on first consideration, to demand all the technological tools that are available. However, laboratory methods are time-consuming and expensive, and they have limited diagnostic utility. The changes in gait due to central neurological diseases are often nonspecific. Consequently, laboratory methods should never be used in lieu of a careful clinical assessment and always must be interpreted in the context of clinical data. The gait laboratory has greatest clinical utility in the assessment of patients before and after orthopedic surgery and orthotic treatment.

Many types of equipment are available for the analysis of gait. The choice of a specific device should be based foremost on the specific aims of the investigator. Cost and technical complexity are major considerations, but these considerations should not result in the selection of equipment that is incapable of accomplishing the required measurements.

A digital computer lies at the core of nearly all motion analysis laboratories. Expensive minicomputers are quickly being supplanted by far less expensive but impressively powerful personal computers. The computer is interfaced with other motion analysis equipment, using an analog-to-digital converter. This device samples continuous voltage signals at specified intervals of time, producing a series of numbers that can be handled by computer software. The sampling frequency must exceed twice the highest frequency in the voltage signal. With regard to body motion, the highest frequencies are due to physiological tremor, which does not exceed 12 Hz except in the finger [14]. Thus, signals from motion transducers, force transducers, and cameras generally are digitized at rates of 25 Hz or more. Electromyography (EMG) falls in the frequency range of 0 to 400 Hz [15]. Therefore, EMG signals usually are low-pass filtered to permit digitization at rates of 500 Hz or less.

ELECTROMYOGRAPHY

Most motion analysis laboratories are equipped with EMG, which is discussed extensively by Basmajian and De Luca [15]. Skin electrodes or intramuscular wire electrodes are arranged in a bipolar fashion and fed to a differential amplifier with high impedance. Skin electrodes are not invasive, record from a large population of motor units, and are easily applied. However, the electrical signal is attenuated and low-pass filtered by the impedance of the skin. Consequently, the frequency range and amplitude of surface EMG is lower (approximately 0–200 Hz) than that of wire EMG (0–400 Hz). Loose skin can make accurate and stable electrode placement difficult or impossible during limb motion, and intramuscular wire electrodes tend to creep from their desired location with repeated muscle contractions. Skin electrodes are not capable of recording electrical activity from deep muscles, and they are more prone to recording "cross-talk" electrical activity from neighboring muscles. Wire electrodes are particularly useful in recording precisely from small and deeper muscles.

EMGs frequently are full-wave rectified and low-pass filtered, with a cutoff frequency of 30 Hz or below (Fig. 8-1). This may be accomplished with analog devices or digitally on a personal computer. Analog filtering is performed conveniently in real time, but artifactual phase delays may impede measurement of EMG latencies. Digital transformations with a short computer program can be accomplished within a few seconds and without phase shift. Most motion analysis laboratories have the capacity to perform both analog and digital filtering. The relationship between rectified-filtered EMG and muscle force is nonlinear, varies with muscle length (i.e., joint angle) [16], and differs among muscles [15]. Therefore, rectified-filtered EMG accurately measures muscle activation but only approximates muscle force.

Like all other measures of gait, the patterns of EMG activation during the gait cycle vary with the velocity of walking. Significant between-subject differences also exist [17]. By contrast, the patterns of EMG activation vary little for a given subject walking at a constant speed.

FORCE PLATES

Several devices for measuring foot-floor ground reaction forces are available commercially [18]. Floor-mounted plates and pressure insoles are available for studying the distribution of pressure beneath the foot during the stance phases of gait, but these devices do not measure anteroposterior and lateral shear forces

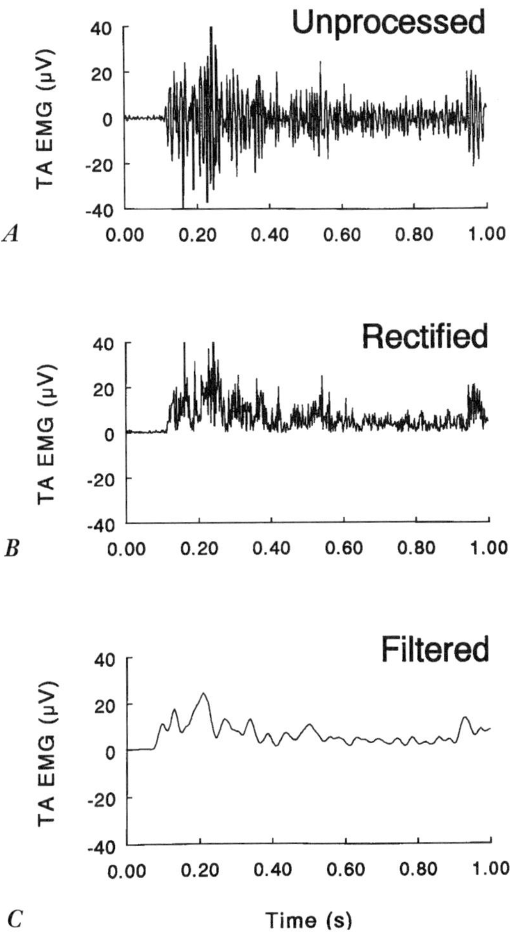

Figure 8-1. Electromyogram (EMG) recorded from the right tibialis anterior (TA) with skin electrodes during the initiation of gait. The unprocessed EMG (*A*) is shown after full-wave rectification (*B*) and subsequent low-pass filtering (*C*) (-3 dB at 15 Hz).

necessary for computing gait dynamics [18]. By contrast, floor-mounted precision force plates are capable of measuring the resultant ground reaction force and its point of application, a measurement needed for computing gait dynamics, but force plates do not reveal the distribution of pressure beneath the foot. Force plates occasionally are used alone in studies of gait and postural sway [19, 20] but most commonly are used in conjunction with other motion analysis equipment.

KINEMATICS

The term *kinematics* pertains to the motion of a body in space, without regard to the forces that cause this motion. Translational motion occurs when all points on a body segment move through space at the same velocity. Points on a rigid body move through space at different velocities when there is rotation. The motion of any rigid body can be regarded as the superposition of translational and rotational motions. A body segment such as the leg moves in three-dimensional space with 6 degrees of freedom: three directions of translation and three angles of rotation. The motion of at least three noncolinear landmarks on a body segment must be measured to compute its translational and rotational motions completely. These landmarks are used to define an "embedded" body segment coordinate system (x, y, z). The embedded coordinate system translates and rotates in space, relative to a general earth-fixed (inertial) coordinate system (X, Y, Z) that is defined somewhere in the motion analysis laboratory. A position vector $\mathbf{P} = (x, y, z)$ and a rotation vector $\Phi = (\Phi_x, \Phi_y, \Phi_z)$ are used to define the position and orientation of the segment coordinate system (i, j, k) relative to the general coordinate system at a particular moment in time (Fig. 8-2). Relative motion of the embedded coordinate systems of two adjoining segments is computed to estimate joint angles. Details of these kinematic computations are described elsewhere [18, 21].

A comprehensive description of limb or body motion is not always necessary. At times, only rotations of a few joints are of interest, as in the evaluation of an arthritic knee during ambulation. Such measurements can be accomplished with

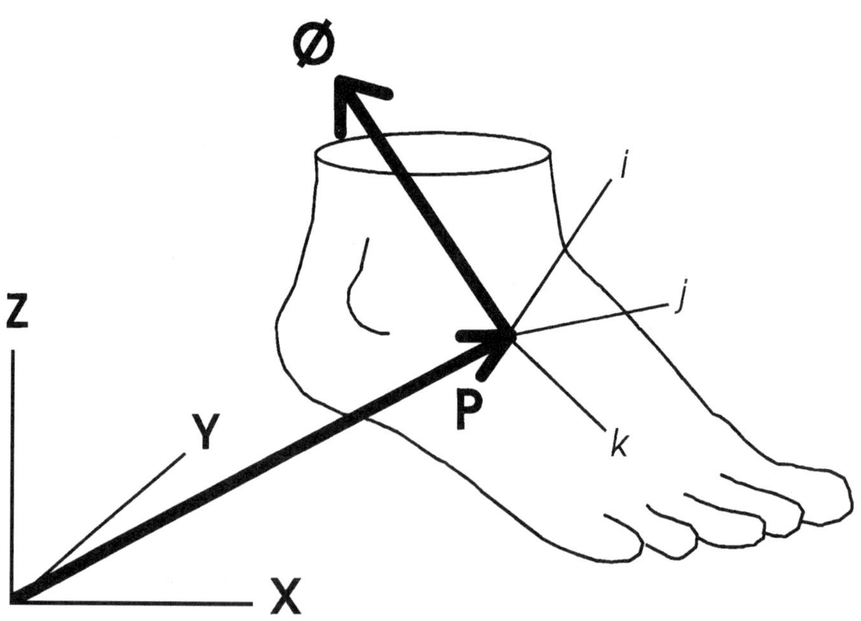

Figure 8-2. Coordinate systems for measuring body segment translation and rotation. A general coordinate system (X, Y, Z) is ground-based and stationary. The embedded coordinate system (i, j, k) is fixed within the body segment (e.g., the foot) and therefore translates and rotates as the segment moves through space. The position and attitude of the segment (i.e., embedded coordinate system) at any time are defined by vectors $\mathbf{P}$ and Φ.

a *goniometer*. The most common goniometers consist of a precision rotational potentiometer that produces a voltage proportional to joint angulation. Goniometric data can be processed quickly and easily with a personal computer, and goniometers are relatively inexpensive and simple to use [22, 23]. However, their mechanical bulk may be restrictive to some patients. Loose flesh and limb deformities impede the proper attachment of goniometers, causing variable and invalid measurements. This is particularly true for abduction-adduction and internal-external joint rotations, the measurement of which requires special triaxial goniometers [23]. Goniometers have no external (ground-based) reference, so they are capable of measuring only relative joint angles between body segments. Such kinematic information is not sufficient for computing joint torques.

Miniature *accelerometers* theoretically are suitable for recording the motion of body segments during gait, but their use in this capacity is impeded by computational problems and mechanical artifact produced by tremor, shock forces during heel strike, and skin motion [24]. A cable of several fine wires from each accelerometer must be fed to a suitable amplifier and a recording system. Walking and other movements are encumbered by the numerous accelerometers (at least six uniaxial accelerometers per body segment) required for comprehensive motion analysis.

Many photogrammetric motion analysis systems are available. The attributes of most commercially available systems are reviewed in the excellent monograph by Vaughan et al. [18]. These systems range widely in sophistication and price. The most popular systems use a set of computer-controlled precision cameras. The cameras of some systems emit stroboscopic infrared light that is reflected from topographical markers back to the cameras (e.g., the VICON system, Oxford Metrics Ltd.: Oxford, England). The center of light from each reflectile ("passive") marker then is computed and recorded at 50 Hz or higher as the marker moves through space. Great care and considerable hands-on interaction with the computer are needed to ensure that all markers are identified accurately and tracked through time and space. Fortunately, increasingly sophisticated computer software is becoming available for expediting this task. Other popular camera systems use "active" topographical markers, which are light-emitting diodes (LEDS) that emit pulses of infrared light (Selspot, Selective Electronics, Inc., Southfield, MI; Watsmart, Northern Digital, Inc., Waterloo, Ontario). Identification of LEDs is not necessary because they are activated sequentially by a computer. The main disadvantage of an active marker system is the encumbered motion produced by the wires from the LEDs to the computer.

Active and passive marker systems vary in their ease of use, spatial resolution, accuracy, and price. Ease of use is a particularly important concern. Data analysis may take days or even weeks, depending on the equipment, software, and quantity of data. The spatial resolution of the X, Y, and Z coordinates of a topographical marker is limited by the optics of the cameras and by the process of computer digitization. The upper limit of the spatial resolution is determined by the resolution of the analog-to-digital converter interfaced with the cameras. The resolutions of 10-bit, 12-bit, and 16-bit analog-to-digital converters are

1 : 1,024, 1 : 4,096, and 1 : 65,536, respectively. For a 2-m^3 viewing volume and 12-bit analog-to-digital conversion, the X, Y, and Z coordinates of a topographical marker are resolved to 0.49 mm, but the accuracy is ±1 to 3 mm for most systems. Competition has forced the major manufacturers of active and passive marker systems to be competitive in price and performance.

Computer-integrated high-speed video systems are available commercially and are far less expensive than the active and passive marker systems discussed thus far (e.g., Peak Performance Technologies, Inc., Englewood CO). Images from two or more video cameras are displayed on a high-resolution 1,000 × 1,000–pixel computer video screen. Landmarks of interest are marked (digitized) by the computer operator with the aid of special computer software. The resolution of the field of view is 1 : 1,000. The accuracy is less and depends on the operator's ability to identify landmarks consistently.

Much attention is paid to the accuracy and resolution of motion analysis systems, but other sources of error in kinematic studies are equally important. The embedded coordinate system for each body segment is defined by an arbitrary set of topographical markers, and these markers are assumed to be located on a rigid body with invariant landmarks. The topographical markers are positioned with the specific aim of defining skeletal motion. Example marker sets are described by Kadaba et al. [25] and by Vaughan et al. [18]. Unfortunately, flexibility of some body segments (e.g., the foot) is significant, and motion of topographical markers on the underlying soft tissue relative to skeletal landmarks may be substantial, particularly in obese individuals and in older individuals with loose skin. These sources of artifactual marker motion produce variability in the embedded coordinate system, which in turn leads to errors in the computation of joint angles. Furthermore, limb and joint anatomy vary among people of all ages, and joint axes usually are estimated by using limited anthropometric data [18], which may be distorted by pathology such as arthritis. Ramakrishnan and Kadaba [21] found that a ±15-degree uncertainty in the extension-flexion axis of the knee produced a ±10-degree uncertainty in the estimated knee abduction-adduction but fortunately caused little uncertainty in extension-flexion. The abduction-adduction uncertainty was even greater in patients with cerebral palsy. Finally, mechanical and electrical noise impedes the computation of velocities and accelerations. Angular and linear velocities and accelerations are computed by numerically differentiating rotations and translations, respectively. Numerical differentiation is used to obtain the first derivative (velocity) and second derivative (acceleration). The velocity of translational or angular noise with amplitude A and frequency ω (radians per second) will have an amplitude Aω. Similarly, the acceleration of such noise will have an amplitude Aω^2. For example, the amplitude of 60-Hz electrical noise would increase by factors of 377 (60 × 2π) and 142,122 after first and second differentiation. Therefore, noise must be filtered prior to differentiation to prevent the obscuration of velocity and acceleration estimates. A simple but effective method of filtering and differentiation is described by Savitzky and Golay [26].

DYNAMICS (KINETICS)

Thus far in this chapter, we have considered only the kinematics of gait, without regard to the forces that caused the motion. Dynamics is the study of these forces. There are two basic types of problems in rigid-body dynamics. The direct dynamics (kinetics) problem begins with a known set of forces, and the motion of the rigid body then is computed using the laws of mechanics. The inverse dynamics problem begins with a complete knowledge of rigid-body motion, and the responsible forces are computed [18, 27]. The inverse dynamics approach is most common in biomechanics. The direct dynamics approach would require the direct measurement of forces and moments of force (torques) acting on each joint, which currently is not possible (but see Krebs [28]). In the inverse approach, body segment parameters (segment moment of inertia, mass, and center of mass), angular and linear kinematics, and the ground reaction forces (force plate data) are used in Newton's laws of motion to compute the forces and torques at the joints between body segments, beginning with the foot and working proximally, segment by segment.

The utility of the inverse dynamics approach is limited by several factors that are topics of ongoing research [28]. The problems in computing linear and angular accelerations already have been discussed. The inverse approach uses Newton's second law of motion as it applies to the translational component of motion (i.e., force = mass × acceleration) and to the rotational component of motion (i.e., torque = moment of inertia × angular acceleration). Hence, the vector sum of the external forces acting on each body segment (e.g., the foot in Fig. 8-3) equals the mass of the segment times the acceleration of the segment's center of mass. Similarly, the vector sum of the external torques (moments of force) acting on a segment about its center of mass equals the angular acceleration of the segment times its moment of inertia [18]. These calculations are impeded by noisy linear and angular acceleration estimates. Errors in the estimation of the joint axes of rotation (joint center) also distort the angular acceleration estimates and, in turn, the estimated joint torques. This is true particularly of abduction-adduction and twisting (internal-external) joint torques, which are frequently of great interest to orthopedists. Estimates of body segment mass, moment of inertia, and center of mass are additional sources of error, because typically they are based on limited anthropometric data [18, 21]. The definition of some body segments, such as the trunk, also is a concern.

The computations of inverse dynamics produce estimates of the resultant joint forces and torques. The resultant joint forces and torques are the net forces and torques across a joint and are produced by the effects of gravity, segment accelerations, passive joint properties (i.e., friction, viscosity, and elasticity), and the muscle contractions. Too few equations of motion can be written to solve for these individual sources of force and torques. For example, bone-on-bone joint pressures (forces) are of great interest to orthopedists but are not attainable [27]. Similarly, cocontraction of antagonistic muscles is a common abnormality in

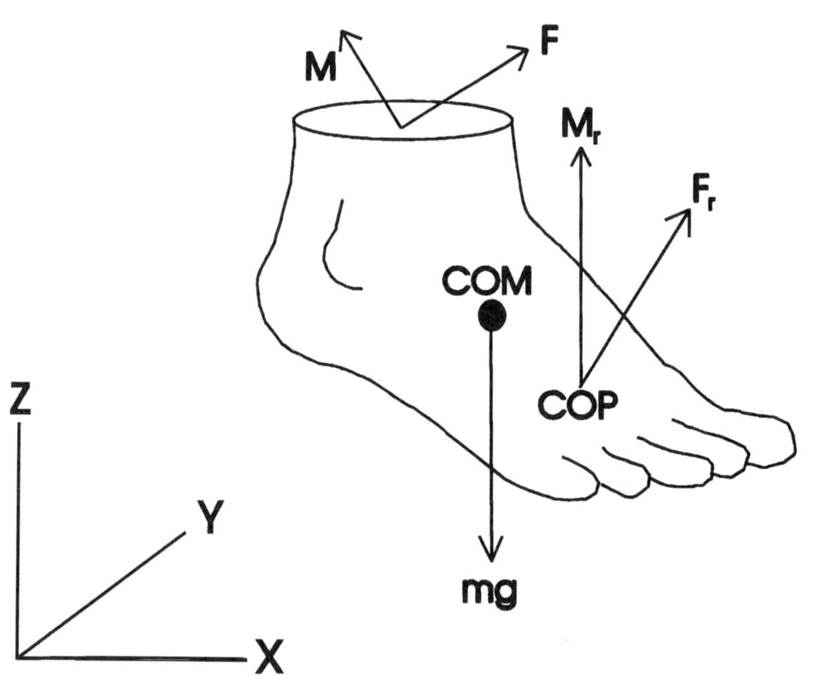

Figure 8-3. Free-body diagram of the foot. The ground-reaction torque and force vectors (M_r and F_r) acting at the center of pressure (COP) are measured with force plates. The center of mass (COM) is approximated, using anthropometric data. Newton's laws of motion are used to solve for the torque and force vectors at the ankle (**M** and **F**). This procedure then is repeated for more proximal segments (e.g., the leg). m = mass of the foot; g = acceleration of gravity; X,Y, Z = general coordinate system.

neurological patients, but the contractions of individual muscles cancel in such a way that they are not reflected in the computed resultant forces and torques.

REPEATABILITY OF MOTION ANALYSIS

The kinematic, EMG, and kinetic variables of gait are sufficiently repeatable at a constant velocity of walking so that the measurement of only a few gait cycles is necessary [29]. Many aspects of modern motion analysis laboratories tend to encumber normal gait, so one or more warm-up walks are advisable before data are recorded. The degree of trial-to-trial variability frequently is examined by computing the ensemble average of gait variables recorded in three or more trials [29].

Some trial-to-trial and day-to-day variability in gait are produced by the biomechanical and neurophysiological complexities of locomotion. The contributions of these biological sources of variability cannot be separated easily from technical sources, such as variability in topographic marker placement and the estimation of joint centers of rotation. These technical sources of variability probably contribute significantly to the between-day variability in joint angle and torque measurements, particularly in the coronal and transverse planes [29]. Other causes of variability, such as the use of shoes, restrictive garments, or a treadmill [30], must be considered in comparing data between studies and laboratories.

SELECTING AN APPROPRIATE METHOD

Clinical rating scales should not be dismissed hastily in favor of alluring, high-tech methods of gait analysis. Comprehensive assessments of locomotor performance are accomplished easily and reliably with available clinical rating scales (e.g., see Table 7-2). These rating scales frequently are supplemented with standard video recordings. Comparable assessments in a motion analysis laboratory would require an immense amount of time and instrumentation. The motion analysis laboratory is needed in situations that require a detailed assessment of gait kinematics, kinetics, or EMG. For example, quantitative motion analysis might be used to assess the forces and moments of force at one or more joints following prosthetic or orthotic treatment of a musculoskeletal deformity [31]. A detailed analysis of limb segment coordination in a patient with cerebellar ataxia is another suitable use. By contrast, the *Get-up-and-go test*, the Tinetti protocol, and other less detailed measures of gait (e.g., velocity, stride, and cadence) will suffice in most clinical therapeutic trials (see chapter 7).

Functional assessment, not clinical diagnosis, is the chief goal of all forms of quantitative gait analysis. Kinematic, kinetic and EMG analyses of gait usually produce no pathognomonic data. This is particularly true for neurological disturbances of gait. Gait analyses must be interpreted in the context of a comprehensive clinical evaluation. Gait analysis reveals changes in performance and biomechanical function that are produced by a disease. Additional data from other sources usually are needed to make a specific diagnosis.

REFERENCES

1. Tinetti ME, Ginter SF. Identifying mobility dysfunctions in elderly patients. *JAMA* 1988; 259:1190–1193.
2. Nutt JG, Marsden CD, Thompson PD. Human walking and higher-level gait disorders, particularly in the elderly. *Neurology* 1993:43:268–279.
3. Tinetti ME, Williams TF, Mayewski R. Fall risk index for elderly patients based on number of chronic disabilities. *Am J Med* 1986;80:429–434.
4. Mathias S, Nayak USL, Isaacs B. Balance in the elderly patient: The "get-up and go" test. *Arch Phys Med Rehabil* 1986;67:387–389.
5. Podsiadlo D, Richardson S. The timed "Up & Go": A test of basic functional mobility for frail elderly persons. *J Am Geriatr Soc* 1991;39:142–148.
6. Craik R. Measuring function in the elderly: Neurologic. *The Eugene Michels Researchers' Forum Proceedings.* Alexandria, VA: American Physical Therapy Association 1988;7–16.

7.   Elble RJ, Thomas SS, Higgins C, Colliver J. Stride-dependent changes in gait of older people. *J Neurol* 1991;238:1–5.

8.   Nakamura R, Handa T, Watanabe S, Morohashi I. Walking cycle after stroke. *Tohoku J Exp Med* 1988;154:241–244.

9.   Smidt GL. Gait Assessment and Training in Clinical Practice. In: Smidt GL, ed. *Gait in Rehabilitation*. New York: Churchill Livingstone, 1990. Pp 301–315.

10. Wade DT, et al. Walking after stroke: Measurement and recovery over the first 3 months. *Scand J Rehabil Med* 1987;19:25–30.

11. Wagenaar RC, Beek WJ. Hemiplegic gait: A kinematic analysis using walking speed as a basis. *J Biomech* 1993;25:1007–1015.

12. Wolfson L, Whipple R, Amerman P, Tobin JN: Gait assessment in the elderly: A gait abnormality rating scale and its relation to falls. *J Gerontol* 1990;45:M12–M19.

13. Eastlack ME, et al. Interrater reliability of videotaped observational gait-analysis assessments. *Phy Ther* 1991; 71:465–472.

14. Elble RJ, Koller WC. *Tremor.* Baltimore: Johns Hopkins University Press, 1990.

15. Basmajian JV, De Luca CJ. *Muscles Alive: Their Functions Revealed by Electromyography,* 5th ed. Baltimore: Williams & Wilkins, 1985.

16. Solomonow M, Baratta RV, D'Ambrosia R. EMG-force relations of a single skeletal muscle acting across a joint: Dependence on joint angle. *J Electromyogr Kinesiol* 1991;1:58–67.

17. Arsenault AB, Winter DA, Marteniuk RG. Is there a 'normal' profile of EMG activity in gait? *Med Biol Eng Comput* 1986;24:337–343.

18. Vaughan CL, Davis BL, O'Connor JC. *Dynamics of Human Gait.* Champaign, IL: Human Kinetics Publishers, 1992.

19. Dichgans J, Mauritz K-H, Allum J-H-J, Brandt Th. Postural sway in normals and atactic patients: Analysis of the stabilizing and destabilizing effects of vision. *Agressologie* 1976;17:15–24.

20. Nilsson J, Thorstensson A. Ground reaction forces at different speeds of human walking and running. *Acta Physiol Scand* 1989;136:217–227.

21. Ramakrishnan HK, Kadaba MP. On the estimation of joint kinematics during gait. *J Biomech* 1991;24:969–977.

22. Ellis M, Howe A. A clinical gait analysis system. *Eng Med* 1987;16:217–220.

23. Isacson J, Gransberg L, Knutsson E. Three-dimensional electrogoniometric gait recording. *J Biomech* 1986;19:627–635.

24. Hayes WC, et al. Leg motion analysis during gait by multiaxial accelerometry: Theoretical foundations and preliminary validations. *J Biomech Eng* 1983;105:283–289.

25. Kadaba MP, Ramakrishnan HK, Wootten ME. Measurement of lower-extremity kinematics during level walking. *J Orthop Res* 1990;8:383–392.

26. Savitzky A, Golay MJE. Smoothing and differentiation of data by simplified least squares procedures. *Anal Chem* 1964;36:1627–1639.

27. Winter DA. *Biomechanics of Motor Control and Human Movement.* New York: Wiley, 1990.

28. Krebs DE. Seize the moment: Dynamics and estimated moments of force in locomotion analysis. *The Eugene Michels Researchers' Forum Proceedings.* Alexandria, VA: American Physical Therapy Association 1992;109–119.

29. Kadaba MP, et al. Repeatability of kinematic, kinetic and elecromyographic data in normal adult gait. *J Orthop Res* 1989;7:849–860.

30. Van Ingen Schenau CJ. Some fundamental aspects of the biomechanics of overground versus treadmill locomotion. *Med Sci Sports Exer* 1980;12:257–261.

31. Smidt GL. Gait in Musculoskeletal Abnormalities. In: Smidt GL, ed. *Gait in Rehabilitation.* New York: Churchill Livingstone, 1990. Pp 199–252.

9. Toward a Nosology of Gait Disorders: Descriptive Classification

C. David Marsden and Philip Thompson

Many patients with neurological diseases first present with walking difficulties. The neurologist's approach to any problem is to classify the impairment and disability according to the level of the nervous system affected. This approach can be applied to gait disorders through a logical examination of a patient's balance and locomotion, based on physiological principles. Observation of balance and gait is supplemented by the traditional neurological examination to detect accompanying signs of neurological impairment. Combining the two analyses allows a gait disorder to be classified according to the level of the nervous system affected, following the terminology of Hughlings Jackson [1]:

1. Lowest-level disorders include musculoskeletal or primary muscles diseases, peripheral neuropathies or radiculopathies, and deafferentation.
2. Middle-level disorders include spastic gaits due to hemiparesis or paraparesis, cerebellar syndromes, and parkinsonian gaits.
3. Highest-level disorders include those gait difficulties that cannot be explained by the problems listed in items 1 and 2 but are due to damage to the cerebral hemispheres or psychogenic problems.

Having defined the gait disorder syndrome in these terms, the next stage is to determine its cause.

Following this plan, first we will summarize the elements of normal walking on which the examination and classification of gait disorders are based. Then we will describe the critical features of examination of gait. Last, we will examine the various syndromes of gait disturbance, with particular emphasis on those occurring in the elderly.

NORMAL WALKING

Two abilities are essential to walking: (1) *equilibrium*, the capacity to assume the upright posture and to maintain balance (see Chapter 3); and (2) *locomotion*, the ability to initiate and maintain rhythmic stepping (see Chapter 4). Table 9-1 summarizes the key features involved in these mechanisms.

Table 9-1. Summary of the basic requirements for walking on two legs and the basic abnormalities in the dissolution of gait

Neural control mechanisms	Physiologic mechanisms	Abnormalities
Equilibrium		
Arise to the erect posture	Righting reactions	Inability to rise
Support upright position	Supporting reactions	Inability to stand
Correct perturbations and adapt to circumstance	Anticipatory postural reactions	Inability to protect upright stance
	Reactive postural responses	
	Rescue reactions	
	Protective reactions	
Locomotion		
Initiate steps	Shift center of gravity	Gait ignition failure
	Start stepping	
Step	Locomotion	Alterations in pattern of stepping
Adapt stepping to circumstances	Voluntary	Inability to perform dexterous stepping
Nonneurologic factors		
The mechanical support system	Bones, joints	Limp
General health (cardiorespiratory)	Exercise tolerance	Slowness

SOURCE: JG Nutt, CD Marsden, PD Thompson. Human walking and higher-level gait disorders, particularly in the elderly. *Neurology* 1993;43:268–279.

Equilibrium

The capacity to assume the upright posture and to maintain balance involves a series of physiological mechanisms. The human must get from the sitting or lying position to the vertical position. This is achieved by *righting reactions*, which consist of coordinated muscle synergies that bring the head and body into an upright position for stance and locomotion. These reflexes are triggered by vestibular, proprioceptive, tactile, and visual stimuli [2], any one of which is normally sufficient to allow an animal to right itself. Once the human is vertical, upright posture is maintained by contraction of antigravity muscles, termed *supporting reactions*. The distribution of such muscle contraction determines body posture; slight changes alter the position of the body.

The stability of vertical posture, with the center of gravity over a narrow base provided by the feet, can be threatened by inherent body sway, by voluntary movement of the limbs and trunk, or by external disturbances. Preservation of balance while standing involves the control of normal body sway. The mechanics of the human body provide some resistance to sway, through the elasticity of ligaments, tendons, and muscles stabilizing joints, particularly at the ankles, knees, and hips. In addition, balance requires active muscle contraction generated by interacting visual, vestibular, and proprioceptive input and by experience and foreknowledge [3].

Balance is threatened at the moment the human moves. The lifting of an arm shifts body mass. Balance is preserved by *anticipatory postural reflexes* [4]. Anticipatory postural reflexes are programmed in advance of the intended voluntary movement in such a way as to alter antigravity muscle contraction, thus setting the stage for the intended movement. Alternatively, if one pulls on the arm of a standing subject, early muscle responses in antigravity postural muscles anticipate the resultant shift of the center of gravity [5] as a result of proprioceptive feedback.

Anticipatory postural reflexes may be insufficient to maintain balance. When the center of gravity shifts beyond a certain point, a series of sequential *reactive postural responses* are brought into operation to maintain balance. The earliest of these are spinal monosynaptic and polysynaptic reflexes. These are not essential for the maintenance of upright posture, as patients with deafferentation can stand. Subsequent functional stretch reflexes appear approximately 120 msec after an ankle displacement and make a major contribution to the preservation of balance [6, 7]. Their long latency allows reflex arcs to the brain stem and cerebrum to be involved. Such functional stretch reflexes are complex, involving strategies of contraction of leg and trunk muscles influenced by visual and vestibular stimuli, by the nature of the support surface, by experience, and by expectation [8, 9].

If anticipatory postural reflexes and reactive postural responses fail, *rescue reactions* involving the arms and legs are brought into play to restore balance. They occur automatically but also are under voluntary control. For instance, an individual whose balance is in peril may take one or two steps, so as to bring the feet back under the shifted center of gravity. If this is insufficient, windmill arm movements are brought into play to try and restore balance. If falling is imminent and unavoidable, a series of *protective reactions* are brought into play to break the fall and minimize injury (e.g., the arms are thrown out automatically, and the head is averted).

Locomotion

Walking involves the initiation of gait followed by the subsequent engagement of rhythmic stepping and the adjustment of locomotion to changing circumstances. *Gait ignition* refers to the act of starting to walk. This involves shifting the center of gravity to one side and then forward as the leading leg is released in advance. The shifts of the center of gravity are achieved by redistribution of contraction in posturally active muscles, in the course of which a starter signal must be issued to initiate or ignite rhythmic locomotion. *Locomotion* then proceeds by alternating, coordinated movements of the legs and trunk. The size, direction, and speed of each step must be adjusted to the terrain or changing circumstances. If balance is threatened in the course of walking, the various mechanisms described above are brought into play to maintain equilibrium.

It is crucial to distinguish between failure of postural reflexes (basal ganglia disease) from locomotor ataxia (cerebellar disease).

EXAMINATION OF BALANCE AND GAIT

Against the physiological background previously described, we suggest that balance and gait can be examined in a rational fashion. Each of the following key elements should be assessed.

1. The ability to rise from a chair (righting reactions). Some patients, particularly those with basal ganglia disease, are unable to get themselves out of a chair into the standing position.
2. The ability to stand unsupported (supporting responses). Even if they can get into the vertical posture, some patients (again, commonly those with basal ganglia disease) may be incapable of maintaining vertical stance: they keel over unless supported. The ability to stand in the vertical posture with the eyes closed (Romberg's test) is a measure of the integrity of proprioceptive (and vestibular) control.
3. Ability to withstand a push. The push test assesses the effectiveness of both reactive postural responses (fore and aft and side-to-side) and, if these are inadequate, whether rescue reactions and protective reactions occur.
4. The ability to initiate walking. Failure of gait ignition manifests as start-hesitation when attempting to begin to walk (i.e., the "slipping-clutch phenomenon" or "magnetic feet"). The patient cannot take the first steps to walk and shuffles on the spot, or the feet appear glued to the floor. If walking is begun, ignition subsequently may fail, so that the patient "freezes" in midstride. Freezing often is precipitated by turning or passing through a narrow space, such as a doorway.
5. The ability to locomote. Particular attention should be given to the width of the base, stride length, foot clearance, arm swing, and cadence. Locomotor difficulty takes two main forms. In locomotor ataxia, the rhythm of stepping is disrupted, steps are irregular in timing and length (too long or too short), are misdirected to one side or the other, or the leg is lifted too high or not high enough. In locomotor hypokinesia, the rhythm is preserved, the direction of stepping is correct, but steps are too short, so that the patient shuffles. Locomotor ataxia usually is accompanied by walking on a wide base, whereas in locomotor hypokinesia, the base is narrow.
6. The ability to negotiate turns. Making a turn poses particular threats to balance and locomotion. Turning may unearth imbalance, with staggering and the need to engage reactive postural responses (and even rescue reactions and protective reactions). Turning also may unearth freezing and subsequent start-hesitation or gait ignition failure.
7. The ability to walk a straight line heel to toe. This test again evaluates balance and may unearth defective reactive postural responses and rescue and protective reactions.

Following these observations of balance and gait, formal neurological examination on the bed must be undertaken in the traditional way. In addition, the patient should be asked to mimic the act of rhythmic leg movements while lying or seated and to draw patterns with the feet. Communication between observers may be improved by such a detailed description of balance and gait and would be enhanced by videotaping of the standard sequence.

CLASSIFICATION OF GAIT DISORDERS

We propose considering gait disorders in terms of the hierarchy of lowest, middle, and highest sensorimotor levels (Table 9-2).

Lowest-Level Gait Disturbances

Lowest-level gait disturbances may be due to either peripheral skeletomotor problems or peripheral sensory problems. The arthritic, myopathic, and peripheral neuropathic gaits generally are recognized easily by clinicians and require no further comment. Likewise, the sensory ataxic, vestibular ataxic, and visual ataxic gaits are relatively easy to diagnose on the basis of the character of the disturbance and associated symptoms and signs. It is important to note the dysfunction at these lowest levels is generally well-compensated if the central nervous system is intact. People who are blind, those who have defective proprioception, or those with artificial limbs can walk.

Gait disturbances due to orthopedic and foot problems are discussed in Chapter 11; those due to peripheral neuropathy and disorders of proprioception are discussed in Chapter 17; and those due to vestibular disorders are discussed in Chapter 16.

Middle-Level Gait Disturbances

Examples of middle-level gait and balance dysfunction include the gaits associated with spasticity (hemiplegia and paraplegic; see Chapter 12), ataxia (see Chapter 16), parkinsonism (see Chapter 13), dystonia, and chorea. Again, neurologists generally have little difficulty in diagnosing these various middle-level gait disturbances on the basis of the character of the abnormalities of balance and locomotion and the associated symptoms and signs.

Disorders of pyramidal, cerebellar, and basal ganglia motor systems cause distortion of appropriate postural and locomotor synergies. In general, the correct postural and locomotor responses are selected, but their execution is faulty.

Highest-Level Gait Disturbances

The highest sensorimotor systems are responsible for choosing the postural and locomotor responses appropriate for the support surface, body position in space, the environment, and the intention of the individual. These highest systems

Table 9-2. Classification of gait syndromes

Lowest-level gait disorders
Peripheral skeletomuscle problems
   Arthritic gait
   Myopathic gait
   Peripheral neuropathic gait
Peripheral sensory problems
   Sensory ataxic gait
   Vestibular ataxic gait
   Visual ataxic gait

Middle-level gait disorders
Hemiplegic gait
Paraplegic gait
Cerebellar ataxic gait
Parkinsonian gait
Choreic gait
Dystonic gait

Highest-level gait disorders
Cautious gait
Subcortical disequilibrium
Frontal disequilibrium
Isolated gait ignition failure
Frontal gait disorder
Psychogenic gait disorder

SOURCE: JG Nutt, CD Marsden, PD Thompson. Human walking and higher-level gait disorders, particularly in the elderly. *Neurology* 1993;43:268–279.

are the least understood and are the greatest cause of clinical confusion. The proposed classification of highest-level gait disorders (see Table 9-2) is based on clinical features. However, before considering the individual syndromes of highest-level gait disorders, one has to take into account the overriding problem of the cautious gait.

The Cautious Gait

The cautious gait is characterized by a normal to mildly widened base, a shortened stride, slowness of walking, and turning en bloc. Anyone whose balance is insecure for whatever reason will attempt to compensate. As a consequence, the final picture of gait in those with disease may be the sum of the deficits in balance and locomotion produced by the underlying disease plus compensatory mechanisms brought into play in an attempt to overcome the impairments. Normal compensation is best illustrated by our natural reaction to walking on ice. The feet are placed apart to widen the base; the body, hips, and knees are bent to place the center of gravity firmly over the widened base; and the arms are held somewhat abducted and flexed in anticipation of unexpected threats to balance. Locomotion proceeds with small steps on this wide base, with a flexed posture. We walk in the same way on the deck of a rolling ship. To a greater or lesser degree, many old people adopt this cautious gait to compensate for arthritis, pain, sensory or vestibular impairment, or all of these or simply because of fear of falling.

The cautious gait pattern is an appropriate response to real or perceived disequilibrium. However, many individuals may adopt an inappropriately cautious gait. Elderly people who trip, fall, and fracture a femur may be unable to walk independently after hip surgery, despite adequate strength and neurological function (the postfall syndrome) [10]. This gait pattern also has been referred to as *stasobasophobia* [11]. At one extreme, it may lead to timid locomotion around the periphery of the room or clutching onto furniture or walls, giving rise to the so-called space phobia [12].

Those with neurological disease and perceived instability also adopt this cautious gait, which initially may mask the underlying neurological deficit. With progression of the disease, however, the characteristic neurological signs of the underlying gait disorder become apparent. Often it is necessary, therefore, to strip away the components of the cautious gait so as to unearth the underlying neurological deficit and gait syndrome.

Such underlying highest-level gait syndromes have been a cause of great nosological confusion. Many terms have been applied: *the senile gait, gait apraxia, marche à petit pas, lower-half parkinsonism,* and so on. In our view, these various disorders can be encompassed within four main categories: (1) subcortical disequilibrium, (2) frontal disequilibrium, (3) isolated gait ignition failure, and (4) frontal gait disorder (see Nutt et al. [1] for review). Table 9-3 shows the various terms used to describe these syndromes and the likely sites of lesions responsible for them.

Subcortical Disequilibrium

Subcortical disequilibrium is characterized by severe impairment of balance postural reflexes. Patients may be unable to stand or walk at all because of the absence of adequate supporting reactions and postural reflexes. If they can stand, they may fall over, usually backward. Postural responses may be inappropriate; for example, the patient may hyperextend the neck and trunk and fall backward. Locomotion primarily is impaired because of the severe disequilibrium. Associated signs include ocular abnormalities (vertical gaze palsies and pupillary defects), dysarthria, and extrapyramidal signs. *Astasia-abasia* is a term used to describe this disturbance of balance and gait, although historically it was employed to describe hysterical gait disturbances.

Subcortical disequilibrium has been reported as an acute phenomenon after thalamic, basal ganglia, or midbrain stroke. Masdeu and Gorelick [13] described a series of patients who could not stand after acute vascular lesions of the thalamus (thalamic astasia), particularly those involving the superior portion of the ventral lateral nucleus. Despite relatively preserved strength and sensation, they fell backward or to the side opposite the lesion. This disturbance of equilibrium improved over a matter of days or weeks. Labadie et al. [14] reported a similar disorder in patients with acute infarction or hemorrhage affecting the putamen (also sometimes involving the globus pallidus). These patients tilted slowly and collapsed to the side opposite the lesion "like a falling log," without appropriate corrective actions. This clinical picture also has been reported following unilateral midbrain lesions [15].

Table 9-3. Comparison of proposed terms used
to describe the clinical patterns of gait in the elderly

Proposed terminology	Previously used terms	Lesions
Cautious	Elderly gait Senile gait	Musculoskeletal Peripheral nervous lesions Central nervous lesions
Subcortical disequilibrium	Tottering Astasia-abasia Thalamic astasia	Midbrain Basal ganglia Thalamus
Frontal disequilibrium	Gait apraxia Frontal ataxia Astasia-abasia	Frontal lobe and white-matter connections
Isolated gait ignition failure	Gait apraxia Magnetic gait Slipping-clutch gait Lower-half parkinsonism Arteriosclerotic parkinsonism Trepidant abasia (Petren's gait)	Frontal lobe, white-matter connections, and basal ganglia
Frontal gait disorder	Marche à petit pas Magnetic gait apraxia Arteriosclerotic parkinsonism Parkinsonian ataxia Lower-half parkinsonism Lower-body parkinsonism	Frontal lobe and white-matter lesions

SOURCE: JG Nutt, CD Marsden, PD Thompson. Human walking and higher-level gait disorders, particularly in the elderly. *Neurology* 1993;43:268–279.

The syndrome of subcortical disequilibrium also is seen early in the course of a number of progressive degenerative Parkinson-plus syndromes, such as progressive supranuclear palsy (Steele-Richardson-Olszewski disease) and multiple system atrophy. Indeed, the early prominence of disequilibrium is one important clue to the recognition of these conditions and their distinction from other akinetic-rigid syndromes, in particular Parkinson's disease. The early loss of postural reflexes in such subcortical degenerations causes falls that may be associated with significant injury, because rescue and protective reactions also are defective. In such degenerative Parkinson-plus syndromes, locomotion (if possible) also is often abnormal, with difficulties in initiating gait, start-hesitation and freezing, and locomotor hypokinesia.

Frontal Disequilibrium

Frontal disequilibrium also is dominated by disequilibrium that can be severe enough to prevent standing or walking. However, most patients can walk, but when they attempt to do so, their steps are inappropriate; their feet frequently cross or move in a direction inappropriate to the center of gravity, and there appears to be a breakdown of the leg movements required for locomotion. As a result, the gait often is bizarre, with crossing of the legs and ineffective propulsion.

In view of the marked disequilibrium, Bruns [16] coined the term *frontal ataxia* to describe this gait in patients with frontal mass lesions. Gerstmann and Schilder [17] distinguished this gait from that of cerebellar ataxia and suggested that the problem represented an apraxia of gait, along the lines of Leipmann's concept of apraxia of arm and hand movement. Van Bogaert and Martin {18] also used the term *apraxia de la marche* to describe the gait of a woman with a frontal abscess who was unsteady and exhibited small steps and bizarre, clumsy movements of the legs, which became tangled and caused her to fall. She also was unable to make purposeful movements of the legs on command, such as bicycling when lying in bed, but might do so spontaneously. They interpreted her abnormality of balance and gait in terms of a disconnection between the idea of walking and the motor programs required to walk. Meyer and Barron [19] also used the term *apraxia of gait* but applied it to a different pattern of gait disturbance (see below).

All these clinical descriptions of frontal disequilibrium have in common a severe disturbance of balance and inappropriate postural responses and locomotor patterns. Dementia, incontinence, perseveration, difficulty with repetitive movements, and frontal release signs further point to a disturbance of function of the frontal lobes and their connections. Indeed, this pattern of frontal disequilibrium has been reported with a variety of structural lesions of the frontal lobes, including tumor, abscess, and infarction or hemorrhage, hydrocephalus, or diffuse white-matter disease.

The use of the term *gait apraxia* to describe this condition is open to a number of objections. First, if gait apraxia is accepted as an entity, equilibrium apraxia also must be accepted because, in many patients, the distortion of postural reflexes and the impairment of balance are the most prominent aspects of their disorder. Second, patients with marked bilateral apraxia for limb movements may walk normally [20]; conversely, many patients with gait disturbances described as apraxic do not have limb apraxia [21].

Isolated Gait Ignition Failure

Isolated gait ignition failure is characterized by an inability to initiate and sustain locomotion. A patient cannot start walking because of hesitation and may freeze in the course of locomotion, particularly on a turn. Balance, however, is preserved. Once locomotion is initiated, steps are short and barely clear the ground to begin with, giving the gait a shuffling appearance. However, with continued stepping, the stride lengthens, foot clearance is normal, and the arms swing normally. Postural responses are normal, stance and gait width usually are normal, and falls are distinctly rare. Tricks such as pretending to kick the bottom of a cane, stepping over the handle of a cane held upside down, or counting repetitively frequently aid the initiation of gait [22].

Petren [23] probably was the first to describe this gait syndrome under the title of *trepidant abasia*. Isolated gait ignition failure may remain as the sole abnormality for many years. There are no other clinical signs and, in particular, there often is no evidence of dementia or parkinsonism. The pathological cause of prolonged isolated gait ignition failure is not clear. Brain imaging excludes tumor, hydrocephalus, or significant vascular disease in the majority of patients. The presumption is that it represents an isolated focal degenerative cortical condition, but this is speculation.

In other patients, their illness may begin with isolated gait ignition failure but, with the passage of time, they develop other abnormalities of gait and additional neurological symptoms and signs indicating a progressive frontal gait disorder (see below). In this situation, cerebrovascular disease, hydrocephalus, or even a frontal lobe tumor may be responsible.

Frontal Gait Disorder

Frontal gait disorder is characterized by a variable base (narrow to wide), difficulty in starting to walk, short steps, shuffling, and hesitation on turns, with freezing and moderate disequilibrium. The frontal gait disorder differs from subcortical and frontal disequilibrium by lesser impairment of postural responses so that ambulation is still achieved. However, with progression, patients with a frontal gait disorder develop increasing imbalance and falls and may evolve into frontal disequilibrium. The frontal gait disorder differs from gait ignition failure in that there is disequilibrium and impaired locomotion. Patients with this gait syndrome frequently have associated cognitive impairment, pseudobulbar signs and dysarthria, frontal release signs, paratonia, pyramidal signs, and urinary disturbances.

This is the gait described as *marche à petit pas* [24], a term that refers to the short-stepped military gait, with an upright trunk posture and stiff legs. As the condition progresses, there is start-hesitation, shuffling, freezing, and increasing disequilibrium. In its complete form, the frontal gait disorder evolves into frontal disequilibrium comprising elements of imbalance with locomotor ataxia of the legs, parkinsonism with locomotor hypokinesia, gait ignition failure, and disequilibrium, with impaired righting reactions with loss of rescue and protective reactions. Patients with this gait syndrome may exhibit surprisingly normal function of the upper limbs and a lively facial expression, which has led to the use of the term *lower-half parkinsonism*. Critchley [25] described this same gait under the title of *arteriosclerotic parkinsonism*, emphasizing the role of diffuse cerebral arterial disease in its causation. Thus, this gait has come to be associated with vascular disease, particularly with subcortical arteriosclerotic encephalopathy and the lacunar state (Binswanger's disease) [21]. A similar syndrome of frontal gait disorder has been described in patients with hydrocephalus [26–28]. Indeed, Fisher [29] attributed the imbalance and short shuffling steps of the elderly gait to hydrocephalus, although his criteria for the diagnosis of hydrocephalus are controversial [30]. In an influential review, Meyer and Barron [19] reported seven patients with a frontal gait disorder due to vascular insults, tumor, or atrophy. All walked slowly on a wide base, with the feet rooted to the ground, employing short shuffling steps and exhibiting freezing. All had disequilibrium and falls. These investigators used the term *apraxia of gait* to describe this frontal gait syndrome, but (as discussed earlier) there are major objections to this notion.

Overlap of These Syndromes

A crucial question is the extent to which these various syndromes of highest-level gait disorders are separate or overlap. Subcortical disequilibrium, frontal disequilibrium, isolated gait ignition failure, and the frontal gait disorder all share common etiologies. In particular, cerebrovascular disease (see Chapter 14) and hydrocephalus (see Chapter 15) can cause any of these patterns of highest-level gait dysfunction. In pure culture, they are quite distinctive, but it must be admitted that the edges are blurred. Elsewhere [1] we have put forward the view that gait disorders are analogous to language disorders; classic Wernicke's and Broca's aphasia are easily distinguishable, but in many aphasic patients, there are elements of both types of language disturbance. Likewise, early dementia may present patterns that suggest predominant frontal, parietal, or subcortical involvement, but with progression, these distinctions are lost, replaced by a picture of global dementia. Similarly, many patients with gait disorders have mixtures of disequilibrium, locomotor abnormalities, and gait ignition difficulties. The classification may resemble stages in the dissolution of gait rather than separate entities. For example, a patient may present initially with a cautious gait pattern, progress to gait ignition failure, then to a frontal gait disorder, and finally develop a full frontal disequilibrium syndrome. Nevertheless, we believe that these clinical syndromes of highest-level gait disturbances are useful categories of description on which further research can be based.

REFERENCES

1. Nutt JG, Marsden CD, Thompson PD. Human walking and higher-level gait disorders, particularly in the elderly. *Neurology* 1993;43:268–279.
2. Magnus R. Physiology of posture. *Lancet* 1926;2:531–536, 585–588.
3. Davidoff RA. Skeletal muscle tone and the misunderstood stretch reflex. *Neurology* 1992;42:951–963.
4. Martin JP. *The Basal Ganglia and Posture*. Philadelphia: Lippincott, 1967.
5. Marsden CD, Merton PM, Morton HB. Human postural responses. *Brain* 1981;104:513–534.
6. Melvill-Jones G, Watt DGD. Observations of the control of stepping and hopping movements in man. *J Physiol [Lond]* 1971;219:709–727.
7. Nashner LM. Fixed patterns of rapid postural responses among leg muscles during stance. *Exp Brain Res* 1977;30:13–24.
8. Horak FB, Nashner LM. Central programming of postural movements: Adaptation to altered support-surface configurations. *J Neurophysiol* 1986;55:1369–1381.
9. Horak FB, Diener HC, Nashner LM. Influence of central set on human postural responses. *J Neurophysiol* 1989;62:841–853.
10. Murphy J, Isaacs B. The post-fall syndrome: A study of 36 elderly patients. *Gerontology* 1982;82:265–270.
11. Garcin R. The Ataxias. In: Vinken PJ, Bruyn GW, eds. *Handbook of Clinical Neurology* (vol 1). Amsterdam: North-Holland, 1969. Pp 309–352.
12. Marks I. Space "phobia," a pseudo-agoraphobic syndrome. *J Neurol Neurosurg Psychiatr* 1981;44:387–391.
13. Masdeu JC, Gorelick PB. Thalamic astasia: Inability to stand after unilateral thalamic lesions. *Ann Neurol* 1988;23:596–603.

14. Labadie EL, Awerbuch GI, Hamilton RH, Rapesak SZ. Falling and postural deficits due to acute unilateral basal ganglia lesions. *Arch Neurol* 1989;45:492–496.

15. Felice KJ, Keilson GR, Schwartz WJ. 'Rubral' gait ataxia. *Neurology* 1990;40:1004–1005.

16. Bruns L. Über sturugen des gleichgewichtes bei stirnhirntumoren. *Otsch Med Wochenschr* 1892;18:138–140.

17. Gerstmann J, Schilder P. Über eine besondere gangstorung bei stirnhirner kranting. *Wien Med Nochenschr* 1926;76:97–107.

18. Van Bogaert L, Martin P. Sur deux signes du syndrome de desequilibration frontale: L'apraxie de la marche et l'antonie statique. *Encephale* 1929;24:11–18.

19. Meyer JS, Barron DW. Apraxia of gait: A cliniophysiological study. *Brain* 1960;83:261–284.

20. Geschwind N. The apraxias: Neural mechanisms of disorders of learned movement. *Am Sci* 1975;63:188–195.

21. Thompson PD, Marsden CD. Gait disorder of subcortical arteriosclerotic encephalopathy: Binswanger's disease. *Mov Disord* 1987;2:1–8.

22. Atchison PR, Thompson PD, Frackowiak RSJ, Marsden CD. The syndrome of gait ignition failure: A report of six cases. *Mov Disord* 1993;8:285–292.

23. Petren K. Veber den Zusammenhang zwischen anatomisch bedingter und fractioneller gangsturung (Besonders in der farn von trepid ander abasie) im Greisenalter. *Arch Psychiatr Nerven* 1901;33:444–489.

24. von Malaise E. Studien uber wese grundlagen senile getstoringen. *Arch Psychiatr* 1910;46:902–1009.

25. Critchley M. Arteriosclerotic parkinsonism. *Brain* 1929;52:23–82.

26. Messert B, Baker NH. Symptoms of progressive spastic ataxia and apraxia associated with occult hydrocephalus. *Neurology* 1966;16:440–452.

27. Adams RD, et al. Symptomatic occult hydrocephalus with "normal" cerebrospinal fluid pressure: A treatable syndrome. *N Engl J Med* 1965;273:117–126.

28. Estanol BV. Gait apraxia in communicating hydrocephalus. *J Neurol Neurosurg Psychiatry* 1981;44:305–308.

29. Fisher CM. Hydrocephalus as a cause of disturbances of gait in the elderly. *Neurology* 1982;32:1358–1363.

30. Koller WC, Glatt SL, Fox JH. Senile gait: A distinct neurologic entity. *Clin Geriatr Med* 1985;1:661–669.

10. Clinical Approach to Gait Disorders of Aging: An Overview

Lewis Sudarsky

Like falls, gait disorders are common and present a problem of enormous heterogeneity. Prevalence and the clinical spectrum vary, depending on the setting and population under consideration. Precise estimates of prevalence have been difficult to establish, as there is no standard definition or criteria. In a community study in Durham, North Carolina, 15% of individuals older than 60 had some degree of difficulty with ambulation [1]. According to studies from Western Europe, 20–25% of people use mechanical aids for walking by age 80 [2]. In East Boston, gait abnormality of an apparently neurological nature (shuffling, difficulty with turns) was identified in 49% of the population over 85 [3].

In an acute-care hospital, 20–30% of patients have some difficulty with ambulation. The disturbance in locomotor function often is transient, related to injury, drug effects, or metabolic disturbances. Prakash and Stern [4] examined 100 admissions to an acute geriatric unit; all were inpatients with no history of neurological disease. They found 70 to be fully independent in ambulation, 8 to be bedbound, and 22 to have gait disorders. "A wide variety of gaits were encountered, most being slow and cautious, but no acceptable comprehensive classification was possible" [4]. Nutt and Marsden [5] collected 43 cases of higher-level gait disorder from a busy geriatric inpatient unit in London, patients with balance and walking problems unexplained by elemental neurological deficits. In a number of these patients, the gait disorder was attributed to cerebrovascular disease.

A somewhat different perspective is obtained in a chronic hospital or nursing home setting, where many patients are nonambulatory, and a cause for their failure may be difficult to establish. Some 40–50% of nursing home patients are unable to walk independently [6]. Depending on the level of the facility, a very different spectrum of illness is encountered. In a frail older patient with a large burden of chronic disease, identifying the cause of impaired mobility and recurrent falls can be a real challenge.

HETEROGENEITY AND CLASSIFICATION

Many different diseases of the nervous system present in the elderly with a failing gait, and often the manifestations are nonspecific. The heterogeneity of gait disorders observed clinically reflects the large amount of anatomy at risk. A network of subcortical systems participate in the coordinated management of postural control and locomotion [7, 8]. Cortical modulation adapts the performance to suit a complex hierarchy of purposes and needs [9]. Balance is particularly dependent on sensory systems that may be vulnerable to age-related change.

In their review of the higher-level gait disorders, Nutt and Marsden [5] approach the classification descriptively, using classical physiological principles. One difficulty with this approach is the lack of specificity and phenomenological overlap encountered when these principles are applied. Many failing gaits look fundamentally similar, even though different mechanisms are at work. This overlap reflects common patterns of adaptation to declining performance. Any gait disorder can be viewed as the product of abnormal physiology and an adaptive response. An alternative approach is to classify these disorders by etiology whenever possible. Although some gait disorders are multifactorial, often it is possible to identify the principal cause. In our experience, only 10–15% of neurological outpatients presenting for gait disturbance cannot be assigned a diagnosis based on clinical evaluation and laboratory tests.

The first step in evaluation is to separate neurological disorders of ambulation from musculoskeletal disorders. A clean separation may not be possible, as many patients have a little of both. Older people frequently have coexistent arthritis, and minor orthopedic deformity is a common source of gait abnormality. There are no good data on how many gait disorders in a community are musculoskeletal and how many reflect underlying neurological disease, but misattribution of neurological gait disorder to arthritis is a well recognized phenomenon [10].

CAUSES OF GAIT DISORDER IN A NEUROLOGICAL REFERRAL PRACTICE

We will consider gait disorders from the perspective of neurological office practice. Our 1983 study [11] provides a point of departure by enumerating some of the frequently encountered disorders. Table 10-1 includes another 70 cases (from 1990–1994), which were referred to a neurologist for undiagnosed gait disorder. Gait problems caused by arthritis and skeletal deformity were excluded from the study, which focused on neurological disease. A highly similar spectrum of illness was observed in a study of gait disorders from a neurological inpatient unit in Taiwan [12]. The principal causes of gait disorder are reviewed briefly in the following sections and are considered in more detail in Chapters 11 through 19.

Myelopathy

Often unrecognized by internists and generalists, myelopathy from cervical spondylosis is a common cause of gait disorder in the elderly. Spinal disease was the cause of gait disturbance in 16.7% of patients in our series and in 22% in the study of Fuh et al. [12] from Taiwan. Studies of prevalence in a general autopsy population suggest that the problem is increasingly common with advanced age [13]. Spondylitic bars and ligamentous hypertrophy narrow the canal, causing mechanical compression and vascular compromise. The core clinical features are spastic paraparesis, together with mild standing imbalance and bladder instabil-

Table 10-1. Classification of gait disorder
in 120 patients, according to etiological cause

	1980–1982	1990–1994	Total	Percentage
Sensory deficits	9	13	22	18.3
Myelopathy	8	12	20	16.7
Multiple infarcts	8	10	18	15.0
Unknown cause	7	10	17	14.2
Parkinsonism	5	9	14	11.7
Cerebellar degeneration	4	4	8	6.7
Hydrocephalus	2	6	8	6.7
Other	3	3	6	5.0
Psychogenic	1	3	4	3.3
Toxic or metabolic	3	0	3	2.5

SOURCE: Data for 1980–1982 from L Sudarsky; M Ronthal. Gait disorders among the elderly patients: A survey study of 50 patients. *Arch Neurol* 1983;40:740–743. Data for 1990–1994 derived from 70 additional patients.

ity (urgency, frequency). Neck pain and radiculopathy often are absent, though some patients complain of "numb clumsy hands." The condition typically is associated with a spastic or spastic and ataxic gait. An occasional patient will experience a discrete worsening in relation to an injury or fall. Magnetic resonance imaging (MRI) has improved the ease of diagnosis, though clinical correlation with the degree of spinal compression is quite imprecise. Plain films with flexion and extension sometimes reveal abnormal mobility about protruding bars when deformation of the cord is not dramatic on MRI. The natural history is quite variable; some patients apparently stabilize, whereas others progress. There is no consensus on the role of spondylosis surgery in an older patient [14]. We have seen a few patients with myelopathy from vitamin B_{12} deficiency and we now obtain B_{12} levels routinely in older patients with this presentation.

Parkinsonsim

Parkinson's disease also is common, affecting 1.5% of the population past 65. The flexed attitude in posture and the festinating gait are distinctive. Older patients sometimes present with axial rigidity and gait disorder, without tremor or slowness in the upper limbs. Some 20–25% of patients presenting with a bradykinetic or rigid syndrome will turn out to have something other than idiopathic Parkinson's disease [15]. The list of causes includes progressive supranuclear palsy, striatonigral degeneration, and corticobasal ganglionic degeneration. These diagnoses should be considered, particularly in patients presenting with postural instability and in those unresponsive to levodopa. Parkinsonian syndromes are discussed in Chapter 13.

Drug-induced parkinsonism is increasingly recognized in ambulatory practice as a cause of impaired gait and balance. It is particularly common in a chronic-care setting. The presence of coexistent tardive dyskinesia may be a diagnostic

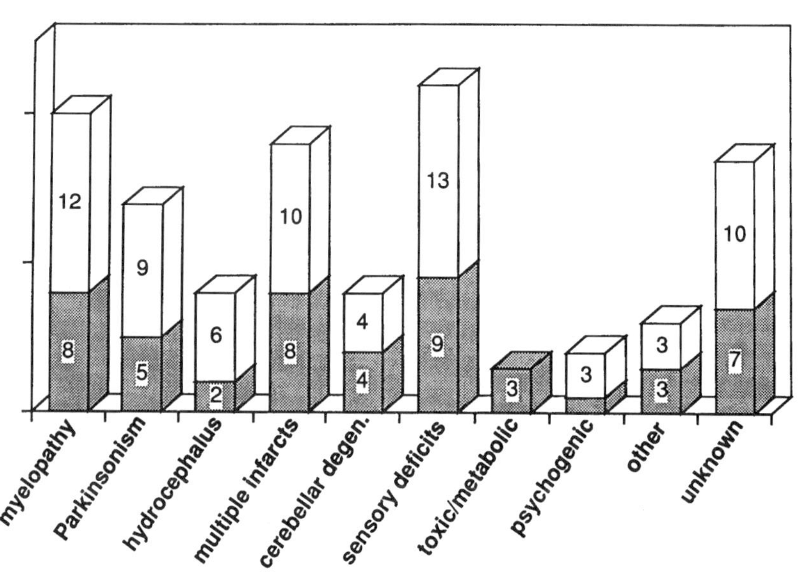

Figure 10-1. Etiologic diagnosis in 120 patients with gait disorder who were referred to a neurologist. Data are based on the study by L Sudarsky, M Ronthal, Gait disorders among elderly patients: A survey study of 50 patients. *Arch Neurol* 1983; 40:740–743, with 70 additional cases from 1990–1994. The original series is represented with stippled bars; more recent cases are on top.

clue. Neuroleptic drugs are known to impair postural support responses and contribute to the risk for falls. The disorder often takes 2–3 months to resolve after the offending medication has been discontinued [16].

Late-Life Hydrocephalus

Since normal-pressure hydrocephalus (NPH) was described by Adams et al. [17], there has been a sense that NPH is uncommon as a cause of reversible dementia. Hydrocephalus in the elderly more often presents with gait disorder as the salient feature [18]. The gait is slowed with start-hesitation, and patients walk with feet "stuck to the floor" [19]. The pathophysiology is not well understood; there is presumably a disconnection of cortical modulation.

Among patients presenting with this type of frontal gait disorder (gait apraxia), it is not unusual to find ventricular enlargement by computed tomography (CT) or MRI. A dynamic test is necessary to confirm the presence of true (as opposed to ex vacuo) hydrocephalus [20]. The literature is quite confusing on predictive tests for shunting; the topic is reviewed in Chapter 15. We use clinical response to the removal of 30 ml cerebrospinal fluid (CSF) as a screening test, understanding that the sensitivity is imperfect and some patients will be missed [21, 22]. MRI-based studies of CSF flow through the aqueduct may help with the evaluation of these patients [23]. Gait improves more consistently than does mental function after a shunt.

Vascular Disease and Gait

Neurological deficits from stroke often contribute to gait impairment, particularly if there is an element of lower-limb paralysis or ataxia. Acutely, stroke can compromise postural control without causing paralysis, particularly if the lesion involves the lateral thalamus (thalamic astasia) or brain-stem tegmentum [24, 25a]. The consequences of multiple infarcts on postural control and locomotion often are substantial, as the network is unable to compensate for multiple lesions. Fifteen percent of neurological outpatients with gait disorder in our study had multiple cerebral infarcts. Such patients comprise 24% of the series of hospitalized patients from the Neurological Institute in Taiwan [12]. The associated clinical syndromes are reviewed in Chapter 14.

Some patients with vascular disease present with a progressive disorder of gait without a clear-cut history of stroke. Parkinsonian features may be correlated with basal ganglia lacunes as evidenced by CT or MRI. Some patients with chronic hypertension have ischemic lesions of the deep white matter, so-called Binswanger's disease. Diagnosis should not be based solely on the radiological picture, which is somewhat nonspecific. The clinical syndrome consists of mental change, dysarthria, pseudobulbar affect, hyperreflexia in the limbs, and a shuffling gait [26]. Patients have difficulty with gait initiation and turns and experience a variable degree of imbalance. The pathophysiology of gait impairment probably is similar to that in hydrocephalus [27].

Cerebellar Disorders

Disorders of quiet stance and dynamic balance are a well-described phenomenon with lesions of the vestibulocerebellum and midline vermis [28]. Patients with lesions of the anterior vermis display increased sway in the anterioposterior direction at 3 Hz and a disturbance in the long-latency postural response (excess amplitude and prolonged response in tibialis anterior to toe-up perturbation). Visual stabilization is preserved, and such patients do not fall often. Patients with disorders of the flocculonodular lobe have a low-frequency, omnidirectional sway ($\leq$ 1 Hz). They are worse with eye closure and often fall laterally.

The ataxic gait is characterized by instability of the trunk and head, poor control of the center of mass, erratic foot placement, a widened stance, and decompensation when attempting to walk on a narrow base. Studies by Hallett et al. [29] demonstrate a lateral drift with progression, and path deviation in individual steps. Poor interlimb coordination is evident in a study of the joint moments. Ground reaction forces have an irregular temporal profile, particularly at the point of weight acceptance.

Inherited and sporadic forms of cerebellar degeneration can occur with late onset. Olivopontocerebellar atrophy is the most commonly recognized syndrome, but other types are described. Molecular markers soon may help with the classification of inherited ataxia. For the present, atrophy of the cerebellum and brain stem can be appreciated by CT or MRI. Other causes of cerebellar atrophy include toxins (alcohol, possibly phenytoin) and paraneoplastic cerebellar degeneration. Chronic alcoholics with anterior vermis atrophy experience primarily truncal ataxia [30].

Sensory Deficits and Gait Instability

A large number of patients present with chronic imbalance due to deficits in sensory afferent systems. Balance depends on high-quality information from the visual system and the vestibular system and on proprioceptive afferents from the lower limbs in contact with the support surface. When this information is lost, standing balance is impaired, and gait instability results. Many patients perceive imbalance and adopt a cautious gait, whereas others lurch about with gross sensory ataxia and an erratic stride. These patients are at particular risk for falls.

Somatosensory deficits sufficient to compromise balance can be appreciated by using Romberg's test and other functional assessment techniques (one-leg stance, tandem stance). The classic example of this phenomenon is the locomotor ataxia of tabetic neurosyphilis, nicely described by Gowers [31] in the nineteenth century. There is erratic foot placement and a tendency to misstep; balance may be lost if a patient attempts to turn too quickly. The abnormality of gait is more evident on attempting to walk with the eyes closed or to walk backward. The most common source of sensory imbalance in contemporary practice is peripheral neuropathy, affecting large-fiber afferents. In the absence of other sensory deficits, neuropathy must be moderately severe before gait and balance are impaired.

Disequilibrium and gait imbalance in the elderly sometimes are manifestations of bilateral vestibular hypofunction [32]. Patients with bilateral vestibular deficits may lack vertigo, and physiological testing often is required to confirm the clinical impression. In a study of 26 patients older than 75 years who presented with standing imbalance and no apparent cause on clinical evaluation, Fife and Baloh [32] observed profound deficits on vestibular testing in 7. Abnormalities included a marked reduction of gain on vestibulo-ocular reflex (VOR) and increased sway on platform posturography. The gait pattern of patients with bilateral vestibular deficits has been studied at the biomotion lab at Massachusetts General Hospital. When self-paced, patients with vestibular deficits choose a longer cycle time, with increased double support time and reduced vertical excursions of the center of gravity and head [33].

Other Causes

It is important to recognize motor manifestations of toxic and metabolic encephalopathies, as these disorders are relatively common and usually treatable. Patients with metabolic encephalopathy often display an insecure gait and may fall over backward if displaced. This phenomenon is particularly dramatic with uremia and hepatic failure, in which asterixis may impair stance. Sedative drugs, especially neuroleptics and long-acting benzodiazepines, affect postural reflexes and increase the risk for falls [34].

A few elderly patients presenting with gait disorder have a mass lesion: primary CNS tumor or metastatic cancer. Subdural hematoma should be ruled out in a patient with subacute evolution and a history of falls.

Psychogenic Gait Disorder

Gait is unconscious and automatic, but walking is nonetheless influenced by psychological state. The cautious gait described by Nutt et al. [5] is a common phenomenon, a nonspecific biomechanical adaptation to perceived imbalance. Patients walk with small steps and a widened base of support, as if walking on a slippery surface. Psychomotor retardation in depression can be manifest in posture and gait [35]. Depressed patients often walk with a slow lifting motion and do not propel themselves forcefully.

Many older persons experience anxiety about their balance and a resultant fear of falling. This results in cocontraction of postural muscles, and can influence the dynamics of postural control [36]. Such patients may have subtle deficits in balance, and it is difficult to sort out cause from effect. Patients with fear of falling can present with a phobic disorder, a pathological variant of the cautious gait. They are extremely timid in stance, abducting the arms as if walking across a slippery surface and clinging to walls or furniture for support.

Hysterical and somatiform disorders of gait occur at all ages. Astasia-abasia was recognized in the nineteenth century, and these disorders were prevalent in Europe during World War I. Contemporary studies by Keane [37] and Lempert et al. [38] emphasize common patterns and phenomenological clues to aid in diagnosis. These include moment-to-moment fluctuations in the level of impairment, extreme slowness (resembling slow motion or "walking through water"), and uneconomical postures with wastage of muscular energy. Exaggerated sway was noted on Romberg's test, with a consistent tendency to fall toward or away from the examiner. Performance can be improved by distraction. These disorders rarely are subtle and usually are apparent to an experienced observer. Dramatic cures can be observed in approximately half of patients.

Gait Disorder Without Identifiable Cause

In many patients (up to 15%), there is no obvious diagnosis after a careful evaluation and workup. These cases sometimes are called *essential senile gait*, though it is unlikely that they represent a true morbid entity [39, 40].

APPROACH TO THE EVALUATION OF GAIT DISORDERS

Evaluation of a patient presenting with a chronically progressive disorder of gait includes three steps: history, neurological examination, and functional assessment of gait and balance. The history from patients with a chronically progressive disorder of gait reiterates certain common themes. First awareness of a balance problem often follows a fall. Many patients limit their activity because of fear of falling. In some patients, the progression is stepwise, suggesting vascular disease. Pain with walking suggests the presence of musculoskeletal disease or lumbar spinal stenosis. (Most of the neurological disorders under consideration are not painful.) It is always important to review the use of alcohol and medications that might influence gait and balance.

As the list of potential diagnoses is lengthy, information on localization derived from the neurological examination can be useful to narrow the search. Neurological examination typically is more informative than is watching a patient walk, though each provides complementary information. Gait observation gives a direct measure of the degree of a patient's disability. Certain distinctive patterns can be recognized; the gait pattern of Parkinson's disease is particularly distinctive. Balance can be examined as the patient stands from a chair or in response to gentle pressure on the sternum. It is helpful to separate patients with locomotor disorders from those with a balance problem.

Brain-Imaging Studies

Brain-imaging tests, such as CT and MRI, frequently are used as an aid in diagnosis. MRI is more informative. Topography of cerebellar degeneration can be appreciated by MRI, whereas it may be inapparent by CT. MRI is an excellent screening test for hydrocephalus, and MRI-based studies of CSF flow may prove useful as a dynamic test. MRI is invaluable in examining cerebral infarcts that contribute to gait disorder, as noted earlier. The issue of clinical correlation is more controversial with respect to white-matter abnormality (leukoaraiosis). Masdeu et al. [41] and others have suggested a relationship between white-matter disease in the elderly and disorders of gait and postural control. MRI is a sensitive investigation, and the appearance of excess water on the T_2-weighted imaging study is both common and nonspecific. Pathological correlation has been problematic when the lesions are slight. Several studies suggest that the phenomenon may be relevant to gait disorder in elderly patients when the lesions are extensive and confluent in the frontal centrum semiovale [42].

Neurophysiology and Posturography

Standard neurophysiological investigations, such as nerve conduction velocity, somatosensory evoked potentials, and electronystagmography occasionally are useful in the evaluation of the patient with standing imbalance and sensory ataxia. Examination of VOR in response to low-frequency sinusoidal rotation is particularly informative in patients with imbalance and fear of falling, as described by Fife and Baloh [32]. A subgroup of such patients have bilateral vestibular hypofunction. Platform tests of balance also are sensitive in patients with mild imbalance and recurrent falls, though the abnormalities observed often are nonspecific, and the test provides little aid in differential diagnosis.

Gait Analysis

Gait analysis has matured as a technology since the first studies in the 1960s, and the cost of the equipment has decreased. There are now over 100 clinical gait laboratories in the United States. The principal focus of interest is in orthopedics and cerebral palsy, but many of these units operate in a rehabilitation context, and they are beginning to address neurological issues. Most gait analysis systems perform kinematic analysis or look at ground reaction forces. The better kinematic systems read dots from video cameras and can reconstruct the trajectory of the body segments in three dimensions. Simultaneous EMG data can be acquired from the trunk and legs.

The principal strength of this technology is in clinical investigation and in monitoring the success of a specific therapeutic intervention. Applications have been limited in diagnosis and clinical decision making (with the possible exception of cerebral palsy). One of the problems is that the studies generate reams of data on numerous parameters so as to characterize the performance. This results in a difficult sifting task to identify the clinically relevant details. Another issue that limits gait analysis as a diagnostic test is its lack of specificity. A few characteristic abnormalities are buried in a mass of nonspecific changes: stride-dependent adjustments and adaptations to declining performance. An experienced clinical eye looks at a few key features but also can take in at a glance an overview of the performance. Does the gait appear parkinsonian? Is the patient limited by fear? These are gestalt issues. Sophistication in pattern recognition must be written into the software before automated systems will begin to perform discriminative analysis at the expert level.

The low-tech alternative is some form of observational gait analysis. Generally we record cadence, velocity, and stride (observations that can be made in the office with a tape measure and a stopwatch). Key characteristics of the performance also can be scored directly or from videotape. We look at the ability to rise from a chair, the postural attitude of the trunk, the stance width and step height (shuffling), erratic foot placement (path deviation), and the facility for gait initiation and turns. Tinetti [43] has scored sixteen aspects of gait and balance function for assessment of falls risk (see Table 7-2, page 114).

WHAT IS TREATABLE?

Our experience suggests that roughly one in four patients will be found to have a treatable disorder. This compares favorably with the yield in dementia evaluation. Most patients are referred for physical therapy, though it is not clear as yet which groups benefit most. One approach to gait rehabilitation features the use of sensory feedback and sensory training to improve balance skills. Another approach described by Fiatarone et al. [44] is to improve muscle strength with conditioning exercises and resistance training.

We also stress the importance of appropriate footwear, assistive devices, and simple interventions to improve safety and reduce risk for falling in the home.

REFERENCES

1. Newman G, Dovermuehle RH, Busse EW. Alterations in neurologic status with age. *J Am Geriatr Soc* 1960;8:915–917.
2. Lundgren-Lindquist B, Aniansson A, Rundgren A. Functional studies in 79-year-olds: III. Walking performance and climbing capacity. *Scand J Rehabil Med* 1983;15:125–31.
3. Odenheimer G, et al. Comparison of neurologic changes in successfully aging persons vs the total aging population. *Arch Neurol* (in press).
4. Prakash C, Stern G. Neurological signs in the elderly. *Age Ageing* 1973;2:24–27.
5. Nutt JG, Marsden CD, Thompson PD. Human walking and higher-level gait disorders, particularly in the elderly. *Neurology* 1993;43:268–279.
6. Tinetti ME, Speechley M, Ginter S. Risk factors for falls among the elderly persons living in the community. *N Engl J Med* 1988;319:1701–1707.
7. Eidelberg E, Walden JG, Nguyen LH. Locomotor control in Macaque monkeys. *Brain* 1981;104:647–663.
8. Mori S. Integration of posture and locomotion in acute decerebrate cats and in awake, freely moving cats. *Prog Neurobiol* 1987;505:66–74.
9. Armstrong DM. The supraspinal control of mammalian locomotion. *J Physiol* 1988;405:1–37 Lond.
10. Rasker JJ, Jansen ENH, Haan J, Oostrom J. Normal-pressure hydrocephalus in rheumatic patients: A diagnostic pitfall. *N Engl J Med* 1985;312:1239–1241.
11. Sudarsky L, Ronthal M. Gait disorders among elderly patients: A survey study of 50 patients. *Arch Neurol* 1983;40:740–743.
12. Fuh JL, et al. Neurologic Disease Presenting with Gait Impairment in the Elderly. In: Woollacott M, Horak F, ed. *Posture and Gait: Control Mechanisms* (vol 2). Eugene: University of Oregon Books, 1992. Pp 71–74.
13. Brownell G, Hughes JT. Necropsy observations on the damage to the nervous system in degenerative disease of the C spine. Fifth International Congress of Neuropathology (Zurich), 1966.
14. Rowland LP. Surgical treatment of cervical spondylotic myelopathy, *Neurology* 1992;42:5–13.
15. Hughes AJ, Daniel SE, Kilford L, Lees AJ. The accuracy of the clinical diagnosis of Parkinson's disease: A clinicopathologic study of 100 cases. *J Neurol Neurosurg Psychiatry* 1992;55:181–184.
16. Stephen PJ, Williamson J. Drug-induced Parkinsonism in the elderly. *Lancet* 1984;2: 1082–1083.
17. Adams RD, et al. Symptomatic occult hydrocephalus with "normal" cerebrospinal fluid pressure: A treatable syndrome. *N Engl J Med* 1965;273:117–126.
18. Fisher CM. Hydocephalus as a cause of disturbances of gait in the elderly. *Neurology* 1982; 32:1358–1363.
19. Sudarsky L, Simon S. Gait disorder in late-life hydrocephalus. *Arch Neurol* 1987;44:263–267.
20. Borgesen SE, Gjerris F. The predictive value of conductance to outflow of CSF in normal-pressure hydrocephalus. *Brain* 1982,105:65–86.
21. Wikkelso C, Anderson H, Blomstrand C, Lindgvist G. The clinical effect of lumbar puncture in normal-pressure hydrocephalus. *J Neurol Neurosurg Psychiatry* 1982;45:64–69.

22. Hanley DF, Borel CO, Herdman S. Normal-Pressure Hydrocephalus. In: Johnson RT, ed. *Current Therapy in Neurological Disease*, 3rd ed. Philadelphia: Decker, 1990. Pp 305–309.

23. Bradley WG, et al. Marked cerebrospinal fluid void: Indicator of successful shunt in patients with suspected normal-pressure hydrocephalus. *Radiology* 1991;178:459–66.

24. Masdeu JC, Gorelick PB. Thalamic astasia: Inability to stand after unilateral thalamic lesions. *Ann Neurol* 1988;23:596–603.

25. Brandt T, Dieterich M. Pathological eye-head coordination in roll: Tonic ocular tilt reaction in mesencephalic and medullary lesions. *Brain* 1987;110:649–666.

25a. Masdeu J, Alampur U, Cavaliere R, Tavoulareas G. Astasia and gait failure with damage of the pontomesencephalic locomotor region. *Ann Neurol* 1994;35:619–621.

26. Babikian V, Ropper AH. Binswanger's disease: A review. *Stroke* 1987;18:2–12.

27. Thompson PD, Marsden CD. Gait disorder of subcortical arteriosclerotic encephalopathy: Binswanger's disease. *Mov Disord* 1987;2:1–8.

28. Diener HC, Dichgans J. Pathophysiology of cerebellar ataxia, *Mov Disord* 1992;7:95–109.

29. Hallett M, Stanhope SJ, Thomas SL, Massaquoi S. Pathophysiology of Posture and Gait in Cerebellar Ataxia. In: *Neurobiological Basis of Human Locomotion*. Shimamura M, Grillner S, Edgerton VR, eds. Tokyo: Japan Scientific Societies Press, 1991.

30. Victor M, Adams FD, Mancall EL. A restricted form of cerebellar cortical degeneration occurring in alcoholic patients. *Arch Neurol* 1959;1:579–688.

31. Gowers WR. *Diseases of the Nervous System*. Philadelphia: Blakiston Press, 1899. Pp 288–291.

32. Fife TD, Baloh RW. Disequilibrium of unknown cause in older people. *Ann Neurol* 1993;34:694–702.

33. Kirkpatrick R, et al. Center of Gravity Control in Normal and Vestibulopathic Gait. In: Woollacott M, Horak F, eds. Eugene, OR: University of Oregon Books, 1992. Pp 260–264.

34. Ray WA, et al. Psychotropic drug use and the risk of hip fracture. *N Engl J Med* 1987;316:363–369.

35. Sloman L, et al. Gait patterns of depressed patients and normal subjects. *Am J Psychiatr* 1982;139:94–97.

36. Maki BE, Holliday PJ, Topper AK. Fear of falling and postural performance in the elderly, *J Gerontol Med Sci* 1991;46:123–131.

37. Keane JR. Hysterical gait disorders: 60 cases. *Neurology* 1989;39:586–589.

38. Lempert T, Brandt T, Dietrich M, Huppert D. How to identify psychogenic disorders of stance and gait. *J Neurol* 1991;238:140–146.

39. Koller WC, Glatt SL, Fox JH. Senile gait: A distinct neurologic entity. *Clin Geriatr Med* 1985;1:661–669.

40. Elble RJ, Hughes L, Higgins C. The syndrome of senile gait. *J Neurol* 1992;239:71–75.

41. Masdeu JC, et al. Brain white matter changes in the elderly prone to falling. *Arch Neurol* 1989;46:1292–1296.

42. Sudarsky L. Frontal Gait Disorder: Clinical Correlation with MRI. In: Woollacott M, Horak F, eds. *Posture and Gait: Control Mechanisms* (vol 2). Eugene, OR: University of Oregon Books, 1992. Pp 156–159.

43. M Tinetti. Performance-oriented assessment of mobility problems in elderly patients. *J Am Geriatr Soc* 1986;34:119–126.

44. Fiatarone M, et al. High-intensity strength training in nonagenarians. *JAMA* 1990;22:3029–3034.

11. Foot and Ankle Disorders Affecting Gait and Balance

Elly Trepman

The functions of the foot and ankle in standing posture and gait include support of the body, balance, shock absorption, adaptation to nonlevel surfaces, and push-off power and direction. Alteration in structure or function resulting from painful conditions or deformity of the foot and ankle may cause disturbances of balance and gait. Changes in weight-bearing patterns may result in other painful conditions within the foot and thereby reduce walking efficiency. Conditions of the foot and ankle may contribute to problems proximally, as in the patient who experiences hip or back pain after a foot injury.

It is essential to review orthopedic disorders of the foot and ankle, with emphasis on the effects on balance and gait in aging individuals. Normal structure and function, pathomechanics of standing and gait, and specific disorders (with respect to effects on standing posture and gait) are considered.

THE FOOT AND ANKLE IN STANDING POSTURE AND GAIT

Functional Anatomy and Biomechanics

The ankle joint is the articulation between the tibia, fibula, and talus (Fig. 11-1). The talus is positioned in the mortise comprising the distal end of the tibia and the medial and lateral malleoli. The ankle may be modeled as a single-axis joint with dorsiflexion and plantar-flexion movement. The axis of motion of the ankle joint lies approximately along a line just distal to the tips of the medial and lateral malleoli [1, 2].

The foot consists of three anatomically and functionally distinct regions: hindfoot, midfoot, and forefoot. The hindfoot includes the talus and calcaneus bones; the midfoot: navicular, cuboid, and cuneiforms; and the forefoot: metatarsals, sesamoids, and phalanges (Fig. 11-2).

In the hindfoot, talocalcaneal (subtalar) joint movement consists primarily of inversion and eversion of the calcaneus under the talus. This movement is important in the adaptation of the weight-bearing foot to both level and nonlevel surfaces.

The hindfoot is connected to the midfoot at the transverse tarsal (Chopart's) articulation, which is comprised of the cup-shaped talonavicular and the saddle-shaped calcaneocuboid joints. The relative motion of these two joints is depen-

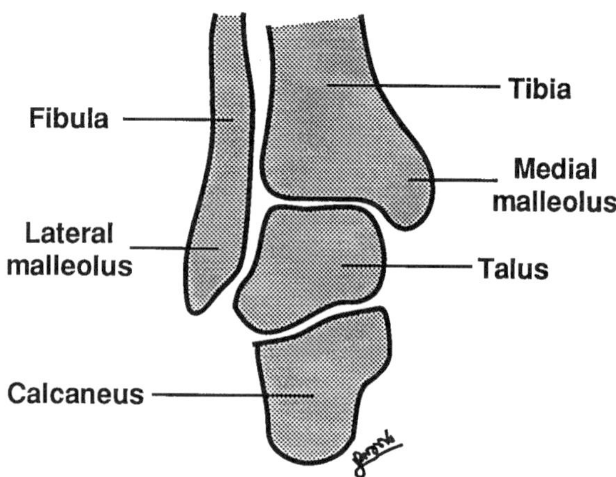

Figure 11-1. The ankle joint. The axis of motion lies along a line just distal to the tips of the medial and lateral malleoli.

dent on hindfoot position; when the calcaneus is everted, the transverse tarsal articulation is flexible; when inverted, it is rigid [3].

In the midfoot, the navicular, cuboid, and three cuneiforms constitute a transverse arch and keystone of the longitudinal arch of the foot. The midfoot bones are stabilized by multiple ligaments and a closely packed bony arrangement. Stability of the bony arch enables the foot to support body weight.

The midfoot is joined to the forefoot at the tarsometatarsal (Lisfranc's) articulation. Some dorsiflexion and plantar-flexion motion is present at the fourth and fifth metatarsal-cuboid joints, which may further facilitate adaptation to nonlevel surfaces.

The forefoot includes the metatarsal bones and phalanges of the toes. The first metatarsophalangeal joint is specialized on the plantar surface by the presence of the sesamoid apparatus, which consists of two sesamoid bones and supporting ligaments. The lesser (second to fifth) metatarsophalangeal joints are supported by a fibrocartilaginous plantar plate (plantar ligament) that inserts into the base of the proximal phalanx and serves as insertion to the flexor tendon sheath and plantar fascia [4, 5]. The metatarsophalangeal joints are further stabilized by collateral ligaments [6].

Active control of joint motion by muscles is determined by the relative location of the tendon and joint axis of motion. The tibialis anterior actively dorsiflexes the ankle. Other muscles, such as the extensor hallucis longus and the extensor digitorum longus also may effect ankle dorsiflexion. The gastrocsoleus plantar flexes the ankle. The tibialis posterior and peroneals are invertors and evertors, respectively, of the subtalar joint.

The plantar aponeurosis (plantar fascia) is a ligamentous structure with origin at the calcaneus and insertion at the plantar plate of the metatarsophalangeal

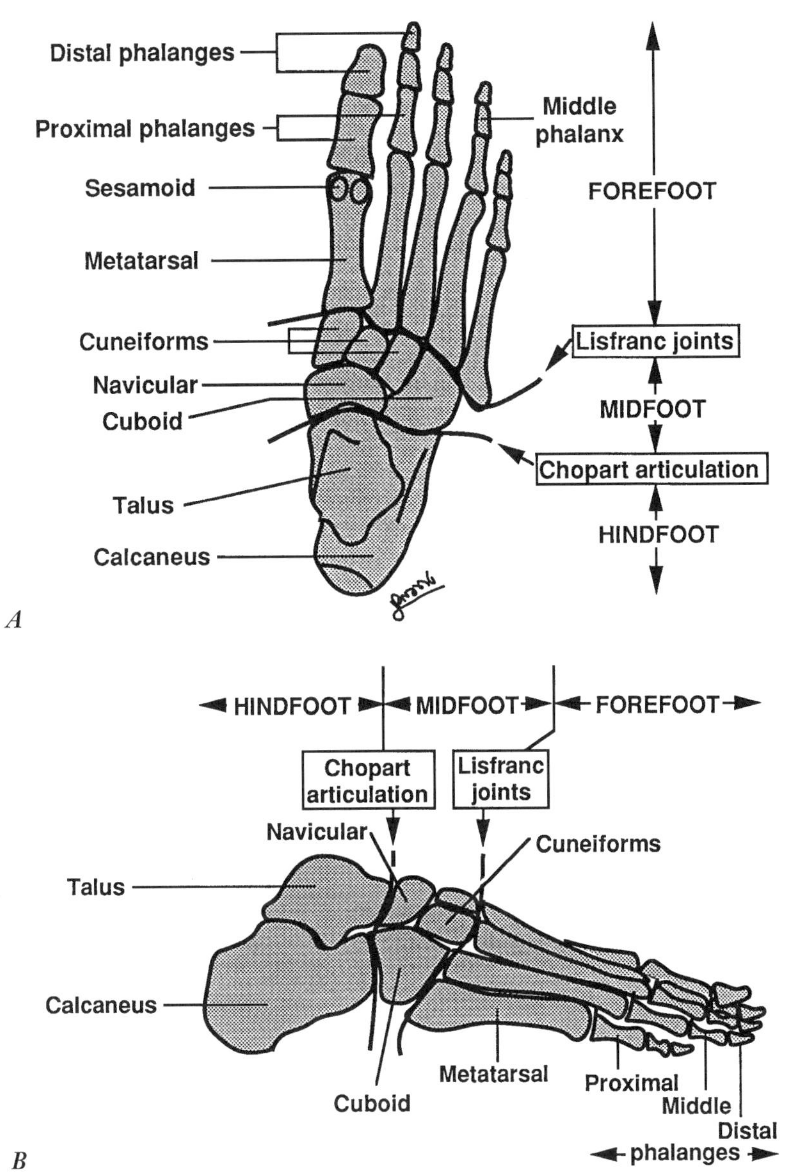

Figure 11-2. Bones and joints of the foot. *A.* Anteroposterior (dorsal to plantar) view. *B.* Lateral view.

joints and base of the proximal phalanges. When the toes are in the dorsiflexed position, increased tension occurs in the plantar aponeurosis, and the arch rises, analogous to a windlass (Fig. 11-3) [7, 8] In this fashion, the plantar aponeurosis contributes to longitudinal arch stability when the heel rises from the ground during walking.

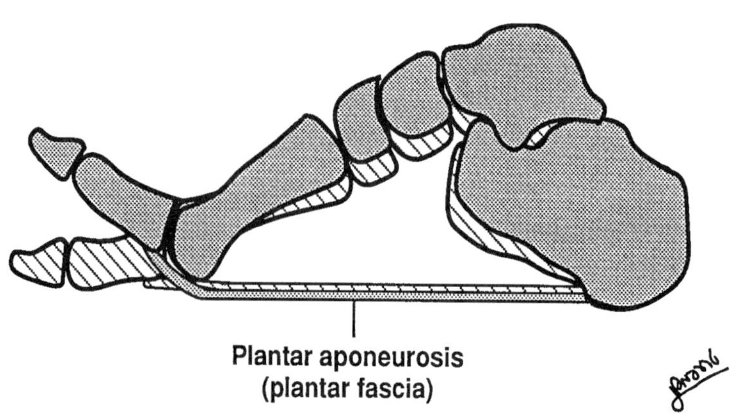

Figure 11-3. The plantar aponeurosis (plantar fascia) and the windlass mechanism. When the toes are in the dorsiflexed position, increased tension in the plantar aponeurosis causes the arch to rise.

The Foot and Ankle in Normal Standing and Gait

During barefoot standing, peak pressures under the heel in the normal foot are 2.6 times greater than under the forefoot [9]. The plantar surface of the heel supports 60.5% of body weight; the forefoot, 28.1%; the midfoot, 7.8%; and the toes, 3.6% [9]. Static balance of the body in neutral position is achieved with minimal activity in the leg muscles. Forward sway during quiet standing results in electromyographic activity in the calf muscles, whereas backward sway causes activity in the tibialis anterior [10]. The intrinsic muscles of the foot are inactive during quiet standing.

The normal gait cycle of a limb consists of swing (62% of gait cycle) and stance (38%) phases. Stride length is the distance from heel-strike to the next ipsilateral heel-strike (one gait cycle); step length is the distance from heel-strike to the following contralateral heel-strike. A period of double-limb support occurs at the beginning (12% of gait cycle) and end (12%) of stance phase, coinciding with the end and beginning, respectively, of contralateral limb stance phase. The foot and ankle during the stance phase undergo a sequence of events from heel-strike to foot-flat (0–7% of gait cycle), foot-flat to heel-off (7–34%), and heel-off to toe-off (34–62%) (Fig. 11-4) [1]. During these periods, changes normally occur in foot and ankle alignment, muscle activity, and pressure distribution on the sole, which may be altered in pathological conditions.

At heel-strike, the subtalar joint is inverted (supinated), which is a reason for the wear pattern of shoes often observed on the lateral heel of the sole. The ankle, initially in slight dorsiflexion, is rapidly plantar flexed as foot-flat is achieved, and is controlled by eccentric contraction of the tibialis anterior. When foot-flat is achieved, the tibialis anterior becomes inactive and remains so throughout the remainder of stance phase.

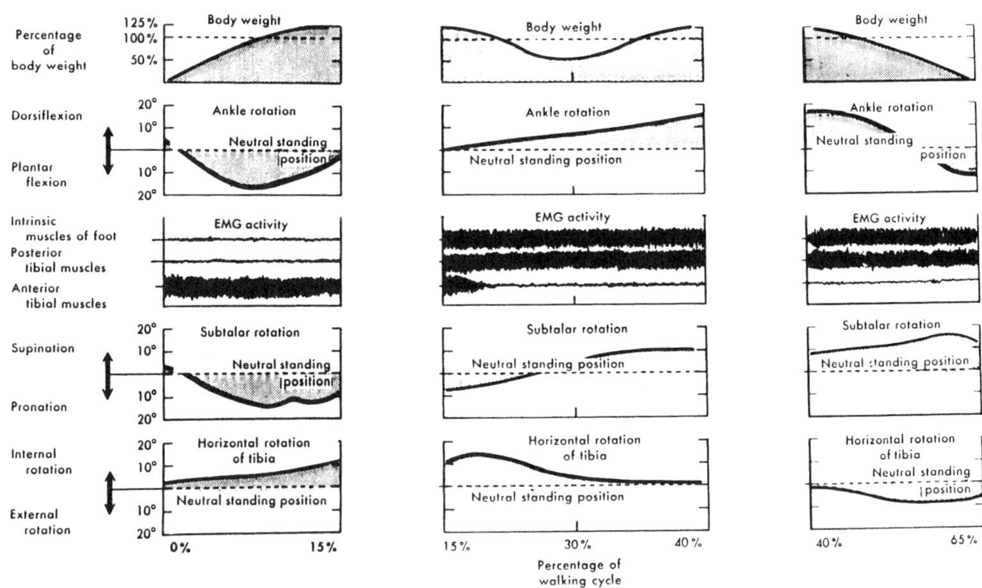

Figure 11-4. Stance phase of gait cycle. *From top to bottom:* Vertical ground reaction force. Ankle rotation. Muscle activity. Subtalar rotation. Tibial rotation. (*Left*) Heel-strike to foot-flat; (*middle*) foot-flat to heel-rise; (*right*) heel-rise to toe-off. (From Mann, RA. Biomechanics of the Foot and Ankle. In: RA Mann, MJ Coughlin, eds. *Surgery of the Foot and Ankle*, 6th ed. St. Louis: Mosby, 1993. Pp 29–31.) Reprinted with permission, Mosby-Year Book Inc.

During foot-flat, the ankle joint is progressively dorsiflexed as the body moves forward over the foot. The posterior calf muscles are active, with eccentric contraction that provides control of forward movement of the body. The tibialis posterior is active, with eccentric contraction that may limit or dampen eversion (pronation) of the subtalar joint [11]. The transverse tarsal articulation is flexible, allowing for adaptation to nonlevel surfaces.

As foot-flat progresses, the subtalar joint is progressively inverted (supinated) out of the maximally everted (pronated) position, with concentric contraction of the tibialis posterior. The intrinsic muscles also are active as supination occurs during foot-flat, with earlier activity noted in flatfooted individuals [12]. Inversion of the subtalar joint results in locking of the transverse tarsal joint so that the foot may serve as a rigid lever for heel-rise.

During early heel-rise, active ankle plantar flexion is effected by concentric gastrocsoleus activity, which then ceases as further plantar flexion occurs as the body continues to move forward. Body weight is transferred to the metatarsal heads and toes, and metatarsophalangeal joint dorsiflexion occurs. The maximum first metatarsophalangeal joint force is 0.8 times body weight [13]. Stability of the midfoot arch is in part a result of the plantar aponeurosis (windlass effect) [7, 8], locking of the transverse tarsal articulation associated with inversion of the subtalar joint [3], intrinsic muscle activity [12], and vertical compression stresses at the talonavicular joint with the foot plantar flexed.

At toe-off, activity of the calf muscles ceases. Ankle joint dorsiflexion occurs by concentric tibialis anterior contraction, which enables clearance of the toes during the swing phase.

During normal gait (in contrast with standing), load-bearing function of the forefoot is three times that of the hindfoot [14]. After heel-strike, a peak of pressure under the forefoot occurs with forefoot impact on the ground as the ankle is plantar flexed and foot-flat is achieved [15]. The center of pressure moves rapidly from the heel to the metatarsal head area, where it remains from 30% to 55% of the gait cycle, and then moves to the great toe. Another peak of pressure under the forefoot occurs during heel-rise and toe-off [15]. Peak pressure is greatest under the first, second, and third metatarsal heads [16, 17]. The toes are important in weight bearing during the last 30% of stance phase [1].

Effect of Aging

Aging-related changes in joint range of motion, muscle strength, and tissue properties may affect gait [18, 19]. Range of motion of lower-extremity joints, including the hip and knee, diminishes with increased age [20]. A small decrease in active range of plantar flexion, abduction, and adduction of the foot and ankle complex as a function of age also has been demonstrated [21]. Progressive muscle atrophy occurs with increased age; total skeletal muscle mass decreases by 40% from ages 24 to 80, with three-fourths of this decline occurring between ages 50 and 80 [22, 23]. Collagen stability increases with age, evidenced by the progressively increased resistance to collagenase digestion of human diaphragm tendon from ages 20 to 80 [24].

Gait patterns differ between younger and older individuals [25–27]. Men aged 60 to 65 have decreased stride and step length and greater out-toeing compared with those aged 20 to 25 years [26], and male subjects from 67 to 87 years have decreased stride length and percentage of time in swing phase [27]. After age 80, other measured gait parameters also are different than in younger individuals, including increased out-toeing and decreased ankle plantar flexion after heel-strike during fast walking [27]. Older women (ages 60–84) also demonstrate decreased stride length, step length, and ankle range of motion when compared to younger subjects (age 20–35 years) [25].

A problem in studies of balance and locomotion is to distinguish changes related to normal aging from those secondary to disease processes. Gait and function may be affected by diseases that have increased prevalence with age. When subjects are carefully selected to exclude those with history, symptoms, or physical signs of disorders that may affect gait, step length is shorter in older subjects; however, no differences in step-to-step variability of gait parameters are observed between older and control subjects [28]. Therefore, clinically observed variability of gait patterns with increased age is not aging-specific but may be a result of pathological processes that are associated with increased age [28]. In the clinical situation, both aging-specific and disease-related effects may be important.

EFFECTS OF FOOT AND ANKLE PROBLEMS ON STANDING AND GAIT

Definitions

By definition, a musculoskeletal deformity is described by the orientation of the distal part relative to the proximal. In a forefoot abduction deformity, the longitudinal axis of the forefoot is in abduction relative to that of the hindfoot. In valgus deformity, the distal part is angulated lateral to the normal position in relation to the proximal structure; in varus deformity, the distal part is angulated medially. Equinus deformity is a plantar-flexion deformity of the foot; in calcaneus deformity, the calcaneus is in a position of greater dorsiflexion than is normal.

Malalignment of the arch may consist of cavus (high-arch), flatfoot (low-arch), or rocker bottom (convex plantar) deformity. On the lateral standing radiograph of the normal foot, the longitudinal axis of the talus is colinear with that of the first metatarsal. In a cavus foot, the first metatarsal is plantar flexed relative to the talus; in flatfoot deformity, the first metatarsal is dorsiflexed relative to the talus because of collapse in the midfoot, and the forefoot is abducted relative to the hindfoot. Flexible flatfoot deformity usually is asymptomatic, and no specific treatment is required. However, a rigid flatfoot (such as from tarsal coalition) or acquired flatfoot (as with posterior tibial tendon rupture) may cause pain and limit function. Evaluation of the cause of the deformity may enable rational treatment.

Pathomechanics: The Effect of Foot and Ankle Conditions on Gait and Balance

General Considerations

Several mechanisms may contribute to changes in gait and balance (Table 11-1). Disease or conditions of the foot and ankle may affect balance and gait by causing limitation of joint motion (stiffness, ankylosis, arthrodesis), alteration of stress patterns (fixed deformity), or muscle weakness (paralysis, nerve injury). For example, with footdrop deformity secondary to tibialis anterior weakness or with fixed equinus deformity resulting from congenital or arthritic condition, increased hip and knee flexion or circumduction may be observed during the swing phase to effect clearance of the foot.

Limited motion or deformity of a joint, such as with degenerative arthritis, orthosis use, or arthrodesis, also may result in increased stresses and secondary degenerative arthritis in adjacent joints. Limitation of ankle range of motion from degenerative arthritis or arthrodesis may result in increased stresses and degenerative changes in the joints of the foot. Limited flexibility resulting from tight

Table 11-1. Factors contributing to changes in gait or balance

Foot structure, deformity, or malalignment
    Varus alignment (distal part medial compared with normal position)
    Valgus alignment (distal part lateral compared with normal position)
    Flatfoot
        Flexible
        Rigid: congenital or acquired
    Cavus foot
    Hallux valgus
    Hammertoes
Limitation of joint motion
Compensatory gait patterns
    Weight shifting, limp
Pain
Limitations in strength
    Acquired (e.g., tendon rupture)
    Atrophy (e.g., immobilization)
Limitations in flexibility
    Achilles tendon
Effects of treatment
    Arthrodesis
    Orthoses (e.g., ankle-foot orthosis, rocker bottom shoe)
Shoe wear
    High heels
    Heel counter support
    Toe box
    Arch support
    Sole

soft-tissue structures, such as Achilles tendon contracture, also may cause increased stresses elsewhere in the foot-ankle complex.

Joint deformity may alter adjacent soft-tissue structures and result in painful conditions. With second metatarsophalangeal joint dislocation dorsally, the plantar fat pad normally beneath the metatarsal head is displaced distally, resulting in increased stresses and a painful callus under the second metatarsal head (Fig. 11-5).

Muscle weakness may contribute to limited muscle function during the gait cycle and thus may lead to compensatory gait patterns and increased stresses on other parts. Tendon rupture also may be associated with secondary deformity because of increased stresses on static structures, such as ligaments and joints, resulting from loss of dynamic musculotendinous stabilizing mechanisms. Posterior tibialis tendon rupture is a major cause of acquired flatfoot deformity.

Painful conditions also may result in altered patterns of gait because of the tendency to avoid moving or stressing the painful part, even in the absence of demonstrable weakness, deformity, or limitation of joint motion. This may result in increased stresses on other parts of the foot and ankle (weight shifting),

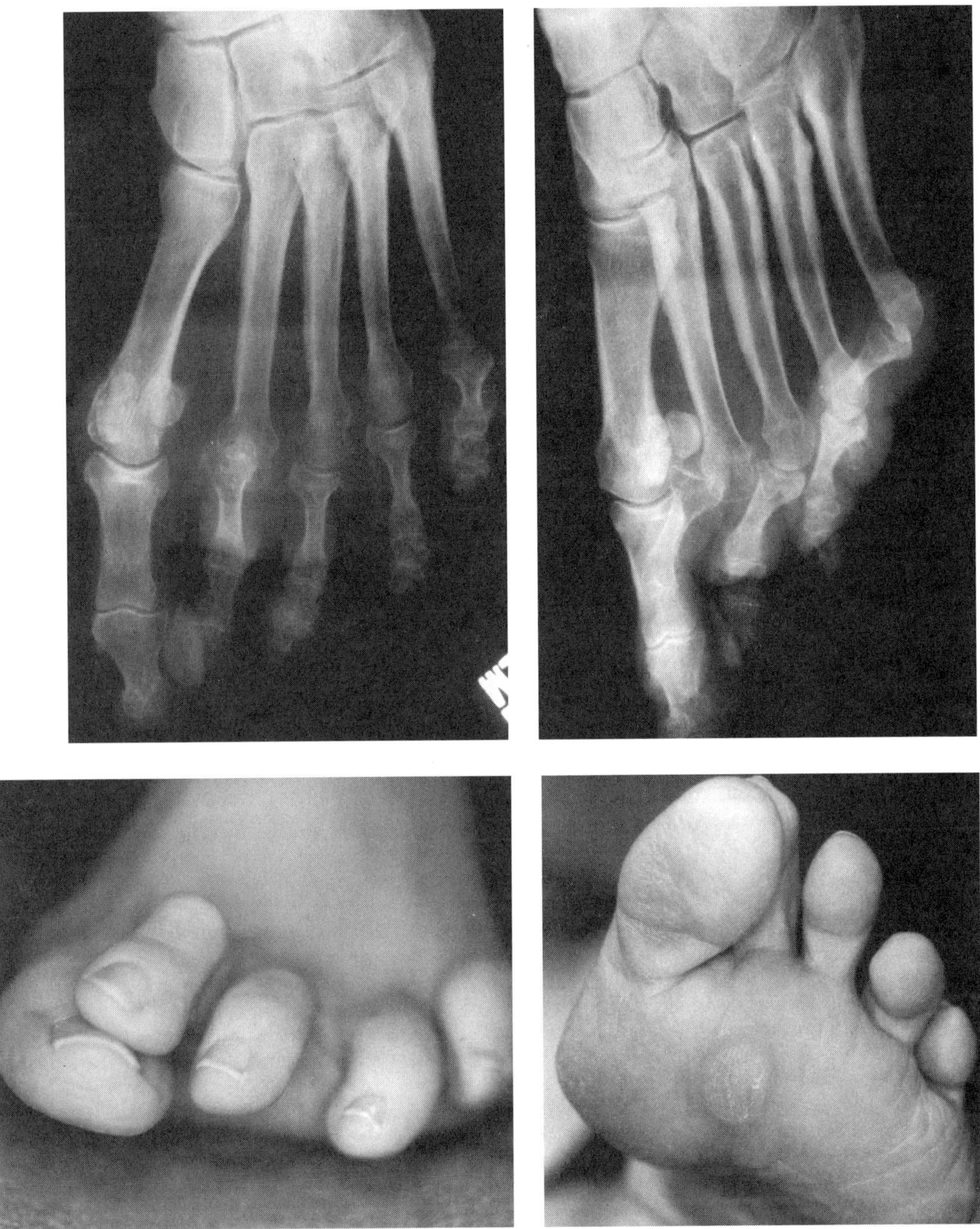

Figure 11-5. Crossover deformity of a 62-year-old woman's second toe. The second metatarsophalangeal joint is dislocated, and a second hammertoe is present. The dorsal position of the toe causes distal migration of the plantar fat pad from under the second metatarsal head, resulting in a localized painful plantar keratosis.

resulting in secondary painful conditions. Some patients with plantar fasciitis seek evaluation for pain under the lateral border of the foot caused by lateral weight shifting to avoid further mechanical irritation of the plantar fascia.

If untreated, weight shifting to avoid the secondary condition may lead to a tertiary condition. In some instances, evaluation of a foot with longstanding pain may reveal several distinct irritated structures, and it may be difficult to establish the identity of the primary condition.

The Ankle

Ankle motion normally occurs throughout the gait cycle (see Fig. 11-4). From heel-strike to foot-flat of the stance phase, progressive ankle plantar flexion occurs as the foot comes flat onto the ground, controlled by eccentric contraction of the tibialis anterior muscle. From foot-flat to heel-off, progressive dorsiflexion occurs as the body moves over the weight-bearing limb. From heel-off to toe-off, ankle plantarflexion occurs. During the swing phase, ankle dorsiflexion, accomplished by concentric tibialis anterior contraction, is required for clearance of the foot.

Stiffness or ankylosis of the ankle joint may affect gait in various ways, depending on the position of the joint. Ankylosis in the plantar-flexed (equinus) position effectively lengthens the lower limb (Fig. 11-6) and may result in (1) decreased stride length; (2) hyperextension of the knee ("back-knee" or genu recurvatum) after foot-flat is achieved and the body moves forward without progressive ankle dorsiflexion, resulting in strain on the knee; (3) early heel-off, with prolonged weight bearing in the forefoot and associated pain under the metatarsal heads; and (4) difficult toe clearance during the swing phase, resulting in toe-drag, compensatory increased hip and knee flexion, or circumduction of the lower limb. Ankylosis of the ankle in the dorsiflexed position is less common and may cause: (1) prolonged weight bearing on the heel in early stance phase, with associated heel pain and balance difficulty because foot-flat is delayed, and (2) difficulty with heel-rise because plantar flexion is limited.

Ankylosis or arthrodesis of the ankle may result in increased dorsiflexion and plantar-flexion stresses on other joints including the subtalar and transverse tarsal joints. Over time, this may result in hypermobility of these joints and associated instability with collapse of the arch or in progressive degenerative joint disease.

Weakness of ankle motors also may affect gait patterns. Tibialis anterior weakness may result in (1) slap-foot gait from heel-strike to foot-flat because of limited eccentric strength, (2) toe-drag or compensatory increased hip and knee flexion during the swing phase (steppage gait) [29], and (3) compensatory use of the long toe extensors (extensor hallucis and digitorum longus) that may result in hammertoe deformity. Gastrocsoleus weakness may result in a vaulting gait pattern because of limited deceleration of forward movement of the body from foot-flat to heel-off, and in limited heel-rise.

Ankle immobilization with an ankle-foot orthosis (AFO), commonly used for stabilization of a footdrop or flail ankle, may improve impaired gait patterns.

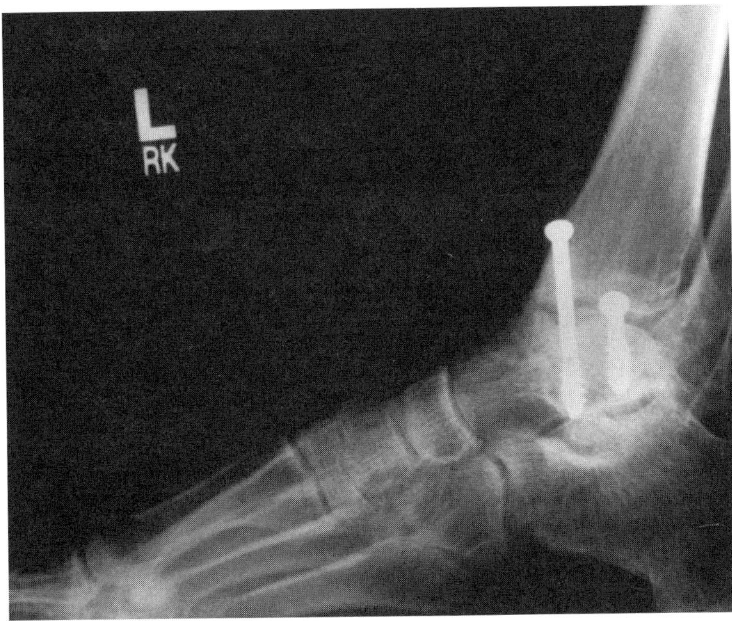

Figure 11-6. Ankylosis of the ankle in plantarflexion. This patient had been treated for an ankle fracture but developed posttraumatic arthritis; subsequent ankle arthrodesis was complicated by painful nonunion, with malposition in plantar-flexion.

With peroneal nerve dysfunction, the decreased time from heel-strike to foot-flat and shortened contralateral step length may be restored to normal with an AFO [29]. Nevertheless, an AFO does not restore efficiency of gait to normal, as is evidenced by residual increased ipsilateral hip and knee flexion during the swing phase [29].

The Subtalar and Transverse Tarsal Joints

At heel-strike, the subtalar joint is inverted (supinated) (see Fig. 11-4). Eversion (pronation) of the subtalar joint occurs through the early foot-flat period, dampened by eccentric contraction of the posterior tibialis muscle. As foot-flat progresses to heel-rise, progressive inversion of the subtalar joint from the maximally everted position occurs with concentric contraction of the posterior tibialis muscle. Inversion of the subtalar joint is maintained after heel-rise until toe-off [30].

Subtalar joint stiffness, ankylosis, or arthrodesis is associated with a reduced agility in walking, particularly on nonlevel surfaces. The coupling of subtalar eversion with tibial internal rotation, and inversion with external rotation (see Fig. 11-4) is not functional when subtalar motion is limited, resulting in altered stress pattern proximally and reduced efficiency of gait. The loss of dynamic unlocking of the transverse tarsal articulation with subtalar eversion in early foot-flat may cause reduced ability to adapt to nonlevel surfaces. Subtalar ankylosis in the inverted position also may limit adaptation to nonlevel surfaces, because the transverse tarsal articulation may be locked when flexibility is required. With subtalar ankylosis in eversion, push-off strength may be limited because the transverse tarsal joint may be flexible so that the foot cannot function as a rigid lever as with subtalar inversion and locking of transverse tarsal joint, and because posterior tibialis muscle action is ineffective in achieving inversion of the subtalar joint and associated support of the arch. Over time, increased stresses on the ankle and transverse tarsal joints, resulting from limited subtalar motion, may cause degenerative changes in these joints, as seen in patients with talocalcaneal coalitions.

Pantalar arthrodesis, which includes fusion of the ankle, subtalar, and transverse tarsal joints, may restrict motion markedly and result in degeneration of joints in the midfoot (Fig. 11-7). Malunion of a pantalar arthrodesis in plantar flexion may be particularly stressful on the midfoot and forefoot; the lower extremity is effectively lengthened, and increased stresses may occur under the forefoot and in the midfoot joints (see Fig. 11-7).

Subtalar joint position is a major determinant of the alignment of the distal regions of the foot. Deformity of the calcaneus or subtalar joint may be associated with weight shifting and associated pain. Varus (inversion) deformity of the hindfoot after calcaneus fracture may result in increased weight bearing and a painful callus under the lateral side of the foot. Varus malunion after subtalar or triple arthrodesis may similarly be associated with lateral heel pain. Valgus (eversion) deformity, resulting from degenerative subtalar joint arthritis or posterior tibial tendon rupture, may cause increased stresses and progressive degenerative arthritis on the medial side of the foot.

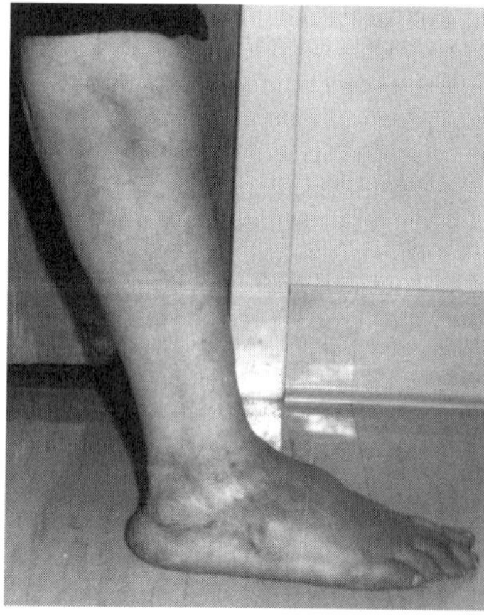
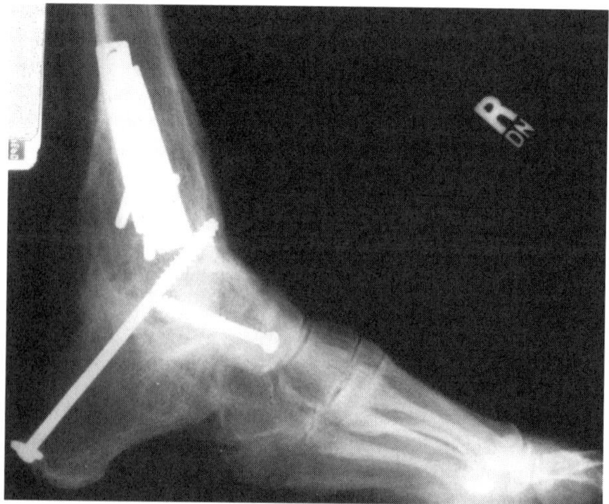

Figure 11-7. Pantalar arthrodesis in plantar-flexed malposition. The plantar flexion deformity subsequently was corrected with distal tibial dorsiflexion osteotomy. The patient later developed painful degenerative changes at the metatarsal-cuneiform joints.

Posterior tibial tendon dysfunction secondary to tendinitis, tenosynovitis, or rupture may cause gait disturbance because of limited active inversion of the subtalar joint and hindfoot support during heel-rise.

The Midfoot

The normal stabilizing functions of the midfoot arch during gait may be absent in conditions that result in abnormal alignment or hypermobility of joints. In the normal foot, force transmission through the talonavicular joint in the direction of the longitudinal axis of the foot occurs during heel-rise; the resulting talonavicular compression is a component of arch stability. In acquired flatfoot deformity secondary to conditions such as posterior tibial tendon rupture, trauma, or degenerative joint disease, subluxation of the talonavicular joint into a dorsiflexed and abducted position may be present, with associated poor push-off power. Limitation of motion at the hindfoot-midfoot junction, such as from a calcaneonavicular coalition, may result in increased stresses on adjacent joints and premature degenerative change.

At the junction between the midfoot and forefoot, hypermobility of the first metatarsal-cuneiform joint may contribute to painful forefoot deformities. Varus malalignment of the first metatarsal secondary to hypermobility may be a contributing factor for some instances of bunion deformity. Increased dorsiflexion of the first metatarsal secondary to degenerative joint disease or ligament insufficiency at the first metatarsal-cuneiform joint, may reduce weight bearing by the first metatarsal head and cause weight shifting to the second metatarsal head, with associated painful callus.

The Forefoot

During normal gait, the functions of the forefoot include weight bearing and balance. The first and second metatarsal heads usually are the most distal, and the fifth is the most proximal. Body weight usually is shared by all the metatarsal heads when the heel is elevated, either while standing or during push-off in gait. The line connecting the second and fifth metatarsal heads forms the metatarsal break, an axis 50 to 70 degrees oblique to the long axis of the foot [31]. During heel-rise, supination and lateral deviation of the foot (primarily due to inversion of the subtalar joint) occurs so that body weight is distributed among the metatarsal heads and toes; balance from heel-rise to toe-off thereby is maximized because all five metatarsal heads are used for weight bearing. Dorsiflexion of the metatarsophalangeal joints occurs, enabling the toes to remain on the floor for balance.

Footwear may markedly alter plantar forefoot pressures. Forefoot impact pressure during the early part of the stance phase may be reduced with training shoes, soft metatarsal pads, or insoles [15, 32] and may be increased with high heels [15, 33]. However, heel height or insoles have little effect on pressure in the forefoot from heel-rise to toe-off [15]. Shoe modification with a rocker bottom sole may reduce peak pressures in the medial and central forefoot and toes by 30% but may result in increased pressures in the heel, midfoot, and lateral forefoot [34].

Postoperative shoes, casts, and cast boots reduce peak forces under the forefoot and heel of normal feet compared with barefoot ambulation [35, 36]. Short-leg walking casts and insoles also reduce shear forces, in addition to vertical forces, under the metatarsal heads of normal feet during walking [36] and may be useful in the treatment of neuropathic ulceration [37]. Patients with diabetic neuropathy and foot deformities may have areas of abnormally high plantar pressure, increasing the risk of plantar ulceration [38, 39]. Both vertical and shear stresses [36] as well as dynamic (gait) and static (standing) pressures [38] may contribute to neuropathic ulceration. These plantar pressures in neuropathic feet may be reduced with shoe modifications, insoles, and casts [39].

Weight shifting may occur in deformities of the forefoot. Amputation of the great toe results in weight bearing more lateral in the forefoot, with center of pressure passing out toward the third toe [40]. In feet with hallux valgus, there is less weight borne by the first and second toes and more by the lateral metatarsals [41]. Lateral weight shifting also has been demonstrated after silicone metatarsophalangeal joint arthroplasty [42] and may result in a painful callus under the second metatarsal head because of the increased load carried by this area. In diabetic neuropathic feet, less load is borne by the toes and more by the first metatarsal head, which may increase the risk of neuropathic ulceration at this site [43]. In patients with a painful forefoot condition, the center of pressure remains near the heel for a longer period and in the metatarsal head area for a shorter period than for those with normal feet [14], and this may result in heel pain syndromes.

Heel Pad

The plantar heel pad is a specialized arrangement of fat chambers separated by septal walls that dissipate impact forces under the calcaneus during heel-strike [44, 45]. Isolated heel pads have greater shock-absorbing capacity than do ethyl vinyl acetate or Sorbothane, synthetic materials used in shoe soles and orthotic inserts [46]. However, heel pads isolated from cadavers vary in shock absorbency by as much as 100% between different specimens [46], suggesting wide clinical variation between individual heels. Blunt trauma to heel pads reduces shock absorbency, presumably because of disruption of the internal architecture. External confinement with casts or cuplike orthoses and padding the heel with silicone rubber heel cushions may improve impact dissipation during heel-strike [46].

The load pattern on the heel may be changed by varus or valgus deformity of the heel resulting from trauma or degenerative conditions. Atrophy of the heel pad may be observed in some elderly individuals with heel pain and is a potential complication of local corticosteroid injection. Occasionally, increased fat pad mobility in response to shear may contribute to heel pain.

Plantar Fascia

The function of the plantar fascia is to stabilize the longitudinal arch, particularly during heel-rise, when the ligament is under increased tension as a result of dorsiflexion of the toes (see Fig. 11-3). Irritation of the plantar fascia may affect gait by resulting in lateral weight shifting and pain along the lateral border of the foot. Stiffness and pain may be noted during the initial steps from resting positions, such as lying in bed or sitting in a chair, because of tension along the adhesions and contracture of the plantar fascia that form with the foot in the plantar-flexed position. A complete tear of the plantar fascia may result in difficulty with gait from heel-rise to toe-off, and progressive hammertoe deformity may occur.

ETIOLOGY OF COMMON FOOT AND ANKLE DISORDERS

Disorders in the foot and ankle can result in disturbances of gait and balance. Such disorders may be caused by a broad range of conditions (Table 11-2).

Trauma

Trauma to the foot and ankle may cause injury to bones, joints, or soft-tissue structures, including tendons, ligaments, or nerves.

Table 11-2. Etiology of foot and ankle disorders

Trauma	Poliomyelitis
Bone (fracture)	Interdigital (Morton's) neuroma
Joint (osteochondral defect, fracture, synovitis)	Traumatic neuromas
Tendon (Achilles, posterior tibial)	Entrapment neuropathies (tarsal tunnel
Ligament (ankle, subtalar, plantar fascia,	syndrome, sural nerve entrapment)
metatarsophalangeal collateral)	Iatrogenic (incisional neuroma)
Heel pad	Reflex sympathetic dystrophy
Degenerative	Congenital
Joints (arthritis)	Tarsal coalition
Hallux rigidus	Clubfoot
Tendon (partial or full-thickness rupture)	Tumor or neoplasm
Posterior tibial tendon	Ganglion cyst
Achilles tendon	Lipoma
Inflammatory (non-rheumatologic)	Malignancy
Plantar fascia	Structural
Idiopathic synovitis	Hallux valgus
Rheumatological	Hammertoe
Rheumatoid arthritis	Mallet toe
Gout	Hard corn
Pseudogout (calcium pyrophosphate	Soft corn
deposition disease)	Sports injury
Reiter's syndrome	Single-impact
Psoriatic arthritis	Repetitive microtrauma (overuse)
Ankylosing spondylitis	Treatment-associated (Iatrogenic)
Lyme disease	Implant arthroplasty
Neuropathic or neurological	Painful scar
Charcot's disease or diabetes	Infectious
Stroke	Bacterial
Traumatic brain injury	Fungal

Single-impact fractures are caused by bending, tension, compression, and twisting forces. When angulation or displacement of the fracture changes the orientation of regions involved in weight bearing, the associated deformity may be a cause of pain and altered gait pattern (Fig. 11-8). If not adequately corrected, a dorsiflexion deformity of a first metatarsal shaft fracture may lead to increased weight bearing and a consequent painful callus under the second metatarsal head.

Fractures extending to joint surfaces and joint dislocations may result in post-traumatic arthritis (Fig. 11-9). The original injury may include direct trauma to the articular hyaline cartilage, and the healed fibrocartilage surface does not have normal long-term durability. An intra-articular fracture may result in irregularity or step-off at the joint surface, which may result in progressive degeneration of the joint (Fig. 11-10). A more subtle joint injury is the osteochondral defect, a fracture of the articular cartilage and underlying subchondral bone. This injury

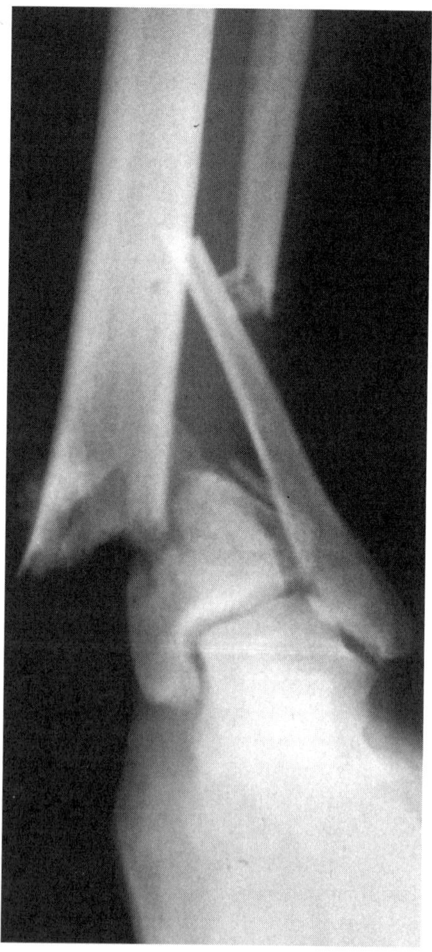

Figure 11-8. Open tibia-fibula fracture in a 55-year-old woman after fall from a stepladder. Treatment included irrigation and debridement of the wound, with reduction and cast immobilization.

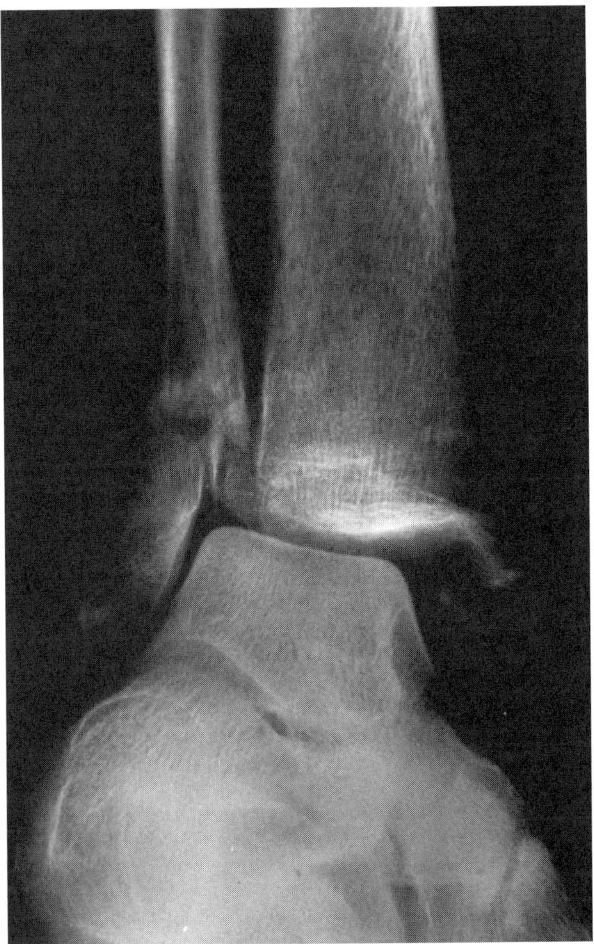

Figure 11-9. Bimalleolar ankle fracture in a 72-year-old man who fell from a ladder. Treatment included open reduction and internal fixation.

may be difficult to visualize on plain-film radiography and may be misdiagnosed initially as a sprain. However, the irregularity of the joint surface may predispose to degenerative arthritis.

Ligament sprains are partial or complete tears of the ligamentous structures that passively stabilize joints. The most common sprain in the ankle involves the lateral ankle ligaments secondary to inversion injury. If the ligaments heal in a lengthened position, joint instability and symptoms of "giving-way," particularly on nonlevel surfaces, may occur. Unrecognized occult fractures also may occur in injuries initially diagnosed as ankle sprain, with residual pain and dysfunction. Some ligament sprains in the foot, such as tears of the supportive ligaments at the tarsometatarsal (Lisfranc's) joints, have a poor prognosis and a high incidence of residual pain.

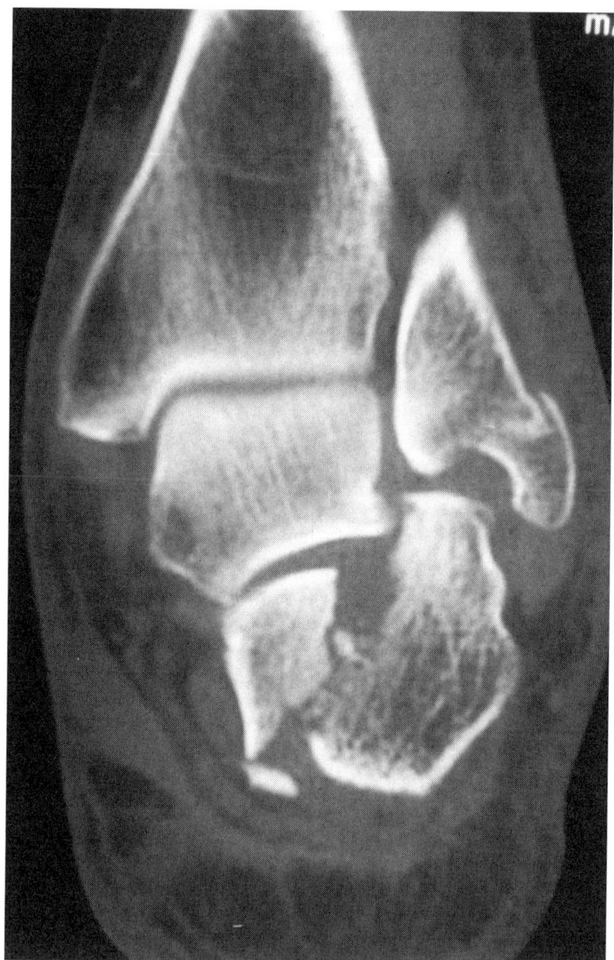

Figure 11-10. Calcaneus fracture in a 69-year-old woman who fell on concrete steps at a swimming pool. Coronal computed tomography scan reveals deformity of the calcaneus including widening of the bone, displacement at the subtalar joint, and impingement of the displaced lateral calcaneus fragment against the distal fibula. A nondisplaced fibular fracture also is present.

Musculotendinous injury includes contusions, strains (partial tears), or complete tendon rupture. Achilles tendon rupture may occur in activities such as basketball or tennis, and the individual may note sudden pain in the posterior leg ("as if kicked by somebody") and difficulty in walking. The diagnosis of this and other complete tendon ruptures may be delayed because radiographs are normal, motor examination is limited by pain, and rupture is unsuspected by the examining clinician.

Contusions of the foot may be problematic because some patients have persistent pain, swelling, and difficulty in walking long after the injury was expected to have resolved. This may occur because large forces may cause injury to various structures and tissues. Contributing factors to poor prognosis include inadequate period of immobilization; contusion to nerves and development of reflex sympathetic dystrophy; unrecognized occult fracture, joint injury, or ligament tear such as a Lisfranc's (tarsometatarsal) injury; or underlying conditions such as diabetes or vascular disease. Contusions of the plantar heel pad or disruption of this structure secondary to a calcaneus fracture may cause chronic pain at heel-strike and associated gait disturbance.

Failure to improve after traumatic injury despite a reasonable period of immobilization should raise the suspicion of the presence of an occult fracture or reflex sympathetic dystrophy, and technetium radionuclide bone scintigraphy may be indicated to evaluate for these possibilities.

Degenerative Change

Primary degenerative arthritis may occur in the ankle, subtalar, talonavicular, tarsometatarsal (Lisfranc's), and first metatarsophalangeal joint. A history of trauma may be present, particularly in the ankle and Lisfranc's regions. Symptoms of degenerative arthritis in the foot and ankle include morning stiffness and pain with weight bearing and motion of the involved joint. Examination may reveal tenderness of the involved joint to palpation, pain with range of motion, swelling, and crepitance. Radiographic changes include joint space narrowing, sclerosis, and osteophytes.

Degenerative arthritis of the first metatarsophalangeal joint (hallux rigidus) is one of the most commonly observed nontraumatic, idiopathic arthritides in the foot (Fig. 11-11). First metatarsophalangeal joint dorsiflexion is important from heel-rise to toe-off, allowing for weight bearing by the great toe during the latter part of the stance phase. With hallux rigidus, heel-rise may be limited because of a limited range of first metatarsophalangeal joint dorsiflexion and because of associated pain. Furthermore, pain resulting from impingement of dorsal osteophytes may limit walking distances and cause lateral weight shifting. Treatment may include shoe modification with a stiff rocker sole to relieve dorsiflexion stresses on the metatarsophalangeal joints. In some patients, debridement of osteophytes (cheilectomy) or first metatarsophalangeal joint arthrodesis (fusion) may provide symptomatic relief.

Ankle joint arthritis may result in decreased stride length during gait because of the limitation of ankle motion required during foot-flat of the stance phase. Orthoses that limit ankle motion may provide adequate pain relief and improvement of gait in many patients (Fig. 11-12). When pain progresses and restricts walking, ankle arthrodesis is a reasonable option.

Degenerative conditions of tendons in the foot and ankle most commonly involve the Achilles and posterior tibial tendons. Irritation or erosion of the Achilles tendon by posterior calcaneal spurs may result in chronic pain or tendon rupture. Symptoms may include posterior heel pain on arising from bed, pain with gait, and aggravation by pressure from the heel counter of shoes. Achilles

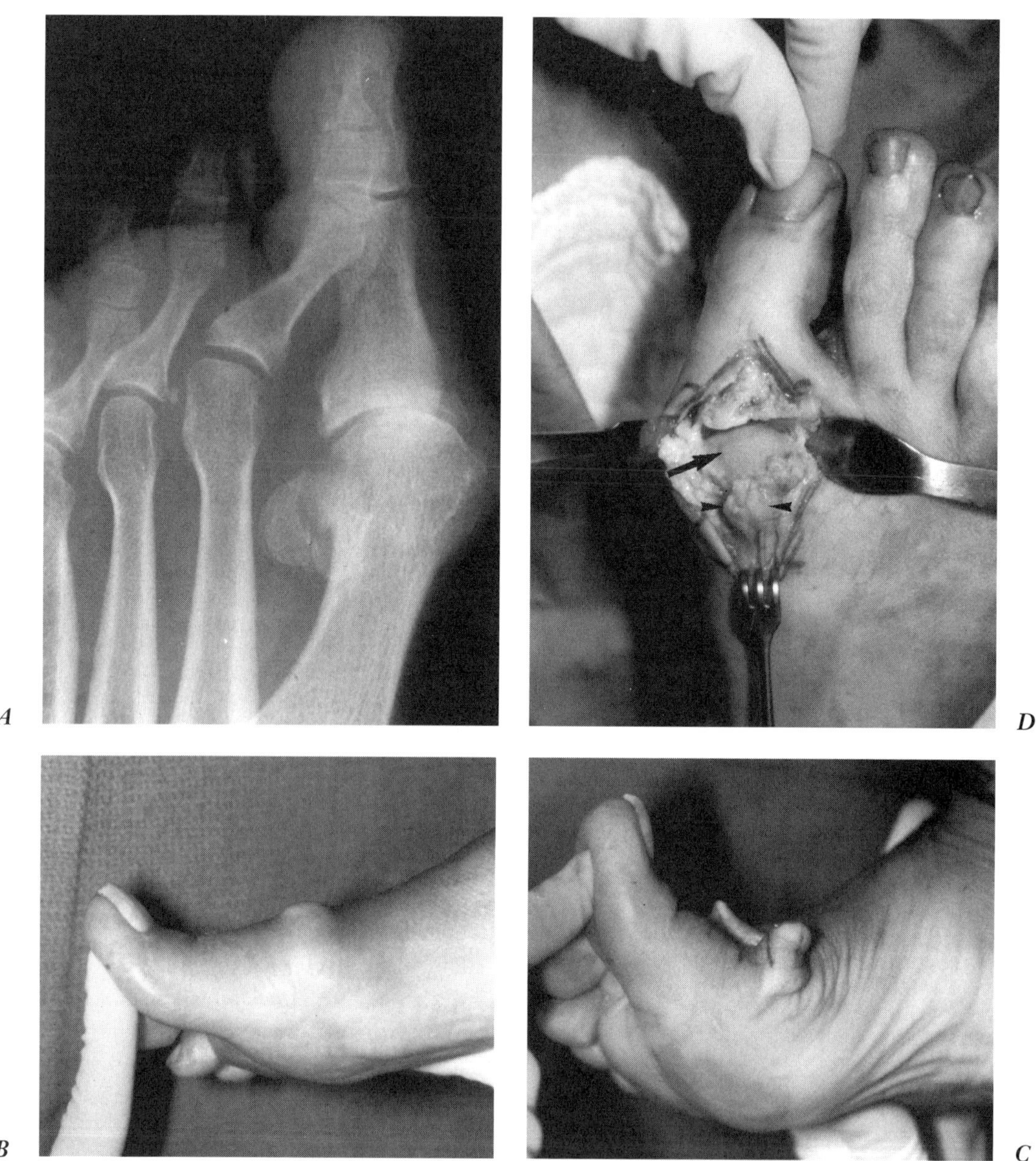

Figure 11-11. Hallux rigidus. *A.* Degenerative changes of the first metatarsophalangeal joint, including joint space narrowing, sclerosis, and osteophytes. *B.* Limitation of passive dorsiflexion. The dorsal osteophyte results in a visible "bump." *C.* Improved passive dorsiflexion after debridement of osteophytes (cheilectomy). *D.* Operative findings in another patient with hallux rigidus, demonstrating flat first metatarsal head (*arrow*), eburnation of joint surface (*arrow*), and large dorsal osteophyte (*arrowheads*).

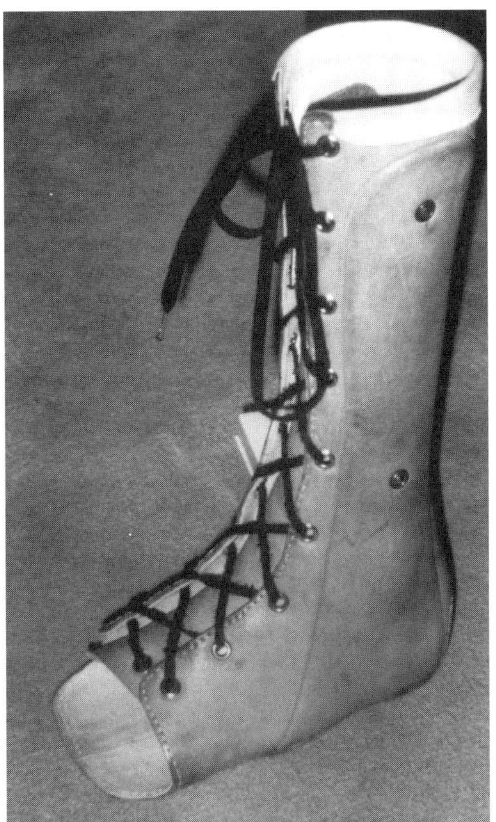

Figure 11-12. Custom-molded leather ankle brace with built-in plastic splinting material rigidly locks the ankle and hindfoot. This may alleviate pain associated with weight bearing in degenerative conditions.

tendon irritation also may involve the tendon proximal to the posterior calcaneal insertion. Full-time immobilization of an irritated tendon in the neutral position using commercially available orthoses for 6 to 12 weeks may decrease pain and increase the ability to walk (Fig. 11-13). It is important that immobilization be continued during the night to avoid contracture with the foot in the plantar-flexed position. Corticosteroid injection is avoided about tendons because it may contribute to the development of tendon rupture. Surgical debridement and repair of degenerated tendon may be indicated, especially if symptoms limit shoe wear or if impending rupture is suspected.

Posterior tibial tendon rupture is one of the most common causes of acquired flatfoot in adults. Rupture occurs most frequently between the medial malleolus and the navicular, and hypovascularity of the tendon in this area may contribute to degeneration or rupture [47]. Obesity and hypertension are associated with posterior tibial tendon rupture, and systemic or local injections of corticosteroid also may contribute to the problem [48]. A patient may have a history of pain and swelling involving the medial hindfoot and ankle. The longitudinal arch gradually collapses, with wear pattern on the medial side of the shoe and progressively increased difficulty in walking. Symptoms are commonly present for greater

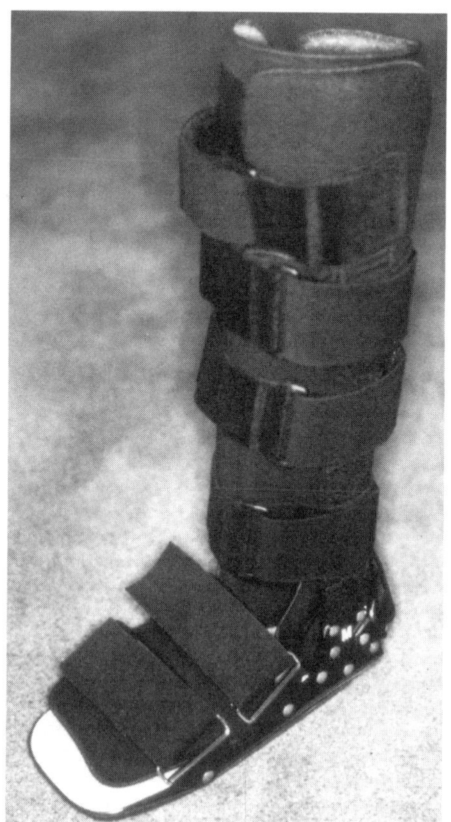

Figure 11-13. Removable short-leg walking cast brace with rocker sole, useful in treating foot and ankle conditions.

than 2 years prior to diagnosis [48]. Physical examination reveals flattening of the arch, medial prominence of the medial malleolus and talar head, forefoot abduction, and eversion (valgus) of the calcaneus, resulting from unopposed action of the peroneus brevis. On tiptoe stance, the patient is not able to invert the calcaneus, and fatigue occurs rapidly. Gait is impaired by pain and limitation of heel-rise. Treatment options include orthoses (see Fig. 11-12), tendon reconstruction, or hindfoot (subtalar, talonavicular, calcaneocuboid) arthrodesis.

Inflammation

Painful, nonrheumatological inflammatory conditions of the foot and ankle are common. Gait and balance may be affected by pain, limitation of function of the painful part, or weight shifting. Mechanical irritation that occurs during standing and walking may cause local inflammation to persist despite nonsteroidal antiinflammatory medication, corticosteroid injection, or physiotherapeutic modalities. For this reason, these conditions may be difficult to treat and may become chronic. Immobilization with shoes or orthoses may limit mechanical stresses, enabling local inflammation to decrease.

Plantar fasciitis is a common problem resulting in heel pain and alteration of gait pattern. Some patients with plantar fasciitis complain of pain in other regions (such as the lateral border of the foot), resulting from weight shifting to avoid the irritated plantar fascia. The plantar fascia is subject to increased irritation from two mechanisms. With each step of walking, dorsiflexion of the toes at heel-rise causes tension stresses on the plantar fascia (windlass mechanism), preventing an inflamed plantar fascia from healing. During resting conditions such as lying in bed or sitting, the foot usually is passively plantar flexed, which may result in adhesions and contracture of the plantar fascia; arising from bed in the morning or from the seated position may result in a sudden stretching or tearing of the adhesions, reirritating the inflamed ligament. Therefore, the patient may notice pain during the first few steps out of bed in the morning, when standing from the seated position, or on exiting a car. Examination may reveal tenderness along the plantar fascia which is increased with the toes in dorsiflexed position. Tenderness may not necessarily be present at the origin of the plantar fascia. The presence of a bony prominence on a lateral radiograph ("heel spur") is not contributory to the diagnosis of plantar fasciitis in most cases, because this finding may be present in asymptomatic individuals or absent in chronic plantar fasciitis. Mechanical methods such as night splints to prevent plantar flexion [49] have been helpful in the treatment of intractable cases.

Idiopathic, nontraumatic synovitis of the lesser metatarsophalangeal joint is a less common condition that may be mistaken for an interdigital neuroma [50]. This condition usually involves the second or third metatarsophalangeal joint. Swelling of the joint and toe, discrete tenderness and fullness of the joint, and occasionally tenderness of the adjacent interdigital nerve may be noted. The condition may be aggravated by dorsiflexion of the joint during heel-rise. Although synovectomy may be required in some cases [50], this condition may be successfully treated in many patients with intra-articular corticosteroid injection in conjunction with a rocker sole shoe for mechanical protection of the joint [51].

Sequelae of inflammatory synovitis of the metatarsophalangeal joints include distention and attenuation of the joint capsule, collateral ligaments, and plantar plate, resulting in metatarsophalangeal joint laxity, subluxation, and dislocation. The abnormal alignment of the tendons about the dislocated metatarsophalangeal joint may result in a hammertoe deformity. The dorsal position of the second toe allows the great toe to migrate laterally, resulting in hallux valgus and crossover deformity [52]. The plantar fat pad normally under the distal ends of the metatarsals is drawn distally, and a painful callus under the metatarsal head may result (see Fig. 11-5).

Tendon irritation may occur as a result of inflammation, as in Achilles or posterior tibial tendinitis. However, in older individuals, degenerative disease of tendons may be present (as noted earlier) and may be difficult to distinguish clinically from a purely inflammatory condition. Nevertheless, treatment options for tendinitis or tenosynovitis are similar to those for degenerative tendinosis without rupture, including immobilization or debridement and tenosynovectomy.

Rheumatism

Rheumatoid arthritis may cause structural and functional changes secondary to chronic synovitis. In the forefoot, synovitis of the metatarsophalangeal joints may result in joint capsule distention, attenuation, and instability (Fig. 11-14). This may result in severe hallux valgus deformity because of forces on the hallux in shoes. Lesser metatarsophalangeal joint dorsal dislocation may occur secondary to dorsiflexion stresses during heel-rise, resulting in distal migration of the plantar metatarsal fat pad and painful callus at the metatarsal heads.

In the midfoot, rheumatoid arthritis may result in fibrosis and ankylosis. However, loss of the longitudinal arch secondary to joint hypermobility and instability may occur. In the hindfoot, progressive destruction of the subtalar and transverse tarsal joints may occur, albeit less commonly and later than in the forefoot [53].

Treatment of the rheumatoid foot is individualized, based on patient symptoms and associated deformity. Patients may benefit from shoes with a wide and deep toe box, soft insoles, and rocker sole. Painful rheumatoid forefoot deformity also may be treated with first-metatarsophalangeal-joint arthrodesis to restore weight-bearing function to the first; lesser metatarsal head resection may allow the plantar metatarsal fat pad to resume the weight-bearing position, with improvement of the painful calluses (see Fig. 11-14). Gait is slower than normal but is improved because of satisfactory pain relief in most cases. In patients with concomitant severe hindfoot deformity, the latter usually is addressed first; realignment of the hindfoot with bracing or arthrodesis may alter stresses in the forefoot, forefoot symptoms, and treatment strategy.

Gout most commonly affects the first metatarsophalangeal joint with sudden, severe pain associated with swelling and erythema. Sodium urate crystals may be identified in joint aspirates examined under polarized light. Treatment includes rest and medical therapy, including indomethacin, colchicine, or allopurinol. Shoe modification with a rocker sole may alleviate dorsiflexion stresses on the metatarsophalangeal joint. In advanced cases, excision of tophaceous deposits may be indicated.

The seronegative spondyloarthropathies—ankylosing spondylitis, psoriatic arthritis, and Reiter's syndrome—may be characterized by heel pain secondary to Achilles tendinitis, plantar fasciitis, or both [54]. Forefoot and toe involvement also may be present in these conditions, especially psoriatic arthritis.

Neuropathy

Neurological conditions may result in deformity and altered gait patterns. Sensory peripheral neuropathy in diabetes is associated with repetitive trauma that contributes to the development of Charcot's arthropathy. In the Charcot foot and ankle, bone and joint destruction may result in severe deformities, including ankle or hindfoot varus or valgus or midfoot arch collapse and rocker bottom deformity (Fig. 11-15). Autonomic neuropathy of diabetes may result in intrinsic

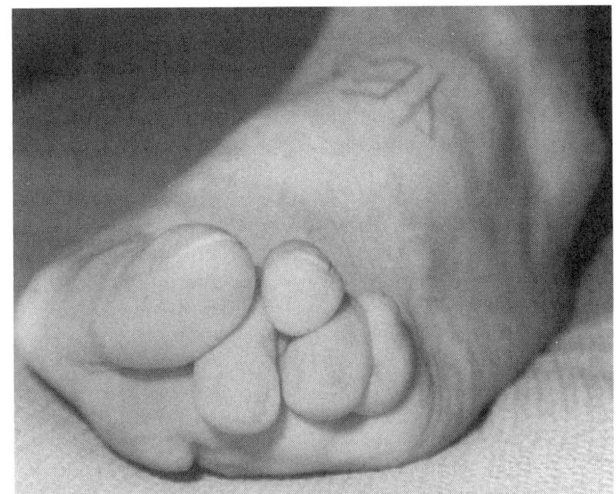

A

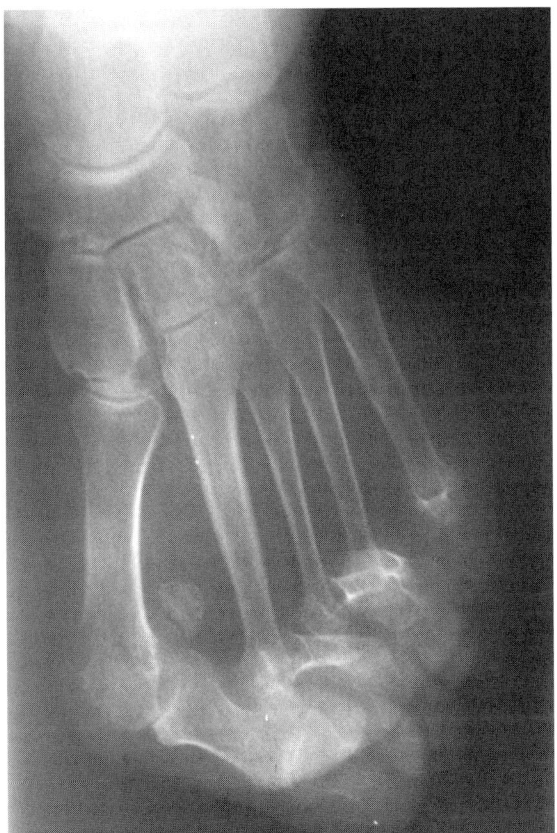

B

Figure 11-14. (A, B) Severe forefoot deformity in a 46-year-old woman with a 10-year history of rheumatoid arthritis. A marked hallux valgus deformity with subluxation of the first metatarsophalangeal joint is present. Dislocation of lesser metatarsophalangeal joints has resulted in distal migration of the plantar metatarsal fat pad and painful calluses under the metatarsal heads.

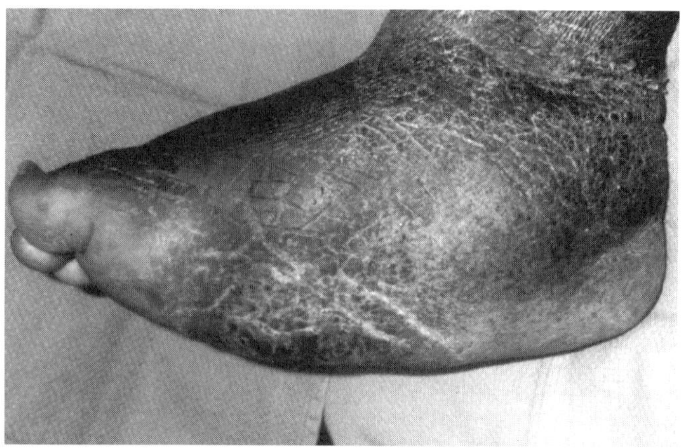
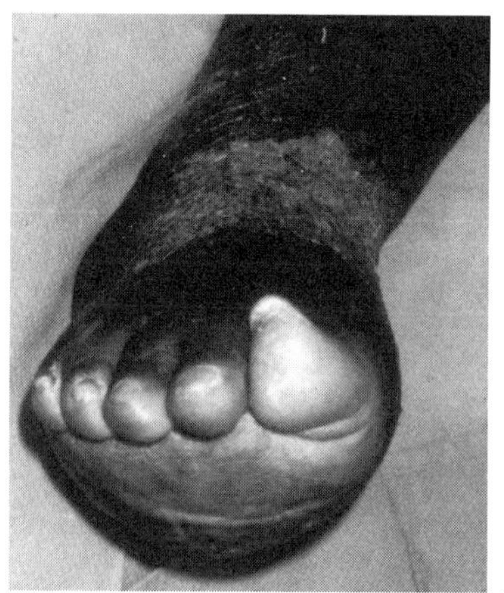

Figure 11-15. (A, B) Severe rocker-bottom and ankle varus deformities resulting from Charcot's arthropathy in a man with insulin-dependent diabetes mellitus. This patient had a good functional result after below-knee amputation.

muscle contracture and claw toes, which may limit weight bearing by the toes during gait.

Cavus foot deformity, as in Charcot-Marie-Tooth disease or poliomyelitis, is a result of muscle imbalance [55]. Movement abnormalities, including dystonia, weakness, spasms, tremor, and increased tone, may occur in reflex sympathetic dystrophy [56].

Congenital Deformity

Congenital deformities may affect gait patterns early in life because of abnormal shape or alignment of bones, resulting in abnormal weight-bearing patterns. Clubfoot with residual deformity and pain despite early treatment may be salvaged with hindfoot arthrodesis. Tarsal coalition is an abnormal nonosseous or bony connection between two bones and may limit normal motion and contribute to pain and degenerative joint disease (Fig. 11-16).

Neoplasm

Neoplastic conditions may cause pain and altered gait patterns because of specific location or treatment required. Plantar fibroma, a nodular growth on the plantar fascia associated with Dupuytren's disease, may cause pain and weight shifting because of tension on the plantar fascia during heel-rise or because of direct pressure on the plantar aspect of the foot. Ganglion cysts or lipomas occasionally may cause pain associated with shoe wear. Bone cysts, if large, may result in pathological fracture. Malignancies of the foot may necessitate amputation.

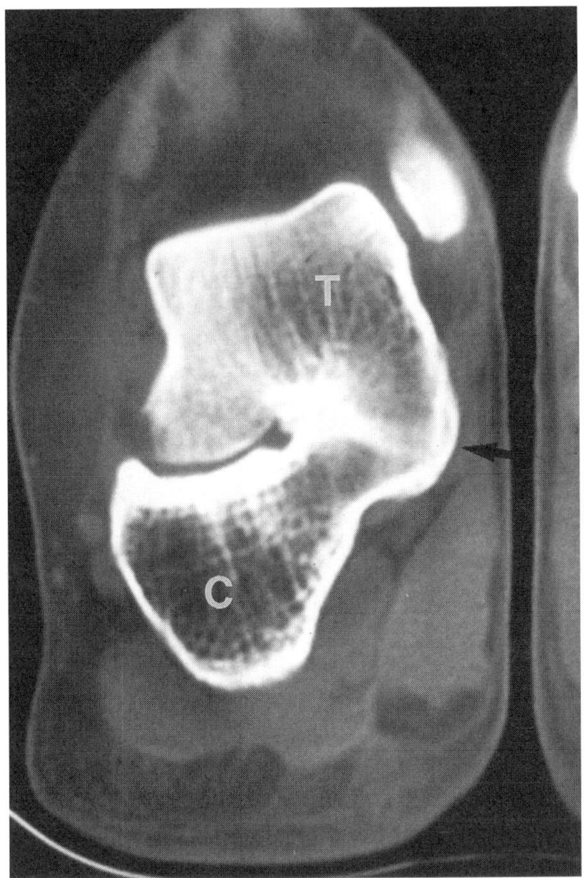

Figure 11-16. Coronal computed tomography scan of the hindfoot, demonstrating subtalar (talocalcaneal) coalition (*arrow*). T = talus; C = calcaneus.

Structural Deformity of the Toes

Hallux Valgus Deformity

Hallux valgus deformity is primarily a result of valgus pressure on the great toe from shoes with a narrow toe box. This may be aggravated by high heels, which tend to drive the forefoot deeper into the toe box. Other factors such as heredity, pes planus, varus alignment of the first metatarsal, and hypermobility of the first metatarsocuneiform joint (resulting from ligament laxity or degenerative changes) also may contribute to the development of hallux valgus deformity.

When hallux valgus develops, the line of action of the flexor tendons to the hallux lies lateral to the metatarsophalangeal joint. Radiographically this is evidenced by a medial shift of the metatarsal head relative to the sesamoids (Fig. 11-17). Once this alignment is established, active flexor activity tends to accentuate the valgus and pronation deformity of the hallux. The medial metatar-

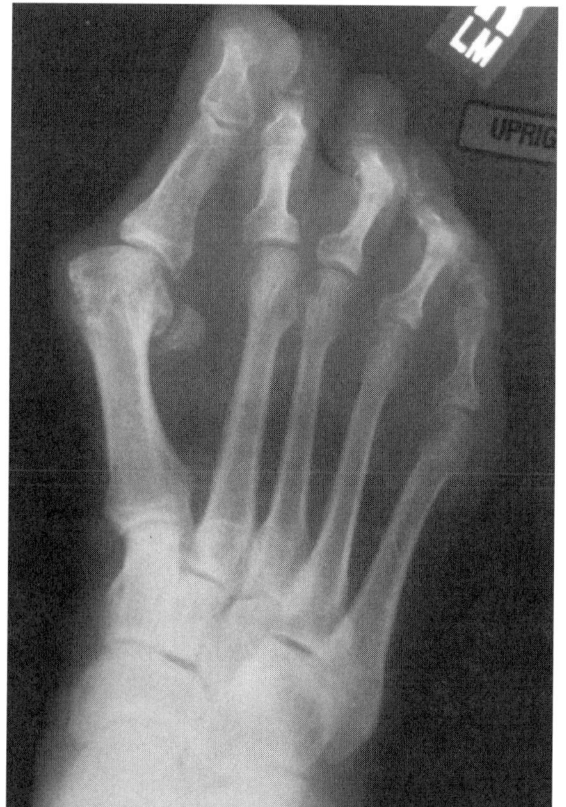

A

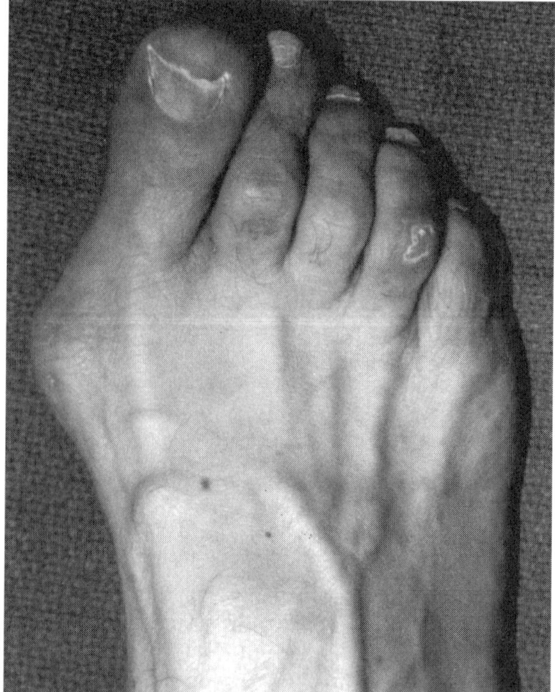

B

Figure 11-17. Progressive forefoot deformity in a 63-year-old man. *A, B.* The hallux valgus deformity includes varus alignment of the first metatarsal, valgus great toe, and medial exostosis. The first metatarsal head is subluxed medially relative to the sesamoids.

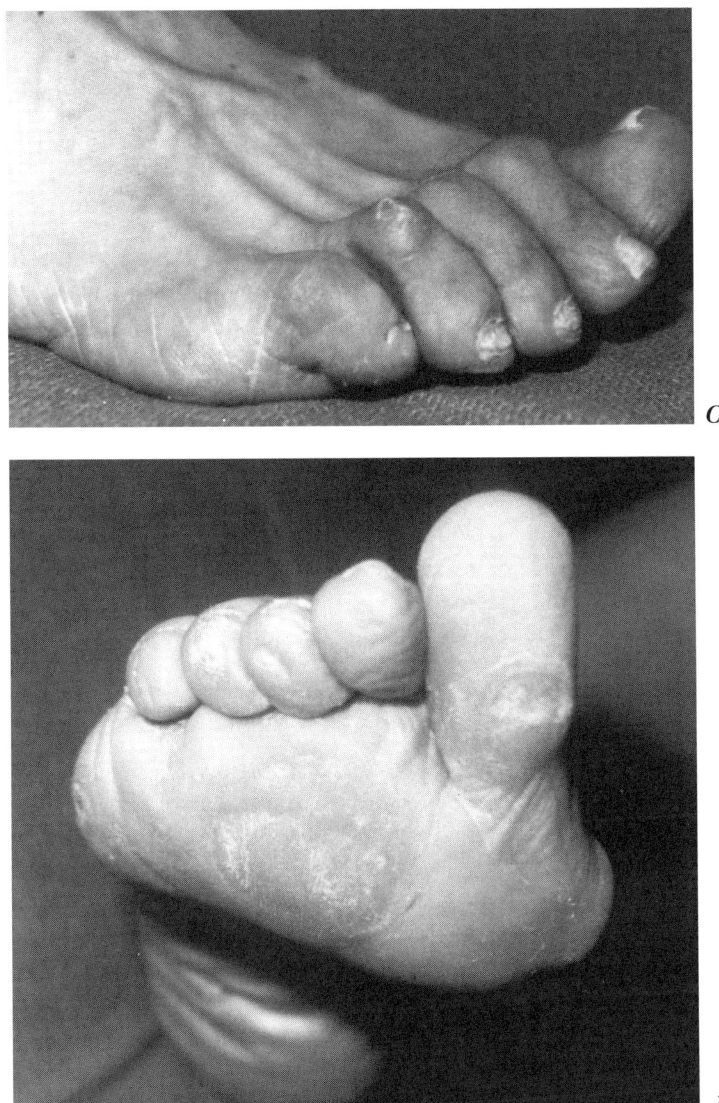

C. Hammertoe deformity resulting in pain at the dorsum of the proximal interphalangeal joints. *D.* Distal migration of the plantar metatarsal fat pad associated with hammertoes, resulting in painful keratosis under the metatarsal heads.

sophalangeal joint capsule becomes stretched out and attenuated. A medial exostosis of the first metatarsal head develops as a result of direct irritation of the bone or as a response to capsular traction.

Symptoms usually include pain as a result of direct pressure of the shoe on the medial exostosis. Nonoperative treatment may include shoes with laces, stretching the medial toe box to alleviate pressure on the bunion, doughnut pads, bunion-last shoes, or open sandals. Operative treatment may involve excision of the medial exostosis and, in most cases, realignment of the first ray using soft-tissue or bony procedures.

Hammertoe

Hammertoe deformity consists of a toe with increased dorsiflexion at the lesser metatarsophalangeal joint and plantar flexion of the proximal interphalangeal joint (see Fig. 11-17). The problem may result from inflammatory conditions of the lesser metatarsophalangeal joints [50, 51], muscle imbalance, use of shoes that are too short, or trauma. The dorsal position of the toe may cause distal migration of the plantar metatarsal fat pad and result in a painful keratosis at the plantar aspect of the metatarsal heads (see Fig. 11-17). A painful corn may develop at the dorsum of the proximal interphalangeal joint as a result of pressure on the toe box (Fig. 11-18) and may break down and become infected.

Treatment includes pressure relief using shoes with laces to allow for a larger toe box, stretching the shoe, corn pads, and soft insoles or metatarsal pads. Surgical correction may be indicated in some patients if nonoperative methods are not satisfactory.

Mallet Toe

A mallet toe is a plantar-flexion deformity of the distal interphalangeal joint of a lesser toe. This may result from degenerative disease of this joint, trauma to the extensor apparatus, or shoe pressure. The distal phalanx is pointed in the plantar direction, and the patient may develop a painful callus at the distal tip of the toe secondary to pressure from nonphysiological weight bearing on the tip, normally a non-weight-bearing area. Treatment may include soft pads and insoles or surgical correction.

Sports Injuries

The increased popularity of exercise programs in the elderly has resulted in a wider recognition of overuse injuries. When the rate of repetitive tissue microtrauma exceeds the rate of healing, macroscopic injury may become evident with pain and soft-tissue swelling. Any tissues subjected to repetitive microtrauma may develop overuse injury, including bone (stress fracture), joint cartilage (chondral defect or chondromalacia), muscle (strain), tendon (tendinitis), ligament (overuse sprain), or periosteum (periostitis). Risk factors contributing to overuse injury include increased frequency or duration of exercise without adequate rest intervals ("too much too soon"), inadequate footwear, poor training surface (e.g., running on concrete or asphalt), or associated conditions that increase musculoskeletal stresses (e.g., arthritis). Initial resting of the injured

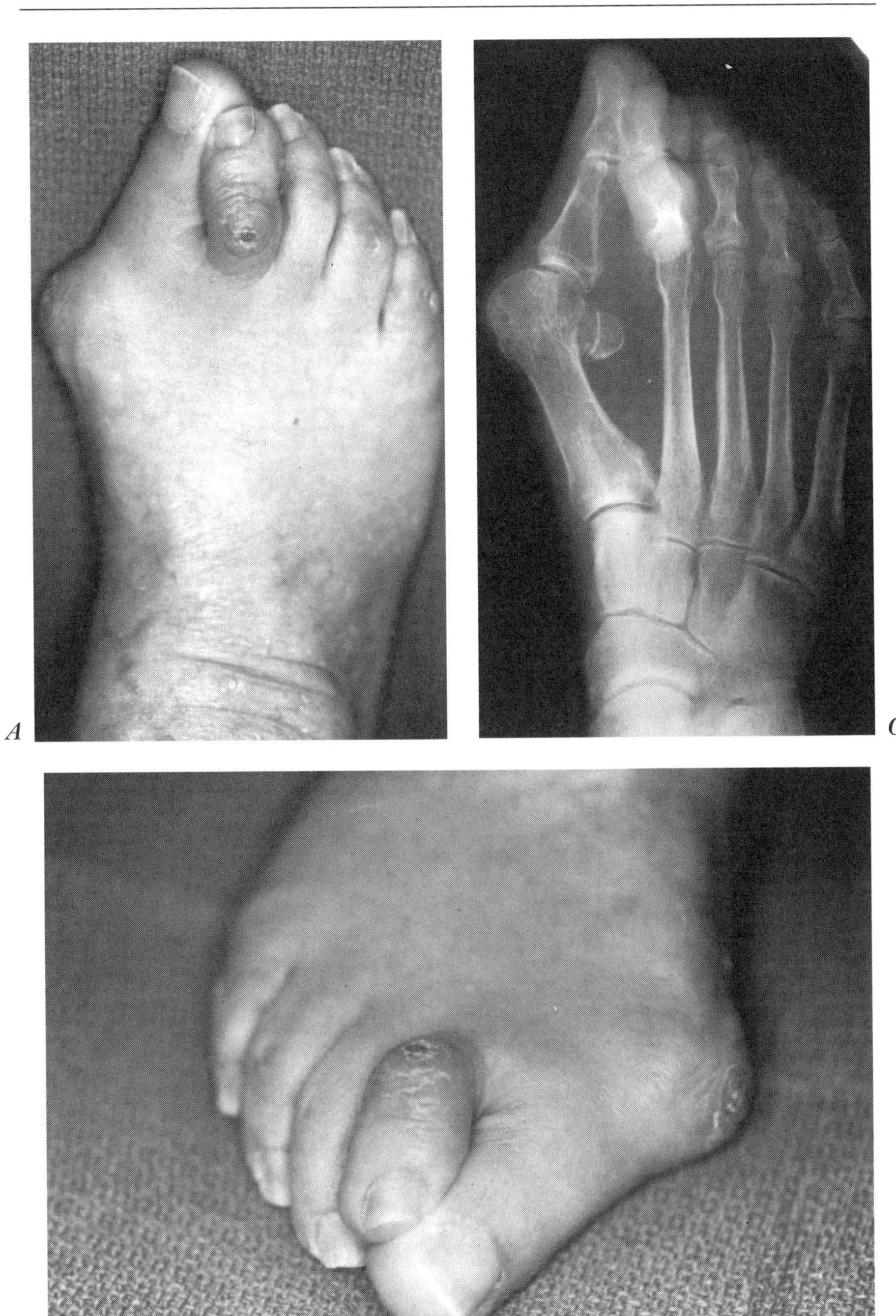

Figure 11-18. *A–C.* Right second hammertoe in an 83-year-old woman. The pain was located at the dorsum of the proximal interphalangeal joint, where a corn was present. A hallux valgus deformity also is present. Note that the first toe touches the third, leaving no room in the plane of the toes for the second.

part followed by a rehabilitation program and gradual return to activity often result in satisfactory resolution of the problem.

Treatment-Associated (Iatrogenic) Causes

Complications of treatment in the foot and ankle may result in pain and deformity that may cause gait disturbance. The Keller procedure for hallux valgus, which includes resection of the base of the hallux proximal phalanx, may be complicated by loss of function of the great toe during heel-rise, weight shifting to the second metatarsal head, and cockup deformity of the great toe. Avascular necrosis of the first metatarsal head is associated with pain and progressive degenerative changes in the first metatarsophalangeal joint; this may result if a distal first metatarsal osteotomy for hallux valgus is performed with extensive soft-tissue stripping and devascularization of the metatarsal head. Steroid use may result in avascular necrosis of the talus, with secondary bony collapse, deformity, and degenerative changes in the ankle joint.

Evaluation and Treatment of Foot and Ankle Deformity

Initial evaluation of painful conditions and deformity of the foot and ankle includes history, physical examination, and radiographic studies. History includes details of single-impact or repetitive trauma, previous treatment, and description of symptoms. Location of pain is determined as precisely as possible by asking the patient to point to or outline the painful areas, using one finger. Character of the pain may be sharp, achy, or dull; paresthesias or burning pain may suggest local nerve irritation or other neuropathic pain. Exacerbating factors may provide clues as to etiology: Pain on getting out of bed or after periods of inactivity (e.g., sitting in a chair) that improves with activity may be a result of inflammation and contracture, whereas night pain may be neuropathic in origin. Pain aggravated by standing or walking may be suggestive of a bone, joint, or soft-tissue process. The history may reveal the presence of risk factors such as diabetes mellitus, rheumatologic conditions, or previous trauma or surgery.

Physical examination of the foot and ankle includes comprehensive assessment of all bones, joints, and soft-tissue structures for possible contribution to pain [57, 58]. Limitation of examination to the stated area of pain may result in failure to identify conditions leading to weight shifting, and incorrect diagnosis and treatment failure may result. Every bone, joint, tendon, and ligament is made to move, and local areas of pain or tenderness are noted. Neurovascular examination includes evaluation of pulses, sensation, and motor strength, including tibialis anterior, gastrocsoleus, tibialis posterior, peroneals, and flexors and extensors of the toes. Each metatarsophalangeal joint and interdigital space is palpated to evaluate for conditions such as synovitis and interdigital neuritis. The plantar fascia is palpated with the toes and ankle in dorsiflexed position, and the

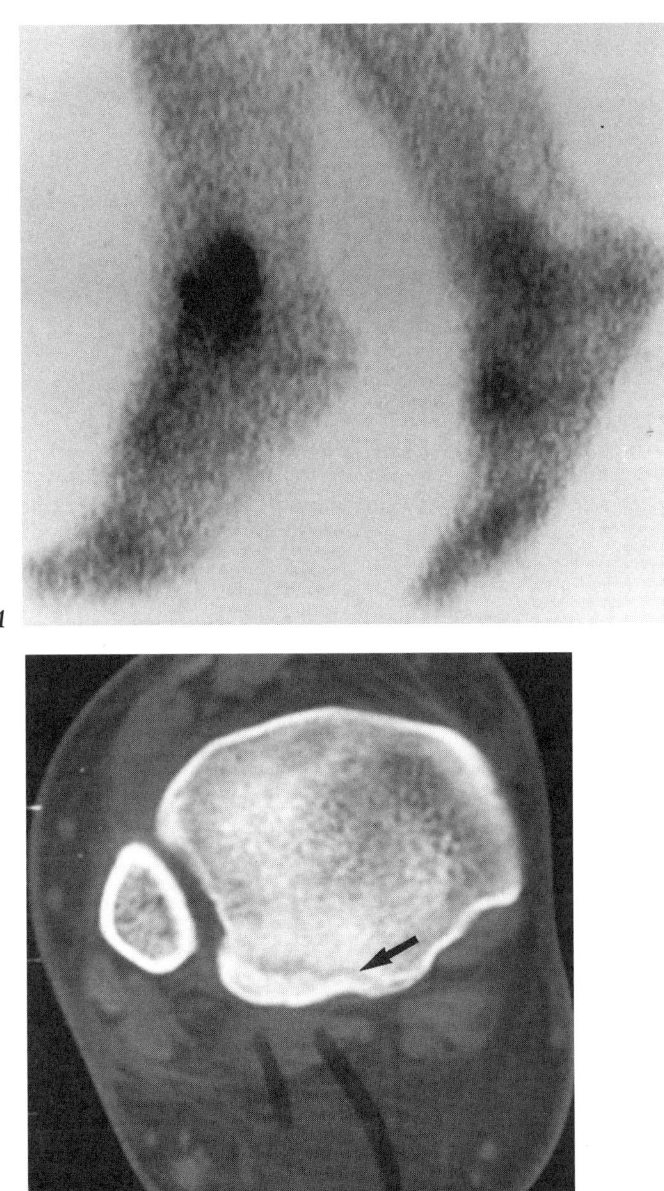

Figure 11-19. Technetium radionuclide bone scintigraphy and computed tomography may be useful in detecting occult fractures. This patient had ongoing right ankle pain 6 months after a "sprain." Plain-film radiography did not reveal any abnormality. *A.* Scintigraphy demonstrating increased activity at the ankle joint. *B.* Axial computed tomography scan of the ankle showing a posterior malleolus ankle fracture (*arrow*).

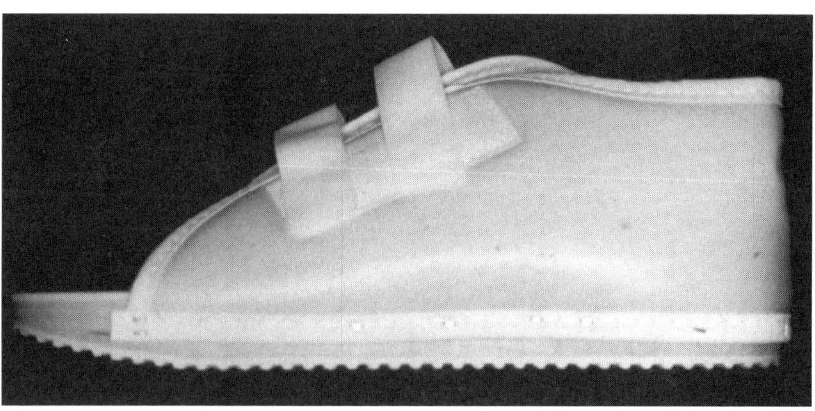

Figure 11-20. A wooden postoperative shoe with rocker sole, useful in treatment of such forefoot conditions as metatarsal fractures or injuries of the metatarsophalangeal joints.

Achilles tendon is palpated with the ankle in dorsiflexion; tenderness in this position, reduced by palpation in plantar-flexed position in which the structure is relaxed, suggests inflammation of the palpated structure. Percussion of the tarsal tunnel area is performed to test for irritation of the posterior tibial nerve.

Depending on location of pain and tenderness, radiographs of the foot, ankle, or both are made. Caution is advised in the evaluation of pain after a twisting injury of the foot and ankle, which may be underdiagnosed as an ankle sprain; palpation and radiography of the foot may reveal a fracture of the fifth metatarsal or calcaneus. Further evaluation of the painful foot may include technetium radionuclide scintigraphy, which may detect occult fractures, early arthritic changes, or reflex sympathetic dystrophy even when plain-film radiography is within normal limits (Fig. 11-19). In special cases, computed tomography or magnetic resonance imaging may be helpful in the detailed evaluation of bone, joint, or soft-tissue abnormality. In some instances where the anatomical source of pain is unclear, injection of local anesthetic with confirmation of position using contrast radiography or arthrography may facilitate localization of the painful structure [59].

Initial treatment of foot and ankle pain, particularly if evaluation suggests local inflammation aggravated by mechanical factors, may include immobilization using braces, casts, shoe modifications, or splints. Removable short-leg casts with rocker bottom soles enable full weight bearing, with reduction of stresses on irritated structures, and allow some painful conditions to resolve. In cases where weight shifting has resulted in secondary and tertiary areas of irritation, immobilization in the short-leg walking, rocker bottom cast brace for 6 to 12 weeks may allow these problems to improve, and the primary condition may become evident (see Fig. 11-13). Other immobilization devices such as night splints may prevent contractures in inflamed plantar fascia or Achilles tendon and may lead gradually to healing of chronic conditions [49]. Activity modification may be necessary to limit mechanical irritation in the foot and ankle.

Failure to improve despite immobilization may suggest conditions that are independent of mechanical factors, such as neurological or rheumatological conditions. Consultation with appropriate specialists may be helpful for cases in which the diagnosis is unclear, multiple problems are present, or anticipated improvement in response to treatment is not achieved.

Goals of treatment for painful conditions of the foot and ankle include alleviation of pain to enable functional gait. In some instances, chronic bracing (see Fig. 11-12), rocker sole shoes (Fig. 11-20), physiotherapy, or surgical intervention may be reasonable options. In situations where several conditions are present, improvement of one may result in amelioration of the other by improved gait pattern and reduction in weight shifting.

REFERENCES

1. Mann RA. Biomechanics of the Foot and Ankle. In: Mann RA, Coughlin MJ, eds. *Surgery of the Foot and Ankle*, 6th ed. St. Louis: Mosby, 1993. Pp 3–43.
2. Inman VT. *The Joints of the Ankle*. Baltimore: Williams & Wilkins, 1976.
3. Elftman H. The transverse tarsal joint and its control. *Clin Orthop* 1960;16:41–45.
4. Bojsen-Møller F, Flagstad KE. Plantar aponeurosis and internal architecture of the ball of the foot. *J Anat* 1976;121:599–611.
5. Johnston RB, Smith J, Daniels T. The plantar plate of the lesser toes: An anatomical study in human cadavers. *Foot Ankle Int* 1994;15:276–282.
6. Sarrafian SK. *Anatomy of the Foot and Ankle*, 2nd ed. Philadelphia: Lippincott, 1993.
7. Hicks JH. The mechanics of the foot: II. The plantar aponeurosis and the arch. *J Anat* 1954;88:25–30.
8. Sarrafian SK. Functional characteristics of the foot and plantar aponeurosis under tibiotalar loading. *Foot Ankle* 1987;8:4–18.
9. Cavanagh PR, Rodgers MM, Iiboshi A. Pressure distribution under symptom-free feet during barefoot standing. *Foot Ankle* 1987;7:262–276.
10. Joseph J. *Man's Posture: Electromyographic Studies*. Springfield, IL: Charles C Thomas, 1960.
11. Basmajian JV, De Luca CJ. *Muscles Alive. Their Functions Revealed by Electromyography*, 5th ed. Baltimore: Williams & Wilkins, 1985.
12. Mann R, Inman VT. Phasic activity of intrinsic muscles of the foot. *J Bone Joint Surg* 1964;46A:469–481.
13. Stokes IAF, Hutton WC, Stott JRR. Forces acting on the metatarsals during normal walking. *J Anat* 1979;129:579–590.
14. Grundy M, Tosh PA, McLeish RD, Smidt L. An investigation of the centres of pressure under the foot while walking. *J Bone Joint Surg* 1975;57B:98–103.
15. Bransby-Zachary MAP, Stother IG, Wilkinson RW. Peak pressures in the forefoot. *J Bone Joint Surg* 1990;72B:718–721.
16. Soames RW. Foot pressure patterns during gait. *J Biomed Eng* 1985;7:120–126.
17. Hughes J, Kriss S, Klenerman L. A clinician's view of foot pressure: A comparison of three different methods of measurement. *Foot Ankle* 1987;7:277–284.
18. Buckwalter JA, Goldberg VM, Woo SL-Y, eds. *Musculoskeletal Soft-Tissue Aging: Impact on Mobility*. Rosemont, IL: American Academy of Orthopaedic Surgeons, 1993.
19. Buckwalter JA, et al. Current concepts review. Soft-tissue aging and musculoskeletal function. *J Bone Joint Surg* 1993;75A:1533–1548.
20. Schultz AB. Biomechanics of Mobility Impairment in the Elderly. In: Buckwalter JA, Goldberg VM, Woo SL-Y, eds. *Musculoskeletal Soft-Tissue Aging: Impact on Mobility*. Rosemont IL: American Academy of Orthopaedic Surgeons, 1993. Pp 23–33.

21.   Nigg BM, et al. Range of motion of the foot as a function of age. *Foot Ankle* 1992;13:336–343.

22.   Booth FW, Weeden SH, Tseng BS. Effect of aging on human skeletal muscle and motor function. *Med Sci Sports Exerc* 1994;26:556–560.

23.   Lexell J, Taylor CC, Sjöström M. What is the cause of the ageing atrophy? Total number, size and proportion of different fiber types studied in whole vastus lateralis muscle from 15- to 83-year-old men. *J Neurol Sci* 1988;84:275–294.

24.   Hamlin CR, Kohn RR. Determination of human chronological age by study of a collagen sample. *Exp Gerontol* 1972;7:377–379.

25.   Hageman PA, Blanke DJ. Comparison of gait of young women and elderly women. *Phys Ther* 1986;66:1382–1387.

26.   Murray MP, Drought AB, Kory RC. Walking patterns of normal men. *J Bone Joint Surg* 1964;46A:335–360.

27.   Murray MP, Kory RC, Clarkson BH. Walking patterns in healthy old men. *J Gerontol* 1969;24:169–178.

28.   Gabell A, Nayak USL. The effect of age on variability in gait. *J Gerontol* 1984;39:662–666.

29.   Lehmann JF, Condon SM, de Lateur BJ, Price R. Gait abnormalities in peroneal nerve paralysis and their corrections by orthoses: a biomechanical study. *Arch Phys Med Rehabil* 1986;67: 380–386.

30.   Wright DG, Desai SM, Henderson WH. Action of the subtalar and ankle-joint complex during the stance phase of walking. *J Bone Joint Surg* 1964;46A:361–382, 464.

31.   Isman RE, Inman VT. Anthropometric studies of the human foot and ankle. *Bull Prosth Res* 1969;10/11:97–129.

32.   Holmes GB, Timmerman L. A quantitative assessment of the effect of metatarsal pads on plantar pressures. *Foot Ankle* 1990;11:141–145.

33.   Snow RE, Williams KR, Holmes GB. The effects of wearing high heeled shoes on pedal pressure in women. *Foot Ankle* 1992;13:85–92.

34.   Schaff PS, Cavanagh PR. Shoes for the insensitive foot: The effect of a "rocker bottom" shoe modification on plantar pressure distribution. *Foot Ankle* 1990;11:129–140.

35.   Shereff MJ, Bregman AM, Kummer FJ. The effect of immobilization devices on the load distribution under the foot. *Clin Orthop Rel Res* 1985;192:260–267.

36.   Pollard JP, Le Quesne LP, Tappin JW. Forces under the foot. *J Biomed Eng* 1983;5:37–40.

37.   Myerson M, Papa J, Eaton K, Wilson K. The total-contact cast for management of neuropathic plantar ulceration of the foot. *J Bone Joint Surg* 1992;74A:261–269.

38.   Duckworth T, et al. Plantar pressure measurements and the prevention of ulceration in the diabetic foot. *J Bone Joint Surg* 1985;67B:79–85.

39.   Bauman JH, Girling JP, Brand PW. Plantar pressures and trophic ulceration. An evaluation of footwear. *J Bone Joint Surg* 1963;45B:652–673.

40.   Mann RA, Poppen NK, O'Konski M. Amputation of the great toe. A clinical and biomechanical study. *Clin Orthop Rel Res* 1988;226:192–205.

41.   Hutton WC, Dhanendran M. The mechanics of normal and hallux valgus feet—A quantitative study. *Clin Orthop Rel Res* 1981;157:7–13.

42.   Beverly MC, Horan FT, Hutton WC. Load cell analysis following silastic arthroplasty of the hallux. *Int Orthop* 1985;9:101–104.

43.   Ctercteko GC, Dhanendran M, Hutton WC, Le Quesne LP. Vertical forces acting on the feet of diabetic patients with neuropathic ulceration. *Br J Surg* 1981;68:608–614.

44.   Jahss MH, et al. Investigations into the fat pads of the sole of the foot: Anatomy and histology. *Foot Ankle* 1992;13:233–242.

45.   Jahss MH, Kummer F, Michelson JD. Investigations into the fat pads of the sole of the foot: Heel pressure studies. *Foot Ankle* 1992;13:227–232.

46.   Jørgensen U, Bojsen-Møller F. Shock absorbency of factors in the shoe/heel interaction-With special focus on role of the heel pad. *Foot Ankle* 1989;9:294–299.

47.   Frey C, Shereff M, Greenidge N. Vascularity of the posterior tibial tendon. *J Bone Joint Surg* 1990;72A:884–888.

48. Holmes GB, Mann RA. Possible epidemiological factors associated with rupture of the posterior tibial tendon. *Foot Ankle* 1992;13:70–79.

49. Wapner KL, Sharkey PF. The use of night splints for treatment of recalcitrant plantar fasciitis. *Foot Ankle* 1991;12:135–137.

50. Mann RA, Mizel MS. Monarticular nontraumatic synovitis of the metatarsophalangeal joint: A new diagnosis? *Foot Ankle* 1985;6:18–21.

51. Trepman E, Yeo S-J. Nonoperative treatment of metatarsophalangeal joint synovitis. *Foot Ankle Int* 1995;16:771–777.

52. Coughlin MJ. Crossover second toe deformity. *Foot Ankle* 1987;8:29–39.

53. Thompson FM, Mann RA. Arthritides. In: Mann RA, Coughlin MJ, eds. *Surgery of the Foot and Ankle*, 6th ed. St. Louis: Mosby, 1993. Pp 615–671.

54. Gerster JC. Plantar fasciitis and Achilles tendinitis among 150 cases of seronegative spondarthritis. *Rheum Rehabil* 1980;19:218–222.

55. Mann RA. Pes Cavus. In: Mann RA, Coughlin MJ, eds. *Surgery of the Foot and Ankle*, 6th ed. St. Louis: Mosby, 1993. Pp 785–801.

56. Schwartzman RJ, Kerrigan J. The movement disorder of reflex sympathetic dystrophy. *Neurology* 1990;40:57–61.

57. Mann RA. Principles of Examination of the Foot and Ankle. In: Mann RA, Coughlin MJ, eds. *Surgery of the Foot and Ankle*, 6th ed. St. Louis: Mosby, 1993. Pp 45–60.

58. Mizel MS. Physical examination of the foot. *Video J Orthop* 1992;7(6).

59. Yodlowski M, Newberg AH, Trepman E, Mizel MS. Subtalar joint arthrography in the diagnosis of hindfoot pain. In: *Abstracts of the Tenth Annual Summer Meeting. Coeur d'Alene, ID:* American Orthopaedic Foot and Ankle Society, July 1994. Pp 17–18.

12. Cervical Spondylotic Myelopathy

Raj Murali and Joseph C. Masdeu

Degenerative disease affecting the cervical spine often is referred to as cervical spondylosis. Cervical spondylosis is an age-related phenomenon and is present almost universally in people older than 65. In advanced cases, degenerative changes of the cervical spine begin to cause compression of the neural elements, such as the spinal cord and nerve roots. Thus, *cervical spondylotic myelopathy* (CSM) may be defined as a slowly progressive neurological disorder of the spinal cord characterized by the development of an upper–motor-neuron type of paralysis of the lower limbs and an upper– or a lower–motor-neuron type of paralysis of the upper limbs. *Cervical spondylosis* itself is defined as a degenerative disorder of the cervical spine, with primary changes starting in the intervertebral discs and resulting in secondary changes in the surrounding bones, joints, and soft tissues [1]. There is loss of flexibility and compliance of the ligaments and cartilage, with thickening and deposition of calcium in those tissues. Eventually, overgrown spinal elements narrow the spinal canal, compressing the cord.

SOME HISTORICAL PERSPECTIVES

Degenerative changes of the cervical spine, especially in relation to age, have been recognized by European anatomists for many centuries. In 1952, Brain [2] finally established CSM as a distinct entity and described the specific anatomical, radiological, and clinical features of this disease. In a landmark article, he described in detail the neurological manifestations of CSM in 45 patients. In 1956, Clarke and Robinson [3] emphasized the importance of making a clear differentiation between the cervical myelopathy caused by acute disc protrusion and the more chronic spinal cord disorder characteristic of spondylotic myelopathy. Pallis [4] pointed out the frequent incidence of cervical spondylosis and a narrowed cervical spinal canal resulting in myelopathy. Robinson and Smith [5] and Cloward [6] described anterior approaches to the cervical spine for removal of discs and osteophytes. Laminectomy for CSM had been performed intermittently since 1930, by Elsberg [7] and Stookey [8]. Spurling and Scoville [9] are credited with establishing the posterior approach firmly and reporting on a large series of patients.

PATHOPHYSIOLOGY OF CSM

The etiology of CSM is multifactorial. The degenerative process usually starts in the intervertebral discs. As the discs degenerate, the disc space height is lost, and

197

the vertical height of the cervical spinal column diminishes, leading to a decrease in the size of the intervertebral foramina. Due to disc degeneration, the vertebral body end plates are subjected to increased stress and strain, resulting in sclerosis and osteophyte formation. Osteophytes, protruding into the anterior aspect of the canal and into the neural foramina, further contribute to the reduction in the size of the spinal canal and neural foramina. Disc space degeneration and narrowing also cause a reciprocal infolding, degenerative swelling, or hypertrophy of the ligamentum flavum. The ligamentum flavum then compresses the posterior aspect of the spinal cord [10]. These circumferential degenerative changes of the cervical spine ultimately lead to progressive narrowing of the canal and to cord compression. In certain positions of the neck (such as hyperextension), the ligamentum flavum bulges anteriorly to cause additional cord compression by pincer effect. Thus, both static and dynamic mechanical factors are important in the development of CSM. The static factors include osteophytes, disc protrusions, and a developmentally narrow canal. The dynamic factors involve the pincer effect [11].

Spinal cords of patients with cervical myeloradiculopathy show several gross and microscopic changes. The spinal cord appears flattened and distorted, molded by the irregular and narrow canal. Demyelination is most prominent in the lateral columns at the levels of the osteophytic bars. Anterior horn cells are diminished in number, and the gray matter may be cavitated. The posterior columns are affected less severely. The spinal nerve roots may be surrounded by fibrotic arachnoid within the dural sleeve.

Vascular factors also are significant [12]. Arterial spasm and thrombosis may occur at the site of narrowing. Blood supply to the spinal cord and nerve roots may be sufficiently reduced to cause ischemia or infarction. Affected patients often are elderly and may have coincidental atheromatous or arteriosclerotic vascular disease or disturbances of the microcirculation, as seen in diabetes. All these factors contribute to the development of myelopathy. Venous drainage from the cord also may be impeded. Some patients thus affected also may fall and sustain hyperextension injuries to the gray matter of the cord, resulting in a central cord syndrome, with weakness in the arms but relatively preserved lower-extremity function.

CLINICAL PRESENTATION

The symptomatology of CSM is complex and patients present a pleomorphic and varied pattern [2]. The myelopathy usually is gradual, slowly progressive, and sometimes punctuated with sudden worsening, especially after trauma. The duration of symptoms often spans many years, with an average of 2 years in the majority of subjects. Initial symptoms include difficulty in getting about due to a combination of stiffness, clumsiness, and unsteadiness of gait, often attributed initially to "rheumatism" or "old age." Symptoms tend to be worse early in the morning and are most noticeable after a period of rest or inactivity. Difficulty in walking briskly, with a tendency to trip, also is commonly reported. The slowly developing paraparesis is described by patients as heaviness of legs, trembling and cramping of thigh and calf muscles, and difficulty in negotiating uneven ground, mounting steps, and getting in and out of vehicles [13].

Motor Findings

Motor findings in CSM classically affect the lower limbs. Usually they consist of weakness associated with spasticity. Upper-limb weakness also is common and could be due to upper– or lower–motor-neuron paralysis. Frank quadriplegia is rare and sometimes follows an injury occurring in a setting of cervical spondylosis. Spastic paraparesis is the most common motor finding in CSM. Sometimes affected patients may have associated lumbar spondylosis causing root compression, which may result in a combination of upper– and lower–motor-neuron paralysis in the lower limbs as well. Spasticity often is more severe than the weakness and results in the classic gait disturbance of CSM: a labored, short-paced gait, with a tendency to drag one or both feet. The degree of leg weakness at times may be asymmetrical, with one limb being more affected than the other. Wasting of the proximal or distal muscles of the upper limb can occur and may not correspond exactly to the area of segmental spinal cord compression. For example, cord compression at the C3–4 level may produce severe weakness and wasting of the intrinsic muscles of the hands. When there is asymmetrical paralysis of the upper limbs, the side of maximal involvement usually is the same in both the upper and lower limbs. The degree of spasticity in upper limbs usually is not as pronounced as in the lower limbs and also is not as constant. Atrophy of the muscles in the upper limb also may be associated with fasciculations. Amyotrophic lateral sclerosis, also more frequent in the older age group, may cause similar motor findings but is unaccompanied by sensory loss.

Sensory Changes

Sensory changes are common in CSM. In severe cases of myelopathy, a clear sensory level can be elicited, usually in the upper thoracic dermatomes. Radicular-type sensory changes also may occur in the upper limbs due to root compression. Diminished vibration sense, especially in the lower limbs, is seen frequently in patients with CSM. Brown-Séquard type sensory changes also are observed in some patients. The degree of sensory changes may be minimal or absent in some patients, even in the presence of profound motor paralysis.

Reflex Changes

Hyperactive deep-tendon reflexes, especially in the lower limbs, are the most common finding in patients with CSM. In severe cases, bilateral ankle clonus and extensor plantar responses also are observed. The reflex changes in the upper limbs are more unpredictable and reflect the balance of upper– and lower–motor-neuron interaction at each segmental level. If myelopathy is caused by a high cervical cord compression, such as at the C3–4 level, the upper-limb reflexes will be uniformly hyperactive, with Hoffman responses. On the other hand, if nerve root compression occurs in addition to cord compression, the reflexes may be diminished or absent at the appropriate segmental level. Absence of forearm flexion, on testing of the radial reflex, and excessive finger flexion have been referred to as the *inverted radial reflex*. This usually is considered to be a highly useful test to confirm CSM, although it has been found to be positive in certain other conditions, such as multiple sclerosis. In his series, Clarke [3] found the following reflex changes: 25% of patients showed a symmetrical increase of upper-limb reflexes, with exaggerated lower-limb reflexes and extensor plantar responses; another 25% showed a hemiparetic pattern of reflex activity; 15% showed normal arm reflexes, with hyperactive lower-limb reflexes; and 33% of patients showed one or more diminished or absent arm reflexes in a setting of exaggerated upper-limb reflexes.

Sphincter Disturbances

Disturbances of bladder and bowel function are rare in CSM. In extremely severe cases presenting with frank quadriplegia, bladder and bowel dysfunction may occur, but this is an exception rather than the rule. Retention of urine, dribbling incontinence, or fecal incontinence almost never is seen in CSM, and their presence should raise a serious doubt regarding the diagnosis.

INVESTIGATIONS

In older individuals, the differential diagnosis of a mild spastic paraparesis and lower–motor-neuron signs in the arms should include amyotrophic lateral sclerosis. Less frequent than CSM, nonetheless it may present in a similar manner, particularly in elderly who may have vibratory sense loss in the feet and mildly impaired proprioception from other causes (as discussed in Chapter 17). Amyotrophic lateral sclerosis will be favored if the radiographic findings in the neck are not severe enough to account for the motor impairment and electromyography shows widespread fasciculations in the legs.

X-rays of the cervical spine obtained in multiple projections are a useful initial study for patients with CSM. X-rays are valuable in determining the shape of the cervical spine, the alignment of the vertebrae, the nature of the bone, the vertical extent of the disease process, the degree of anterior and posterior osteophytes, and the nature of the disc spaces (Fig. 12-1A). X-rays also are useful as a baseline for comparison with postoperative x-rays when surgery is being considered. In considering the etiology of gait impairment, degenerative changes on x-rays should be interpreted with caution. Irvine et al. [14] found spondylosis on x-rays in 70% of women and 85% of men by age 59 and in 97% of the men and 93% of the women past age 70.

Imaging modalities such as magnetic resonance imaging (MRI) and computerized tomography (CT) have made a tremendous difference in facilitating the clear understanding of the nature and degree of cord compression in patients with CSM. MRI scan of the cervical spine is recommended after plain x-rays, as an initial test. The sagittal images obtained with both T_1 and T_2 pulse sequences offer a lot of information about the size of the canal, the spinal cord, and the surrounding subarachnoid space (see Fig. 12-1B). However, MRI scan is not as good at showing osteophytes or ossification of the posterior longitudinal ligament. CT scan of the cervical spine is superior in this regard and will give more information in the axial projection. If surgical treatment is contemplated, thin CT slices of the cervical spine after the intrathecal introduction of a nonionic water-soluble contrast material are of great help (see Figs. 12-1C, D). MRI scan, CT scan, and CT myelography are complementary tests and not mutually exclusive. CT myelography is most valuable when surgical decisions, such as anterior versus posterior approach, are being made. CT myelography also allows for accurate measurement of the spinal canal in the axial, sagittal, and coronal planes. A canal diameter of less than 12 mm in the anteroposterior plane is considered stenotic. MRI scan may show, within the spinal cord itself, changes due to chronic compression, such as syrinx formation, atrophy, and myelomalacia. MRI scan also is of great value in the differential diagnosis of myelopathy, because conditions such as tumor and infection can be ruled out easily. In multiple sclerosis, an abnormal signal corresponding to plaques of demyelination may be found in the spinal cord and often in the brain as well. Ossification of the posterior longitudinal ligament sometimes is found in patients with CSM. This ossification may be segmental or continuous in the cervical spine. CT myelography is particularly useful for diagnosing this entity, which has significant bearing on the type of surgical procedure to be performed (Fig. 12-2).

METHODS OF TREATMENT

CSM often occurs in elderly patients who may have other serious coexisting illnesses, such as diabetes mellitus, osteoporosis, and cardiovascular disease. Mild to moderate CSM in elderly patients with one or more of these complicating factors often can be treated conservatively with periodic reevaluation. Age by itself is not a contraindication to surgical treatment, as many elderly patients have undergone successful surgery.

Conservative Treatment

Conservative treatment, usually carried out under the supervision of a physiatrist, includes the management of pain, limb mobility, gait impairment, and risk of falling. (The treatment of gait impairment and risk of falling is discussed extensively in Chapsters 20–24.) Pain, either in the neck or in the limbs, is managed with analgesics or nonsteroidal antiinflammatory agents. If neck pain or stiffness is prominent, a cervical collar may be necessary. Patients with walking difficulty are given a walking aid and are instructed to be careful while walking

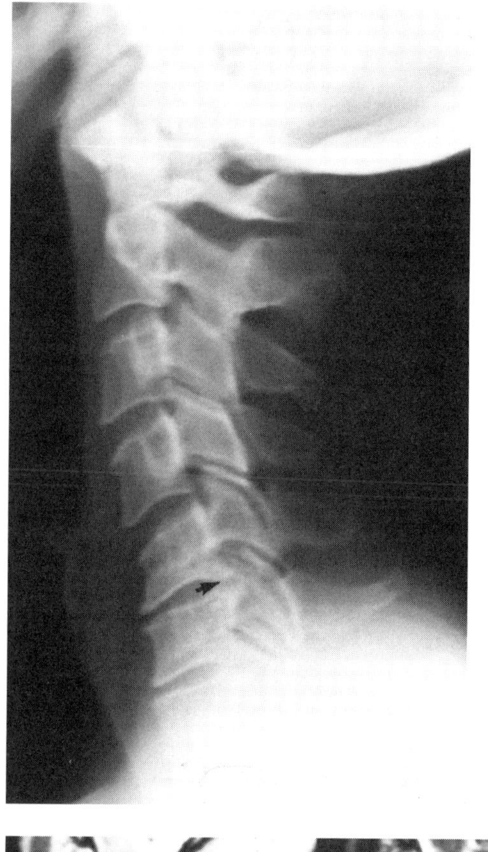

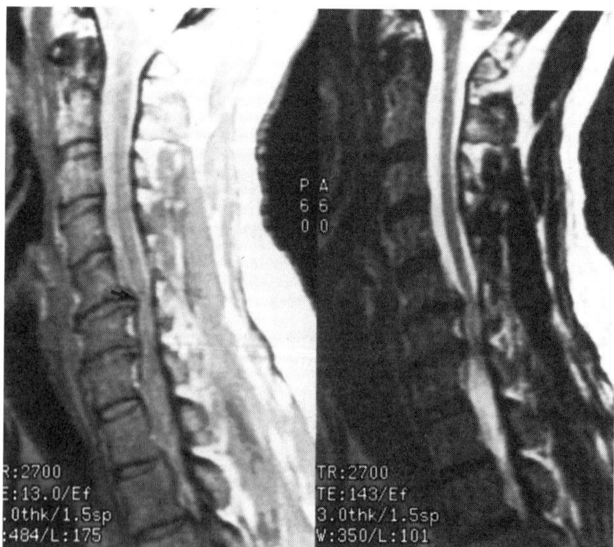

Figure 12-1. *A.* Plain x-ray of the cervical spine, showing the absence of cervical lordosis, slight angulation at C5-6, marked osteophyte formation at C5-6, narrow disc spaces at C5-6 and C6-7 levels, and canal stenosis. *B.* MRI scan of the same patient, showing severe spinal cord compression at C5-6 and C6-7 levels due to a combination of osteophytes, herniated discs, and narrow canal.

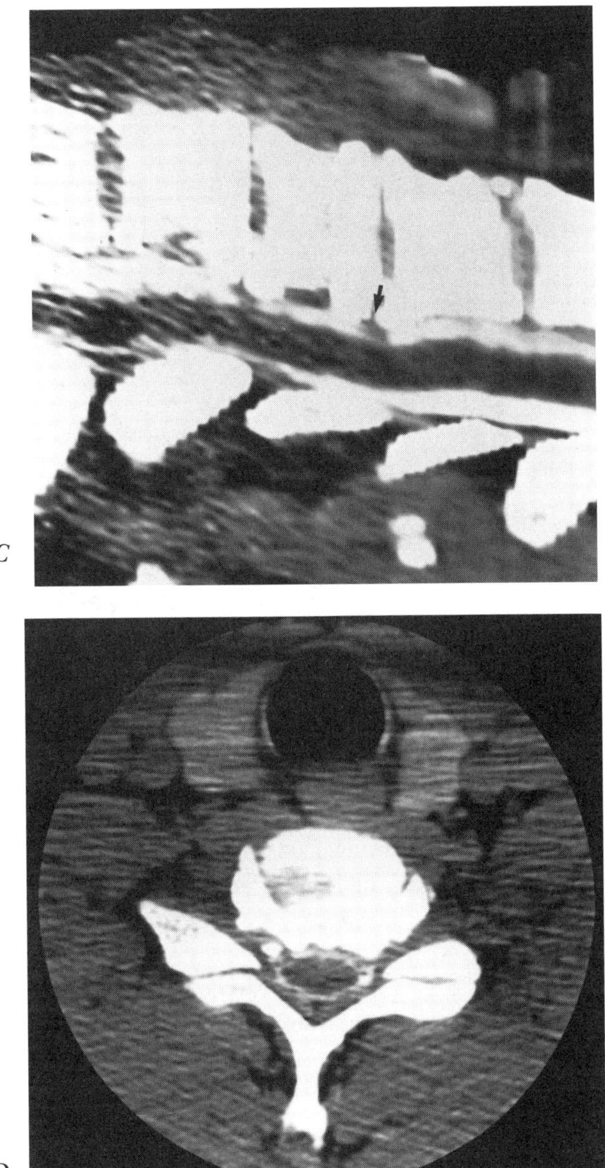

Figure 12-1. *Cont. C.* CT myelogram with sagittal reconstruction of the same patient, showing the main cause of cord compression to be osteophytes and a narrow canal at the C5-6 and C6-7 levels. *D.* CT myelogram in the axial projection of the same patient, showing cord compression due to osteophyte and narrow canal.

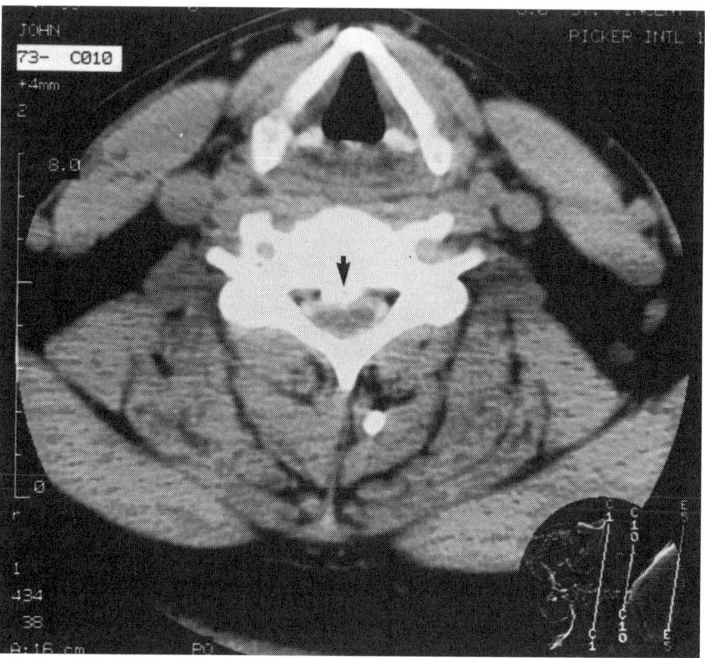

Figure 12-2. CT myelogram in the axial projection, showing ossification of the posterior longitudinal ligament in the midline of the dorsal aspect of the vertebral body, with cord compression (*arrow*).

to avoid falls that can be catastrophic; a severe paraparesis may result from sudden cord compression. Physical therapy is given to the limbs to improve range of motion and strength. Functional assessment is performed, and the patients are given appropriate aids at home to facilitate activities of daily living. Specific weakness of the foot or knee can be addressed by appropriate orthosis. Finally, patients receiving conservative therapy should be evaluated periodically from the neurological standpoint; if there is significant deterioration of neurological function, surgery should be reconsidered.

Surgical Treatment

The main aim of surgery for patients with CSM is adequate decompression of the spinal cord and nerve roots in the cervical spine. This may require anterior or posterior decompression or, in some cases, a combination of both. Extensive decompression, especially when carried out from the anterior approach, always must be supplemented with stabilization. Multilevel posterior decompression by laminectomy and partial facetectomy usually can be performed without stabilization. Multilevel anterior decompression, usually consisting of median corpectomy and discectomy, always requires stabilization. The question of anterior versus posterior decompression is one of the great controversies of neurosurgery, and although there are strong advocates for both methods of treatment, statistical proof does not exist to support the superiority of one over the other.

Anterior Approaches to the Cervical Spine

The ideal indication for anterior cervical decompression and fusion is cord compression at one or two levels. Since the pathology in most cases of CSM is located anteriorly, an anterior approach is logical. In this procedure, the affected cervical discs and adjacent vertebral bodies above and below are drilled down to the level of the dura and removed. The spine then is stabilized with an iliac crest strut graft. When the pathology affects three or more segments of the cervical spine, a more extensive procedure is required. Multilevel anterior and middle-column decompression can be performed by means of median corpectomy whereby the vertebral bodies and the intervening discs are removed totally, thoroughly decompressing the dura. It is possible to perform an anterior median corpectomy from C2 to C7 and to stablize the spine with a cadaver fibular graft as a strut in the midline (Fig. 12-3A, B). Saunders [15] reports an 89.7% success rate using corpectomy for CSM in a series of more than 100 patients. The complications of anterior surgery to the cervical spine include damage to prevertebral soft-tissue structures (e.g., esophagus and recurrent laryngeal nerve), problems with the bone graft (including slippage or fracture), and spinal cord damage from surgical trauma. Multilevel anterior decompression with fibular graft fusion also is a more technically demanding procedure and may not be tolerated well by elderly patients. Postoperative halo stabilization also may be necessary in some of these patients to prevent graft slippage. Saunders [15] also has reported an approximately 15% incidence of delayed postoperative radiculopathy in the anterior corpectomy series. Though these are some of the principles of anterior decompression, it is beyond the scope of this chapter to elaborate on the finer details of this operation.

Posterior Approach to the Cervical Spine

The posterior approach to the cervical spine consists of cervical laminectomy and partial facetectomy. It has been shown quite clearly that the extent of decompression must be both wide and long. The decompression should extend at least two levels above and two levels below the site of maximal cord compression, and this usually means a laminectomy from C3 to C7. This should be accompanied with bilateral partial facetectomy, foraminotomy to decompress the nerve roots, and possibly removal of osteophytes located laterally. Because the anterior and middle columns are intact, stabilization rarely is necessary. Tarlov [16] has noted 56% improvement, 30% stabilization, and 10% worsening of myelopathy in patients treated with posterior decompression. Cervical laminectomy and decompression is technically easier to perform than is multilevel anterior corpectomy and is well tolerated even by elderly patients. However, meticulous attention to detail is necessary to prevent surgical trauma to an already compromised spinal cord.

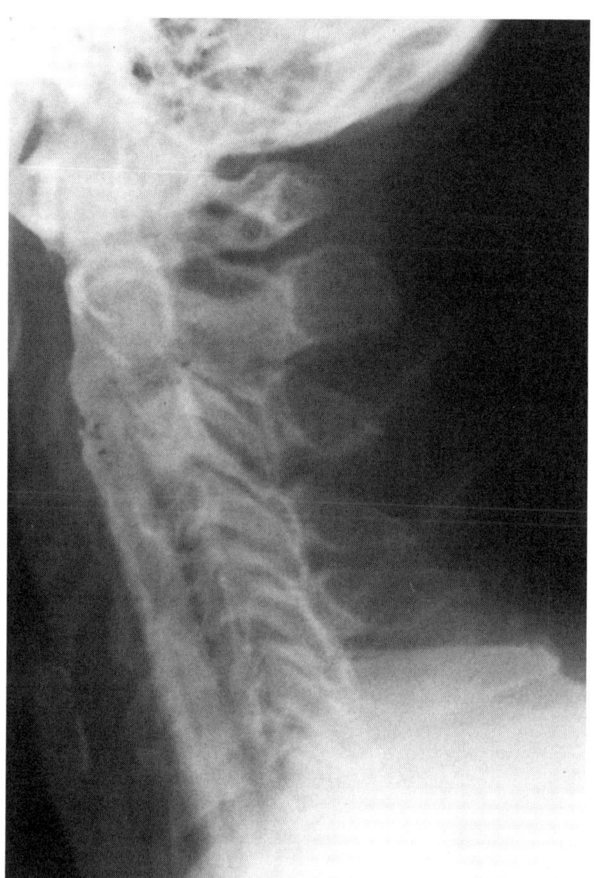

A

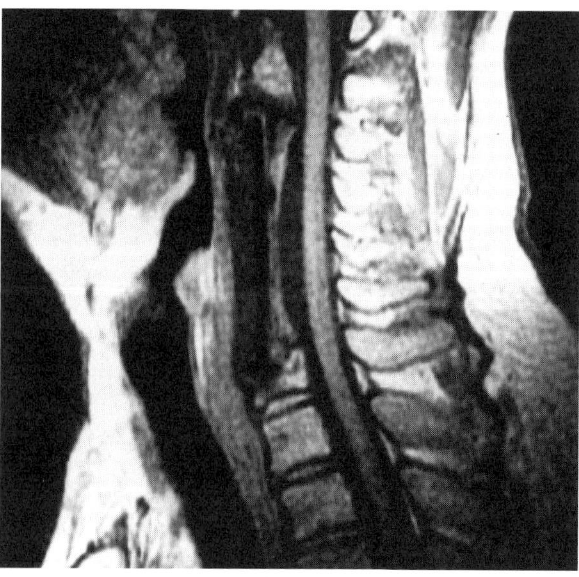

B

Figure 12-3. *A.* Plain x-ray of the cervical spine in the lateral projection following multilevel anterior median corpectomy and fibular graft fusion from C2 to C7. Note the long fibular strut graft in front of the cervical spine. *B.* Postoperative magnetic resonance imaging scan of the same patient as in Figure 3A, showing excellent decompression of the spinal cord from C2 to C7. The fibular graft itself is seen as a black strut in this image.

Results of Surgery

Irrespective of the approach used to decompress the spinal cord, the main aim of surgery is adequate decompression of the spinal cord in all three dimensions: sagittal, coronal, and axial. The series by Saunders [15] on multilevel anterior cervical decompression for CSM showing an overall improvement of 89.7% is perhaps the best of those reported to date.

Several prognostic factors have been found to be important in predicting the outcome of treatment. Long-standing severe neurological deficits (including spasticity in the lower limbs and atrophy of the small muscles of the hand) indicate a poor prognosis, and patients thus affected may not improve significantly with any method of treatment. In such patients, surgical treatment may prevent only further worsening. Other poor prognostic factors include cord atrophy or a bright spot in the spinal cord on T_2-weighted images of the MRI scan [17]. Patients with the combination of paraparesis and clumsy, numb hands have done well after surgery, but the number reported is too small to generalize [18].

Although, as indicated earlier, surgery is favored currently for the treatment of progressive spondylotic myelopathy, some have argued that the benefit of surgery has not been proved [19]. In asking for the organization of a controlled therapeutic trial, these authors point to the lack of studies documenting the natural history of the disease, the risk of surgery, and the lack of definitive predictors of outcome. Most of the surgical studies summarized in Figure 12-4 are more recent than the trials of conservative therapy, perhaps indicating a current preference for surgery.

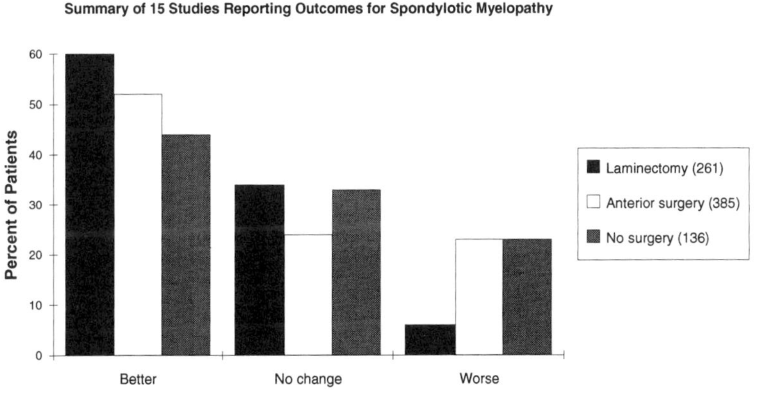

Figure 12-4. Summary of 15 studies reporting outcomes in spondylotic myelopathy [19]. The numbers in parentheses after each type of management approach correspond to the total number of patients reported. Patient characteristics and approaches vary among studies, precluding a reliable statistical analysis.

CONCLUSION

CSM is seen increasingly in our aging population. Patients with CSM can present to a variety of specialists, all of whom have to be aware of this entity. Early clinical diagnosis can lead to appropriate imaging studies that will confirm the disorder. Usually, prompt surgical treatment before the onset of severe neurological deficits will reverse or at least arrest the process.

REFERENCES

1. Wilkinson M. *Cervical Spondylosis: Its Early Diagnosis and Treatment.* Philadelphia: Saunders, 1971.
2. Brain R, Northfield D, Wilkinson M. Neurological manifestations of cervical spondylosis. *Brain* 1952;75:187–225.
3. Clarke E, Robinson PK. Cervical myelopathy: A complication of cervical spondylosis. *Brain* 1956;79:483–510.
4. Pallis C, Jones AM, Spillane JD. Cervical spondylosis. *Brain* 1954;77:274.
5. Robinson RA, Smith GW. Anterolateral cervical disc removal and interbody fusion for cervical disc syndrome [abstract]. *Bull Johns Hopkins Hosp* 1955;96:223–224.
6. Cloward RB. The anterior approach for removal of ruptured cervical discs. *J Neurosurg* 1958;15:602–614.
7. Elsberg GA. The extradural ventral chondromas (ecchondroses), their favorite sites, the spinal cord and root symptoms they produce and their surgical treatment. *Bull Neurol Inst NY* 1931;1:350–388.
8. Stookey B. Compression of spinal cord and nerve roots by herniation of the nucleus pulposus in the cervical region. *Arch Surg* 1940;40:417–432.
9. Spurling RG, Scoville WB. Lateral rupture of the cervical intervertebral discs: A common cause of shoulder and arm pain. *Surg Gynecol Onst* 1944;78:350–358.
10. Burrows EH. The sagittal diameter of the spinal canal in cervical spondylosis. *Clin Radiol* 1963;14:77–86.
11. Penning L. Some aspects of plain radiography of the cervical spine in chronic myelopathy. *Neurology* 1962;12:513–519.
12. Taylor AR. Vascular factors in the myelopathy associated with cervical spondylosis. *Neurology* 1964;14:62–68.
13. Spillance JD, Lloyd GHT. The diagnosis of lesions of the spinal cord in association with osteoarthritic disease of the cervical spine. *Brain* 1952;75:177.
14. Irvine D, Foster J, Newell D, Klukvin R. Prevalence of cervical spondylosis in a general practice. *Lancet* 1965;2:1089–1092.
15. Saunders RL. *Anterior and Middle Column Decompression.* In: Saunders RL, Bernini PM, eds. *Cervical Spondylitic Myelopathy.* Boston: Blackwell, 1992.
16. Tarlov EC. *Posterior Column Decompression in Cervical Spondylotic Myelopathy,* Saunders RL, Bernini PM, eds. Boston: Blackwell, 1992.
17. Mehalic TF, Pezzuti RT, Applebaum BI. Magnetic resonance imaging and cervical spondylotic myelopathy. *Neurosurgery* 1990;26:217–227.
18. Voskuhl R, Hinton R. Sensory impairment in the hands secondary to spondylotic compression of the cervical spinal cord. *Arch Neurol* 1990;47:309–311.
19. Rowland LP. Surgical treatment of cervical spondylotic myelopathy: Time for a controlled trial. *Neurology* 1992;42:5–13.

13. Gait Disorders in Parkinsonism and Other Movement Disorders

Rajesh Pahwa and William C. Koller

Gait disorders and immobility are the second most common neurological accompaniment of aging [1]. Significant mortality and morbidity are associated with immobility, and this often results in nursing home placement [2]. There are multiple causes of gait disturbances in the elderly, and patients can experience more than one cause for the gait disturbance (see Chapter 10). In this chapter we discuss movement disorders causing gait disturbances in the elderly: Parkinson's disease (PD), parkinsonsim-plus syndromes, secondary parkinsonism (including senile gait), and orthostatic tremor.

PARKINSON'S DISEASE

Epidemiology

PD is a common degenerative disease of the nervous system [3]. It is rare before age 30, and only 5–10% of the cases present before age 40 [4]. The mean age of onset is approximately 62 years [5]. The incidence of PD increases with advancing age up to 70 to 79 years; at very high ages (older than 90 years), incidence rates indicate a decline [6]. The mean age of PD patients living in the community is 67 to 69 years, with 75–80% being 60 to 79 years [7]. The average annual incidence is 20 cases per 100,000 [8]. Both genders are affected equally [5]. The current data indicate that whites are at a greater risk for PD than are blacks and Asians [9, 10].

Clinical Features

Resting tremor, rigidity, bradykinesia, and postural instability are the cardinal signs of PD. Often, tremor is the most common initial symptom that results in neurological consultation. Other early manifestations include loss of dexterity of finger movements (e.g., buttoning a shirt), infrequent blinking of the eyelids, lack of facial expression, micrographia, flexed posture of the trunk, poverty of associated movement, dragging of a leg, and the sensation of tightness, stiffness, and aching in the limbs [11]. Gait abnormalities are very common in PD. Although postural instability and falls often are seen in the late stages of PD, usually they are not the presenting symptoms. In fact, early postural instability and falls are not typical of PD and suggest alternative diagnoses, such as the parkinsonism-plus syndromes.

In 1817, in *An Essay on the Shaking Palsy* [12], James Parkinson described gait abnormality as follows:

> The propensity to lean forward becomes invincible, and the patient is thereby forced to step on the toes and fore part of the feet, whilst the upper part of the body is thrown so far forward as to render it difficult to avoid falling on the face. In some cases, when this state of the malady is attained, the patient can no longer exercise himself by walking in his usual manner, but is thrown on the toes and forepart of the feet; being, at the same time, irresistibly impelled to take much quicker and shorter steps, and thereby to adopt unwillingly a running pace. In some cases it is found necessary entirely to substitute running for walking; since otherwise the patient, on proceeding only a very few paces, would inevitably fall.

Gait abnormalities are the presenting complaint in 12–18% of PD patients [5, 13]. Early in the disease, when one side is affected, the patient appears to drag a leg during ambulation. When the opposite leg also is involved, the steps are short, and the feet appear barely to clear the floor, giving the impression of a shuffling gait (*marche à petits pas*). Parkinsonian patients have great difficulty with taking the first step (start-hesitation). As the disease progresses, the patient develops a stooped posture, with flexion of the shoulders, neck, and trunk. The center of gravity is shifted forward and, during ambulation, the flexed trunk precedes the lower limbs, leading the patient to take increasingly frequent, short steps, often ending with the patient falling. This phenomenon is known as *festination* and is one of the characteristics of advanced PD. Instead of the propulsive gait, a patient might develop retropulsion, a tendency to fall backward or to take increasingly frequent, short backward steps. Resting tremor often is exacerbated while walking.

When gait abnormalities are present, a patient turns with small steps and moves the trunk in a rigid manner (*en bloc turning*). There is little associated body movement. The arm swing is decreased or may be absent. "Freezing" may be seen, a phenomenon referring to the patient's feet appearing stuck to the ground while walking, rendering the patient unable to initiate movements of the lower limbs. This is seen especially in doorways and elevators and on turns. After a few seconds to minutes, the patient may be able to walk again, first taking multiple small steps and then resuming normal stride. Freezing episodes and related phenomena in general often are called *motor blocks*. Giladi et al. [14] reported that 32% of their 990 PD patients had motor blocks. Start-hesitation occurred in 86%, blocking on turning in 45%, and blocking in narrow spaces in 25% of patients. When the initial symptoms of PD occur in the upper body, there is less likelihood of motor blocks. Giladi et al. also reported that a longer duration of the disease, a higher Hoehn and Yahr stage, and a longer duration of levodopa therapy were significantly associated with the presence of motor blocks.

Normally during walking, the heel strikes the ground before the forefoot.

Hughes et al. [15] studied foot-strike in PD patients and healthy controls. In controls, 16% of the strikes were made simultaneously by heel and forefoot, but in no instance did the forefoot precede the heel. The strikes with forefoot alone are not uncommon in PD.

Falling is another major disability in PD. Although multiple causes of falling occur in this disease, the most important ones include mental status changes, difficulties in sitting and rising, orthostatic hypotension, dyskinesias, postural instability, age-related physical changes, and gait abnormalities [16–20]. Gait abnormalities such as start-hesitation, festination, retropulsion, and freezing also can lead to falls. At times, the patient may trip or stumble over rough surfaces because each step is too small to clear the obstacle. In the later stages of the disease, frequent falling often is caused by postural instability [21].

Treatment

Early gait difficulties in PD may be helped with antiparkinsonian medications. Although anticholinergics are suggested to be most effective in the treatment of tremor and rigidity, in some patients with severe gait disorder and postural reflex impairment, there might be some degree of benefit from these drugs [22]. Anticholinergics should be used cautiously in the elderly because of significant cognitive adverse effects. Walker et al. [23] reported the beneficial effects of amantadine monotherapy in 42 PD patients, reporting significant improvement in 10 of the 19 tests of strength and posture and in all tests of coordination and gait.

Similarly, levodopa therapy in parkinsonian patients has been shown to increase maximum velocity as well as stride length at maximum velocity [24]. Blin et al. [25] performed quantitative analysis of gait in 20 parkinsonians before and after administration of levodopa. They found that certain parameters, such as stride length and swing velocity and peak velocity, were levodopa-sensitive, whereas stride and swing duration and stride duration variability were levodopa-resistant.

Gait improvement has been reported in clinical trials with such dopamine agonists as bromocriptine and pergolide [26–29]. Weiner et al. [30] studied the use of ciladopa (a troponylpiperazine derivative) in 32 parkinsonian patients and found significant improvement in gait scores and in total disability scores. However, this drug presently is not available.

Unfortunately, the treatment of motor blocks in PD is very disappointing. Giladi et al. [14] have proposed that motor blocks can occur due to disease progression or as short-term or long-term side effects of levodopa treatment. Hence, the initial drug management of motor blocks should include changes in dopaminergic therapy. Some Japanese investigators have reported marked improvement in the freezing phenomenon with L- and DL-threodihydroxyphenylserine [31, 32]; however, these findings could not be confirmed by other investigators [33, 34]. When drugs have no benefit in motor blocks, behavioral therapy may be considered. Motor and sensory tricks can help the patient to combat freezing for a short time [35]. It is believed that the use of sensory inputs will force the use of motor skills that require attention and will help to relieve motor blocks. Dunne et al. [36] reported three parkinsonian patients who discovered that their gait was facilitated by inverting a walking stick and using the handle as a visual cue to step over and initiate walking. Similarly, placing strips on the floor [37] over which to step and marching in place are other techniques that should be considered.

Postural instability responds poorly to drug therapy. Klawans and Topel [38] studied 11 parkinsonian patients with loss of postural reflexes and reported that all 11 patients responded to amantadine or levodopa but not to anticholinergics. However, Koller et al. [21] did not find any benefit by changing levodopa dosage or by adding bromocriptine. It is a general opinion of Parkinson's disease experts that postural instability does not respond to present pharmacological treatment.

Some patients who had undergone autologous adrenal implants had improvement in gait and postural instability [39–41]. However, this form of therapy presently has been abandoned. Similarly, gait improvement has been reported following human fetal mesencephalic tissue transplantation [42, 43]. However, this procedure still is under investigation. Significant gait improvement also has been reported with stereotactic surgery for PD [44].

Recently, Burleigh et al. [45] conducted a study to evaluate balance improvements in a patient who had PD and had undergone thalamic stimulation for control of left upper-extremity tremor. These researchers used electromyograms (EMGs) and forceplate recordings to quantify the benefits of thalamic stimulation on tremor and lower-extremity postural muscle activations for quiet-stance, step initiation, and equilibrium responses. Their results suggested that thalamic stimulation improved the balance by reducing tremor and by increasing burst duration and magnitude of the tibialis anterior, which functions as the postural prime mover for step initiation and balance tasks.

At times, patients with PD do not respond to antiparkinsonian medications or cannot tolerate these medications because of the adverse effects. Electroconvulsive therapy used for treatment of depression has been shown to improve gait in PD [46].

Gait training and physical therapy are other forms of treatment that might be of benefit in PD. However, scientific data regarding the use of these forms of therapy are lacking. Although physical and occupational therapy is used routinely in PD patients, Gibbard et al. [47] did not find any benefit from these therapies in PD patients on stable doses of antiparkinsonian medications. Similarly, Pedersen et al. [48] studied 10 patients with mild to moderate parkinsonism before and after a 12-week training program and found no improvement in gait. However, Palmer et al. [49] assessed two groups of PD patients with two different 12-week exercise programs. They showed that the majority of patients in both groups improved in gait, tremor, grip strength, and motor coordination. In the later stages of the disease, patients may be forced to use a wheelchair to prevent morbidity from falls. The use of physical and occupational therapy is discussed in detail in Chapters 20 through 24.

OTHER MOVEMENT DISORDERS THAT CAUSE GAIT IMPAIRMENT IN THE ELDERLY

Other causes of parkinsonism (Table 13-1) and basal ganglia lesions, frontal lobe dysfunction, diffuse white matter disease, and advancing age may also cause similar gait disturbances. Parkinsonism-plus syndromes, (Table 13-2) initially may be difficult to differentiate from PD. However, the fully developed syndromes have distinctive clinical characteristics.

Progressive supranuclear palsy (PSP) is a neurodegenerative disease of unknown etiology; occurs at a rate of 0.3 per 100,000 [50] and its prevalence is 1.46 per 100,000 [51]. The mean age of onset of symptoms is 62 years [51]. Clinical features include bradykinesia, rigidity, supranuclear gaze palsy, pseudobulbar signs, and severe gait difficulty. Other important features include dementia, axial extensor dystonia, poor response to levodopa, and a more rapid course than untreated PD [52]. Gait disturbances are the most common presenting complaints in PSP [53, 54]. Those affected also have marked postural instability that leads to falls early in the disease. Jankovic et al. [55] suggested that the instability was due to visual-vestibular impairment, axial rigidity, and bradykinesia. The gait in PSP is different from that in PD. PSP patients have a stiff, broad-based gait with ataxic quality. Instead of turning en bloc, these patients pivot and also often fall backward while pivoting or backing to a chair [50].

The drug treatment of PSP has been disappointing, though levodopa therapy may produce modest improvement in parkinsonian signs early in the disease. In a review of the literature [52], Jankovic reported that 30 of 59 patients treated with levodopa had improvement in parkinsonian or pseudobulbar signs. Dopamine agonists, amantadine, and anticholinergics have been reported to produce an inconsistent response [56, 57]. Amitriptyline improved gait and rigidity in three of four patients [58]. Similar benefit was reported with desipramine [50]. Ghika et al. [59] studied the use of idazoxan in PSP and found a significant benefit in mobility, balance, gait, and measures of digital dexterity. However, due to sympathetic side effects, further development of this drug has been abandoned [50]. Physical therapy and gait training might benefit these patients in early disease.

Striatonigral degeneration (SND) is a condition with diffuse neuronal degeneration of the putamen and substantia nigra. The average age of onset is 58 years [60]. Clinical features of SND are similar to those of PD. The gait is slow and shuffling, with festination and decreased arm swing. In contrast to those with PD, patients with SND manifest a tendency to fall early in the course of the disease. Other atypical features include decreased incidence of resting tremor, absence of response to levodopa, and severe dysphonia or dysphagia [60].

The initial clinical presentation of *olivopontocerebellar atrophies* (OPCA) is ataxia of gait, with kinetic tremor and dysarthria. Initial gait manifestations might include imbalance or occasional stumbling. This might progress to wide-based staggering gait. Affected patients might tend to lurch from side to side or

Table 13-1. Secondary causes of parkinsonism

Causes	Comments
Infectious	Onset in young adults; history of encephalitis
Toxins	
Manganese	Chronic exposure required; initial presentation neuropsychiatric symptoms; later parkinsonism; action rather than rest tremor; cerebellar dysfunction
Carbon monoxide	History of exposure; diffuse nervous system dysfunction with parkinsonism; CT of the head: bilateral globus pallidus necrosis
Carbon disulphide	Parkinsonism, dementia, neuropathies seen with chronic exposure
Cyanide	Parkinsonism in cyanide poisoning survivors
MPTP*	In young adults; use of intravenous drugs purported to be synthetic heroin
Pharmacological causes	Various drugs can cause parkinsonism (e.g., neuroleptics, reserpine, tetrabenazine, alpha-methyldopa)
Parkinsonism-plus syndromes	See Table 13-2
Other degenerative conditions	
Primary pallidal atrophy	Juvenile onset, progressive parkinsonism with chorea and dystonia
Idiopathic dystonia-parkinsonism	Juvenile and adult onset; diurnal fluctuations of parkinsonism, dystonia
CBGD*	Onset in midlife; clinical features of cortical and basal ganglia involvement; unilaterality
Hemiparkinsonism	Late complication of hemiatrophy due to injury in early life
ALS-parkinsonism-dementia	Endemic occurrence in Guam; signs of ALS, parkinsonism, and dementia
Alzheimer's and Pick's	Primary dementing conditions, parkinsonism possibly seen in later stages of the disease
Atherosclerotic	See text
CJD*	Dementing condition with subacute onset and rapid course; many regions of central nervous system involvement, including basal ganglia
GSSD*	Onset in midlife; ataxia, pyramidal signs, dementia, later parkinsonism
Central nervous disorders	
NPH*	See text
Brain tumors	Parkinsonism possibly seen with brain tumors; neuroimaging diagnostic
Trauma	Rare, chronic traumatic encephalopathy of boxers
Metabolic causes	
Hypoparathyroidism and basal ganglia calcification	Disorders of calcium metabolism possibly resulting in basal ganglia calcification and sometimes parkinsonism
Chronic hepatocerebral degeneration	Seen in some patients with repeated episodes of hepatic coma
Hereditary disease	
Wilson's disease	Onset in adolescence; decreased serum ceruloplasmin and copper and increased 24-hr excretion of copper diagnostic
Huntington's chorea	Hyperkinetic disorder; juvenile onset possibly with primary parkinsonian features

*MPTP = 1-methyl-4-phenyl-1,2,3,6-tetrahydropyridine; CBGD = corticobasal ganglionic degeneration; ALS = amyotrophic lateral sclerosis; CJD = Creutzfeldt-Jakob disease; GSSD = Gerstmann-Sträussler-Scheinker disease; NPH = normal-pressure hydrocephalus.

Table 13-2. Parkinsonism-plus syndromes

	PD	PSP	SND	OPCA	SDS
Rest tremor	+	±	±	−	+
Kinetic tremor	−	−	−	+	+
Rigidity	+	+	+	+	+
Postural instability	+	+	+	+	+
Pyramidal signs	−	±	−	+	+
Cerebellar signs	−	±	−	+	+
Autonomic dysfunction	±	±	±	±	+
Dementia	±	+	±	+	±
Axial and nuchal rigidity	−	+	−	−	−
Supranuclear gaze palsy	−	+	−	−	−
Response to levodopa	+	±	−	±	±

PD = Parkinson's disease; PSP = progressive supranuclear palsy; SND = striatonigral degeneration; OPCA = olivopontocerebellar atrophy; SDS = Shy-Drager syndrome.
+, present; −, absent; ±, may be present.

drift to one side while walking. Parkinsonian features may present in later stages of the disease, and the gait may change to slow and shuffling, wide-based gait with decreased arm swing. The age of onset varies from infancy into the seventh decade [61].

There are patients who do not fit any category of PSP, SND or OPCA. These patients have drug-resistant parkinsonism along with upper– or lower–motor-neuron signs and (often) with autonomic failure. These patients' disorders are classified as *multi system atrophy* or *Shy-Drager syndrome* (if associated with autonomic failure) [62]. Gait abnormalities include unsteadiness of gait, slow shuffling gait, wide-based ataxic gait, or (rarely) spastic gait. Some patients may have a combination of these features.

Diffuse Lewy-body disease (DLBD) is being increasingly recognized in patients with degenerative dementing illnesses. Although the clinical presentation is variable, most patients have a combination of dementia and parkinsonism. Some investigators have suggested that prominent gait impairment with mild dementia early in the disease might be a distinguishing feature of DLBD [63]. Gait abnormalities are similar to those seen with PD and include slow shuffling gait with festination. Pathological features include changes of PD along with considerable number of Lewy bodies in the cortex. In addition, patients may have Alzheimer-type changes (senile plaques and neurofibrillary tangles) [63].

Corticobasal ganglionic degeneration (CBGD) is a disease characterized by marked asymmetry of clinical presentation and course [65]. The symptoms usually begin in one upper limb and remain limited for a few years before they become generalized. When the symptoms are limited to the upper limb, the gait abnormality present is decreased arm swing or dystonic posturing of the affected arm while walking. Rarely, gait abnormality, postural instability, or falls can be the presenting feature of this disease.

Pure akinesia is a rare syndrome of progressive akinesia of gait, speech, and handwriting without rigidity, tremor, or dementia [65]. The majority of cases are reported from Japan. Gait difficulties include trouble in initiating walking with either leg, festination, freezing, and dysequilibrium that leads to frequent falling [65].

Atherosclerotic parkinsonism differs from PD by the absence of tremor, symmetrical involvement, older age, and presence of hypertension [66]. A shuffling gait similar to that in PD is present in atherosclerotic parkinsonism; however, these patients have persistent freezing as opposed to transient freezing with PD. There is a lack of festination and the presence of a full arm swing in these patients (see Chapter 14).

The term *gait apraxia* is used to describe gait abnormalities in patients with frontal lobe disease and in normal-pressure hydrocephalus (NPH). Gait apraxia is defined as inability to walk despite no abnormalities in motor strength, coordination, or sensory function [67]. NPH is a syndrome of progressive dementia, gait difficulty, and urinary incontinence. The gait difficulty has some resemblance to that of PD [68]. Similar to freezing seen in PD, on attempting to walk, patients with NPH appear to be glued to the floor and are unable to take any steps. Walking produces short, shuffling steps, with poor balance leading to falls (see Chapter 15).

The term *senile gait* refers to severe walking difficulty in elderly patients in whom no underlying cause can be found [69]. Critchley [71] defined senile gait as gradual onset of a broad-based gait, with small steps associated with diminished arm swing, stooped posture, flexion of hips and knees, uncertainty and stiffness in turning, occasional difficulty in initiating steps, or a tendency toward falling. Such patients have difficulty in starting to walk, they often shuffle, or their feet appear to be glued to the floor. Once they begin, they may walk fairly well. Koller et al. [69] studied 16 patients with senile gait and reported the following abnormalities: inability to perform tandem gait, 100%; wide-based gait, 88%; poor truncal stability, 75%; gait dysrhythmia, 69%; flexed attitude, 63%; shortened steps, 63%; bradykinesia, 50%; loss of associated arm movement, 31%; diminished ability to advance steps, 25%; gait apraxia, 13%; and broad base, 6%. CT of the head may show dilatation of the lateral and third ventricle without changes in cerebral atrophy. The etiology of senile gait is unknown, and it is unclear whether there are multiple types of senile gait or whether it is a single progressive disorder. Senile gait has been suggested to be a manifestation of extrapyramidal dysfunction [70], frontal lobe disease [71], or cerebellar dysfunction [72] or to be secondary to sensory abnormalities [72] or hydrocephalus. However, none of these conditions causes senile gait. At times, senile gait may be difficult to differentiate from PD. However, symmetrical signs, absence of tremor, and poor response to levodopa are present only in senile gait. There is no pharmacological treatment that has benefited senile gait. Physical therapy and gait training are the only options available.

Orthostatic tremor may present as a gait disorder in the eldery. Since Heilman's[1] description of this entity in three patients, there have been several reports[2] of this distinctive tremor. The patients, generally middle-aged or elderly persons, complain of shakiness or tremulousness on standing causing the patients to fall unless they sit or walk, when the tremor markedly decreases or disappears. Thus, the characteristic clinical feature is its presence in the legs only on standing or pressing the feet against the foot end of the bed in the supine position. In the strictest sense, orthostatic tremor is a disorder of station rather than the gait. Orthostatic tremor shows distinctive physiological characteristics[3,4]. It occurs at a fast rate of 14-18 Hz with an average of 16 Hz synchronously in the homologous lower limbs and may be synchronous or alternating between agonist and antagonist muscles of the same limb. Peripheral perturbations (e.g., electrical stimulation of the peroneal or tibial nerves) do not reset or disrupt the leg tremor. Although patients do not complain of tremor in the upper extremities, electrophysiologic recordings in the forearm muscles of the outstretched upper limbs often display a tremor with similar frequency as in the lower limbs[4]. The patients generally do not have a voice or head tremor. The relationship between orthostatic tremor and essential-familial tremor remains controversial. Some investigators consider orthostatic tremor as a variant of essential tremor[2,5,6] but there are striking differences between these two entities in terms of clinical presentation, physiologic findings and pharmacologic responses[7]. The presence of tremor in the legs only on standing and not on walking, a frequency of 16 Hz, synchronicity between the homologous limbs, a failure of resetting of the tremor following peripheral perturbation, generally good response to clonazepam and not to beta blockers or alcohol differentiate orthostatic tremor from essential tremor. On the other hand, some findings may be cited to support the theory that orthostatic tremor is a variant of essential tremor, as follows: (1) the presence of similar tremor in the outstretched upper extremities[4,7], (2) reports of leg tremors only on standing and responding to clonazepam in some family members of essential tremor[5], (3) occasional reports of change of frequency of tremor from 16 Hz to 8 Hz tremor during physiologic recordings in orthostatic tremor patients;[3] and (4) a rare report of voice tremor in patients with orthostatic tremor. Until molecular genetic analysis identifies a specific gene for essential tremor or orthostatic tremor patients, it seems best to consider orthostatic tremor as a distinct entity separate from essential tremor and treat it accordingly with clonazepam with success in most of the cases.

SUMMARY

Gait abnormalities are common problems in PD. The parkinsonian gait is slow and shuffling, with periodic freezing. The patient turns en bloc. Postural instability and falling are other major gait problems in PD. Similar gait disturbances may be seen with other causes of parkinsonism. Early gait difficulties respond to dopaminergic therapy. In the later stages of the disease, one can offer physical therapy and gait training.

REFERENCES

1. Drachman D. An Approach to the Neurology of Aging. In: Birren J, Sloan R, eds. *Handbook of Mental Health and Aging*. Englewood Cliffs, NJ: Prentice-Hall, 1980. P 501.

2. Sudarsky L, Ronthal M. Gait disorders among elderly patients: A survey study of 50 patients. *Arch Neurol* 1983;40:740–743.

3. Koller WC. *Handbook of Parkinson's Disease*. New York: Marcel Dekker, 1993.

4. Teravainen H, et al. The age of onset of Parkinson's disease: Etiological implications. *Can J Neurol Sci* 1986;13:317–319.

5. Hoehn MM, Yahr MD. Parkinsonism: Onset, progression and mortality. *Neurology* 1967;17:427–442.

6. Marttila RJ, Rinne UK. Epidemiology of Parkinson's disease in Finland. *Acta Neurol Scand* 1976;53:81–102.

7. Martilla RJ. Epidemiology. In: Koller WC, ed. *Handbook of Parkinson's Disease*, 2nd ed. New York: Marcel Dekker, 1993. Pp 35–57.

8. Tanner CM. Epidemiology of Parkinson's disease. *Neurol Clin* 1992;10:317–329.

9. Osuntokun BO. The pattern of neurological illness in tropical Africa: Experience at Ibadan, Nigeria. *J Neurol Sci* 1971;12:417.

10. Okada K, Kobayashi S, Tsunematsu T. Prevalence of Parkinson's disease in Izumo City, Japan. *Gerontology* 1990;36:340–344.

11. Weiner WW, Lang AE. Parkinson's Disease. In: Weiner WW, Lang AE, eds. *Movement Disorders, a Comprehensive Survey*. New York: Futura, 1989. Pp 23–116.

12. Parkinson J. *An Essay on the Shaking Palsy*. London: Sherwood, Neely, and Jones, 1817.

13. Martin WE, Loewenson RB, Resch JA, Baker AB. Parkinson's disease. Clinical analysis of 100 patients. *Neurology* 1973;23:783–790.

14. Giladi N, et al. Motor blocks in Parkinson's disease. *Neurology* 1992;42:333–339.

15. Hughes JR, et al. Parkinsonian abnormality of foot strike: A phenomenon of aging and/or one responsive to levodopa therapy. *Br J Clin Pharmacol* 1990;29:179–186.

16. Purdon-Martin J. *The Basal Ganglia and Posture*. Philadelphia: Lippincott, 1967.

17. Reichert WH, Doolittle J, McDowell FH. Vestibular dysfunction in Parkinson's disease. *Neurology* 1982;32:1133–1138.

18. Traub MM, Rothwell JC, Marsden CD. Anticipatory postural reflexes in Parkinson's disease and other akinetic-rigid syndromes and in cerebellar ataxia. *Brain* 1980;103:393–412.

19. Weiner WJ, Nora LM, Wentz RH. Elderly inpatients: Postural reflex impairment. *Neurology* 1984;34:945–946.

20. Jankovic J. Pathophysiology and Clinical Assessment of Motor Symptoms in Parkinson's Disease. In: Koller WC, ed. *Handbook of Parkinson's Disease*, 2nd ed. New York: Marcel Dekker, 1993. Pp 129–157.

21. Koller WC, Glatt S. Vetere-Overfield B, Hassanein R. Falls and Parkinson's disease. *Clin Neuropharmacol* 1989;12:98–105.

22. Comella CL, Tanner CM. Anticholinergic Drugs in the Treatment of Parkinson's Disease. In: Koller WC, Paulson G, eds. *Therapy of Parkinson's Disease*. New York: Marcel Dekker, 1990. Pp 123–141.

23. Walker JE, et al. A qualitative and quantitative evaluation of amantadine in the treatment of Parkinson's disease. *J Chron Dis* 1972;25:149–182.

24. Pedersen SW, Eriksson T, Öberg B. Effects of withdrawal of antiparkinson medication on gait and clinical score in the Parkinson patient. *Acta Neurol Scand* 1991;84:7–13.

25. Blin O, Ferrandez AM, Pailhous J, Serratrice G. Dopa-sensitive and dopa-resistant gait parameters in Parkinson's disease. *J Neurol Sci* 1991;103:41–54.

26. Lieberman A, Kupersmith M, Gopinathan G. Bromocriptine in Parkinson's disease: Further studies. *Neurology* 1979;29:363–369.

27. Corsini GU, Bonuccelli U, Rainer E, Del Zompo M. Therapeutic efficacy of a partial

dopamine agonist in drug-free parkinsonian patients. *J Neural Transm Park Dis Dement Sec* 1985;64:105–111.

28. Sage JI, Duvoisin RC. Pergolide therapy in Parkinson's disease: A double-blind placebo-controlled study. *Clin Neuropharmacol* 1985;8:260–265.

29. Langtry HD, Clissold SP. Pergolide. A review of its pharmacological properties and therapeutic potential in Parkinson's disease. *Drugs* 1990;39:491–506.

30. Weiner WJ, Factor SA, Sanchez-Ramos J, Berger J. A double-blind evaluation of ciladopa in Parkinson's disease. *Mov Disord* 1987;2:211–217.

31. Narabayashi H, et al. L-Threo-3,4-Dihydroxyphenylserine for Freezing Phenomenon of Parkinsonism. In: Yahr MD, ed. *Current Concepts in Parkinson's Disease.* Amsterdam: Elsevier, 1983. Pp 152–158.

32. Yamamato M, Ujike H, Ogawa N. Effective treatment of pure akinesia with L-threo-3,4-dihydroxyphenylserine (DOPS): Report of a case, with pharmacological considerations. *Clin Neuropharmacol* 1985;8:334–342.

33. Quinn NP, Perlmutter JS, Marsden CD. Acute administration of DL-threo-DOPS does not affect the freezing phenomena in parkinsonian patients. *Neurology* 1984;34(suppl 1):149A.

34. Suzuki T, Sakoda S, Veji M, et al. Treatment of parkinsonism with L-threo-dihydroxyphenylserine. *Neurology* 1984;34:1446–1450.

35. Stern GM, Lander CM, Lees AJ. Akinetic freezing and trick movements in Parkinson's disease. *J Neural Transm Park Dis Dement Sec* 1980;16(suppl):137–141.

36. Dunne JW, Hankey GJ, Edis RH. Parkinsonism: Upturned walking stick as an aid to locomotion. *Arch Phys Med Rehabil* 1987;68:380–381.

37. Martin JP. Disorder of Locomotion Associated with Disease of the Basal Ganglia. In: *The Basal Ganglia and Posture.* Philadelphia: Lippincott, 1967. Pp 24–35.

38. Klawans HL, Topel JL. Parkinsonism as a falling sickness. *JAMA* 1974;230:1555–1557.

39. Goetz CG, et al. Multicenter study of autologous adrenal medullary transplantation to the corpus striatum in patients with advanced Parkinson's disease. *N Engl J Med* 1989;320:337–341.

40. Allen GS, Burns RS, Tulipan NB, Parker RA. Adrenal medullary transplantation to the caudate nucleus in Parkinson's disease. *Arch Neurol* 1989;46:487–491.

41. Olanow CW, et al. Autologous transplantation of adrenal medulla in Parkinson's disease: 18-month results. *Arch Neurol* 1990;47:1286–1289.

42. Spencer DD, et al. Unilateral transplantation of human fetal mesencephalic tissue into the caudate nucleus of patients with Parkinson's disease. *N Engl J Med* 1992;327:1541–1548.

43. Freed CR, et al. Survival of implanted fetal dopamine cells and neurologic improvement 12 to 46 months after transplantation for Parkinson's disease. *N Engl J Med* 1992;327:1549–1555.

44. Laitinen LV, Bergenheim AT, Hariz MI. Leksell's posteroventral pallidotomy in the treatment of Parkinson's disease. *J Neurosurg* 1992;76:53–61.

45. Burleigh AL, Horak FB, Burchiel KJ, Nutt JG. Effects of thalamic stimulation on tremor, balance, and step initiation: A single subject study. *Mov Disord* 1993;8:519–524.

46. Levy LA, Savit JM, Hodes M. Parkinsonism: Improvement by electroconvulsive therapy. *Arch Phys Med Rehabil* 1983;64:432–433.

47. Gibbard FB, et al. Controlled trial of physiotherapy and occupational therapy for Parkinson's disease. *Br Med J* 1981;282:1196.

48. Pedersen SW, Oberg B, Insulander A, Vretman M. Group training in parkinsonism: Quantitative measurements of treatment. *Scand J Rehabil Med* 1990;22:207–211.

49. Palmer SS, et al. Exercise therapy for Parkinson's disease. *Arch Phys Med Rehabil* 1986;67:741–745.

50. Golbe LI. Progressive Supranuclear Palsy. In: Stern MB, Koller WC, eds. *Handbook of Parkinsonian Syndromes.* New York: Marcel Dekker, 1993. Pp 227–247.

51. Golbe LI, Davis PH. Progressive Supranuclear Palsy. Recent Advances. In: Jankovic J, Tolosa E, eds. *Parkinson's Disease and Movement Disorders.* Baltimore: Urban and Schwarzenberg, 1988. Pp 121–130.

52. Jankovic J. Progressive supranuclear palsy: Clinical and pharmacological update. *Neurol Clin* 1984;2:473–486.

53. Maher ER, Lees AJ. The clinical features and natural history of the Steele-Richardson-Olszewski syndrome (progressive supranuclear palsy). *Neurology* 1986;36:1005–1008.

54. Golbe LI, Davis PH, Schoenberg BS, Duvoisin RC. Prevalence and natural history of progressive supranuclear palsy. *Neurology* 1988;38:1031–1034.

55. Jankovic J, Friedman DI, Pirozzolo FJ, McCrary JA. Progressive supranuclear palsy: Motor, neurobehavioral, and neuro-ophthalmic findings. *Adv Neurol* 1990;53:293.

56. Jankovic J. Controlled trial of pergolide mesylate in Parkinson's disease and progressive supranuclear palsy. *Neurology* 1983;33:505–507.

57. Lieberman AN, Goldstein M, et al. The use of lisuride, a potent dopamine and serotonin agonist, in the treatment of progressive supranuclear palsy. *J Neurol Neurosurg Psychiatr* 1982;45:261–263.

58. Newman CG. Treatment of progressive supranuclear palsy with tricyclic antidepressants. *Neurology* 1985;35:1189–1193.

59. Ghika J, et al. Idazoxan treatment in progressive supranuclear palsy. *Neurology* 1991;41:986–991.

60. Fearnley JM, Lees AJ. Striatonigral degeneration. A clinicopathological study. *Brain* 1990;113:1823–1842.

61. Mark MH, Sage JI. Olivopontocerebellar Degeneration. In: Stern MB, Koller WC, eds. *Handbook of Parkinsonian Syndromes*. New York: Marcel Dekker, 1993. Pp 43–68.

62. Fazzini E. Multiple-System Atrophy Associated with Progressive Autonomic Failure: The Shy-Drager Syndrome: A New Classification Scheme. In: Stern MB, Koller WC, eds. *Parkinsonian Syndrome*. New York: Marcel Dekker, 1993. Pp 69–78.

63. Crystal HA, et al. Antemortem diagnosis of diffuse Lewy body disease. *Neurology* 1990;40:1523–1528.

64. Riley DE, et al. Cortical-basal ganglionic degeneration. *Neurology* 1990;40:1203–1212.

65. Riley DE, Fogt N, Leigh JR. The syndrome of "pure akinesia" and its relationship to progressive supranuclear palsy. *Neurology* 1994;44:1025–1029.

66. Hurtig HI. Vascular Parkinsonism. In: Stern MB, Koller WC, eds. *Handbook of Parkinsonian Syndromes*. New York: Marcel Dekker, 1993. Pp 81–93.

67. Estanol BV. Gait apraxia in communicating hydrocephalus. *J Neurol Neurosurg Psychiatr* 1981;44:305–308.

68. Messert B, Wanamaker BB. Reappraisal of the adult hydrocephalus syndrome. *Neurology* 1974;24:224–231.

69. Koller W, et al. Senile gait: Correlation with computed tomographic scan. *Ann Neurol* 1983;13:343–344.

70. Critchley M. Senile disorders of gait. *Geriatrics* 1948;3:364–370.

71. Meyer J, Barrow D. Apraxia of gait: A clinico-physiological study. *Brain* 1960;83:761–784.

72. Greenhouse AH. Neurologic Disability in Normal Aging. In: Joynt RJ, ed. *Seminars in Neurology*. New York: Thieme-Stratton, 1981. Pp 13–21.

73. Fisher CM. The role of hydrocephalus in unexplained late life gait disorders. *Ann Neurol* 1980;8:91–92.74. Heilman K. Orthostatic tremor. Arch Neurol 1984; 41:880-881.

75. Cleeves L, Findley LJ, Marsden CD. Odd tremors. In: Marsden CD, Fahn S (eds). Movement Disorders 3. Oxford: Butterworth-Heinemann, 1994; 434-458.

76. Thompson PD, Rothwell JC, Day BL, et al. The physiology of orthostatic tremor. Arch Neurol 1986; 43:584-588.

77. Tavoulareas G, Chokroverty S, Sander H, et al. Orthostatic tremor: An electrophysiologic analysis. Neurology 1996; 46(2):A 390-391.

78. Wee AS, Subramony SH, Currier RD. Orthostatic tremor in familial-essential tremor. Neurology 1986; 36:1241-1245.

79. Papa SM, Gershanik OS. Orthostatic tremor: An essential tremor variant? Mov Disord 1988; 3:97-108.

80. Britton TC, Thompson PD, Van der Kamp W, et al. Primary orthostatic tremor: Further obervations in six cases. J Neurol 1992; 239:209-217.

14. Cerebrovascular Disorders

Joseph C. Masdeu

Cerebrovascular disorders are very common in older people. They are the third most common cause of death in the United States, after cardiovascular disease and stroke. The majority of the approximately 175,000 yearly fatalities caused by cerebrovascular disease occur in people older than 65 [1]. The term *cerebrovascular disease* designates any abnormality of the brain resulting from a pathological process in its vascular supply. Approximately 85% of instances of cerebrovascular disease result from ischemia following occlusion of brain vessels; the rest are due to hemorrhage from arterial rupture. Approximately 30% of ischemic cases result from atheromatous deposits in the larger arteries, from the carotid bifurcation to the middle cerebral artery. In another 30%, an embolus from the heart, the ascending aorta, or a neck artery occludes a more distal portion of the arterial tree. Arteriolsclerosis of the distal arteries causes approximately 20% of ischemic vascular disease in the form of lacunar infarcts, which are small but often affect multiple areas of the brain. The balance of ischemic strokes are caused by a variety of diseases, or their etiology remains unclear. Typically, cerebrovascular disease causes the clinical syndrome of stroke, with the sudden onset of obvious hemiparesis or aphasia. However, vascular disease of the brain can present as a disorder of gait or equilibrium, with little or no weakness of isometric strength.

This chapter reviews the evidence for vascular disease causing ambulation impairment in older people and indicates the most frequent types of pathology and localization. A summary of therapeutic approaches is provided, but detailed descriptions of the management of cerebrovascular disease can be found in other publications [1, 2].

HISTORICAL PERSPECTIVE

Gait impairment in the elderly as the result of lacunar disease was described by Lhermitte [3] in a monograph on "senile paraplegia" published in 1907. In 1948, Critchley [4] described a common gait abnormality of aging and ascribed it to vascular disease of the brain, reflecting the views of the time. He stated:

> There exists a large group of cases where the gait in old people becomes considerably disordered, although the motor power of the legs is comparatively well preserved. A paradoxical state of affairs is the result: testing of the individual movements of the legs while the patient reclines upon the couch shows little, if any, reduction in the strength. The tonus may not be grossly altered and the reflexes may betray only minor deviations. Sensory tests show no unusual features. But when the patient is instructed to get out of bed and to walk, remarkable defects may

be witnessed. The patient, first of all, appears most reluctant to make the attempt. His stance is bowed and uncertain. He props himself against the end of the bed and seeks the aid of the bystanders. Encouraged to take a few steps, he advances warily and hesitatingly. Clutching the arms of two supporters, he takes short, shuffling steps. The legs tend to crumble by giving way suddenly at the knee joints. Progression, as far as it is possible, is slow and tottery. The patient veers to one side or the other. Frequently the legs cross, so that one foot gets in the way of the other.

In the 1960s and 1970s, the characterization of Parkinson's disease turned the attention of neurologists to dopaminergic dysfunction to explain syndromes of the elderly resembling Critchley's masterly description. Even recently, the term *lower-body parkinsonism* has been coined to designate a similar gait pattern in patients who probably do not suffer from nigral deficiency but have vascular disease of the brain [5, 6]. Despite its decline in diagnostic popularity, stroke still can be listed among the most frequent and yet often forgotten causes of impaired gait and balance. What is overlooked is not sizeable infarction resulting in sudden leg weakness but the accumulation over time of the effect of chronic ischemia or minor episodes of vascular disease of the brain, giving rise to the more subtle and progressive changes in ambulation described by Critchley. Gait impairment may be the consequence of the ischemic white-matter disorder that has been termed *Binswanger's disease* [7]. In addition, in recent years lacunar strokes or acute hemorrhage have been recognized to cause acute impairment of the ability to stand and walk but with little or no change in volitional isometric strength of the muscles of the lower extremities [8].

Neuropathologic and Topographic Classification of Vascular Brain Disease

Ischemic brain disease tends to follow one of three patterns discernible by clinical evaluation and with the help of neuroimaging procedures: (1) cortical infarcts, most often related to embolic disease; (2) subcortical disease, often in the form of widespread lacunes and white-matter changes, most often related to arteriolar disease; and (3) a mixture of the two patterns, often related to atheromatous disease of the major vessels [1, 2]. The second and third of these types of cerebrovascular disease tend to cause gait and balance impairment early in the course of the disease. Strategically located subcortical infarcts may impair equilibrium and gait, with little or no limb weakness on isometric testing. Lacunar events, easily imaged with CT or MRI in the chronic stage, albeit elusive acutely, often are responsible for the sudden onset of impaired balance and gait in an older individual. These lesions tend to affect structures with a critical role in gait and balance mechanisms. Well-known are the disturbances of mobility caused by cerebellar or vestibular cerebrovascular lesions. Recently, striking abnormalities of gait and balance have been described with lesions in the thalamus, in the basal ganglia, and in the pedunculopontine region of the infratentorial compartment [8–10]. These recently recognized syndromes will be described in greater detail.

In addition to acute vascular events, ischemic disease of the brain may cause loss of neurons and oligodendrocytes over time. Unlike the tempo of acute stroke, this type of disorder evolves slowly over several years [11]. Ischemic disease of the white matter will be discussed in detail because it may represent a cause of gait impairment in the elderly [7].

ACUTE VASCULAR DISEASE

In the past few years, several vascular syndromes have been described in which the patients had pronounced abnormalities of their ability to stand and walk, despite having strong leg muscles. These patients' gait differed somewhat from cerebellar gait in that it was not, or was only minimally, broad-based. The outstanding feature was unsteadiness or disequilibrium. Patients tended to topple over after their knees suddenly buckled under them, or they fell like a log, without activating ankle or hip strategies to break the fall. Because most of the lesions involved subcortical structures, this disorder has been called *subcortical disequilibrium* [12]. Lesions of the thalamus, suprathalamic white matter, and basal ganglia may cause this syndrome (Fig. 14-1).

Thalamic Astasia

Inability to stand or walk despite minimal weakness has been recorded with thalamic infarction [13, 14] and hemorrhage [15, 16]. It also has been reported in patients who had lesions in the internal capsule or corona radiata and had the syndrome of unilateral ataxia and crural paresis (ataxic hemiparesis) [17–20].

Masdeu and Gorelick [8] described 15 patients with thalamic lesions (13 of a

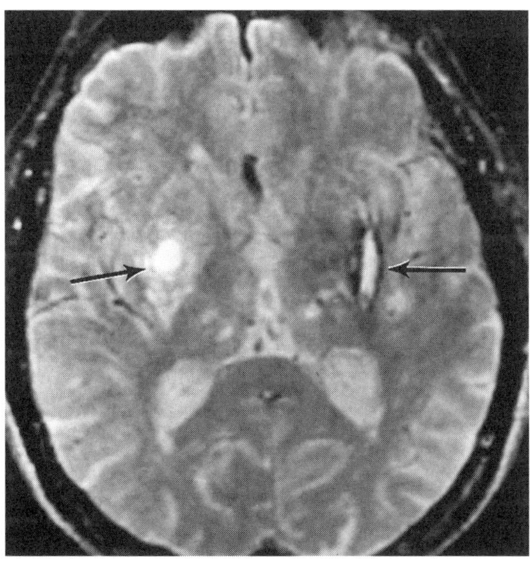

Figure 14-1. Lacunar disease. MRI of a 73-year-old chronic hypertensive man, with a transient episode of mild left-sided weakness but progressive gait impairment. The patient was unsteady on his feet and had sustained multiple falls. In addition to multiple thalamic lacunes and a larger infarct in the right lenticular nucleus, there is an organizing hematoma, surrounded by a dark ring from hemosiderin deposition, in the left external capsular region (*right arrow*).

vascular nature) causing a syndrome of "thalamic astasia." Alert, possessing normal or near normal strength on isometric muscle testing, and with a variable degree of sensory loss, these patients could not stand, and seven of them could not sit up unassisted. They fell backward or toward the side contralateral to the lesion. They appeared to have a deficit of overlearned motor activity of an axial and postural nature. Postural activation of axial muscles, recorded with surface electromyography, was impaired on the side opposite the lesion. Unless supported, the patients fell to either side or backward like a log, failing to perform corrective movements.

A similar situation took place when they tried to sit up in bed: They pulled themselves up by holding onto the side rails but could not sit up unsupported, falling generally backward. Remarkably, they could sit up unsupported if they tried to push forward with the upper part of their chest against the examiner's hand. This discrepancy between preserved volitional strength and poor automatic postural reflexes translated into many other motor behaviors. When asked to push themselves up in bed while lying supine, these patients would not use the limbs contralateral to the lesion, giving the impression that they were hemiplegic. However, they could raise the affected arm or leg on command, often with normal isometric strength. When the lesions were smaller, or in the process of recovery, the patients could stand and walk almost normally for as long as they attended to their gait. As soon as they were distracted, they would become prone to falling by a lack of proper activation of motor synergies involved in automatic walking or even standing. Unexpected, sudden knee buckling, as previously described by Critchley [4], was one of the mechanisms leading to falls. In the 13 vascular cases, the deficit improved in a few days or weeks (Fig. 14-2). However, these patients had a tendency to sustain falls during the rehabilitation period. The lesions were clustered mainly in the superior portion of the ventrolateral nucleus of the thalamus, often involving the suprathalamic white matter (Fig. 14-3).

The propensity of thalamic lesions to cause balance and gait impairment is understood easily by reviewing thalamic connectivity. The ventrolateral nucleus of the thalamus consists of two portions [21, 22]: the smaller anterior portion (VLa) receives projections from the medial globus pallidus via the thalamic fasciculus and projects to area 6 of the frontal cortex (including the supplementary motor area); the larger posterior portion (VLp) receives cerebellar, spinothalamic, and vestibular afferents and projects in a somatotopic fashion to area 4 of the precentral gyrus [21]. Laterosuperior neurons project to the anterior portion of the paracentral lobule in the medial aspect of the frontal lobe, where the trunk and leg are represented. Fibers destined for the leg region course in the posterior limb of the internal capsule and then ascend in the more medial portion of the corona radiata, near the wall of the lateral ventricle. Impairment of gait in the elderly with periventricular white-matter disease might be related to involvement of this pathway [7]. Through the fastigial projection, VLp receives information from the vestibulocerebellum [23]. Bilateral representation of this projection may be one of the factors explaining the transient nature of balance impairment when only one side is affected. Bilateral involvement of these structures by lacu-

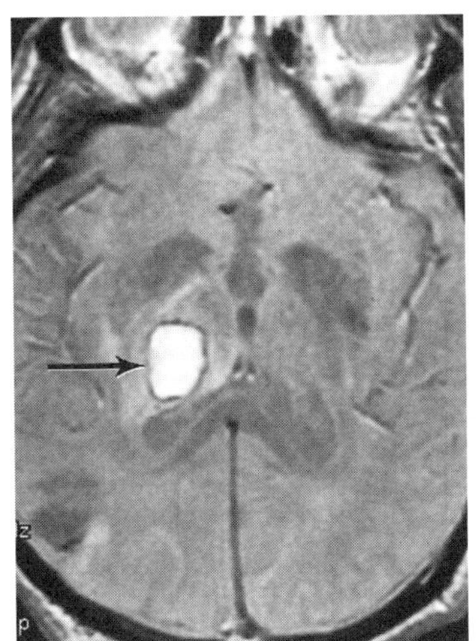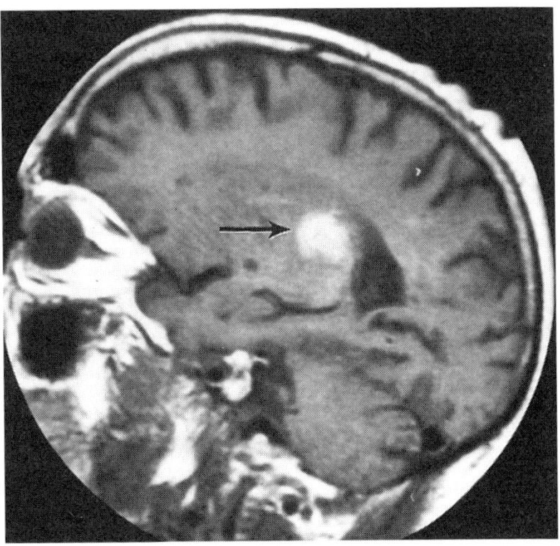

A   *B*

Figure 14-2. Thalamic hematoma. MRI of an 86-year-old man with a transient mild left hemiparesis but with inability to walk for 8 weeks, despite recovery of isometric strength. Gait was unsteady, with the characteristics of "subcortical disequilibrium." A right thalamic hematoma (*arrow*) involves the ventrolateral and ventral posterior nuclei, as well as the pulvinar. Displayed on axial (*A*) and sagittal sections (*B*).

nar disease or disease of the white matter may result in permanent impairment of gait and balance.

Capsular and Basal Ganglia Lesions

A tendency to fall despite good strength was recorded by Groothuis et al. [24] in a patient with a small medial capsular hemorrhage involving the most lateral portion of the ventrolateral nucleus of the thalamus, and by Labadie et al. [9] in patients with acute lesions in the basal ganglia. Multiple bilateral lacunes involving the basal ganglia can be attended by gait impairment (see Fig. 14-1). The impairment of balance resembles the syndrome after lesions of the ventrolateral nucleus of the thalamus. Acutely, such patients fall with a slow, tilting motion (like a falling log) in a lateral or diagonal trajectory. The patients are not aware that they are about to fall and make no protective movements. Within a few days after the acute event, the patients will realize that they are falling when they fall but are unable to perform full corrective movements, such as tilting their body, moving their feet or arms, or reaching for nearby objects. As in the thalamic cases, these patients recovered their ability to ambulate independently in 3 to 6 weeks. Recovery was slower when patients had bilateral basal ganglionic lesions.

Lesions of the putamen interrupt one of the major control loops of the motor system. Starting in the motor and somatosensory areas of the cortex, this pathway projects to the putamen. The putamen projects through the globus pallidus to the ventrolateral and ventral anterior thalamic nuclei, which in turn project to

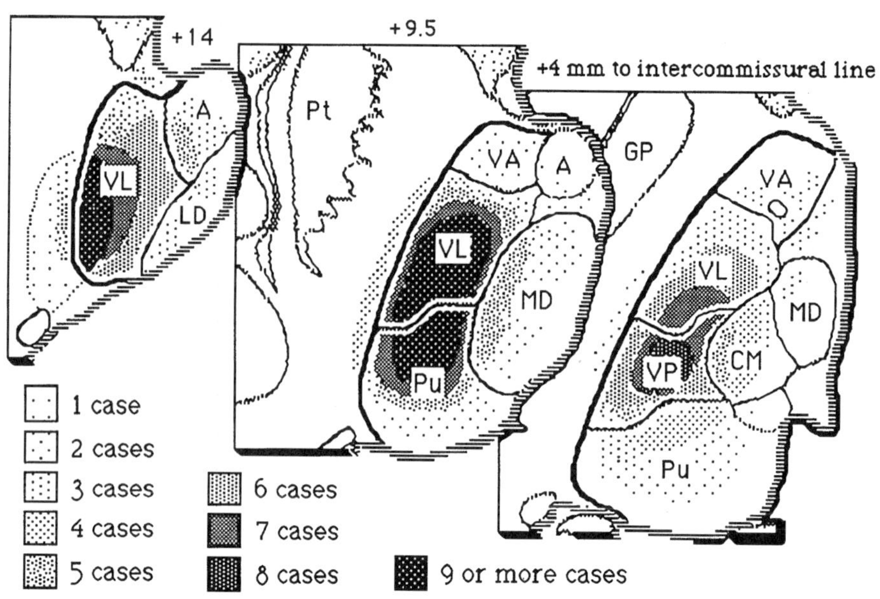

Figure 14-3. Thalamic astasia. Horizontal sections of the thalamus showing the regional frequency distribution of lesions in the patients with thalamic astasia reported by Masdeu and Gorelick [8]. Note that anterior is on top, posterior at the bottom, medial to the right, and lateral to the left. The most rostral section is at the left and the most caudal at the right. Heavier shading indicates a greater number of cases where that region was involved. The code is at the bottom of the figure. A = anterior nuclear group; CM = centromedial nucleus; DM = dorsomedial nucleus; GP = globus pallidus; LD = latero-dorsal nucleus; Pt = putamen; Pu = pulvinar; VA = ventral anterior nucleus; VL = ventrolateral nucleus; VP = ventral posterior nucleus.

the precentral gyrus, supplementary motor area, and premotor cortex of the frontal lobe. Lesions in this pathway are likely to cause impairment of over-learned motor behavior, such as standing or walking, mediated predominantly by proximal muscles.

Pontomesencephalic Gait Failure

The laterodorsal region of the midbrain contains the mesencephalic locomotor region, which plays an important role in locomotion in animals [25]. Stimulation of this region in cats induces rapid walking, followed by running. This area contains the nucleus cuneiformis and the cholinergic pedunculopontine nucleus. In humans, loss of neurons in the pedunculopontine nucleus has been found in progressive supranuclear palsy and Parkinson's disease but not in patients with Alzheimer's disease, implying perhaps a role of this nucleus in ambulatory mechanisms (Fig. 14-4) [26]. The patient who had a hemorrhage in the area of the pedunculopontine nucleus (and whose MRI is shown in Fig. 14-5) had the acute onset of inability to walk, without hemiparesis or sensory loss [10]. She was waiting for a bus after her weekly 6 hours of casino playing when she became nause-

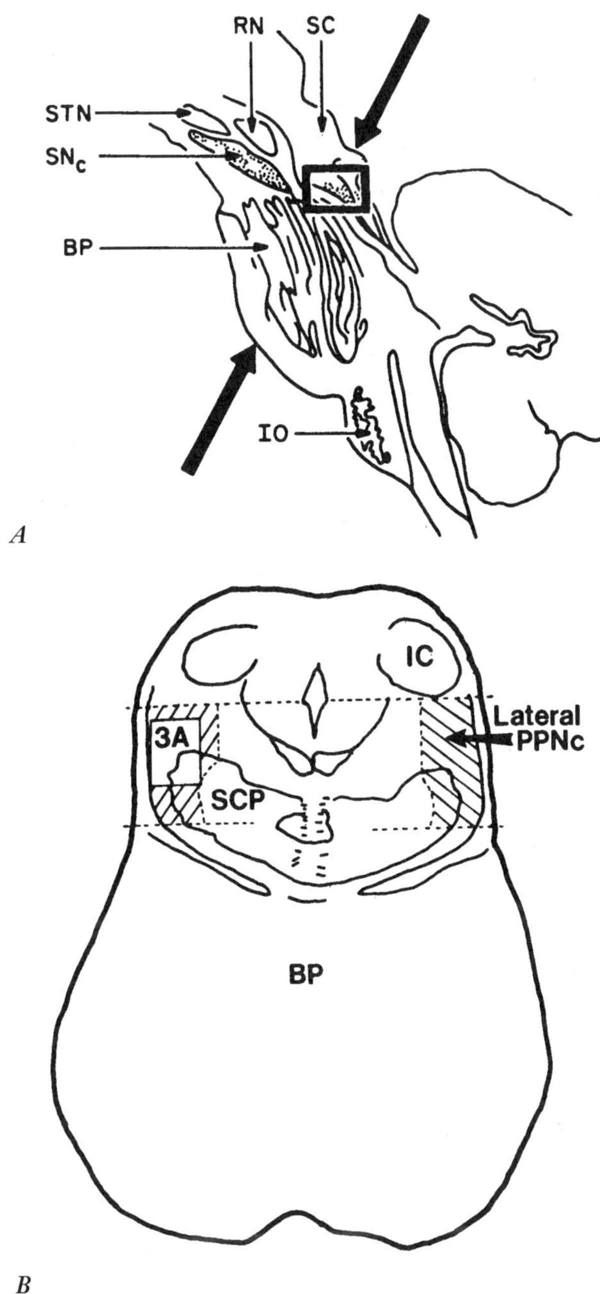

Figure 14-4. Location of the pedunculopontine nucleus (PPN) in the human brain stem, at the junction of the pons and midbrain. *A.* Parasagittal section of a human brain stem through the pedunculopontine nucleus pars compacta (PPNc). Large arrows define approximate level of section *B. B.* Axial section of the brain stem through the lateral PPNc. Shaded areas correspond to lateral PPNc. BP = basis points; IC = inferior colliculus; IO = inferior olive; LL = lateral lemniscus; RN = red nucleus; SC = superior colliculus; SCP = superior cerebellar peduncle; Snc = substantia nigra pars compacta; STN = subthalamic nucleus. (From R Zweig et al. Pedunculopontine cholinergic neurons in progressive supranuclear palsy. *Ann Neurol* 1987; 22:18-25.)

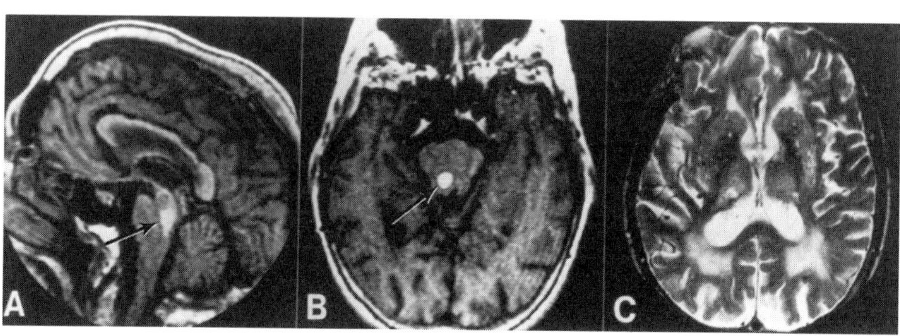

Figure 14-5. Pedunculopontine gait failure. MRI of an 83-year-old woman with gait failure after a hemorrhage in the locomotor mesencephalic region. Lesion is shown in sagittal (*A*) and coronal (*B*) planes. In addition, periventricular white-matter changes and small thalamic lacunes were present in this chronic hypertensive individual (**C**). (From J Masdeu, U Alampur, R Cavaliere, G Tavoulareas. Astasia and gait failure with damage of the pontomesencephalic locomotor region. *Ann Neurol* 1994;35:619–621.

ated and fell to the floor, alert but unable to stand or walk. She could draw a circle with either leg when sitting down but did not generate regular stepping movements with her feet and was unable to stand without support. Holding on to a walker and stooped forward, she walked with short, shuffling, irregular steps. Her base of ambulation was only minimally wide. Regular stepping was not initiated either in attempted walking or in response to loss of her balance. The steps were of irregular amplitude and direction, sometimes directed laterally. The left foot seemed to step less readily than the right. Often there would be two steps with one foot while the other remained motionless. There was no cadence or rhythm in this patient's gait. Her performance bore striking resemblance to the gait failure experienced by many elderly individuals, which in most cases does not have a clear anatomical correlate [12]. Such individuals lack the ability to generate spontaneous, rhythmic stepping movements.

The connectivity of the pedunculopontine region suggests an important role in motor behavior for this area. It receives projections from the deep cerebellar nuclei, substantia nigra, globus pallidus, nucleus locus coeruleus and the raphe nuclei, and projects to the substantia nigra, globus pallidus, subthalamic nucleus, ventrolateral nucleus of the thalamus, motor cortex, and to pontomedullary reticular nuclei known to influence the pattern generators in the spinal cord [25, 27, 28]. In addition to the effects of electrical stimulation mentioned earlier, the results of injection in this area of putative neurotransmitters suggest a role for the pedunculopontine area in locomotion. Spontaneous locomotion, which occurs in the precollicular-premamillary transected cat, can be blocked by the injection of GABA. In contrast, by giving increasing amounts of GABA antagonists or substance P, the step cycle frequency can be increased from a walk to a trot to a gallop [29]. Lesions of the pedunculopontine nucleus lead to a reduction of locomotor activity in experimental animals [30].

Imaging studies in patients with sudden dysfunction of the mesencephalic locomotor center have shown hemorrhagic or ischemic lesions [31–33]. Like the woman described earlier, these patients generally are hypertensive, with small-vessel disease causing white-matter changes and lacunes in the basal ganglia and thalami. Therefore, their impairment could be caused by damage of several overlapping brain mechanisms subserving gait and balance in the human brain.

Vestibular Vascular Disease

Vestibular involvement occurs in the lateral medullary syndrome (Wallenberg's), which is caused by infarction in the territory of the vertebral or the posteroinferior cerebellar arteries. Affected patients tend to fall to the side of the infarct. Their gait is broad-based and lurching. Removal of vision by environmental darkness or impaired eye-sight negatively affects their ability to ambulate and predisposes them to falls. Initially, most of these patients have a prominent headache and are nauseated. In addition to the impairment of balance and to ataxia ipsilateral to the lesion, they have a crossed sensory loss (on the ipsilateral face and contralateral body), an ipsilateral Horner's syndrome, and ipsilateral palatal weakness, with hoarseness and dysphagia. These findings reflect involvement of the vestibular nuclei and inferior cerebellar peduncle, trigeminal pathways, spinothalamic tract, sympathetic pathways projecting from the hypothalamus to the low cervical segments, and nucleus ambiguus of the glossopharyngeal and vagus nerves. Also, they have central vestibular nystagmus or oculoparetic nystagmus if the lesion extends upward into the lower pons.

Atherosclerotic vascular disease of the vertebral or posteroinferior cerebellar arteries may occlude these vessels and is responsible for this syndrome in approximately half of such cases (Fig. 14-6) [34]. Vascular reconstruction may help

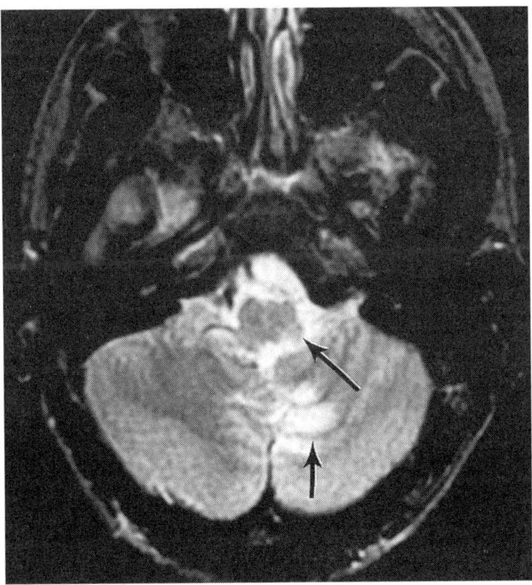

Figure 14-6. Wallenberg's syndrome. MRI showing an infarct in the distribution of the posteroinferior cerebellar artery that involves the laterodorsal medulla and the medial tonsillar region of the cerebellum (*arrows*).

some of these patients [35]. Most of the rest are due to cardiogenic emboli. Spontaneous dissection of the arterial wall is a frequent cause in younger patients [36], but not in older patients, where *temporal arteritis* should be suspected, particularly in the very old with a high sedimentation rate [37]. In a small autopsy series of patients with temporal or giant-cell arteritis, the vertebral arteries were found to be affected in all cases [38]. Polymyalgia rheumatica may be present but is not a universal finding. The superficial temporal arteries often are tender and swollen, with a faint pulse. Temporal arteritis responds to treatment with steroids or other immunomodulators. Oral prednisone often works well. Dose will depend on the response, but patients on starting doses of 40 mg/day or less have fewer complications [39]. Long-term therapy often is needed.

More controversial in the genesis of brain stem ischemia is the role played by compression of the vertebral arteries by overgrown bone as the arteries transverse the vertebral foramina of the cervical vertebrae. Sheehan et al. [40] popularized this mechanism by publishing a study of 26 patients with angiographic demonstration of kinking or stenosis of the vertebral artery at the vertebral foramina. Many of their patients had dizziness evoked by head turning or extension, in addition to frank strokes at different levels of the neuraxis. Localization was based on the clinical findings because this study antedated CT. For this reason, and given the frequency of spondylotic narrowing of the vertebral foramina and of peripheral vestibular disease causing dizziness in older individuals with or without strokes, the cause and effect of the angiographic changes to the production of ischemic damage are far from proved. Recent studies on this topic are scant. Sakai et al. [41] reported on a 58-year-old man who, on single-photon emission computed tomography had reduced perfusion in the left cerebellum and the right occipital region during an attack of vertebrobasilar insufficiency. Angiography demonstrated compression of the left vertebral artery by osteophytes when the patient turned his head to the left. Unless this mechanism of ischemia is proved clearly for an individual patient, surgical decompression of the vertebral artery at the vertebral foramina is not recommended [1].

Cerebellar Vascular Disease

Cerebellar infarction or hemorrhage, particularly when affecting the flocculonodular lobe (or vestibulocerebellum) can present with acute or progressive impairment of balance and gait. Although most often patients with cerebellar lesions tend to fall to the side of the lesion, some patients with lesions in the tonsillar area develop increased tone (and increased reflexes) in the ipsilateral side and fall to the contralateral side. This was the case with the 64-year-old whose CT is shown in Figure 14-7. Gait impairment is the most frequent presentation of infarcts in the territory of the superior cerebellar artery [34].

In the older age group, infarction in the territory of the posteroinferior cerebellar artery is caused by atheromatous vascular disease as often as by embolic disease. Presumed cerebral embolism was the predominant stroke mechanism in patients with superior cerebellar artery distribution infarcts [34].

Daily medication with aspirin, 325 mg, may reduce the risk of additional

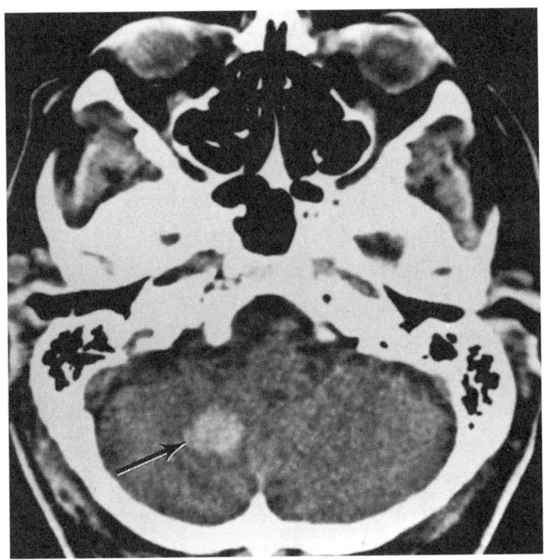

Figure 14-7. Cerebellar hematoma. CT of a 64-year-old man with sudden onset of inability to walk and a tendency to fall to the left side. A hemorrhage involves the right supratonsillar region (*arrows*).

strokes in patients with atherothrombotic disease [42] unless the patient is cognitively impaired or at risk for falls. Chronic anticoagulation is indicated for patients at risk of repeated embolic events from a cardiac source, such as those with lone atrial fibrillation [42].

The clinical presentation of cerebellar hemorrhage may be acute, subacute, or chronic [43, 44]. Variations in location, size, and development of the hematoma; brain-stem compression; fourth ventricular penetration; and development of hydrocephalus result in variations in the mode of presentation of cerebellar hemorrhage. These hemorrhages most frequently occur in the region of the dentate nucleus. Patients present with occipital or frontal headache, dizziness, vertigo, nausea, repeated vomiting, and inability to stand or walk. Often they have truncal or limb ataxia, ipsilateral-gaze palsy, and small reactive pupils. Horizontal-gaze paresis, paretic nystagmus, and facial weakness also are frequent. Frank hemiparesis is absent. Ocular bobbing and skew deviation may be present. Not all patients present such a dramatic picture. Those with small cerebellar hematomas (usually less than 3 cm in diameter) may present only with vomiting and with no headaches, gait instability, or limb ataxia.

Hypertension is the predominant risk factor for cerebellar hemorrhage, particularly in the elderly. The management of hypertension is discussed later (see White-Matter Disease in the Elderly). Cavernous angioma, a more common lesion in younger patients seldom is responsible for intracerebellar hemorrhages in the elderly. Its surgical management is described by Ojemann et al. [45].

Management of Lacunar Stroke

Blood pressure should not be lowered aggressively in a patient with acute ischemic stroke. Often there is a mild to moderate transient rise in blood pressure after stroke, which may have a protective effect on perfusion of the ischemic area [42]. The motor deficit is managed with early physical therapy, as discussed in Chapter 21. The physical therapist should be mindful of the particular kind of deficit these patients have. Strategies that rely on the volitional control of motor activity (e.g., standing and walking) normally not under the control of the will are likely to be successful. With small unilateral lesions, even automatic strategies will recover eventually.

Progression of the gait impairment in these patients is predicated on the basis of accumulation of lacunes. Over the course of years, small-vessel disease of the brain tends to produce additional lacunar infarcts distributed in the subcortical regions. Whereas the patients recover easily from a single lesion, they become increasingly unsteady as lesions accumulate, particularly when they affect parallel critical areas of both hemispheres. For this reason, the medical interventions addressed to these patients involve mainly prevention of risk factors for lacunar stroke. Control of hypertension is discussed later (see White-Matter Disease in the Elderly). Cigarette smoking should be discontinued, and excessive alcohol consumption should be eliminated. Hyperlipedemia should be treated as recommended for the management of coronary artery disease [42]. An active lifestyle with physical exercise protects from both coronary artery disease and stroke. Postmenopausal women need not discontinue estrogen intake [42].

Although we know that antithrombotic therapy is effective for the prevention of stroke, no prospective trials have addressed lacunar stroke specifically. A subgroup analysis in the French aspirin and dipyridamole trial suggested a benefit of aspirin in these patients [42]. The recommended dose of aspirin is a tablet (325 mg) per day. Ticlopidine (250 mg bid) is a useful alternative in patients who cannot take aspirin or who continue to have small strokes on aspirin. Gastric dysfunction is less frequent with ticlopidine than with aspirin, but ticlopidine causes diarrhea in approximately 12% of patients and severe neutropenia in approximately 1%. For this reason, periodic blood counts have to be conducted in the first 90 days of treatment with ticlopidine. Because patients with lacunar strokes also are predisposed to hemorrhagic stroke, these recommendations are made with some trepidation. Nothing definite can be said until more data are available in this area.

White-Matter Disease in the Elderly

Since the advent of CT and, particularly, MRI, the ubiquitous changes observed in the white matter of older individuals have mesmerized both clinicians and radiologists. The clinical significance of these changes is still to be fully elucidated, but the best data point to gait and balance impairment rather than to cognitive deterioration as the main clinical correlates of white-matter disease of the elderly.

Neuroimaging Findings
Neuroimaging findings are considered before clinical findings because they alert clinicians to the presence of this disorder and are paramount for the diagnosis.

The clinical significance of white-matter changes on CT or MRI still is being elucidated. White-matter changes on CT or MRI are very frequent in older people. On MRI, some degree of white-matter change is present in approximately 30% of subjects past age 65 [46]. Because these changes are unusual before age 50 and their severity and prevalence increase with age, it is clear that they are related somehow to the aging process [47–51]. On CT, the density of the centrum semiovale decreases with age [52].

White-matter hypodensity of the elderly, subtle on CT, has striking visual characteristics when imaged by MRI [47, 53–55]. Areas of the periventricular white matter that are hypodense on CT appear markedly hyperintense on T_2-weighted images and hypointense on T_1-weighted images (Fig. 14-8). However, high-intensity areas on T_2-weighted MRI often are undetected on CT. On T_2-weighted MRI, it may be difficult to distinguish between functionally normal areas of increased water content (due to dilation of perivascular spaces with normal aging or transependymal CSF absorption) and areas of tissue damage, because both have increased intensity values [55–57]. On proton-density images, areas of increased water content appear isointense or slightly hypointense, whereas areas of gliosis are hyperintense. For this reason, it seems preferable to make the diagnosis of white-matter disease only when the abnormalities are visible not only on T_2-weighted images but also on proton-density or T_1-weighted images. However, there are no data available exploring the functional significance of white-matter changes on only T_2-weighted images versus changes on all pulse sequences.

Clinical Correlates

Although many reports (often negative) have addressed the possible correlation of CT-MRI white-matter changes with the presence of dementia [58], few have commented on gait disturbances [59]. However, there is ample evidence that white-matter disease causes gait impairment more often than does dementia. Disorders of gait were pronounced among 41 well-documented cases of progressive arteriopathic white-matter disease described with histology from 1978 to 1987 (men = 23; women = 18; mean age of onset, 60 ± 9.7 years; mean length of illness, 5.8 ± 4.2 years) [48, 60–65]. Impairment of ambulation preceded cognitive impairment in 43% of the cases, whereas in only 17% dementia developed before gait impairment, in 20% they evolved simultaneously, and in 20% insufficient data precluded timing of gait abnormality versus dementia. Two of the cases where dementia occurred first had amyloid angiopathy and senile changes in the cortex [61]. Steingart et al. [66] found an abnormal gait more often among subjects with leukoaraiosis. In two other CT series, most subjects with hypodense periventricular white matter had impaired gait [67, 68]. Comparing demented elderly subjects with controls for dementia, George et al. [69] and Hendrie et al. [70] failed to find a significant correlation between white-matter disease and dementia, but white-matter disease was associated with gait impairment. In a series of patients with mild vascular dementia, Hennerici et al. [71] found a correlation between white-matter changes and impaired gait. Periven-

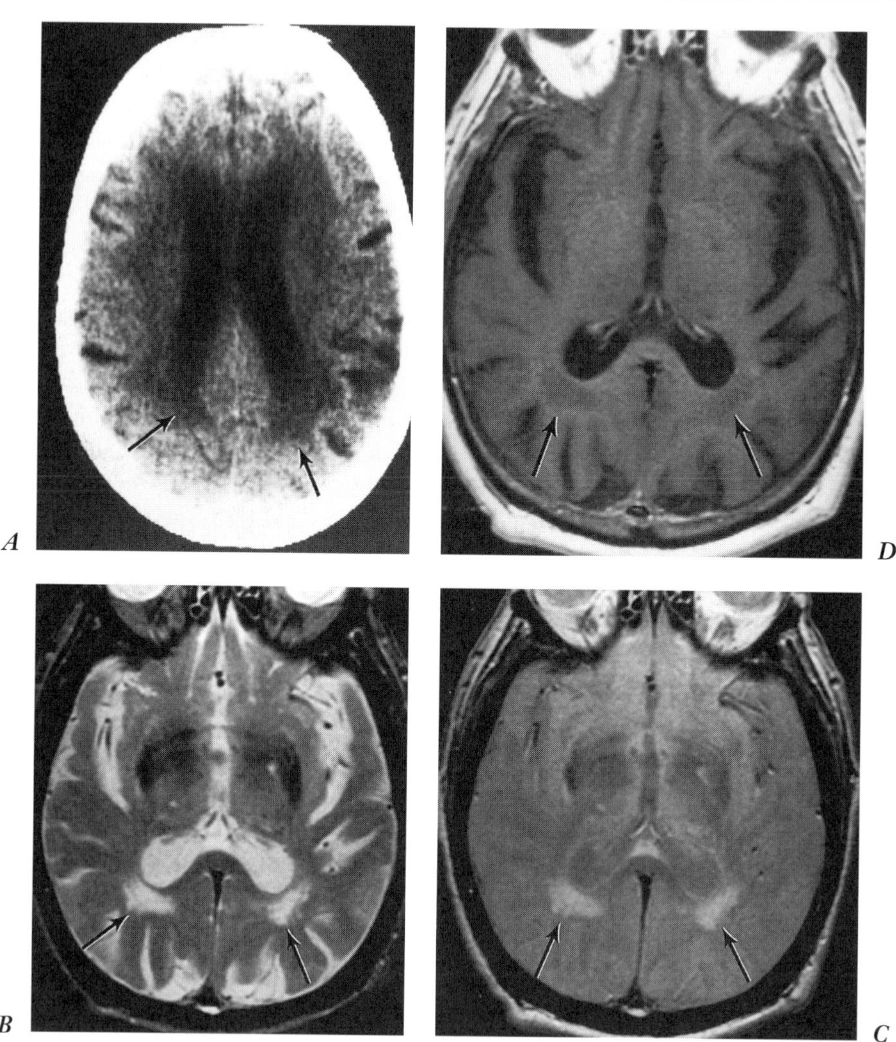

Figure 14-8. White-matter changes of the elderly. CT and MRI of a normotensive 79-year-old woman with normal mentation but slow, hesitating gait and a propensity for falling. Areas of low density on CT (*A*), particularly in the periatrial white matter (*arrows*), appear to be of high intensity on T_2-weighted MRI (*B*) and proton-density MRI (*C*) and of low intensity on T_1-weighted MRI (*D*).

tricular white-matter changes were present in the cases of "lower-body parkinsonism" described in elderly subjects by Thompson and Marsden [59] and by FitzGerald and Jankovic [5]. In a controlled study of elderly prone to falling, we found that impaired gait and balance, as well as a tendency to fall, correlated with the presence of white-matter disease on CT [7].

Characteristically, patients with severe white-matter changes have an unsteady gait, with features of parkinsonism and ataxia [5, 59]. However, unlike patients with cerebellar ataxia, they seldom broaden their base of support on standing or walking. Their performance resembles that in Critchley's description (see Historical Perspective) of the gait of some elderly people [4]. Disequilibrium dominates the clinical picture and predisposes these patients to falls [7, 71]. Though they have difficulty in walking or even in standing, often they are able to use their feet on finer volitional tasks, such as drawing a cross or a circle. Long-tract findings, including Babinski signs and hyperreflexia, are not necessarily present. Paratonia is generally pronounced in the legs, less so in the upper extremities.

Pathology, Pathogenesis, and Risk Factors

Because the histology underlying white-matter neuroimaging changes remains elusive, Hachinski proposed the descriptive term *leukoaraiosis* for the CT findings. Several authors have reported normal histology, but vascular or ischemic disease has been present in cases with pronounced changes on MRI or CT [65, 67, 73–77]. Pronounced white-matter changes on T_1-weighted MRI and CT most often correspond to ischemic changes similar to the findings in subcortical arteriosclerotic encephalopathy or Binswanger's disease [65, 67, 73–78].

The mechanisms by which periventricular white-matter disease may interfere with normal gait and balance need further clarification. Long-loop reflexes, essential for adequate gait and balance, are mediated by ascending fibers from the ventrolateral nucleus of the thalamus to the paracentral lobule and by descending corticospinal fibers. These fibers may be affected as they traverse the periventricular region. With arteriolosclerotic or amyloid arteriopathic disease of the white matter, the periventricular fibers are affected predominantly [61]. The periventricular region represents the arterial end and border zone for the perforating medullary vessels [79]. Thus, it can sustain acute or chronic ischemic damage as a result of arteriolar disease, hemorrheologic factors, anoxia, or hypotension. The subcortical U fibers generally are spared because their angioarchitecture is part of the cortical rather than of the deep medullary supply [80].

Cerebrovascular disease and hypertension are frequent correlates of subcortical arteriosclerotic encephalopathy [53, 81, 82]. In elderly patients, isolated systolic hypertension is common. Isolated systolic hypertension is defined by systolic readings of greater than or equal to 160 and diastolic readings of less than 90 mm Hg. Caused by a reduction in connective-tissue elasticity of large blood vessels, the prevalence of isolated systolic hypertension is approximately 7% in those past age 60 and increases with age to nearly 20% in those past 80 [83]. Prevalence is higher in women and nonwhites.

Although in both cases the white matter is affected, subcortical arteriosclerotic encephalopathy or Binswanger's disease may differ pathogenetically from white-matter hypodensity in the elderly [72]. Hypertension or left ventricular hypertrophy, commonly reported in association with subcortical arteriosclerotic encephalopathy in patients in their 60s, may not be present in subjects in their

80s, with white-matter changes [7]. Severely hypertensive patients may suffer a greater degree of white-matter disease earlier in life and may not survive into their 80s. Factors other than hypertension may be important in the genesis of white-matter disease in the more advanced decades. Cerebral hypoperfusion from episodic hypotension or cardiac dysrhythmias has been incriminated [84, 85]. Plasma viscosity was increased in a group of eight patients with CT diagnosis of subcortical arteriosclerotic encephalopathy (mean age, 62 years) [86]. Cardiovascular and hematological risk factors should be explored in an effort to identify potentially treatable causes of white-matter disease of the elderly.

Amyloid angiopathy has been recently described in the genesis of white-matter disease in some elderly individuals [61, 63]. In addition to white-matter changes, amyloid angiopathy results in subcortical or thalamic hemorrhages. Most of these individuals were normotensive.

Particularly when asymmetrical, white-matter disease can be related to chronic hypoperfusion from carotid artery stenosis. Affected patients typically have a history of several episodes of mild unilateral weakness and may have frank infarcts in the distal territory of the middle cerebral artery, particularly in the white matter lateral to the head of the caudate nucleus or in the white matter underlying the middle frontal and superior temporal gyri.

Treatment

As discussed earlier, chronic hypertension may be a risk factor for ischemic white-matter disease. There is no direct evidence that blood pressure control lessens the progression of white-matter changes in the elderly, but treated hypertensives may have fewer white-matter changes than do untreated hypertensives [87]. Clearly, treatment of hypertension prevents ischemic brain disease, even in the elderly. Hypertension control in patients aged 40 to 69 at the start of follow-up effected stroke reduction in a large longitudinal study [88]. In the Systolic Hypertension in the Elderly Program, treated subjects past age 60 with isolated systolic hypertension had a 36% reduction in stroke risk compared with those in the placebo group [42].

In the treatment of hypertension, the mean perfusion pressure must be monitored carefully in older patients. Daily fluctuations in blood pressure, such as postprandial hypotension, may result in unwanted hypotensive episodes with overtreatment [89]. Chronic hypotension may cause selective necrosis of oligodendrocytes because these cells are particularly prone to ischemic injury [90]. Precautions for detection and evaluation of hypertension in the elderly include multiple blood pressure measurements in the fasting state and sitting and supine blood pressure measurements before and during therapy. Pseudohypertension due to stress may be recorded in a doctor's office in older patients with denervation supersensitivity of sympathetic receptors. For this reason, 24-hour ambulatory blood pressure monitoring can be used to obtain a more accurate picture of the response to medication [91].

In the treatment of hypertension, the decision to treat must be made on an individual patient basis. The "low and slow" approach to therapy is helpful in minimizing adverse effects. In ordinary hypertension, the goal is to maintain a diastolic blood pressure below 90 mm Hg. For isolated systolic hypertension, a reasonable goal is a 20-mm Hg reduction in systolic pressure, as long as hypotension is avoided [83].

Low-dose diuretics have been documented to be effective in blood pressure control. Chlorthalidone, 12.5 or 25 mg/day, is suggested. Other agents, such as beta-blockers, reserpine, angiotensin-converting enzyme (ACE) inhibitors, and calcium channel blockers, are best used as step 2 agents [83, 91, 92].

A greater than 70% carotid stenosis should be considered an indication for carotid endarterectomy in symptomatic patients [93]. This study proved the benefit of therapy in patients with definite transient ischemic attacks or stroke, but patients with only slowly progressive gait impairment were not included. More doubtful is the role of carotid endarterectomy in asymptomatic patients. It may help 1 of 19 patients with carotid stenosis greater than 60%, as long as the combined morbidity from angiography and surgery at a given institution does not exceed 3% [94].

DROP ATTACKS

Drop attacks often are mentioned in the geriatric literature as a major cause of falls and as a common event affecting older people [95]. Generally they are ascribed to vertebrobasilar insufficiency. This notion merits revision. The term *drop attack* originally was used by Sheldon [96] to describe what happens to an otherwise healthy older person who suddenly and without warning falls to the ground without loss of consciousness. Although fully alert, the victim frequently experiences difficulty in standing again and needs help to do so. Why this delay in recovering? In addition to the demands on postural mechanisms required to arise from the ground to the standing position, some of these patients may have more than a brief loss of postural tone. As described by these authors, "[T]he sudden loss of strength and muscle tone in the legs and trunk may last several hours"[95]. Injuries are common.

Vertebrobasilar ischemia as a major cause of drop attacks received particular support from the work of Sheehan et al. [40], published before CT became available. They reported brain-stem ischemia due to osteophyte encroachment on the vertebral arteries at the vertebral foramina. Of 26 patients with angiographic demonstration of kinking or stenosis of the vertebral artery at the vertebral foramina, 6 had drop attacks. These patients had other neurological findings, and most of them had clinical findings reminiscent of the lacunar or hemorrhagic syndromes described earlier. For instance, a 63-year-old severely hypertensive man fell without losing consciousness. He got to his feet, but for some time he was noted to "stagger around" and had to hold onto the furniture while walking. Eventually, he improved, but 10 years later he collapsed while walking on the street, remaining alert but unable to walk. Eventual clinical outcome was not described.

Another patient, a 68-year-old diabetic woman, fell without losing consciousness and was unable to get up. Shortly after admission to the hospital, she became able to walk but was ataxic for several days. Because of the lack of modern neuroimaging techniques or autopsy verification, the responsible lesions could not be localized anatomically. In reporting these cases, Sheehan et al. [40] emphasized the presence of dizziness with head turning and of vertebral changes on angiography. Dizziness with head turning more likely is related to peripheral vestibular dysfunction (common in the elderly) than to brain-stem ischemia, in which dizziness is generally accompanied by diplopia or other brain-stem findings. Cervical spondylosis occurs regularly with aging. Therefore, the link between vertebrobasilar ischemia and drop attacks, as reported by Sheehan et al. [40], remains unproved.

In rare cases, drop attacks are due to ischemia of the pyramids and may herald infarction in the vertebrobasilar territory. One such case was described by Brust et al. [97]. Two episodes of sudden unexpected falls without associated neurological findings preceded infarction of the corticospinal tracts at the pons and medulla and eventual death. At autopsy, there was bilateral vertebral artery occlusion. This was an unusual case because ischemia in the vertebrobasilar territory usually presents with other neurological manifestations (e.g., numbness, diplopia, or vertigo) in addition to sudden loss of postural tone in the legs. In terms of cerebrovascular disease, lacunar strokes of the basal ganglia, thalamus, or suprathalamic white matter are much more likely to cause sudden inability to stand or walk (as described earlier), because these lesions are much more common than ischemia of the pyramids.

Many events meeting the clinical definition of drop attacks are not caused by vascular disease of the brain. Meissner et al. [98] reviewed 108 patients diagnosed with drop attacks at the Mayo Clinic between 1976 and 1983. Mean age was 70 years. In the majority (64%), the mechanism was unknown. Some patients may have had falls on the basis of pathology predisposing to loss of postural control, such as peripheral neuropathy, dopamine deficiency, or one of the vascular syndromes described earlier in this chapter, which were poorly recognized until recently. Cardiac causes were present in 12%, clear-cut cerebrovascular insufficiency in 8%, combined cardiac and cerebrovascular disease in 7%, seizures in 5%, vestibular disease in 3% and, in one case, the falls were believed to be psychogenic. Among the patients with cerebrovascular disease, the two with persistent drop attacks had carotid artery disease. Approximately 80% of the patients were symptom-free at a mean follow-up of 6.5 years. Neurological findings on examination, cardiac arrhythmias, and congestive heart failure increased the risk of death on follow-up. The stroke rate in the overall group, approximately 0.5% per year, was not significantly different from that in a normal age- and gender-matched population. However, small-vessel disease and disease of the white matter evolve over a period longer than that covered in this study.

In addition, these disorders may not have been classified as cerebrovascular disease, because they often present with gait or balance impairment but without hemiparesis or other of the classic features of stroke and because brain imaging was not used regularly in this series. Rare causes of drop attacks include hydrocephalus and intraventricular tumors [99].

Vertebrobasilar ischemia is not accepted currently as a frequent cause of drop attacks. Two recent editions of standard stroke manuals do not even list drop attack in their index [2, 100], and another lists the term only to argue against its purported vertebrobasilar basis [1]. Many of the causes of postural impairment described in Chapters 9 through 19 result in instability. A sudden demand on a system that is marginal may trigger a drop attack. Often, the patient cannot explain how the fall came about. In addition, the vascular syndromes previously described (including white-matter ischemic disease and lacunar or hemorrhagic stroke of the basal ganglia, thalamus, or suprathalamic white matter) result in disequilibrium with a propensity to falling. Falls often are precipitated by sudden buckling of the knees, mimicking a drop attack. In many instances, there is no history of stroke, despite the evidence on neuroimaging studies. It is likely that at least some of the patients described previously as having drop attacks probably had a propensity to falling on the basis of subcortical disequilibrium, caused by one of the vascular syndromes described earlier.

SUMMARY

Several vascular brain syndromes causing gait or balance impairment have been described in the past few years. Some give rise to slow deterioration, such as white-matter ischemic disease or the accumulation of small lacunes. Others, including lacunar or hemorrhagic stroke of the basal ganglia, the ventrolateral nucleus of the thalamus or suprathalamic white matter, the pedunculopontine area at the junction of pons and midbrain, or the cerebellovestibular region, tend to cause sudden impairment from which there is partial recovery. However, affected patients are left with a propensity to falling, particularly as additional ischemic events occur. Prevention of ischemic or hemorrhagic disease is effected through hypertension control, elimination of other stroke risk factors and, for ischemic disease, the use of antithrombotic agents (or steroids in the case of temporal arteritis).

REFERENCES

1. Barnett H, Mohr J, Stein B, Yatsu F. *Stroke, Pathophysiology, Diagnosis and Management*, 2nd ed. New York: Churchill Livingstone, 1992. P 1270.
2. Caplan L. *Stroke. A Clinical Approach*, 2nd ed. Boston: Butterworth-Heinemann, 1993. P 562.
3. Lhermitte J. *Étude sur la Paraplégies des Viellards*. Paris: Maretheux, 1907.

4. Critchley M. On senile disorders of gait, including the so-called "senile paraplegia." *Geriatrics* 1948;3:364–370.

5. FitzGerald P, Jankovic J. Lower body parkinsonism: Evidence for vascular etiology. *Mov Disord* 1987;4:249–260.

6. Masdeu J, Wolfson L. Lower body (vascular) parkinsonism. *Arch Neurol* 1990;47:748.

7. Masdeu J, et al. White matter disease in the elderly prone to falling. *Arch Neurol* 1989;46:1292–1296.

8. Masdeu J, Gorelick P. Thalamic astasia: Inability to stand after unilateral thalamic lesions. *Ann Neurol* 1988;23:596–603.

9. Labadie E, Awerbuch G, Hamilton R, Rapcsak S. Falling and postural deficits due to acute unilateral basal ganglia lesions. *Arch Neurol* 1989;261:492–496.

10. Masdeu J, Alampur U, Cavaliere R, Tavoulareas G. Astasia and gait failure with damage of the pontomesencephalic locomotor region. *Ann Neurol* 1994;35:619–621.

11. Roman GC, et al. Vascular dementia: Diagnostic criteria for research studies. Report of the NINDS-AIREN International Workshop. *Neurology* 1993;43:250–60.

12. Nutt J, Marsden C, Thompson P. Human walking and higher-level gait disorders, particularly in the elderly. *Neurology* 1993;43:268–279.

13. Cambier J, Elghozi D. Strube E. Lésions du thalamus droit avec syndrome de l'hémisphère mineur. Discussion du concept de négligence thalamique. *Rev Neurol* 1980;136:105–116.

14. Laplane D, et al. La négligence motrice d'origine thalamique. A propos de deux cas. *Rev Neurol* (Paris) 1982;138:201–211.

15. Jenkyn L, Alberti A, Peters J. Language dysfunction, somasthetic hemi-inattention, and thalamic hemorrhage in the dominant hemisphere. *Neurology* 1981;31:1202.

16. Verma A, Maheshwari M. Hypesthetic-ataxic-hemiparesis in thalamic hemorrhage. *Stroke* 1986;17:49–51.

17. Fisher C, Cole M. Homolateral ataxia and crural paresis; a vascular syndrome. *J Neurol Neurosurg Psychiatry* 1965;28:48–55.

18. Huang C, Lui F. Ataxic-hemiparesis, localization and clinical features. *Stroke* 1984;15:363–366.

19. Iragui V, McCutchen C. Capsular ataxic hemiparesis. *Arch Neurol* 1982;39:528–529.

20. Sage J, Lepore F. Ataxic hemiparesis from lesions of the corona radiata. *Arch Neurol* 1983;40:449–450.

21. Jones E. *The Thalamus.* New York: Plenum, 1985.

22. Van Buren J, Borke R. *Variations and Connections of the Human Thalamus.* Berlin: Springer, 1972.

23. Asanuma C, Thach W, Jones E. Distribution of cerebellar terminations and their relation to other afferent terminations in the thalamic ventral lateral region of the monkey. *Brain Res Rev* 1983;5:237–265.

24. Groothuis D, Duncan G, Fisher C. The human thalamocortical sensory path in the internal capsule: Evidence from a small capsular hemorrhage causing a pure sensory stroke. *Ann Neurol* 1977;2:328–333.

25. Garcia-Rill E. The pedunculopontine nucleus. *Prog Neurobiol* 1991;36:363–89.

26. Zweig R, et al. The pedunculopontine nucleus in Parkinson's disease. *Ann Neurol* 1989;25:41–46.

27. Hazrati LN, Parent A. Projection from the deep cerebellar nuclei to the pedunculopontine nucleus in the squirrel monkey. *Brain Res* 1992;585:267–271.

28. Morizumi T, Hattori T. Separate neuronal populations of the rat globus pallidus projecting to the subthalamic nucleus, auditory cortex and pedunculopontine tegmental area. *Neuroscience* 1992;46:701–710.

29. Skinner R, Garcia-Rill E. Brainstem Modulation of Rhythmic Functions and Behaviors. In: Klemm W, Vertes R, eds. *Brainstem Mechanisms and Behavior.* New York: Wiley, 1990. Pp 465–496.

30. Mogenson G, Wu M, Brudzynski S. The role of pedunculopontine nucleus in locomotor activity. *Neurosci Abstr* 1990;16:753.

31. Caplan L, Goodwin J. Lateral tegmental brainstem hemorrhage. *Neurology* 1982;32:252–260.

32. Felice K, Keilson G, Schwartz W. 'Rubral' gait ataxia. *Neurology* 1990;40:1004–1005.

33. Sand J, et al. Partial dorsal mesencephalic hemorrhages: Report of three cases. *Neurology* 1986;36:529–533.

34. Kase CS, et al. Cerebellar infarction. Clinical and anatomic observations in 66 cases. *Stroke* 1993;24:76–83.

35. Van-Schil PE, et al. Long-term clinical and duplex follow-up after proximal vertebral artery reconstruction. *Angiology* 1992;43:961–968.

36. Mokri B, Houser OW, Sandok BA, Piepgras DG. Spontaneous dissections of the vertebral arteries. *Neurology* 1988;38:880.

37. Reich KA, Giansiracusa DF, Strongwater SL. Neurologic manifestations of giant cell arteritis. *Am J Med* 1990;89:67–72.

38. Wilkinson I, Russell R. Arteries of the head and neck in giant cell arteritis. *Arch Neurol* 1972;27:378–391.

39. Nesher G, Sonnenblick M, Friedlander Y. Analysis of steroid related complications and mortality in temporal arteritis: A 15-year survey of 43 patients. *J Rheumatol* 1994;21:1283–1286.

40. Sheehan S, Bauer R, Meyer J. Vertebral artery compression in cervical spondylosis. Arteriographic demonstration during life of vertebral artery insufficiency due to rotation and extension of the neck. *Neurology* 1960;10:968–986.

41. Sakai F, et al. Regional cerebral blood flow during an attack of vertebrobasilar insufficiency. *Stroke* 1988;19:1426–1430.

42. Feinberg WM, et al. Guidelines for the management of transient ischemic attacks. From the Ad Hoc Committee on Guidelines for the Management of Transient Ischemic Attacks of the Stroke Council of the American Heart Association. *Circulation* 1994;89:2950–2965.

43. Brennan RW, Bergland RM. Acute cerebellar hemorrhage. Analysis of clinical findings and outcome in 12 cases. *Neurology* 1977;27:527.

44. Marshall J. Cerebellar Vascular Syndromes. In: Toole J, ed. *Vascular Diseases* (part III). In: Vinken PJ, Bruyn GW, eds. *Handbook of Clinical Neurology*: Vol 11. New York: Elsevier, 1989. Pp 89–94.

45. Ojemann RG, Crowell RM, Ogilvy CS. Management of cranial and spinal cavernous angiomas (honored guest lecture). *Clin Neurosurg* 1993;40:98–123.

46. Fazekas F, et al. White matter signal abnormalities in normal individuals: Correlation with carotid ultrasonography, cerebral blood flow measurements, and cerebrovascular risk factors. *Stroke* 1988;19:1285–1288.

47. Gerard G, Weisberg L. MRI periventricular lesions in adults. *Neurology* 1986;36:998–1001.

48. Goto K, Ishii N, Fukasawa H. Diffuse white-matter disease in the geriatric population: A clinical, neuropathological, and CT study. *Radiology* 1981;141:687–695.

49. McQuinn B, O'Leary D. CT periventricular lucencies: Association with systemic disease states and with sub-acute arteriosclerotic encephalopathy (SAE, "Binswanger's disease"). *Stroke* 1986;17:135.

50. Pullicino P, Eskin T, Ketonen L. Prevalence of Binswanger's disease. *Lancet* 1983;1:939.

51. Meyer JS, Kawamura J, Terayama Y. White matter lesions in the elderly. *J Neurol Sci* 1992;110:1–7.

52. Zatz L, Jernigan T, Ahumada AJ. White matter changes in cerebral computed tomography related to aging. *J Comput Assist Tomogr* 1982;6:19–23.

53. Awad I, et al. Incidental subcortical lesions identified on magnetic resonance imaging in the elderly. I. Correlation with age and cerebrovascular risk factors. *Stroke* 1986;17:1084–1089.

54. Brant-Zawadzki M, et al. MR imaging of the aging brain: Patchy white-matter lesions and dementia. *AJNR* 1985;6:675–682.

55. Zimmerman R, et al. Periventricular hyperintensity as seen by magnetic resonance: Prevalence and significance. *Am J Radiol* 1986;146:443–450.

56. Awad I, Johnson P, Spetzler R, Hodak J. Incidental subcortical lesions identified on magnetic resonance imaging in the elderly. II. Postmortem pathological correlations. *Stroke* 1986;17:1090–1097.

57. Kirkpatrick J, Hayman L. White-matter lesions on MR imaging of clinically healthy brains of elderly subjects: Possible pathologic basis. *Radiology* 1987;162:509–511.

58. Almkvist O, et al. White-matter hyperintensity and neuropsychological function in dementia and healthy aging. *Arch Neurol* 1992;49:626–632.

59. Thompson P, Marsden C. Gait disorder of subcortical arteriosclerotic encephalopathy: Binswanger's disease. *Mov Disord* 1987;2:1–8.

60. Caplan L, Schoene W. Clinical features of subcortical arteriosclerotic encephalopathy (Binswanger disease). *Neurology* 1978;28:1206–1215.

61. Dubas F, Gray F, Roullet E, Escourolle R. Leucoencéphalopathies artériopathiques (17 cas anatomo-clinques). *Rev Neurol* (Paris) 1985;141:93–108.

62. Dupuis M, Brucher J, Gonsette R. Obsevation anatomo-clinque d'une encéphalopathie sous-corticale artérioscléreuse ("maladie de Binswanger") avec hypodensité de la substance blanche au scanner cérébral. *Acta Neurol Belg* 1984;84:131–140.

63. Gray F, Dubas F, Roullet E, Escourolle R. Leukoencephalopathy in diffuse hemorrhagic cerebral amyloid angiopathy. *Ann Neurol* 1985;18:54–59.

64. Janota I. Dementia, deep white matter damage and hypertension: 'Binswanger's disease.' *Psychol Med* 1981;11:39–48.

65. Rosenberg G, Kornfeld M, Stovring J, Bicknell J. Subcortical arteriosclerotic encephalopathy (Binswanger): Computerized tomography. *Neurology* 1979;29:1102–1106.

66. Steingart A, Hachinski V, Lau C. Cognitive and neurologic findings in subjects with diffuse white matter lucencies on computed tomographic scan (leuko-araiosis). *Arch Neurol* 1987;44:32–35.

67. Kinkel W, et al. Subcortical arteriosclerotic encephalopathy (Biswanger's disease). Computed tomographic, nuclear magnetic resonance, and clinical correlations. *Arch Neurol* 1985;42:951–959.

68. Loizou L, Kendall B, Marshall J. Subcortical arteriosclerotic encephalopathy: A clinical and radiological investigation. *J Neurol Neurosurg Psychiatry* 1981;44:294–304.

69. George A, et al. Leukoencephalopathy in normal and pathologic aging: CT of brain lucencies. *AJNR* 1986;7:561–566.

70. Hendrie H, et al. Foci of increased T2 signal intensity on brain MR scans of healthy elderly subjects. *Am J Neuroradiol* 1989;10:703–707.

71. Hennerici MG, et al. Are gait disturbances and white matter degeneration early indicators of vascular dementia? *Dementia* 1994;5:197–202.

72. Hachinski V, Potter P, Merskey H. Leuko-araiosis. *Arch Neurol* 1987;44:21–23.

73. Braffman B, et al. Pathologic correlation with gross and histopathology: 2. Hyperintense white-matter foci in the elderly. *Am J Neuroradiol* 1988;9:629–636.

74. Johnson K, et al. Comparison of magnetic resonance and roentgen ray computed tomography in dementia. *Arch Neurol* 1987;44:1075–1080.

75. Lotz P, Ballinger W, Quisling R. Subcortical arteriosclerotic encephalopathy: CT spectrum and pathologic correlation. *Am J Radiol* 1986;147:1209–1214.

76. Marshall V, et al. Deep white matter infarction: Correlation of MR imaging and histopathologic findings. *Radiology* 1988;167:517–522.

77. Rezek D, Morris J, Fulling K, Gado M. Periventricular white matter lucencies in senile dementia of the Alzheimer type and in normal aging. *Neurology* 1987;37:1365–1368.

78. Yamanouchi H. Loss of white matter oligodendrocytes and astrocytes in progressive subcortical vascular encephalopathy of Binswanger type. *Acta Neurol Scand* 1991;83:301–305.

79. De-Reuck J, et al. Pathogenesis of Binswanger chronic progressive subcortical encephalopathy. *Neurology* 1980;30:920–928.

80. De-Reuck J. The cortico-subcortical arterial angioarchitecture in the human brain. *Acta Neurol Belg* 1972;72:323–329.

81. Skoog I. Risk factors for vascular dementia: A review. *Dementia* 1994;5:137–44.

82. van Swieten JC, et al. Hypertension in the elderly is associated with white matter lesions and cognitive decline. *Ann Neurol* 1991;30:825–830.

83. Probstfield JL, Furberg CD. Systolic hypertension in the elderly: Controlled or uncontrolled. *Cardiovasc Clin* 1990;20:65–84.

84. Brun A, Englund E. A white matter disorder in dementia of the Alzheimer type: A pathoanatomical study. *Ann Neurol* 1986;16:253–262.

85. Harrison M, Marshall J. Hypoperfusion in the aetiology of subcortical arteriosclerotic encephalopathy (Binswanger type). *J Neurol Neurosurg Psychiatry* 1984;47:754.

86. Schneider R, et al. Do different ischemic brain lesions have different hemorrheological profiles? *Klin Wochenschr* 1986;64:357–361.

87. Fukuda H, Kitani M. Differences between treated and untreated hypertensives in the severity of periventricular hyperintensities observed on brain MRI. *Stroke* 1995;26:1593–1597.

88. Lindbald U, Rastam L, Ranstam J. Stroke morbidity in patients treated for hypertension—The Skaraborg Hypertension Project. *J Intern Med* 1993;233:155–163.

89. Jansen RW, Lipsitz LA. Postprandial hypotension: Epidemiology, pathophysiology, and clinical management. *Ann Intern Med* 1995;122:286–295.

90. Utzschneider DA, Kocsis JD, Waxman SG. Differential sensitivity to hypoxia of the peripheral versus central trajectory of primary afferent axons. *Brain Res* 1991;551:136–141.

91. Furberg CD, Berglund G, Manolio TA, Psaty BM. Overtreatment and undertreatment of hypertension. *J Intern Med* 1994;235:387–397.

92. Kendall MJ, Tse WY, Head A. The treatment of elderly hypertensive patients. *J Clin Pharm Ther* 1993;18:9–14.

93. North American Symptomatic Carotid Endarterectomy Trial Collaborators. Beneficial effect of carotid endarterectomy in symptomatic patients with high-grade carotid stenosis. *N Engl J Med* 1991;325:445–453.

94. Executive Committee for the Asymptomatic Carotid Atherosclerosis Study. Endarterectomy for asymptomatic carotid artery stenosis. *JAMA* 1995;273:1421–1428.

95. Lipsitz LA. The drop attack: A common geriatric symptom. *J Am Geriatr Soc* 1983;31:617–620.

96. Sheldon J. On the natural history of falls in old age. *Br Med J [Clin Res]* 1960;2:1685–1690.

97. Brust JC, Plank CR, Healton EB, Sanchez GF. The pathology of drop attacks: A case report. *Neurology* 1979;29:786–790.

98. Meissner I, Weibers DO, Swanson JW, O'Fallon WM. The natural history of drop attacks. *Neurology* 1986;36:1029–1034.

99. Criscuolo GR, Symon L. Intraventricular meningioma. A review of 10 cases of the National Hospital, Queen Square (1974–1985), with reference to the literature. *Acta Neurochir Wien* 1986;83:83–91.

100. Toole J. *Cerebrovascular Disorders*, 4th ed. New York: Raven, 1990. P 553.

101. Zweig R, et al. Pedunculopontine cholinergic neurons in progressive supranuclear palsy. *Ann Neurol* 1987;22:18–25.

15. A Clinical Approach to Symptomatic Hydrocephalus in the Elderly

Neill R. Graff-Radford and John C. Godersky

Patients with possible symptomatic hydrocephalus (also termed *normal-pressure hydrocephalus* or NPH) often are encountered in clinical practice and may comprise up to 6% of patients in some dementia studies [1]. For the neurologist, the commonly asked question is, Which patients with the clinical triad of gait abnormality, dementia, and incontinence of urine and the radiological finding of hydrocephalus should be recommended for shunt surgery? The basis for this question is that only half of the individuals with this constellation of findings improve with surgery [2, 3]; moreover, shunt surgery has a long-term complication rate of approximately 30–40% [4, 5]. An important corollary question is, Why do half the patients with the clinical triad and hydrocephalus fail to improve with surgery? One of the answers to the latter question is that each of the clinical findings associated with symptomatic hydrocephalus is common in the elderly and may have multiple causes. Severe dementia may occur in up to 5% of people past age 65, and a milder form may be present in many more [6]. Incontinence occurs in 15% of women and 10% of men past age 70 [7]. Gait abnormality also is common in the elderly and has been shown to have multiple etiologies [8]. In our opinion, the gait abnormality found in patients with symptomatic hydrocephalus is nonspecific. Its features are (1) difficulty in standing from a seated position, (2) imbalance while walking, (3) slowed speed, (4) smaller step size, and (5) difficulty in turning, which often is completed in a piecemeal fashion rather than with the normal pivot; difficulty in turning is the earliest finding. In addition, approximately half of such patients have a wide-base gait, and the patient collapses into the chair when sitting. Many neurologists would say the gait appears parkinsonian. The cerebral ventricles increase in size with age [9], and ventriculomegaly is a common accompaniment of Alzheimer's disease [10]. Because none of its cardinal findings is specific to symptomatic hydrocephalus, it is not surprising that a patient can exhibit the typical clinical triad as well as hydrocephalus on CT, and yet not respond to surgery. How can the neurologist best make the decision regarding recommendation for surgery? There is useful information already in the literature.

SELECTING APPROPRIATE PATIENTS FOR SHUNT SURGERY

History

There are several important questions that should be asked when obtaining a history from NPH patients and their families:

1. *How long has the patient been demented?* If the period is more than 2 years, it is less likely that the patient will respond to surgery [5, 11]. Note that the question is not how long the patient has had gait abnormality but how long the patient has been demented. Table 15-1 demonstrates how reliable this information was in predicting surgical outcome in our series [11].
2. *Which started first, gait abnormality or dementia?* If the gait abnormality began before or at the same time as dementia, then there is a better chance for suc-

Table 15-1. Variables predicting surgical outcome in symptomatic hydrocephalus

Variable	No. of patients	Odds ratio	p value[a]	95% confidence interval for odds ratio[b]	Correct classification	
					Unimproved	Improved
Age	30	1.031	0.59	0.919–1.157		
Education	30	0.906	0.41	0.716–1.146		
Gender	30	4.615	0.215[c]	0.423–233.0		
Gait abnormality (yr)	30	1.133	0.51	0.789–1.626		
Incontinence (yr)	30	1.441	0.402	0.614–3.408		
Dementia (yr)	30	9.002	< 0.001	1.542–52.56	5/7	21/23
Order of onset (gait versus dementia)	30	0	0.009[c]	0–0.425	3/7	23/23
% time B-waves present	28	0.969	0.04	0.937–1.001	2/6	22/22
% time pressure > 15 mm Hg	28	0.968	0.055	0.930–1.006	0/6	22/22
% time pressure > 20 mm Hg	28	0.979	0.23	0.940–1.020		
Visual naming test	25	0.941	0.093	0.875–1.013	2/7	17/18
Visual naming, pass or fail	25	8.750	0.058[c]	0.887–113.3	5/7	14/18
Cerebral blood flow (anterior-posterior ratio slice 4)	30	1.120	< 0.001	1.026–1.224	5/7	22/23
CSF conductance	23	0.254	0.956	0–infinity		
CSF conductance, 0.08 as cutoff value	23	1.071	1.00[c]	0.065–67.354		

[a] Probability value based on likelihood ratio test.
[b] Based on Wald test (which is slightly different from likelihood ratio test) and on Fisher's exact test when this test was used.
[c] Probability value based on Fisher's exact test.
SOURCE: From NR Graff-Radford, JC Godersky. Variables predicting surgical outcome in symptomatic hydrocephalus in the elderly. *Neurology* 1989;39:1601–1604.

cessful surgery, whereas, if dementia started before gait abnormality, shunting is less likely to help (see Table 15-1) [11–13].

3. *Is there a history of alcohol abuse?* Alcohol abuse is a poor prognostic indicator [14].

4. *Is there a secondary cause of hydrocephalus?* Examples are subarachnoid hemorrhage, meningitis, previous brain surgery and head injury. If any of these are present, the chances of improvement with surgery are better [5, 15, 16].

Examination

On examination, the following issues should be addressed:

1. *Measure the head circumference.* If it is greater than 59 cm in men or 57.5 cm in women (i.e., greater than the ninety-eighth percentile for head circumference), the patient could have congenital hydrocephalus that has become symptomatic in later life [16, 18]. The CT or MRI in these instances usually does not show much CSF leakage around the ventricles (i.e., transependymal flow on CT and increased periventricular signal on the T_2-weighted images on MRI).

2. *Exclude diseases that may mimic symptomatic hydrocephalus* (e.g. Parkinson's disease, cervical spondylosis with spinal cord compression, progressive supranuclear palsy, multisystem degenerative disorder, phenothiazine use, Alzheimer's disease with extrapyramidal features, and multiple subcortical infarctions). Sometimes this is more easily said than done, but keeping this differential diagnosis in mind during the examination is helpful.

3. *Characterize the gait abnormality.* In our opinion, the gait abnormality is not specific in these patients. They have difficulty in standing from the sitting position, inertia in initiating walking, a slower walking speed, a shorter stride length, less foot-lift height from the ground, less arm swing, unsteadiness, and (most importantly), difficulty in turning. Often, a turn is made in a piecemeal fashion. In the moderate to severe stages, the patients' feet may seem to stick to the ground as they initiate walking. The gait is not festinating, and in only 25% to 50% it is wide-based. When they sit down, they may seem to collapse into the chair.

Neuropsychology

Look for evidence of aphasia. Evidence of aphasia (e.g., anomia) is a poor prognostic indicator for surgical success (see Table 15-1) [11, 14, 19].

CSF Drainage Procedures

If the patient's gait improves after removing a large quantity of CSF by lumbar puncture (e.g., 30–50 ml repeated daily), this person may be a good candidate for shunt surgery [20, 21].

A modification of this technique (i.e., continuous CSF drainage/via a catheter placed in the lumbar CSF space) also has been reported [22, 23]. This technique involves placing a thin subarachnoid catheter in the lumbar CSF space and leading it into a drainage bag. The height of the drainage bag is adjusted to allow drainage of 5 to 10 ml/hr while avoiding CSF hypotensive symptoms of headache in the patient. This is a closed system and allows an average drainage of 150 ml/day. The closed system helps to prevent infection, and the thin tube prevents rapid CSF drainage, thus decreasing the risk of subdural hemorrhage.

Hanley et al. [23] use a larger (16-gauge) catheter through which CSF pressure can also be monitored. They pay attention to the level of the drainage bag, with a goal of draining 240 ml/day. To minimize infection, the drainage system is kept in for 2 to 5 days. If symptoms of headache and nausea develop, too much CSF is being drained.

Improvement of gait after CSF drainage may not always be a clear indicator of the likelihood of surgical improvement. We have seen patients who underwent CSF drainage eventually respond to shunt surgery but saw no obvious improvement for the first postsurgical week. The drainage test could have given a false-negative result in these patients. During this test, a patient may appear improved for the duration of the test (the placebo effect) but not maintain response, leading to a false-positive result. In addition, meningitis and subdural hematoma are possible complications of the continuous CSF drainage procedures.

CT and MRI

Certain factors should be addressed when analyzing CT or MRI:

1. *Hydrocephalus must be present.* The modified Evans ratio (maximum width of the frontal horns/measure of the inner table at the same place) should be greater than 3.1 [16].
2. *It must be determined whether cortical atrophy is prominent.* Extensive cortical atrophy reduces but does not eliminate the chance of improvement with surgery [5, 16, 24].
3. *Pattern of atrophy.* The pattern of atrophy may be useful diagnostically (e.g., it might involve the medial temporal lobes as is seen in Alzheimer's disease). Although data on this point are lacking, it may be that prominent medial temporal cortical atrophy lessens the chances for surgical improvement because these patients may have Alzheimer's disease [25–27].
4. *Evidence of congenital hydrocephalus.* For example is there aqueductal stenosis or an Arnold-Chiari malformation [17, 18]?

Newer MRI techniques, such as cine-MRI, involving the analysis of a CSF flow void in the aqueduct of Sylvius may be helpful in predicting who will respond to a shunt [28–31]. Bradley et al. [29] recently have shown that this parameter on MRI correlates with a good or excellent long-term response to surgery. They recommend that, if the patient fulfills the clinical criteria for symptomatic hydrocephalus and has a flow void in the cerebral aqueduct on MRI, the patient should be considered for surgery.

Regional Cerebral Blood Flow

It has been reported that regional cerebral blood flow (rCBF) is decreased in the frontal areas in hydrocephalus [32], and in the parietotemporal areas in Alzheimer's disease [33]. Assuming that many of the group that did not improve with shunt surgery had Alzheimer's disease (which we have confirmed in two who came to autopsy), we tried to differentiate those who would respond to shunt surgery from those who would not, based on the pattern of preoperative regional cerebral blood flow [34]. To do so, we calculated the ratio of frontal to posterior regional blood flow, expecting a lower frontal-posterior ratio in true symptomatic hydrocephalus and a higher ratio in pseudosymptomatic hydrocephalus patients who have Alzheimer's disease. In fact, this has been a good method for predicting surgical outcome: The ratio predicted 5 of 7 unimproved and 22 of 23 improved patients in our series (see Table 15-1) [11].

Cisternography

Our experience with cisternography is limited, but the literature suggests that there are numerous patients who have a positive test (radioisotope seen within the ventricles 48–72 hours after being injected in the lumbar area) and do not improve with surgery, and many patients who have equivocal or negative tests and do improve.

Further, the test itself may be difficult to interpret. In a review of their experience with this test, Black et al. [15], found the following: Of 11 patients who had a positive test, 9 improved and 2 did not; of 6 patients who had mixed results, 3 improved and 3 did not; and of 6 who had negative results, 4 improved and 2 did not. These researchers suggest that a positive test is helpful but that an equivocal or negative test is not. A recent study by Vanneste et al. [35] reported that "cisternography did not improve the accuracy of combined clinical and computerized tomography in patients with presumed normal-pressure hydrocephalus." Specifically, of the 65 patients who had communicating hydrocephalus and were shunted, cisternography added no predictive value to clinical and CT evaluation. In 17, there was a better prediction by cisternography than by clinical and CT evaluation, but in 23, there was a worse prediction. We do not recommend cisternography as a routine diagnostic test for symptomatic hydrocephalus.

CSF Pressure Monitoring

There have been reports of a significant relationship between measures of intracranial CSF pressure monitoring and surgical outcome for symptomatic hydrocephalus. In the Borgesen and Gjerris study [16] and in our study [11], the greater the percentage of time that B-waves were present, the greater was the chance of a good outcome. Also, in our series, the longer the pressure was more than 15 mm Hg, the better was the chance of successful surgery (see Table 15-1). This implies that increased pressure may be pathogenetic in symptomatic hydrocephalus.

These data raise the issue about what is meant by NPH. Does it mean normal pressure at one spinal tap or does it imply that the pressure remains normal all the time? We do not know what 24-hour CSF pressure recordings in normal people would show. It follows that we do not know whether the pressure is normal or abnormal in those who respond to surgery but have CSF pressures greater than 15 mm Hg for a given period of time. For this reason, at present we prefer the term *symptomatic hydrocephalus* over NPH.

A continuous printout over 24 to 72 hours, with a paper speed of between 50 and 150 mm/hr is needed to assess the overall intracranial pressure and presence of B-waves. Sedation may be helpful at night to reduce the frequency of artifact in the recording.

Infusion Tests

Borgesen and Gjerris [16] described the CSF conductance test, in which CSF absorption is measured at different CSF pressures. In their series, they reported a greater than 90% accuracy in predicting short-term prognosis following shunt surgery and accuracy of approximately 85% in predicting long-term prognosis. The concept is that the greater the pressure needed to obtain an amount of absorption, the better the chances of that patient improving with shunt surgery. Absorption is calculated by infusing fluid through a lumbar puncture needle for a given time (5 min) while catching the overflow from a ventricular catheter. There is some evidence to show that the amount of CSF produced does not vary greatly at different CSF pressures and is approximately 0.4/ml/min. Because one knows how much is infused through the lumbar puncture needle and how much overflows through the ventricular catheter, one can calculate the amount produced in this period. The following equation gives absorption:

$$\text{Absorption} = \text{Infused} + \text{produced} - \text{overflow}$$

The overflow pressure for the ventricular catheter then is raised and absorption is calculated at this new pressure. Between six and eight absorption and pressure measures are obtained in this way; then absorption is plotted against pressure, and the slope of the line is calculated (i.e., absorption÷pressure). The slope of this line is called the *conductance*. Borgesen and Gjerris [16] reported that a conductance of less than 0.08 predicted a favorable outcome.

In our study [11], we found no significant correlation between CSF conductance and improvement (see Table 15-1). However, we chose our patients based on the conductance result, so this was not an independent variable. In addition, most of our patients had idiopathic hydrocephalus, whereas many of Borgesen and Gjerris's patients had secondary hydrocephalus [16]. The conductance test, which relates to CSF absorption, may be a better predictor of outcome in secondary hydrocephalus, in which an absorption defect may be causative.

RECOMMENDING PATIENTS FOR SURGERY

Bearing in mind the aforementioned information, we recommend the following procedure to determine the appropriateness of surgery:

1. Take a careful history from patient and family. Try to establish time of onset of dementia and gait abnormality by asking questions such as: How did the patient walk last Christmas or on the last birthday?
2. Noting the differential diagnoses mentioned earlier, ask appropriate questions to determine other causes of the constellation of findings. For example, has the patient had cervical spondylosis or a previous neck injury; has the patient been a heavy drinker; is there another cause for urinary difficulty (such as prostatism or the birth of multiple children); what medications does the patient take; are there symptoms of autonomic dysfunction (such as postural hypotension); is there a secondary cause for hydrocephalus (such as a head injury, meningitis, or subarachnoid hemorrhage); has the patient had a large head since childhood; or does the patient have symptoms of Parkinson's disease involving the hands (such as micrographia or tremor)?
3. On examination, measure the head size and postural blood pressure, look for signs of Parkinson's disease involving the arms (making Parkinsonism more likely), look for vertical-gaze paresis (unusual in symptomatic hydrocephalus in the elderly), and look for upper–motor neuron signs in the legs or lower–motor neuron signs in the arms (raising suspicion of cervical spondylosis).
4. Perform formal psychometric testing, looking for evidence of aphasia (especially anomia).
5. Order a head CT or MRI, and analyze the results, keeping in mind the points previously mentioned regarding CT and MRI. If necessary, order a cervical MRI.
6. Make a videotape of the patient walking perhaps 20 yards, turning, and walking back. At this time, you may be able to make a decision regarding surgery. If uncertainty persists, perform daily serial lumbar punctures for 3 to 5 days, videotaping the patient before and after. If the patient improves, surgery is likely to help. If there is no improvement, it is possible the patient still might improve, so continue to follow the patient.

Before recommending surgery, be certain to explain to the patient that complications occur in some 30% of patients undergoing shunt surgery. Also, tell the patient and family that even if the patient improves, a return to normal is not likely. In those who respond favorably, gait and incontinence usually improve, but cognition only improves in 50%. These are important improvements and may prevent a patient's being placed in a nursing home, but the patient and family should have realistic expectations. If at this stage you are still unsure of what to do, you can defer the decision and have the patient return in 3 months, repeating the videotape at that time. Longitudinal information documenting whether the problem is stable or progressive may factor into your decision. Alternative diagnostic tests (e.g., cerebral blood flow, CSF pressure monitoring, infusion studies, and continuous CSF drainage studies) are not universally available but can be used as adjunctive information in the centers that use these tests.

SHUNTS

General Information

The function of any shunt device is to provide a pathway for egress of CSF. These devices, therefore, connect a CSF space (cerebral ventricle or lumbar subarachnoid space) with a terminus for absorption (peritoneal cavity or right atrium). Ventriculoperitoneal shunts are the most frequently employed type. The ventricular end may be placed frontally or through a parietal access, with the catheter tip lying in the frontal horn of the lateral ventricle. The peritoneal cavity provides an extensive absorptive surface, and complications with this portion of the shunt are infrequent. In individuals who have undergone multiple abdominal surgery and have peritoneal adhesions, another termination point may be used. Approximately 5–10% of shunts are of the ventriculoatrial type, with the distal catheter entering a vein in the neck and terminating in the right atrium. A third type of shunt, which may be used to manage those with symptomatic adult hydrocephalus of the communicating type, is a lumboperitoneal shunt. In this case, the proximal end of the shunt enters the lumbar subarachnoid space and terminates in the peritoneal cavity. A wide variety of shunt designs are available for use. In general, they consist of a ventricular catheter, reservoir (or CSF holding chamber), valve, and distal catheter (peritoneal or atrial). Other components may be used infrequently (i.e., on-off valves, antisiphon devices). The valves are constructed with different closing pressures: high, medium, and low. The closing pressure is the ventricular pressure at which the valve shuts off and fluid stops flowing until this pressure is again exceeded. We have used medium-pressure valves in the treatment of adult hydrocephalus. The purpose of the shunt and valve is to allow venting of CSF during periods of episodic intracranial pressure excess. The intracranial pressure need not be lowered below normal but only prevented from rising above normal.

Complications

Shunt complication, both major and minor, unfortunately occurs in some 30% of patients [4, 5]. These include intraoperative complications related to general anesthesia in an elderly population, intracranial hemorrhage from ventricular catheter placement, intraabdominal injury (rare), and arrhythmias from incorrect ventriculoatrial distal catheter placement. Perioperative complications include infection (3–8% of cases), CSF hypotensive headaches, and the development of subdural effusions or hematomas. The latter problem is more likely to occur in those with marked reduction in ventricular size after shunting and is more common when low-pressure valves are used for treatment of these effusions. Depending on symptoms, conservative or surgical therapy may be indicated. Long-term complications are related primarily to shunt occlusion or catheter breakage. Infection after the first 2 months is unusual.

Checking Shunt Function

In 22 patients, preoperatively and postoperatively we measured the surface area of the lateral ventricles as a ratio of the inner table of the skull. In 21 instances, the ventricles were smaller postoperatively than preoperatively (Fig. 15-1) [34]. We believe that this surface area ratio can be used as an indicator of shunt patency. However, we should caution that simple inspection of preoperative and postoperative CTs may not be as accurate as measuring the surface area. Some have reported that patients may improve after shunt surgery without the ventricles decreasing in size (as seen on CT). We have seen this in one case.

If it is necessary to determine whether the shunt is functional because of clinical changes, a head CT scan is the first step, as described earlier. If ventricular volume is smaller postoperatively than preoperatively, the shunt probably is functional. In those systems with a reservoir, CSF aspiration following sterile skin preparation can easily assess proximal patency. There are various methods to assess distal patency; they include injecting positive contrast agents or radioactive materials into the shunt system and following their progress to the site of termination. Remember that any time the shunt system is accessed, there is a risk of introducing infection. The shunt valve may be compressed to assess its function; this has some validity for those experienced with the procedure but is not infallible. Invasive shunt testing should be left to the neurosurgeon.

Assessment of Patient Improvement

Traditionally, patient improvement has been assessed on a five-point rating scale [4, 16]. This may be problematic, because levels on the scale overlap, and it is a subjective judgment as to which level the patient occupies. We have tried to develop more objective measures, and we use several.

Serial Videotaping of the Patient's Gait

Preoperatively and at 2 and 6 months postoperatively, we videotape the patient's neurological examination, including walking. Scales have been developed and published to measure both qualitatively and quantitatively the patient's gait performance [11, 13]. We have used the two published scales [13] in previous studies. In the qualitative method, the postoperative videotapes were compared to the preoperative ones and rated on a performance scale of *same, better,* or *worse* on the following five items: standing from a seated position, initiating walking, step size, speed, and turning.

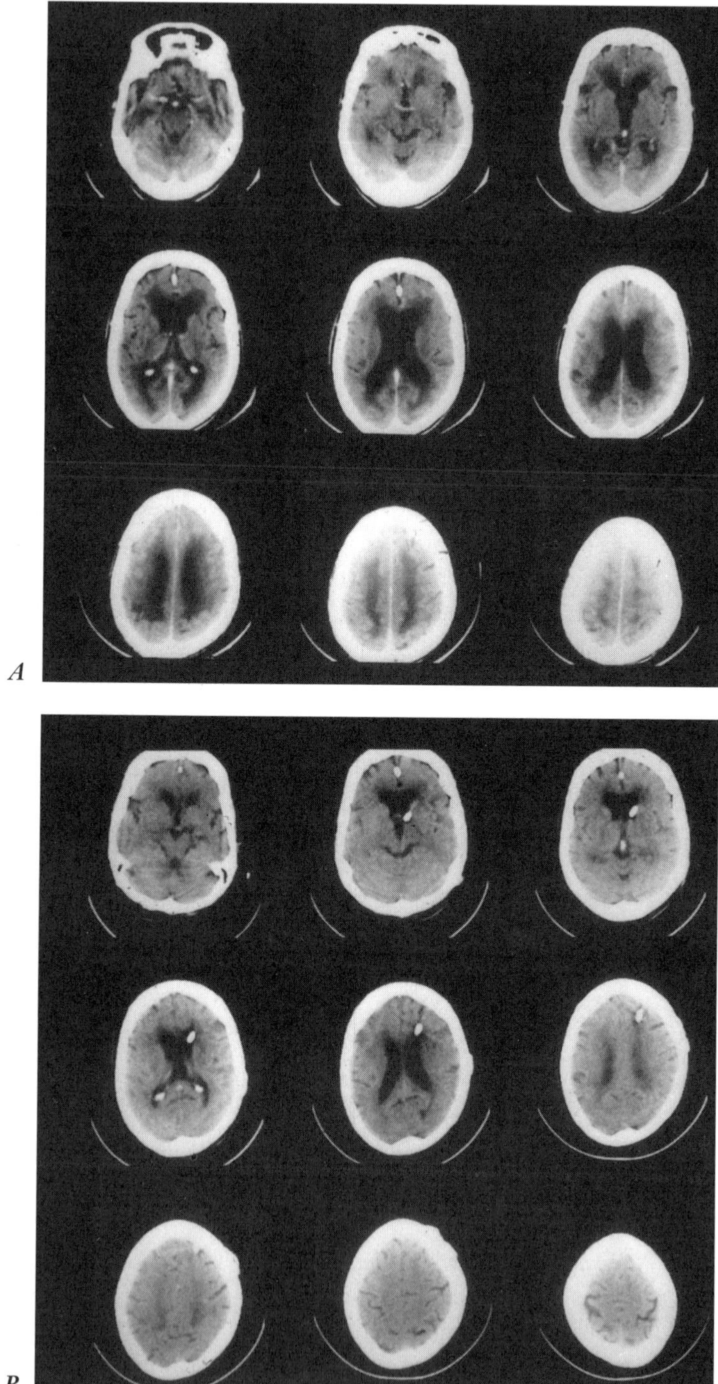

Figure 15-1. (*A*) Preoperative computed tomography of patient with symptomatic hydrocephalus. (*B*) Postoperative computed tomography of the same patient. This patient improved with surgery. Note that the ventricles are smaller after surgery. Sometimes, this decrease in ventricle size is not as obvious even in patients who improve.

The quantitative method uses a numerical score, which is given for the patient's overall performance:

1 = Cannot walk even with help
2 = Can walk with significant support
3 = Walks unsteadily and needs minor support
4 = Walks independently but is markedly unsteady and has difficulty in turning
5 = Walks independently but is mildly unsteady and has difficulty in turning
6 = Walks almost normally but has significant difficulty in turning
7 = Walks normally but has minor difficulty in turning
8 = Walks normally

Two evaluators independently rated the videotapes, and a test of interrater reliability was excellent. The gait was considered improved if the raters agreed that the patient had improved on both scales: the qualitative (better on at least two items without worsening on any of the other items) and the quantitative (an increase of at least one level on the numerical scale).

Katz Index of Activities of Daily Living

This scale rates a patient on six items: bathing, dressing, toileting, transferring, continence, and feeding [36]. The worst score for each item is 3, and the best is 1. Thus, the worst obtainable score is 18, and the best is 6. There is a written description for each score in each item. We regard a change of 2 or more in this index as significant. This allows measurements of small but functionally important changes. An example of a 2-point improvement on this index might be as follows: a change from "occasional urinary accidents" to "controls urination and bowel movements completely by self" (1-point improvement) plus "moves in and out of bed or chair with assistance" to "moves in and out of bed as well as chair without assistance" (1-point improvement).

Neuropsychological Testing

Our patients receive a battery of neuropsychological tests preoperatively and at 2 and 6 months postoperatively [11]. These tests sample orientation, intelligence, verbal and visual acuity, memory, language, visuospatial functioning, and executive control. We judge a patient neuropsychologically improved when there has been a signficant increase in the test scores in two or more neuropsychological areas, provided there is no decline in another area. Only approximately 50% of those responding to shunt surgery improve cognitively by the above criteria.

THE RELATIONSHIP OF IDIOPATHIC SYMPTOMATIC HYDROCEPHALUS AND SYSTEMIC HYPERTENSION

Several lines of evidence in the literature now point to a relationship between hydrocephalus and systemic hypertension. A number of postmortem examinations of NPH patients have found associated hypertensive cerebrovascular changes [37–39]. In our own series [40], a significantly higher prevalence of systemic hypertension was found in idiopathic NPH patients compared with matched, demented controls and to the published prevalence of hypertension in the US population, matched for age.

Another line of evidence showing that systemic hypertension and hydrocephalus may be related comes from the Cooperative Aneurysm Study [41]. In more than 3,000 patients with subarachnoid hemorrhage, it was found that a preoperative history of hypertension, the admission blood pressure measurement, and sustained hypertension during hospitalization after surgery were significantly related to patients developing hydrocephalus. Greitz et al. [42] found a high prevalence of hypertension in patients with hydrocephalus from aqueductal stenosis.

This observation of the association of hypertension and hydrocephalus is corroborated by reports in the animal literature. Ritter and Dinh [43] showed that the spontaneously hypertensive rat develops hydrocephalus. Portnoy et al. [44] showed in dogs that infusing dopamine and norepinephrine led to increased systemic blood pressure, which, in turn, resulted in an increase of CSF pressure and pulse pressure. Experimentally creating an increased pulse pressure with an inflatable balloon in the lateral ventricle of sheep leads to hydrocephalus [45]. In their classic work on dogs, Bering and Salibi [46] concluded that the mechanism involved in the ventricular enlargement seemed to be a combination of at least two factors: "One was the possible failure of CSF absorption in the face of increased superior sagittal sinus venous pressure, and the other the increased intraventricular pulse pressure from the choroid plexus."

Thus, an accumulating body of information positing that systemic hypertension and hydrocephalus probably are associated. If this proves to be true, it remains to be shown whether hypertension causes hydrocephalus or hydrocephalus causes hypertension, or that they cause each other.

FACTORS ASSOCIATED WITH THE PATHOGENESIS OF HYDROCEPHALUS IN THE ELDERLY

Regarding the etiology and pathogenesis of symptomatic hydrocephalus in the elderly, there are several important factors to be considered:

1. *Congenital hydrocephalus.* This becomes symptomatic in the elderly; this made up approximately 10% of our series [17].
2. *Impaired CSF absorption.* There are many lines of evidence supporting this factor (e.g., in the cooperative subarachnoid hemorrhage study [41], items associated with the development of hydrocephalus were intraventricular hemorrhage, diffuse subarachnoid blood, and thick focal accumulation of blood, whereas thin accumulation of blood and intracerebral hematoma were not associated with hydrocephalus. Patients with posterior circulation aneurysms (near the foramina of Luschka and Magendie and thus interfering with

CSF egress from the fourth ventricle) have a significantly higher incidence of hydrocephalus, whereas patients with middle cerebral aneurysms have a significantly lower incidence of hydrocephalus.

3. *Increasing age*. The evidence in favor of this factor is that this is a disease of older individuals. Further, in the cooperative subarachnoid aneurysm study, increasing age was significantly associated with the development of hydrocephalus [41]. Systemic hypertension is present (see earlier section on this subject).

SPECULATION AS TO THE CAUSE OF GAIT ABNORMALITY IN HYDROCEPHALUS

Yakovlev [47] showed that the fibers from the leg area are stretched as they course around the dilated ventricles, a condition that could conceivably interfere with gait. Further, in some patients, on MRI, there is periventricular high signal around the ventricles, indicating excessive water in this area. It is possible that this could also affect the leg fibers.

REFERENCES

1. Wells CE. Diagnosis of dementia. *Psychosomatics* 1979;20:517–522.
2. Katzman R. Normal Pressure Hydrocephalus. In: Katzman R, Terry R Bick KC, eds. *Alzheimer's Disease: Senile Dementia and Related Disorders (Aging)*. New York: Raven, 1978. Pp 115–124.
3. Hughes CP, et al. Adult idiopathic communicating hydrocephalus with and without shunting. *J Neurol Neurosurg Psychiatry* 1978;41:961–971.
4. Black PMcL. Idiopathic normal pressure hydrocephalus. *Neurosurgery* 1980;52:371–377.
5. Peterson RC, Mokri B, Laws ER. Surgical treatment of idiopathic hydrocephalus in elderly patients. *Neurology* 1985;35:307–311.
6. Mortimer JA, Shuman LM, French LR. Epidemiology of Dementing Illness. In: Mortimer JA, Shuman LM, eds. *The Epidemiology of Dementia*. New York: Oxford University Press, 1981.
7. Yarnell JW, St Leger AS. The prevalence, severity, and factors associated with urinary incontinence in a random sample of the elderly. *Age Ageing* 1979;8:81–85.
8. Sudarsky L, Ronthal M. Gait disorders among elderly patients. A survey of 50 patients. *Arch Neurol* 1983;40:740–743.
9. Barron SA, Jacobs L, Kinkel W. Changes in size of normal lateral ventricles during aging determined by computerized tomography. *Neurology* 1976;26:1011–1013.
10. Damasio H, et al. Quantitive computed tomographic analysis in the diagnosis of dementia. *Arch Neurol* 1983;40:715–719.
11. Graff-Radford NR, Godersky JC, Jones MP. Variables predicting outcome in symptomatic hydrocephalus in the elderly. *Neurology* 1989;39:1601–1604.
12. Fisher CM. The clinical picture in occult hydrocephalus. *Clin Neurosurg* 1977;24:270–315.
13. Graff-Radford NR, Godersky JC. Normal pressure hydrocephalus: Onset of gait abnormality before dementia predicts a good surgical outcome. *Arch Neurol* 1986;43:940–942.
14. Demol J. Facteurs pronostiques du resultat therapeutique dans l'hydrocephalie a pression normale. *Acta Neurol Belg* 1985;85:13–29.
15. Black PMcL, Ojemann RG, Tzouras A. CSF shunts for dementia, incontinence, and gait disturbance. *Clin Neurosurg* 1985;32:632–656.

16. Borgesen SE, Gjerris F. The predictive value of conductance to outflow of CSF in NPH. *Brain* 1982;105:65–86.

17. Graff-Radford NR, Godersky JC. Symptomatic congenital hydrocephalus in the elderly simulating normal pressure hydrocephalus. *Neurology* 1989;39:1596–1600.

18. McHugh PR. Occult hydrocephalus. *Q J Med* 1964;130:297–308.

19. Graff-Radford NR, et al. Neuropsychological Testing in Normal Pressure Hydrocephalus. In: Hoff JT, Betz AL, eds. *Intracranial Pressure*, vol. 7. Berlin: Springer, 1989. Pp 422–424.

20. Wikkelsö C, et al. The clinical effect of lumbar puncture in NPH. *J Neurol Neurosurg Psychiatr* 1982;45:64–69.

21. Wikkelsö C, et al. Normal pressure hydrocephalus. Predictive value of the cerebrospinal fluid tap-test. *Acta Neurol Scand* 1986;73:566–573.

22. Haan J, Thormeer RTWM. Predictive value of temporary external lumbar drainage in normal pressure hydrocephalus. *Neurosurgery* 1988;22:388–391.

23. Hanley DF, Borel CO, Herdman S. Normal-Pressure Hydrocephalus. In: Johnson RT, ed. *Current Therapy in Neurological Disease*, 3rd ed. Philadelphia: BC Decker, 1990. Pp 305–309.

24. Huckman MS. Normal pressure hydrocephalus: Evaluation of diagnosis and prognostic tests. *AJNR* 1981;2:385–395.

25. George AE, et al. CT diagnostic features of Alzheimer's disease: Importance of the choroidal/hippocampal fissure complex. *AJNR* 1990;11:101–107.

26. Kido DK, et al. Temporal lobe atrophy in patients with Alzheimer's disease: A CT study. *AJNR* 1989;10:551–555.

27. Sandor T, Albert M, Stafford J, Harpley S. Use of computerized analysis to discriminate between Alzheimer patients and normal control subjects. *AJNR* 1988;9:1181–1187.

28. Bradley WG, Kortman KE, Burgoyne B. Flowing cerebrospinal fluid in normal and hydrocephalic states: Appearance on MR images. *Radiology* 1989;159:611–616.

29. Bradley WG, et al. Marked cerebrospinal fluid void: Indicator of successful shunt in patients with suspected normal-pressure hydrocephalus. *Radiology* 1991;178:459–466.

30. Enzmann DR, Pelc NJ. Normal flow patterns of intracranial and spinal cerebrospinal fluid defined with phase-contrast CINE-MRI imaging. *Radiology* 1991;178:467–474.

31. Jack CR, et al. MR findings in normal-pressure hydrocephalus: Significance and comparison with other forms of dementia. *J Comput Assist Tomogr* 1987;11:923–931.

32. Foster NL, et al. Alzheimer's disease: Focal cortical changes shown by positron emission tomography. *Neurology* 33:1983;961–965.

33. Jagust WJ, Friedland RP, Budinger TF. Positron emission tomography with (^{18}F)-fluodeoxyyglucose differentiates normal pressure hydrocephalus from Alzheimer-type dementia. *J Neurol Neurosurg Psychiatry* 1985;48:1091–1096.

34. Graff-Radford NR, et al. Regional cerebral blood flow in normal pressure hydrocephalus. *J Neurol Neurosurg Psychiatry* 1987;50:1589–1596.

35. Vanneste J, et al. Normal-pressure hydrocephalus. *Arch Neurol* 1992;49:366–370.

36. Kane RA, Kane RL. *Assessing the Elderly. A Practice Guide to Measurements.* Lexington, MA: Lexington Books, 1981.

37. Koto A, et al. Syndrome of normal pressure hydrocephalus: Possible relation to hypertensive arteriosclerotic vasculopathy. *J Neurol Neurosurg Psychiatry* 1977;40:73–79.

38. Earnest MP, Fahn S, Karp JH, Rowland LP. Normal pressure hydrocephalus and hypertensive cerebrovascular disease. *Arch Neurol* 1974;31:262–266.

39. Coblentz JM, et al. Presenile dementia. *Arch Neurol* 1973;29:299–308.

40. Graff-Radford NR, Godersky JC. Idiopathic normal pressure hydrocephalus and systemic hypertension. *Neurology* 1987;37:868–71.

41. Graff-Radford NR, Torner J, Adams HP, Kassell NF. Factors associated with hydrocephalus after subarachnoid hemorrhage. A report of the Cooperative Aneurysm Study. *Arch Neurol* 1989;46:744–752.

42. Greitz T, Levander BE, Lopez J. High blood pressure and epilepsy in hydrocephalus due to stenosis of the aqueduct of Sylvius. *Acta Neurochir (Wien)* 1971;24:201–206.

43. Ritter S, Dinh TT. Progressive postnatal dilatation of brain ventricles in spontaneously hypertensive rats. *Brain Res* 1986;370:327–332.
44. Portnoy HD, Chopp M, Branch C. Hydraulic model of myogenic autoregulation and the cerebrovascular bed: The effects of altering systemic arterial pressure. *Neurosurgery* 1983;13:482–498.
45. Peltarossi VE, et al. Communicating hydrocephalus induced by mechanically increased amplitude of the intraventricular cerebrospinal fluid pulse pressure: Rationale and method. *Exp Neurol* 1978;59:30–39.
46. Bering RA Jr, Salibi B. Production of hydrocephalus by increased cephalic-venous pressure. *Arch Neurol Psychiatr* 1959;81:693–698.
47. Yakovlev PI. Paraplegias of hydrocephalics. *Am J Men Def* 1947;51:561–576.

16. Vestibular and Cerebellar Disorders of Equilibrium and Gait

Hans Christoph Diener and John G. Nutt

VESTIBULAR DISORDERS
Physiology of the Vestibulospinal System in Humans

The maintenance of upright stance in humans requires the integration of visual, proprioceptive, labyrinthine, and otolithic information about the body's position in space. The role of the vestibular system among the three afferent control loops for postural control in humans is still rather obscure. Furthermore, the proportional contributions of otoliths and semicircular canals to balance are unknown. Most of the assumptions concerning the gain and working range of the receptors of the canals and otoliths are based on analogies from animal experiments and, therefore, do not necessarily hold for humans. Experiments performed in humans indicate that the working ranges of the visual, proprioceptive, and vestibular systems partly overlap, supplying redundant information [1–3]. Therefore, visual and proprioceptive systems can generally compensate for the loss of both graviception and canal-dependent vestibular input [4].

In the elderly, aging results in a reduction of hair cells and neurons of the sacculus and utriculus [5] and in fewer eighth nerve fibers [6]. Therefore, less vestibular information is available for the control of stance and gait [7]. The situation is aggravated by a reduction of proprioceptive sensory input by age-related peripheral nerve loss and by declining visual acuity.

Early investigations of vestibular functions in humans used dynamic vestibular stimuli, such as vertical falls, to stimulate the otoliths. These stimuli evoked electromyography (EMG) responses in leg muscles within 60 to 80 msec [8], indicating that the vestibulospinal pathways in humans have short latencies and fast conduction times. Similar latencies for vestibulospinal reflexes have been observed in a patient with a Tullio's phenomenon—the production of dizziness by loud noises [9].

The influence of vestibulospinal inputs on human postural control is now generally investigated by imposing external perturbations on the body by displacements of a platform on which a subject stands. Early reflexlike EMG responses in leg, trunk, and neck muscles can be observed after linear displacements of the platform or treadmill [10–14]. The platform displacement simulates natural situations, such as when a standing subject in a bus or train suddenly is exposed to acceleration or deceleration or hits bumps. Both linear and rotatory (toes-up or toes-down) displacement of the platform stimulates vestibular receptors because of the linear movement of the head and body in space and produces a powerful proprioceptive input from the stretched leg muscles, joints, and skin. The linear displacement and the tilting of the platform produce different patterns of afferent input: A backward linear displacement of the support surface results in a forward sway of the body. Afferent information results from the stretch of the triceps surae muscle (but also upper-leg, trunk, and neck muscles) and the forward displacement of the head in space. A toe-up rotation around the ankle joint leads to a similar proprioceptive input from the triceps surae muscle but results in a backward displacement of the head.

Either type of platform movement elicits short (55–75 msec), medium (75–95 msec), and long (95–140 msec) latency EMG responses in leg muscles [15–17]. The short latency response corresponds to the spinal stretch reflex, the medium latency response represents a polysynaptic spinal reflex, and the long latency response signals a supraspinally generated motor response with powerful contributions from sensorimotor cortex and the cerebellum. The long latency responses appear to generate the automatic postural responses; the short- and medium-duration responses produce little movement around joints. The important difference between the linear and rotational displacements is a practical one: With rotation, it is easier to evoke a spinal stretch reflex and collect information on the status of the short latency response. With linear displacements, the medium latency response cannot be separated from the long latency response. With rotation, medium latency response is in the stretched muscle, and long latency response is in the shortened muscle. This makes it easy to differentiate the end of medium latency response from the start of long latency response.

Dietz et al. [18] induced sudden head tilts in normal subjects during quiet standing, balancing, undisturbed walking, and walking during which unexpected perturbations occurred. A backward-directed head tilt was followed by tonic tibialis anterior activation with a latency of 55 msec, followed by EMG activity in the gastrocnemius muscle with a latency of 95 msec. The size of these EMG responses was, however, small compared to the responses recorded during balancing, walking, and responding to perturbations. These results indicate that under physiological conditions in normal individuals, vestibulospinal reflexes contribute only in a very limited way to postural stabilization.

We investigated the relative contribution of vestibular information on postural control during fast toe-up and toe-down platform displacements and during slow continuous sinusoidal movements of the platform [3]. In subjects standing upright, the head was either in its normal position, tilted forward by 30 degrees (putting the utricle in its optimal working position), extended backward by 45 degrees (decreased sensitivity and gain of the utricles), or tilted to the right or left shoulder by 45 degrees. The different head positions resulted neither in a change of latency nor in a change of amplitude of short, medium, and long latency EMG responses in leg muscles to fast rotations. Head position, however, profoundly affected body stabilization during continuous sinusoidal movements of the platform [3]. One may conclude from these results that fast transient disturbances are compensated by fixed reflexlike motor patterns that are not immediately modified by (and possibly are not even accessible to) inputs from the vestibular and visual systems or from parts of the proprioceptive system, whereas slow continuous displacements of the body are highly dependent on vestibular (and visual and proprioceptive) feedback [19].

Postural Stabilization with Reduced or Absent Vestibular Input

The cause of acute vestibular disfunction in elderly people differs from that in younger people. The most prevalent causes of acute peripheral vestibular dysfunction in younger people are benign paroxysmal positional vertigo and neuritis of the eighth nerve, whereas older people suffer from Meniere's disease and vascular disease of the labyrinth. Often, central vestibular disturbances are due to multiple sclerosis between ages 20 to 40, whereas stroke and tumors are the leading causes in the elderly. Acute vestibular loss results in severe rotational vertigo, horizontal rotatory nystagmus, falling to the side ipsilateral to the lesion, nausea, and vomiting. Tachycardia, sweating, and hypotension are frequent. The vertigo is not influenced by position or positional changes. Central compensation starts within hours or days but is slower in the elderly. With compensation comes a reduction of vertigo and autonomic disturbances. Vertigo still can be provoked in situations with powerful vestibular input (strong acceleration or deceleration) or in conditions of nonphysiological or conflicting sensory stimuli. Examples include vertigo (1) when the neck is extended, reducing vestibular input due to nonphysiological working range of otoliths and reduced input from muscle spindles in shortened neck muscles; (2) with the development of cataracts and reduction of visual spatial information; and (3) with polyneuropathy and reduced somatosensory information.

In addition to causing vertigo and nausea, central vestibular lesions cause other brain-stem symptoms and signs (e.g., sensory disturbances in the face, dysarthria, dysphagia, diplopia, or ataxia). Vertigo and spontaneous rotatory, horizontal, and vertical nystagmus may be position-dependent and do not habituate with repeated positional changes.

Aging, degenerative processes, or toxins affecting the labyrinth and eighth nerves may lead to gradual vestibular dysfunction, allowing for development of central compensatory strategies to overcome the deficit. If there are central lesions as well (e.g., cerebellar dysfunction), compensation will be less.

Patients with bilateral vestibular loss stand with a broad base (to increase the area of stance support) and with their head bent forward (to use visual information from movement with respect to the ground). Cervical muscles are tender because they are fixing the head with respect to the trunk to reduce inappropriate sensory input caused by impaired vestibuloocular reflexes. Stance becomes unstable when visual and proprioceptive systems are also disturbed or absent (e.g., having the eyes closed and standing on a moving or tilting surface) [1].

The role of vestibular input for the compensation of external displacements has been investigated in patients with unilateral and bilateral vestibular deficits. Horstmann and Dietz [20] showed that early leg muscle EMG responses evoked through head movements were absent in patients without vestibular function. The deficit in vestibulospinal input, however, causes only a 10% (biomechanically irrelevant) reduction of EMG amplitudes in leg muscles after linear displacements of the support surface. In contrast, responses to rotational platform movements are more sensitive to vestibular deficits than are responses to linear displacements. With toe-up platform tilt, patients with bilateral vestibular deficit had delayed (120-msec) responses and a 50% decrease in EMG responses in tibialis anterior and soleus [21]. This reduced the torque at the ankle, and patients fell backward when tested with eyes closed [22, 23]. These results suggest that human vestibulospinal reflexes contribute to upright stance and balance when visual and proprioceptive input is reduced, absent, or inappropriate.

The Role of Conflicting Sensory Input in Vestibular Disease

Mismatches between visual and vestibular afferent information produce disorientation, vertigo, and sometimes motion sickness [24]. Such conflicting stimuli can be used to unmask compensated vestibular dysfunction in patients. Both Nashner [1] and Black [25] developed functional platform tests (often referred to as *posturography*) that separate normal individuals from patients with vestibular deficiencies and "distortions" (e.g., benign paroxysmal positional nystagmus).

In posturography studies, patients stand on a movable platform with a wraparound screen that completely fills the subjects' visual fields (see Chapter 3, page 47). In the first three test conditions, the platform surface is fixed, and the eyes are open (condition 1), closed (condition 2), or open but with the visual surround moved in conjunction with the body to eliminate visual clues to position in space (condition 3). Condition 3 creates a conflict between the proprioceptive and vestibular input signaling body motion and the visual perception of no movement. In the next three conditions, the platform is moved in proportion to body sway angle to minimize movement at the ankle and thereby to reduce appropriate proprioceptive input. The moving platform conditions are combined with the three different kinds of visual feedback (producing conditions 4–6). Patients with unilaterally or bilaterally reduced or absent vestibular function are posturally stable with variations in visual input, as long as the platform remains stable. This observation indicates that the classic Romberg test will not detect compensated vestibular deficits. However, vestibular patients lose balance when somatosensory input and vision are disrupted simultaneously, because these senses no longer can compensate for the vestibular deficit. The conflicting sensory information of conditions 5 and 6 renders them helpful tests for monitoring improvement of motor performance objectively after acute vestibular loss [26] or for monitoring the success of rehabilitation therapy [27].

Pyykkö et al. [28] investigated the influence of inappropriate proprioceptive input elicited by vibration applied to the calf or neck muscles in patients with peripheral or central vestibular lesions. Patients with compensated peripheral vestibular lesions were able to counteract the deviations of the body center of mass elicited by the proprioceptive stimulation. In contrast, patients with central vestibular lesions were unable to protect the center of mass during inappropriate proprioceptive input, even when visual input was available.

Effect of Vestibular Function on Choice of Motor Strategy

A fundamental question concerning the organization of postural reactions to external disturbances is whether muscle responses are determined exclusively by spinal or supraspinal reflex loops or are centrally programmed and released according to prior experience. Nashner and McCollum [29] proposed a model in which the central nervous system preprograms a limited number of postural EMG patterns. One such preprogrammed postural response is muscle activity, beginning in muscles acting on the ankle, then on the knee, and finally on the hip, to compensate for body sway induced by linear displacements of the support surface. This pattern of muscle activation results in body sway around the ankle joint and therefore is termed *ankle strategy* [13]. When it is impossible to exert an adequate amount of torque around the ankle joint (e.g., when standing on a narrow beam), subjects will switch to another preprogrammed postural response, the hip strategy, which consists of a proximal-to-distal motor sequence and stabilizes posture by counterphase leg and trunk movements around the hip, keeping the center of mass over the beam.

Patients with completely absent vestibular function used an ankle strategy with normal latencies and EMG patterns when standing on a flat surface [30]. When these patients were placed on a narrow support surface, they continued to use an ankle strategy even though it was ineffective in maintaining balance [29]. However, the hip strategy was used by vestibular patients when the eyes were closed. It seems that the patients with bilateral vestibular loss try to minimize inappropriate visual information caused by inadequate vestibuloocular reflexes by keeping the head stable in space as long as the eyes are open [31]. Head displacements are much smaller with the ankle than with the hip strategy.

Gait in Vestibular Disorders

Gait in patients with vestibular disorders is due to disequilibrium affecting stance and walking, not to disturbances in locomotor synergies or in limb kinematics [32].

With acute vestibular disturbances, the gait may be broad-based, staggering, leaning to one side or backward, and veering from the intended path. Occasionally, the gait may be narrow-based with scissoring steps, as though the patient were reacting to external pushes [32]. The patient may fall toward the diseased labyrinth; the direction of the fall can be altered by changing the position of the head. For example, a patient with a left labyrinth lesion will tend to fall to the left when the head is in neutral position but will fall forward if the chin is turned to the right shoulder.

With long-standing total vestibular loss in an otherwise healthy person, the gait may be completely normal. Only the "sharpened Romberg" (standing in tandem position with eyes closed) or tandem gait with eyes closed may reveal unsteadiness. However, in the elderly (perhaps because of aging or subclinical pathology in other sensory and motor systems), vestibular loss may disturb gait. Fife and Baloh [33] described elderly patients who had vestibular loss and no other peripheral or central neurological pathology, in whom gait was characterized by slightly widened base, unsteady turns, staggering when pushed, increased axial sway, and veering when walking.

Summary of Vestibular Disorders Affecting Equilibrium and Gait

The vestibular system clearly participates in the control of upright posture in humans, but its influence in normal people is masked largely by redundant sensory control through vision and proprioception. The detection of vestibular dysfunction requires either external perturbations of the body or conflicting sensory inputs. The loss of vestibular function also may influence the selection of higher motor synergies. Acute vestibular lesions cause a weaving, unsteady gait; chronic lesions do not disturb gait, except perhaps in the elderly.

CEREBELLAR DISORDERS

Cerebellar Influences on Posture

Two regions of the cerebellum, the vestibulocerebellum and the spinocerebellum, are of particular importance to balance. The analysis of human stance on a force-measuring platform quantifies the clinical Romberg test (Fig. 16-1A-D) and has allowed vestibulocerebellar and spinocerebellar lesions to be distinguished according to their pattern of postural instability [17, 34, 35]. Lesions of the spinocerebellar part of the anterior lobe, most commonly observed in chronic alcoholics, cause a 3-Hz anteroposterior body sway (see Fig. 16-1D). The tremor is provoked by eye closure. Patients rarely fall due to the fact that the body tremor is opposite in phase in head, trunk, and legs, thus resulting in a minimal shift of the center of gravity. Visual stabilization of posture is preserved.

Lesions of the vestibulocerebellum or flocculonodular lobe, most commonly due to tumors, ischemia, or hemorrhage, cause postural tremor of head and trunk in sitting, standing, and walking patients. Postural sway is omnidirectional and contains frequency components below 1 Hz. Visual stabilization (as evaluated by comparing sway with eyes closed and sway with eyes open) is less than in the other groups of cerebellar patients (see Fig. 16-1B).

Bronstein et al. [36] investigated control of balance in patients with cerebellar disease with eyes open and with eyes closed and in response to visual stimuli generated by lateral displacements of a moveable room. Cerebellar lesions spared the visuopostural loop and also spared the ability to shift from visual to proprioceptive control of postural sway.

Long latency responses in stretched muscles can be recorded easily with surface electrodes, and they offer the opportunity to quantify cerebellar dysfunction

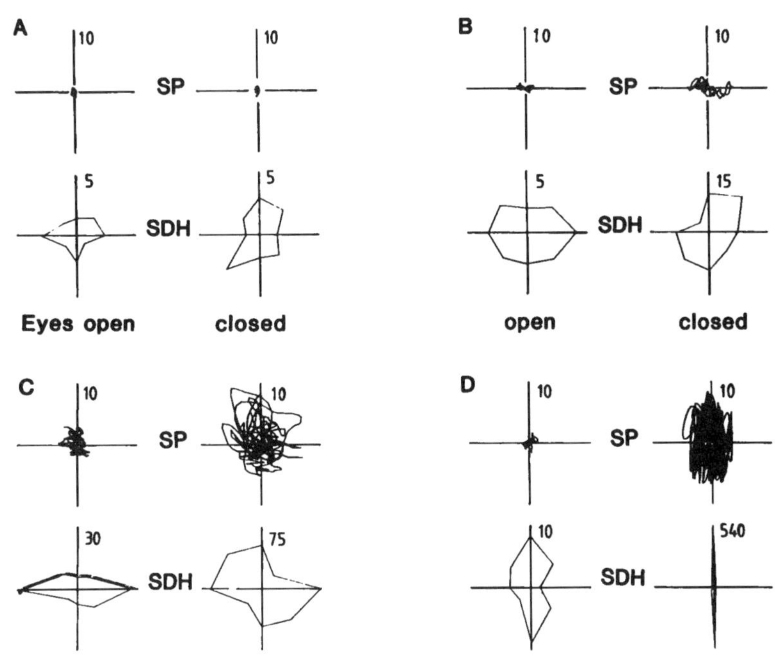

Figure 16-1. Recording of sway path (SP) in anterioposterior and lateral direction and the calculated sway direction histogram (SDH). *A*. Normal subject. *B*. Increased omnidirectional sway in a patient with hemorrhage or the vestibulocerebellar vermis. *C*. Predominantly lateral sway in a patient with Friedreich's ataxia. *D*. Predominantly anterioposterior sway in a chronic alcoholic with atrophy of the anterior lobe. Note the different scalings (*A* versus *B–D*) of the axis of the sway direction histogram, summing the instantaneous sway directions within each of the eight directional bins.

in limb muscles. Friedemann et al. [37] and Diener et al. [38] investigated EMG responses to stretch of hand muscles (first dorsal interosseus) and leg muscles (triceps surae, tibialis anterior) in patients with cerebellar disorders. Latencies of early, medium, and late EMG responses were normal. The cerebellum is, therefore, unlikely to be the primary generator of these muscle responses to stretch. However, duration and intensity of long latency responses were increased in upper and lower extremities, whereas the intensity and duration of short and medium latency responses were normal (Fig. 16-2). These results indicate that the cerebellum has a modulatory influence on the size and duration (and therefore force) of long latency responses.

EMG responses from leg and trunk muscles in response to variations in amplitude and velocity of platform displacement have shown abnormal gain control in cerebellar patients [39, 40]. Reflex responses had normal latencies, and postural synergies basically were normal. However, the gain of EMG response versus platform movement amplitude were increased, and the gain of EMG response versus platform velocity was reduced. This caused dysmetrical postural responses to platform displacements. The abnormal control of amplitude and

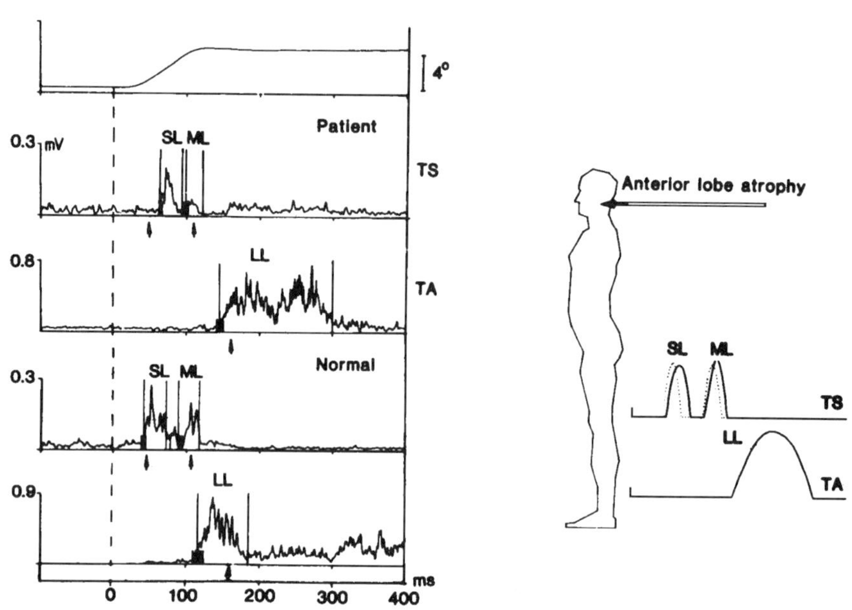

Figure 16-2. Postural reflexes evoked through a platform tilt toe-up in a standing subject; rectified and averaged electromyography responses from triceps surae (TS) and anterior tibial muscle (TA); short (SL) and medium (ML) latency responses in TS and stabilizing long latency response (LL) in TA. The patient with anterior-lobe atrophy exhibits a prolonged activity in anterior tibial muscle. The right side of the figure shows mean latencies, durations, and integrals of SL, ML, and LL in a normal population (*dotted lines*) and in a population of 42 patients with anterior lobe atrophy due to chronic alcoholism. Note the increased duration and integral of LL in TA.

duration of long-loop reflexes may be one of the constituents of postural tremor in cerebellar patients.

Cerebellar Diseases in the Elderly

The most frequent causes of cerebellar dysfunction in the elderly are ischemic strokes and hemorrhages. Hemorrhages lead to sudden headache; vomiting; ataxia of stance, gait, and sitting; and dysarthria. Occlusion of the posteroinferior cerebellar artery leads to ipsilateral ataxia of stance and gait, falling to the ipsilateral side, nystagmus, dysarthria, and ataxia of limb movements. Brain-stem symptoms include ipsilateral disturbances of temperature and pain sensation in the face, contralateral disturbances in the trunk, Horner's syndrome, and swallowing problems. Ischemia in the territory of the inferoanterior cerebellar artery results in acute deafness, peripheral vestibular loss, facial palsy, Horner's syndrome, limb ataxia, and hypotonia but intact stabilization of the trunk.

Degenerative diseases of the cerebellum include disease restricted to the cerebellum and diseases with extracerebellar involvement (e.g., olivopontocerebellar ataxia or multisystem atrophies. Spinocerebellar degenerations typically begin at a younger age.

Paraneoplastic cerebellar syndromes can be seen in bronchial, breast, and ovarian cancer. The symptoms include ataxia of gait and stance, limb ataxia, terminal tremor, gaze-evoked nystagmus, and disturbed smooth-pursuit eye movements.

Toxic cerebellar syndromes in the elderly frequently are due to slower drug metabolism and reduced tolerance. All centrally acting drugs may lead to cerebellar disturbances of stance and gait. The drugs most frequently responsible for toxic disturbances include alcohol, antiepileptics, barbiturates, lithium, and tranquilizers.

Gait Disturbances in Cerebellar Disorders

Cerebellar lesions may affect gait by causing disequilibrium and by altering limb and trunk kinematics and interlimb coordination. The cerebellum does not appear to actually generate postural and gait synergies, because these automatic responses are present in dogs with total cerebellectomies; the execution of these automatic responses is, however, very dysmetric [41].

The effects of cerebellar lesions depend on the area of the cerebellum that is damaged; different syndromes are described for the flocculonodular lobe or vestibulocerebellum, the anterior vermis or spinocerebellum, and the lateral lobes or frontopontocerebellum. In clinical practice, often it is difficult to distinguish which parts of the cerebellum are diseased, and some investigators question whether damage to vestibulocerebellum, spinocerebellum, and corticopontocerebellum can be reliably differentiated [42]. The mode of onset (sudden or gradual) and the acuteness or chronicity of the lesion also affect the symptoms and signs. Finally, the presence of other nervous system lesions may modify a person's ability to compensate for cerebellar lesions.

Lesions of the flocculonodular lobe can produce balance and gait disturbances that resemble those caused by acute vestibular lesions. Given the intimate relationship between labyrinths and the flocculonodular lobe, this makes sense. The acute surgical removal of the flocculonodular lobe in monkeys causes marked disequilibrium that prevents them from walking, much like that caused by acute vestibular lesions. Limb dysmetria is not apparent. Moreover, as with acute vestibular lesions, the monkeys recover fully from flocculonodular ablation and can walk on narrow bars blindfolded [43]. In humans, tremor of the head and trunk, truncal imbalance, and swaying and falling in all directions are characteristic of vestibulocerebellar lesions. Medulloblastomas frequently are used as an example of flocculonodular lobe lesions in humans, but these tumors often cause hydrocephalus and brain-stem signs; thus, it is difficult to attribute all the signs of these lesions to flocculonodular lobe dysfunction.

The clinical syndrome caused by lesions of the spinocerebellum is best characterized by that associated with alcoholic cerebellar degeneration, which primarily affects the anterior cerebellum but also involves the olivary complex and the vestibular nuclei [44]. Patients with alcoholic cerebellar degeneration have a widened base, instability of the trunk, slow and halting gait with irregular steps, and superimposed lurching. The gait abnormalities are accentuated at the initiation of gait, with turns, and with changes in gait speed. It is important to note that such patients may have severe gait ataxia without nystagmus, dysarthria, or arm dysmetria. Even the heel-to-shin test may give little inkling of the severity of the gait disturbance. Interestingly, if patients stop drinking and have adequate nutrition, the gait improves such that the steps are no longer irregular, and tandem walking or sudden movements are necessary to demonstrate the gait ataxia [44].

Lesions of the lateral lobes or frontopontocerebellum cause dysmetria of legs that is similar to that seen in the arms. Specifically, the legs demonstrate irregular timing, force, and cadence, leading to inaccurate and variable stepping [45]. Examination of motor function of the individual limbs is a better indicator of the gait impairment in frontopontocerebellar lesions than it is in vestibulocerebellar and spinocerebellar lesions. In contrast to vestibulocerebellar lesions that appear to produce disequilibrium because of decreased or distorted processing of vestibular input, frontopontocerebellar lesions appear to cause disequilibrium and gait abnormalities because of dysmetrical execution of appropriate balance and locomotor synergies.

REFERENCES

1. Nashner LM, Black FO, Wall C. Adaptation to altered support and visual conditions during stance: Patients with vestibular deficits. *J Neurosci* 1982;2:536–544.
2. Diener HC, Dichgans J. On the role of vestibular, visual and somatosensory information for dynamic postural control in humans. *Prog Brain Res* 1988;76:253–262.
3. Diener HC, Dichgans J, Guschlbauer B, Bacher M. Role of visual and static vestibular influences on dynamic posture control. *Hum Neurobiol* 1986;5:105–113.
4. Paulus W, Straube A, Brandt T. Visual postural performance after loss of somatosensory and vestibular function. *J Neurol Neurosurg Psychiatry* 1987;50:1542–1545.
5. Rosenthal U. Degenerative changes in the aging human vestibular neuro-epithelia. *Acta Otolaryngol* 1973;76:208–220.
6. Bergström B. Morphology of the vestibular nerve: II. The number of myelinated vestibular nerve fibres in man at various ages. *Acta Otolaryngol* 1973;76:173–179.
7. Norre ME, Forrez G, Beckers A. Vestibular dysfunction causing instability in aged patients. *Acta Otolaryngol (Stockh)* 1987;104:50–55.
8. Melville Jones G, Watt DGD. Muscular control of landing from unexpected falls in man. *J Physiol* (Lond) 1971;219:729–737.
9. Fries W, Dieterich M, Brandt T. Otolithic control of posture: Vestibulo-spinal reflexes in a patient with a Tullio phenomenon. *Adv Otol Rhinol Laryngol* 1988;42:162–165.
10. Berger W, Dietz V, Quintern J. Corrective reactions to stumbling in man: Neuronal coordination of bilateral leg muscle activity during gait. *J Physiol* (Lond) 1984;357:109–125.
11. Diener HC, Horak FB, Nashner LM. Influence of stimulus parameters on human postural responses. *J Neurophysiol* 1988;59:1888–1905.
12. Dietz V, Quintern J, Sillem M. Stumbling reactions in man: Significance of proprioceptive and pre-programmed mechanisms. *J Physiol* (Lond) 1987;386:149–163.
13. Horak FB, Nashner LM. Central programming of postural movements: Adaptation to altered support surface configurations. *J Neurophysiol* 1986;55:1369–1381.

14. Nashner LM. Adapting reflexes controlling the human posture. *Exp Brain Res* 1976;26:59–72.
15. Diener HC, Bootz F, Dichgans J, Bruzek W. Variability of postural "reflexes" in humans. *Exp Brain Res* 1983;52:423–428.
16. Diener HC, Dichgans J, Bootz F. Early stabilization of human posture after a sudden disturbance: Influence of rate and amplitude of displacement. *Exp Brain Res* 1989;56:126–134.
17. Diener HC, Dichgans J. Long Loop Reflexes in Posture. In: Bles W, Brandt Th, eds. *Disorders of Posture and Gait*. Amsterdam: Elsevier, 1986. Pp 41–51.
18. Dietz V, Horstmann A, Berger W. Fast head tilt has only a minor effect on quick compensatory reactions during the regulation of stance and gait. *Exp Brain Res* 1988;73:470–476.
19. Diener HC, Dichgans J, Guschlbauer B, Mau H. The significance of proprioception on postural stabilization as assessed by ischemia. *Brain Res* 1984;296:103–109.
20. Horstmann GA, Dietz V. The contribution of vestibular input to the stabilization of human posture: A new experimental approach. *Neurosci Lett* 1988;95:179–184.
21. Allum JHJ, Keshner EA, Honegger F, Pfaltz CR. Indicators of the influence a peripheral vestibular deficit has on vestibulo-spinal reflex responses controlling postural stability. *Acta Otolaryngol* 1988;106:252–263.
22. Allum JHJ, Honegger F, Schicks H. Vestibular and proprioceptive modulation of postural synergies in normal subjects. *J Vestib Res* 1993;3:59–85.
23. Allum JHJ, Honegger F, Schicks H. The influence of a bilateral peripheral vestibular deficit on postural synergies. *J Vestib Res* 1994;4:59–70.
24. Dichgans J, Brandt T. Visual-Vestibular Interaction: Effects on Self-Motion Perception and Postural Control. In: Held R, Leibowitz HW, Teuber H-L, eds. *Handbook of Sensory Physiology*, vol 8: *Perception*. Berlin: Springer, 1978. Pp 755–804.
25. Black FO, Nashner LM. Postural disturbances in patients with benign paroxysmal positional nystagmus. *Ann Otol Rhinol Laryngol* 1984;93:595–599.
26. Cass SP, Kartush JM, Graham MD. Clinical assessment of postural stability following vestibular nerve section. *Laryngoscope* 1991;101:1056–1059.
27. Shepard NT, Telian SA, Smith-Wheelock M, Raj A. Vestibular and balance rehabilitation therapy. *Ann Otol Rhinol Laryngol* 1993;102:198–205.
28. Pyykkö I, Enbom H, Magnusson M, Schalen L. Effect of proprioceptor stimulation on postural stability in patients with peripheral or central vestibular lesion. *Acta Otol Laryngol* 1991;111:27–35.
29. Nashner LM, McCollum G. The organization of human postural movements. A formal basis and experimental synthesis. *Behav Brain Sci* 1985;8:135–172.
30. Black FO, Shupert CL, Horak FB, Nashner LM. Abnormal Postural Control Associated with Peripheral Vestibular Disorders. In: Pompeiano O, Allum JHJ, eds. *Vestibulo-Spinal Control of Posture and Locomotion*. Amsterdam: Elsevier, 1988. Pp 263–275.
31. Horak FB, Nashner LM, Diener HC. Postural strategies associated with somatosensory and vestibular loss. *Exp Brain Res* 1990;82:167–177.
32. Garcin R. The Ataxias. In: Vinken PJ, Bruyn GW, eds. *Handbook of Clinical Neurology*, vol. 2. Amsterdam: North Holland Publishing Company, 1969. Pp 309–355.
33. Fife TD, Baloh RW. Disequilibrium of unknown cause in older people. *Ann Neurol* 1993;34:694–702.
34. Dichgans J, Mauritz KH, Allum JHJ, Brandt T. Postural sway in normals and ataxic patients. *Aggressologie* 1976;17C:15–24.
35. Mauritz KH, Dichgans J, Hufschmidt A. Quantitative analysis of stance in late cortical cerebellar atrophy of the anterior lobe and other forms of cerebellar ataxia. *Brain* 1979;102:461–482.
36. Bronstein AM, Hood JD, Gresty MA, Panagi C. Visual control of balance in cerebellar and Parkinsonian syndromes. *Brain* 1990;113:767–779.
37. Friedemann HH, Noth J, Diener HC, Bacher M. Long latency EMG responses in hand and leg muscles: Cerebellar disorders. *J Neurol Neurosurg Psychiatry*, 1987;50:71–77.
38. Diener HC, Dichgans J, Bacher M, Guschlbauer B. Characteristic alterations of long loop "re-

flexes" in patients with Friedreich's ataxia and late atrophy of the anterior cerebellar lobe. *J Neurol Neurosurg Psychiatry* 1984;47:679–685.

39. Horak FB, Diener HC, Nashner LM. Abnormal scaling of postural responses in cerebellar patients. *Soc Neurosci Abstr* 1986;12:1419.

40. Horak FB, Diener HC. Cerebellar control of postural scaling and central set in stance. *J Neurophysiol* 1994;72:479–493.

41. Rademaker GGJ. *The Physiology of Standing (Das Stehen)*. Denny-Brown D, ed. Minneapolis: University of Minnesota Press, 1980.

42. Gilman S, Bloedel JR, Lechtenberg R. *Disorders of the Cerebellum*. Philadelphia: Davis, 1981.

43. Dow R. Effects of lesions in the vestibular part of the cerebellum in primates. *Arch Neurol Psychiatr* 1938;49:500–520.

44. Victor M, Adams RD, Mancall EL. A restricted form of cerebellar cortical degenerative occurring in alcoholic patients. *Arch Neurol* 1959;1:579–688.

45. Hallett M, Stanhope ST, Thomas SL, Massaquoi S. Pathophysiology of Posture and Gait in Cerebellar Ataxia. Shimamura M, Grillner S, Edgerton VR, eds. In: *Neurobiological Basis of Human Locomotion*. Tokyo: Japan Scientific Societies Press, 1991. Pp 275–283.

17. Peripheral Neuropathy: Disorders of Proprioception

Thomas D. Sabin

Most of this book is devoted to the motor mechanisms involved with walking. However, afferent information vital to this motor performance is monopolized within peripheral nerves and roots before becoming widely dispersed on entry into the spinal cord. Deafferentation in experimental animals by extensive dorsal rhizotomies leads to a devastating disability, even greater than transection of any single afferent path within the cord, including the dorsal columns [1]. Therefore, a possible role for peripheral nerve disfunction in aging is explored in this chapter.

In practice, gait disorders in the elderly often are multifactorial, and any chronic sensory neuropathy (along with visual or vestibular impairments) may conspire to critically decrease the requisite afference for successful motility. Diabetic neuropathy is most frequent. The practitioner should be especially alert for treatable entities such as alcohol-nutritional deficiency, vitamin B_{12} or folate deficiency, Lyme disease, vasculitis, and toxic drug–related polyneuropathies. Some cases of neuropathy with monoclonal gammopathy, especially with anti–myelin-associated glycoprotein (MAG) antibodies also may be found in these patients. Among the toxic causes, arsenic and thallium have become rare, but drug-related sensory neuropathy has increased in frequency: almitrine, chloramphenicol, isoniazid, metronidazole, misonidazole, megadose pyridoxine, and vincristine have been implicated. However, we focus on the neuropathies that cause sensory ataxia as their chief manifestation in an otherwise intact patient.

ATAXIC NEUROPATHIES

The neuropathies that most consistently produce a severe ataxia are those that involve the dorsal root ganglion cells (DRGCs) and their axons. Dorsal root ganglia may be especially vulnerable to certain toxins and immunological attack because they do not share in the vascular barrier that protects the roots, peripheral nerves, and central nervous system.

Types of Ataxic Neuropathies

Carcinomatous Sensory Neuropathy
Carcinomatous sensory neuropathy, or ganglionopathy, is an example of such a disorder. Paresthesias or dysesthesias generally move from a distal to a proximal

direction, but some cases have shown early sensory change in proximal areas, including the face. Position and vibration sense are the most severely affected sensory modalities, with consequent severe sensory ataxia as well as pseudoathetosis in the outstretched limbs [2]. There is early, widespread absence of reflexes. The associated neoplasm most often is a small-cell cancer of the lung. The neuropathy may precede the clinical appearance of the carcinoma for longer than 3 years (but more often by only a few months). The neuropathy often progresses in a subacute fashion but then may level off. Although treatment of the underlying neoplasm usually has no effect on the neuropathy, there are some rather dramatic single cases associated with reversal after effective treatment of the primary neoplasm. Pathological observations show a lymphocytic infiltration of dorsal root ganglia, with a marked depopulation of dorsal root ganglion cells and Nageotte nodules. The peripheral sensory axons degenerate, but there also is degeneration in the centrally directed axon because the dorsal columns (particularly the gracile sectors) are affected severely. This type of carcinomatous neuropathy often is associated with cerebrospinal fluid and serum antibodies that react with dorsal root ganglia (IgG anti-Hu antibodies). These antibodies are also known to react with a brain nuclear protein and an identical antigen highly specific for small-cell lung cancer [3]. The spinal fluid of these patients often shows a few mononuclear cells (5–50/mm^3) with modest elevations of protein but occasionally as high as several grams.

Cisplatin Neurotoxicity

Cisplatin neurotoxicity produces a similar clinical picture. Cisplatin is an antineoplastic agent used in some cases of ovarian, testicular, and germ-cell tumors as well as in small-cell lung cancer and melanomas. The disease begins with widespread paresthesias; Lhermitte's sign sometimes is present, and there is again a severe sensory ataxia with pseudoathetosis in association with absent deep-tendon reflexes and loss of vibration followed by position sense. This syndrome begins after a dose of more than 300–500 mg/m^2 of cisplatin, and the neuropathy may progress for days or weeks after the last administration of the drug [4]. As in carcinomatous sensory ganglionopathy, sensory nerve potentials are absent, but motor conduction velocities are normal. Histological evaluation of peripheral nerve shows axonal neuropathy with loss of large fibers as well as occasional segmental demyelination. Recovery takes many months after discontinuation of cisplatin.

Sjögren's Disease

There is a rare variety of neuropathy in Sjögren's disease in which there is a dorsal root ganglionitis. In these cases, biopsies of dorsal ganglia have shown infiltration with T lymphocytes and macrophages [5]. Large-fiber-type sensory deficits dominate the clinical picture, producing prominent sensory ataxia and pseudochorea with areflexia. This diagnosis is supported by finding the SSA-LA, SSD-RO serum autoantibodies and demonstrating lymphocytic infiltration of a minor salivary gland along with the sicca syndrome.

Pyridoxine-Related Neuropathy

Chronic ingestion of megadoses (2–6 g/day) of pyridoxine also has been associated with an ataxic peripheral neuropathy. Both proximal and distal parts of the body are affected simultaneously by sensory loss of the large-fiber modalities. The other major clinical features are ataxia and pseudoathetosis without severe weakness. Sensory loss may be heralded by Lhermitte's sign, severe paresthesias, or dysesthesias [6]. Experimental pyridoxine intoxication causes a degeneration of DRGCs and their sensory neurons, particularly those associated with large fibers. In experimental pyridoxine neuropathy, an important effect of dose has been observed [7]. Very large doses result in immediate necrosis of the dorsal root ganglian cells, with rapid secondary degeneration in both the peripherally and centrally directed axons. Lower toxic doses first cause a disturbance in the distal part of both the peripherally and the centrally directed axons, but the DRGCs themselves survive. These observations suggest that the lower amount of pyridoxine sufficiently impairs the function of dorsal root ganglion cells so that they are unable to support their axonal processes, though still capable of recovery and orchestration of axonal regeneration when excessive pyridoxine is eliminated.

Nitrous Oxide–Related Neuropathy

Nitrous oxide abuse occasionally is noted (especially in dentists who use the substance for self-treatment of hangovers) and has been associated with a myeloneuropathy. Affected patients may have severe sensory ataxia along with Lhermitte's sign, a positive Romberg test, widespread areflexia, and loss of large-fiber sensory modalities. In addition to the neuropathy, there is clinical evidence of mild pyramidal motor signs. Electrophysiological studies show evidence of an axonal sensory and mild motor neuropathy. Discontinuance of nitrous oxide abuse allows recovery to occur over a period of many months. A mechanism suggesting interference with vitamin B_{12} metabolism has been suggested [8].

Idiopathic Acute Sensory Neuropathy

Idiopathic acute sensory neuropathy begins abruptly, often after a general illness that has required the use of synthetic penicillins for approximately 4 days [9]. The sensory loss does not obey the usual distal-to-proximal pattern and may even begin on the face, but rapidly it becomes extensive. There is a loss of all the deep-tendon reflexes and a profound loss of large-fiber modalities, with a severe gait abnormality associated with difficulty in controlling both the limb and axial musculature, including the upper extremities. Electrophysiological studies reveal no abnormality within the motor fibers, but no sensory potentials are obtainable. Prognosis for this neuropathy often is poor, with permanent disability being the rule.

Chronic Ataxic Sensory Neuropathy

In the chronic ataxic sensory neuropathy, there is a slowly progressive illness with ultimate severe proprioception loss, paresthesia, and kinesthesia with absent deep-tendon reflexes. A significant percentage of these patients have a polyclonal monoclonal or gammopathy [10]. They remain disabled for years due to their ataxia. Often, they have very uncomfortable paresthesias, with a severe loss of balance in the dark. The ataxia is accompanied by pseudoathetosis. Electrophysiological studies show normal motor conduction velocities and electromyographic findings but no sensory potentials. Biopsy of the sural nerve shows loss of large, heavily myelinated fibers. Despite the presence of monoclonal gammopathy, such patients tend to be resistant to steroids, immunosuppression, or plasmapheresis, but (rarely) patients do appear to respond to suppression of the immune response.

The pathogenesis of these forms of sensory ataxia may depend in part on a selective vulnerability of the DRGCs and their axons, perhaps because these cells are not protected by a vascular barrier. Because there may be degeneration of both the peripherally directed and the centrally directed axons, these illnesses may be associated with Lhermitte's sign because of involvement of the DRGCs' centrally directed axons within the dorsal columns. Lhermitte's sign has been noted in pyridoxine megadoses, carcinomatous sensory neuropathy, and nitrous oxide myeloneuropathy.

The severe degree of disability that some of these patients suffer is puzzling. Such patients' motor performances seem far worse off than do the primates that were denervated experimentally by cutting all the dorsal roots [11]. Although many previously learned movements are possible in the extremities, it has been observed that there is an absence of automatic reflex correction of volitional movements and either inability or difficulty in keeping the required amount of muscle contraction constant long enough to carry out required tasks without close visual feedback [12]. The author has assessed several patients who had sensory ganglionopathies and complained bitterly of very uncomfortable "pulling" and "stretching" sensations when they tried to move about and, as a result, confine themselves to bed and chair existence.

Vitamin B₁₂ Deficiency

Pernicious anemia with deficient production of intrinsic factor is the most common cause of B_{12} deficiency, many cases of which occur in older people. B_{12} deficiency also is observed due to chronic intestinal malabsorption and rarely to dietary deficiency. The daily requirement for B_{12} is only 5 µg/day. B_{12} deficiency can produce neuropathy and myelopathy (subacute combined systems degeneration), often without hematological manifestations.

The onset is insidious, beginning with distal paresthesias, weakness, and unsteadiness of gait—particularly difficulty in walking in the dark. Proprioceptive loss in the legs and sensory ataxia can grow quite severe. Lhermitte's sign often is present, as there is degeneration of the dorsal columns as well as of the sensory nerves. Tendon reflexes typically range from depressed to absent. Typically, an extensor plantar response is observed and, with time, a spastic-ataxic gait.

B_{12} assay is used for screening; a Schilling test confirms true addisonian pernicious anemia. It is important to recognize this disorder, as it is encountered occasionally in the elderly and is a treatable cause of imbalance and gait disorder.

Gait improves fully in a majority of patients with duration of neurological signs of less than 3 months.

Spindle Syndromes

All these neuropathies have easily detectable, severe position-sense loss. Is it possible to have gait difficulty due to a disturbance of afferent input without obvious position-sense loss? Though the information regarding tonic and phasic muscle stretch is of major importance in the central elaboration of motor control, the muscle spindle information is not assessed readily by standard bedside techniques. The power of input from spindles can be demonstrated by the production of postural swaying and illusory movements in healthy subjects [13–15]. Isolated alterations in spindle input (even from a single muscle group) can induce derangements in posture and balance affecting the whole body. Very complex, repeatable, and highly specific sensations of movement can be induced by simultaneous stimulation of several muscle groups [16].

The large, heavily myelinated nerve IA fibers that arise from the nuclear bag portion of spindles rapidly conduct muscle stretch information to the central nervous system. A message results in spinal reflexes that cause the contraction of the stretched muscle and an inhibition of its antagonist. This phasic information from IA afferents originally was considered to be an unconscious error-detecting mechanism until evidence emerged that, in addition to the spinal segmental effects of IA afferents, there is a powerful conscious perception of movement derived from spindles [17]. Cortical evoked potentials from spindle input have been documented, and preservation of small-joint kinesthesia occurs when impulses from joint afferents are blocked [15].

One simple and compelling proof of the conscious appreciation of IA afferent information can be demonstrated simply by vibrating a muscle or its tendon. The low-viscosity nuclear bag portion of the muscle spindle is able to follow the rapid distortion-restoration sequence imposed on it by the vibrator, and this results in bursts of firing of IA afferent impulses [18]. These volleys of IA afference induced by the vibrator are misinterpreted as actual muscle stretch. Single-fiber recording of the dorsal roots of experimental animals during muscle vibration shows the occurrence of a selective input from I afferents. A vibrator placed on the biceps of a blindfolded normal individual with outstretched arms will cause involuntary flexion at the elbow. If the person is asked to match the position of the vibrated limb with the other side, there is a constant error of 8 degrees or more with less elbow flexion in the nonstimulated limb [15]. This deception can be exaggerated by stretching the vibrated muscle passively in normal subjects [14]. When the forearm is extended passively during biceps vibration, blindfolded subjects tend to report large errors in perceived position. Some subjects report a perception of anatomically impossible hyperextension of the elbow, often with the autonomic accompaniments of pain, although actual discomfort does not occur. Other subjects experience reduplication of their forearm, one forearm in the anatomically impossible position and one in the actual position. These observations on the effects of muscle vibration indicate that normal perception of limb position is made by an analysis of at least two different types of afferent information. The joint and tendon receptors along with nuclear chain spindles provide a constant measure of joint angle, and the phasic IA spindle afferents contribute to the sensation of movement.

The power of kinesthetic input thus is demonstrated readily in normal subjects, but no proved disorder of this mechanism producing a clinical syndrome in peripheral nerve disease has been documented. The ataxic neuropathies are associated with severe position-sense loss, which confounds the isolation of the possible role of spindles in these ataxias. Simple moderate loss of spindle afferents may not be a sufficient cause, because one would expect ataxia as part of numerous other neuropathies. There are several speculative, more elaborate conditions that produce ataxia:

1. Isolated loss of spindle afferents as in-parallel sensors, while "in-series" muscle stretch receptors remain intact. This condition might cause a constantly varying mismatch between muscle length and tension information that compromises motor tasks (i.e., spindle vertigo).
2. The development of spontaneous-impulse generators or ephaptic cross-talk in the heavily myelinated afferents (i.e., large-fiber causalgia).
3. Loss of the LA component that contributes to the inhibition of antagonists of stretched muscles in the alpha-gamma coactivation schema sufficient to disturb the complex sequencing aspect of ambulation.

Peripheral mechanisms have been implicated in the pathogenesis of heredofamilial essential tremor and the tremor that resembles it in chronic idiopathic ataxic neuropathy with IgM paraproteinemia, in some patients with chronic inflammatory demyelinating polyneuropathy (CIDP), in variant cases of the Roussy-Lévy type, and in some cases of type I hereditary motor sensory neuropathy [9, 19, 20]. Posttraumatic focal dystonia (sometimes also accompanied by tremor) has also been suspected of having a peripheral pathogenesis [21].

The Romberg sign, which is considered a result of loss of position sense, often becomes positive in early cases of tabes dorsalis (a posterior root disease) before detectable loss of position sense [22]. Another clinical phenomenon that raises the possibility of ataxia due to loss of afferent input occurs in the Guillain-Barré syndrome (GBS). Hyperacute GBS is misdiagnosed in the emergency room when a healthy-appearing patient is observed to stagger about with a bizarre ataxia and complains only of tingling paresthesia. Examination reveals good strength that may be sustained only in irregular bursts and also reveals dampened reflexes and normal sensation as tested in the usual way. The patient often is released from the emergency room with a diagnosis of hysteria, but hours later may require emergency care for evolving widespread flaccid paralysis. This early ataxic phase of GBS might also be due to a physiological effect of large-fiber demyelination, which is concentrated in the posterior roots. Some patients recovering from GBS go through a phase of ataxia out of proportion to loss of strength or position sense. The Miller-Fisher variant of GBS consists of ophthalmoplegia associated with severe areflexic ataxia, with nearly normal sensation and strength. There is a rise in cerebrospinal fluid protein and electrophysiological evidence of sensory radiculoneuropathy, but the issue of a central nervous system explanation for the ataxia has not been put to rest entirely. This variety of ataxia also might represent an intriguing gait disorder related to an abnormality of IA afferent input [23].

Animal models of spindle ataxia may occur. In acrylamide neuropathy induced in cats, there is a stage in which the animals are described as ataxic, often dragging their hind legs and exhibiting areflexia but demonstrating good strength, as evidenced by pulling the limb from a pinch. Physiological studies at this stage document extensive dysfunction in IA afferents [24]. The sensory neuropathy induced in rats by administering high doses of pyridoxine also causes a degeneration in primary sensory endings of the nuclear bag portion of spindles, which coincides with the onset of ataxia [25].

PERIPHERAL FACTORS IN THE DETERIORATION OF GAIT WITH AGING

With aging alone, there appears to be a clear deterioration in gait observed as part of everyday life and even is captured by the skillful actor playing the role of an elderly individual. At some point, the gait disorder renders a patient more liable to falls, triggering a neurological evaluation (e.g., the "old-old" in their late seventies and eighties who are considered healthy but do have some widespread age-related changes including those in the visual, vestibular, and posterior column pathways). This type of elderly patient, in whom no definite neurological disease can be diagnosed, shows the following features: Dementia or frontal lobe signs and elementary neurological findings are absent. The gait is cautious, often with extra steps on turning—as if walking on ice. Sometimes the gait disorder is exacerbated acutely by enforced bed rest, as with an intercurrent illness, but may be brought back up to baseline with brief practice or rehabilitation. These patients most often attribute their gait difficulty to weakness but, when confronted with adequate strength during their examination, go on to say that they are fearful of walking or have a dizziness or unsteadiness. The patient experiences a tendency to fall backward; the examiner can readily displace the standing patient backward but finds normal resistance to forward displacement. Vibration threshold in the lower extremities is elevated, and the ankle jerks are dampened compared to the other deep-tendon reflexes. The vibration thresholds in the toes of the elderly may be five times that of the thresholds in the fingers [26]. Position-sense testing in the toes, performed in the usual way with small, rapid, angular deviations and reporting of directions, is normal, but steady displacement of the toe may escape notice. Tracing of large figures on paper with the great toe while supine is normal. Such patients retain dextrous use of the hands, and patients with considerable gait difficulty may write well and play a musical instrument capably. The loss of ankle jerks and elevation of vibratory thresholds in the feet have been viewed as normal findings in the elderly, yet they are suggestive of a large-fiber distal peripheral neuropathy and justify a search for the role of peripheral mechanism in senile gait disorder [16, 27].

The peripheral neuropathy of aging is measurable as a slowly progressive loss of nerve fibers, a decrease in conduction velocities, and a decrease in average internodal lengths. There are daunting technical difficulties, especially in assessing whether there is a specific loss of large fibers or a shrinkage of the entire spectrum of fibers. Pure aging effects are not separated easily from the long-term accumulation of repeated trauma, vascular injuries, or minor bouts of demyelination. The overall result is a loss of the longest, largest-diameter fibers.

A fallout of 5–8% of fibers per decade past age 40 has been observed [28, 30]. Morphometrical analysis of fascicles of the deep peroneal nerve showed a mean internodal length of 1,135 μm in a 46-year-old, whereas the same nerve in a 70-year-old had a mean internodal length of 774 μm [31]. Motor conduction velocities decline at a rate of 0.1 to 0.18 m/sec/yr in aging [32, 33]. Spinal cord sensory conduction velocity (which in part represents the activity of the DRGCs' centrally directed axons) is well maintained until age 60, when a decline of -0.24 m/sec/yr occurs [33]. Magnetic stimulation also is now available to assess age-related changes in the peripheral nerves and their central processes [34].

An elderly individual with a large-fiber neuropathy and some impairment of vision and subclinical loss of precision of joint and tendon sensibility (without information describing muscle stretch during movement) may have to recalculate position after each step and may be particularly vulnerable to a spindle syndrome. If the spindle system plays a role in compensating for the mechanical properties of tissues of the legs, the impairment of the fastest phasic messages in this servo system may result in an inadequate compensation for the increased viscoelastic resistance in the aged musculoskeletal system [35].

A feature common to distal polyneuropathies might explain the tendency to fall backward in such patients. If the neuropathy of aging progresses in a distal-to-proximal mode, as most neuropathies do and as the clinical and electrophysiological evidence suggests, there would be a prolonged period in which the anterior tibial compartment would be denervated while the posterior tibial compartment would remain innervated due to the 10- to 12-cm difference in the length of the nerves innervating these two compartments [36]. This could result in a situation in which, when the patient attempts to stand and stabilize stance by cocontracting the two compartments, a volley of IA afferents from the gastrocnemius-soleus group reflexly stimulates contraction in these muscles but, because there is no corresponding volley arising from the anterior tibial compartment, the patient tends to be drawn backward. In normal standing individuals whose eyes are closed, this situation has been imitated by placing a stick across both Achilles tendons and placing a vibrator on the stick [13]. Such subjects tend to sway backward. Furthermore, they sway backward without any attempt to compensate for the potential fall by extending their arms out in front of them. Normal individuals also can be induced to sway forward if, while they stand slightly pigeon-toed, the vibrating stick is placed across both anterior tibial compartments. This latter feature contrasts with our anecdotal observation of elderly individuals with mild gait disorders who fall backward regardless of whether one vibrates the posterior or the anterior compartments of the legs, which suggests that an asymmetrical postural mechanism is present at some level of neural organization. There is a problem in proving that this relates to a disorder of IA afferents, in part due to the difficulty in measuring activity in the IA afferents in a highly specific manner using electrophysiological techniques [37].

Regardless of the actual mechanism of their gait disorder, these patients may improve their mobility by wearing ankle-high boots. Basketball shoes with inflatable cuffs offer excellent stabilization at the ankle joints. We have also suggested that such patients obtain "walking" eyeglasses made entirely with the distance prescription (i.e., the lower part of the bifocal) removed. Many elderly patients are pleased to know a hypothesis exists that does not rely totally on brain degeneration as a cause of their gait problems. If a peripheral mechanism exists, certain biomedical engineering devices, selective nerve blockades, or other local approaches might be exploited to improve gait.

Neurologists should consider the routine examination of patients' tonic muscular vibratory responses in various disorders so as to assess the role of spindle function, which otherwise eludes observation in the routine neurological examination.

REFERENCES

1. Gilman S, Denny-Brown D. Disorders of movement and behavior following dorsal column lesions. *Brain* 1966;89:397–418.
2. Denny-Brown D. Primary sensory neuropathy with muscular changes associated with carcinoma. *J Neurol Neurosurg Psychiatry* 1948;11:73.
3. Anderson NE, et al. Auto antibodies in paraneoplastic syndromes associated with small-cell lung cancer. *Neurology* 1988;38:1391.
4. Roelofs RI, Hrushesky W, Rogin J, Rosenberg L. Peripheral sensory neuropathy and cisplatin chemotherapy. *Neurology* 1984;34:9348.
5. Griffin JW, et al. Ataxic sensory neuropathy and dorsal root ganglionitis associated with Sjögren's syndrome. *Ann Neurol* 1990;27:30415.
6. Albin RL, et al. Acute sensory neuropathy-neuronopathy from pyridoxine overdose. *Neurology* 1987;37:1729–1732.
7. Xu Yue, Sladky JT, Brown MJ. Dose-dependent expression of neuronopathy after experimental pyridoxine intoxication. *Neurology* 1989;39:1077–1083.
8. Blanco G, Peters HA. Myeloneuropathy and macrocytosis associated with nitrous oxide abuse. *Arch Neurol* 1983;40:416–418.
9. Sterman, AB, Schaumburg H, Asbury AK. The acute sensory neuropathy syndrome: A distinct clinical entity. *Ann Neurol* 1980;7:354–358.
10. Dalakas MC. Chronic idiopathic ataxic neuropathy. *Ann Neurol* 1986;19:545–554.
11. Taub E. Movement in nonhuman primates deprived of somatosensory feedback. *Exerc Sports Sc Rev* 1976;4:335–374.
12. Rothwell JC, et al. Manual motor performance in a deafferented man. *Brain* 1982;105:515–542.
13. Eklund G. Influence of muscle vibration on balance in man. *Acta Soc Med Uppsala* 1969;74:113–117.
14. Craske B. Perception of impossible limb positions induced by tendon vibration. *Science* 1977;196:71–73.
15. Goodwin GM, McClosky DI, Matthews PBC. The contribution of muscle afferents to kinas-

thesia shown by vibrating induced illusions of movement and by the effects of paralyzing joint afferents. *Brain* 1972;95:705–748.

16. Roll JP, Hay L, Quoniam C, Roll R. Muscle proprioception: A powerful sensory input for postural adaptation in man. In: Vellas B, et al., eds. *Falls, Balance and Gait Disorders in the Elderly.* Paris: Elsevier, 1992.

17. Granit R. Constant errors in the execution and appreciation of movement. *Brain* 1972;95:649–660.

18. Bianconi R, van der Meulen JP. The response to vibration of the end organs of mammalian muscle spindles. *J Neurophysiol* 1963;26:177–190.

19. Adams RD, Shahani BT, Young RR. Tremor in association with polyneuropathy. *Trans Am Neurol Assoc* 1972;97:44.

20. Shahani BT, Young RR. Action tremors: A clinical neurophysiological review. In: Desmedt JE, ed. *Physiological Tremor, Pathological Tremors and Clonus.* Basel: Karger, 1978. Pp 129–137.

21. Jankovic J, Van Der Linden C. Dystonia and tremor induced by peripheral trauma: predisposing factors. *J Neurol Neurosurg Psychiatry* 1988;51:1512–1519.

22. Garcin R. *The Ataxias.* In: Vinken PJ, Bruyn GW, eds. *The Handbook of Neurology,* vol. 1. New York: Elsevier, 1969. P 312.

23. Weiss JA, White JC. Correlation of IA afferent conduction with the ataxia of Fisher Syndrome. *Muscle Nerve* 1986;9:327.

24. Sumner AJ, Asbury AK. Physiological studies of the dying-back phenomenon. *Brain* 1975;98: 91–100.

25. Krinke G, Heid J, Bittiger H, Hess R. Sensory denervation of the plantar lumbrical muscle spindles in pyridoxine neuropathy. *Acta Neuropathol* 1978;43:213–216.

26. Pearson GHJ. Effect of age on vibratory sensibility. *Arch Neurol* 1928;20:482–4966.

27. Sabin TD. Biological aspects of falls and mobility limitations in the elderly. *J Am Geriatr Soc* 1982;30:51–58.

28. Ochoa J, Mair WGP. The normal sural nerve in man: II. Changes in the axons and Schwann cells due to aging. *Acta Neuropathol* (Berl) 1969;13:217–239.

29. Swallow M. Fiber size and content of the anterior tibial nerve in the foot. *J Neurol Neurosurg Psychiatry* 1966;29:205–213.

30. O'Sullivan DJ, Swallow M. The fiber size and content of the radial and sural nerves. *J Neurol Neurosurg Psychiatry* 1968;31:464–470.

31. Stevens JC, Lofgren EP, Dyck JP. Histometric evaluation of branches of peroneal nerve. *Brain Res* 1973;52:37–59.

32. Behse F, Buchthal F. Normal sensory conduction in the nerves of the leg in man. *J Neurol Neurosurg Psychiatry* 1971;34:404–414.

33. Dorfman LJ, Bosley TM. Age related changes in peripheral central nerve conduction in man. *Neurology* 1979;29:38–44.

34. Bouche P, et al. Clinical and electrophysiological study of the peripheral nervous system in the elderly. *J Neurol* 1993;240(5):263–268.

35. Nichols TR, Houk JC. Reflex compensation for variations in the mechanical properties of a muscle. *Science* 1973;181:182–184.

36. Sunderland S. *Nerves and Nerve Injuries,* 2nd ed. Edinburgh: Churchill Livingstone, 1978. Pp 927–930.

37. Macefield G, Gandevia SC, Burke D. Conduction velocities of muscle and cutaneous afferents in the upper and lower limbs of human subjects. *Brain* 1989;112:1519–1532.

18. The Cautious Gait, Fear of Falling, and Psychogenic Gait Disorders

Lewis Sudarsky and Rein Tideiksaar

Gait is an unconscious, automatic performance, something that we do every day without thought. Yet experience tells us that walking can be influenced by the psychological state. There is a spring in our step when we are happy. The burden of our worries is at times apparent in our carriage and stride. Motivational factors influence gait as readily as does mood.

Falls are common in the elderly, and fear of falling is widely prevalent. Anxiety and fear can profoundly influence motor performance, resulting in a timid gait. Many older persons voluntarily restrict their activity because of concerns about mobility [1].

In this chapter, we review some of the defensive adaptations that occur in relation to concern about balance, and the phenomenon of the cautious gait. We conclude with a discussion of the more dramatic gait disturbances seen in patients with hysteria and somatiform disorders.

THE CAUTIOUS GAIT

Murray [2], in a study of walking patterns of healthy old men published in 1969, was the first to call attention to the phenomenon of the cautious gait. Kinematic studies of older people generally demonstrate a reduction in velocity and a shorter, broader stride [3, 4]. There is a consistent tendency of self-paced older subjects to choose a slower walking speed [5]. Murray [2] described elements of a distinct walking style, not resembling that of patients with neurological disease:

> Rather, the walking performance of the older men gave the impression of a guarded or restrained type of walking in attempt to obtain maximum stability and security. The walking of older men resembled that of someone walking on a slippery surface.

The slightly crouched postural attitude of the older subjects (hyperextension at the shoulder, flexion of the elbow, and lowered head position) suggests a guarded or careful manner of progression (Fig. 18-1). Murray [2] noted among his oldest subjects an unexpected increase in foot-floor clearance during the early swing phase. This step is very unlike the shuffling of a patient with cerebral pathology; it appears to provide additional security against tripping.

In recent studies on the biomechanics of walking, Winter [6] commented on

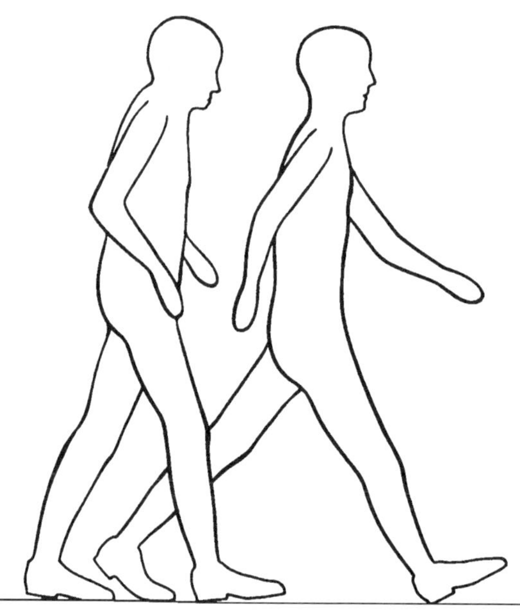

Figure 18-1. Adaptation of posture and stride in the gait of older men, as described by Murray, Kory, and Clarkson [2].

reduction in stride length, increased stance, and double support time in older subjects as adaptations providing a safer gait. His elderly volunteers exhibited a less vigorous plantar flexion, thereby generating less force as the toe pushed off at the end of stance.

Elements of this pattern were noted by Elble et al. [7] in kinematic studies of patients older than age 70 who exhibited various disturbances of gait. They describe a tendency toward stooped posture, reduced stride, and loss of the normal heel-to-toe sequence of foot-floor contact. Elble et al. [7] refer to this common kinematic profile as *senile gait*, though the pattern is somewhat nonspecific and is not restricted to the elderly. Patients with neurological disease were unable to increase their velocity substantially on request, a characteristic feature of many older patients with impaired walking. This reduction in dynamic range may reflect a problem with higher neural control and poses a practical problem for older pedestrians trying to make their way across a signaled intersection [8]. To paraphrase Ecclesiastes, there is a time for caution and a time to get out of harm's way.

The term *cautious gait* was coined by Nutt et al. [9] in a review of higher-level gait disorders observed in a geriatric inpatient unit. The cautious gait is, in a sense, an exaggeration of this adapted style of walking. The cautious gait is encountered frequently when examining patients with gait and balance disorders. Nutt et al. [9] identified aspects of cautious walking in 16 of the 43 patients they surveyed, many of whom explicitly expressed the need for caution to adjust for imbalance and to help avoid falls.

Clinical Presentation

The characteristic features of the cautious gait include a slightly widened base of support, reduced stride length, and slowed progression, with increase in the stance phase and double-limb support. Foot placement is altered, with diminished heel elevation and less forceful push-off of the toe. The foot-floor clearance is not diminished, and the feet do not shuffle along the floor. There is neither difficulty with gait initiation nor freezing. There may be some tendency to turn in segments (en bloc) rather than by making a smooth pivot, a strategy that reduces the angular velocity of turns. The center of mass is lowered slightly in stance. The entire picture evokes the image of someone trying to progress across a slippery surface. Many patients experience imbalance subjectively, though direct examination may reveal little apparent deficit in postural control.

Factors Underlying the Cautious Gait

Nutt et al. [9] suggest that the cautious gait is a compensatory adaptation, "an appropriate response to real or perceived disequilibrium." The shorter, broader stride provides a better base of support for maintenance of dynamic balance. Elble et al. [7] also suggest that the disorder is a compensatory change driven by insecurity and reductions in stride length. Any gait disorder can be viewed as the product of disturbed physiology and of an adaptive response. In the case of the cautious gait, the adaptive response is the salient characteristic.

Understandably, the phenomenon is somewhat nonspecific. A patient may respond appropriately in this manner if threatened by poor traction or a mild postural instability. An arthritic deformity, a sensory disorder, or a subtle change in motor performance thus can result in a cautious gait. It may be somewhat difficult to distinguish these disorders by watching a patient walk, as the defining features of the underlying abnormality are obscured by the common pattern of adaptive response. In some individuals, this gait is a response to anxiety or to an exaggerated sense of disequilibrium. The inappropriately cautious gait typically is seen in association with fear of falling. Walking may become extremely timid, with abduction of the arms and clutching at the furniture and walls for support.

FEAR OF FALLING

Fear of falling is a common problem for older persons, affecting those who never fall as well as those who do. Up to 50% of individuals with a history of recent falls express fear of falling [10–13]. This fear may emerge as a major concern among older people living in the community. Walker et al. [11] found that fear of falling was rated greater than the fears of robbery, forgetting an important appointment, or experiencing financial difficulties. Although fear of falling is strongly associated with a history of recent falls [14], 33% of people with no history of falls admit to a fear of falling [10, 12]. There is controversy about whether the phenomenon is more prevalent in women [10, 11, 14, 15]. The true extent of the problem is unknown and may be underestimated, as it is not always recognized.

Definition

The most obvious explanation for fear of falling is that it represents a rational response to danger. In older persons with a history of falling, it provides motivation to avoid situations to which they are no longer equal, to recognize their physical limitations, and to adjust their behavior accordingly. In this sense, fear works to a person's advantage; it functions as a protective mechanism to reduce fall risk and represents a normal response. In appropriate measures and situations, fear of falling can help maintain safe performance and may protect an individual from further falling episodes; too little caution can lead to carelessness and increase the risk of falls.

However, fear of falling can take a more pathological turn and negate its survival value. Some older people become so frightened and preoccupied with fall avoidance that they limit their everyday activities. Tinetti et al. [12] found that 26% of those who fall chronically acknowledged avoiding activities, as did 13% of those who do not fall regularly. In a prospective study of falls, Nevitt et al. [16] found that 10% of those experiencing recurrent falls reported avoiding activities because of fear of falling. Vellas et al. [17] described a 41% decline in activity over a 1-year period among those who fell, compared with a 23% decline among those who did not fall. They attributed this decline largely to fear of falling. As a consequence, fear of falling becomes detrimental, adversely affecting an individual's mobility and independence.

Underlying Factors

Falls that result in physical injury, functional loss, or prolonged postfall lie times (i.e., a person is unable to rise independently from the ground) are most likely to be associated with significant fear of falling [15]. In persons without a history of falls, fear can be precipitated by episodes of near-falls (i.e., events in which persons lose balance but avert coming to rest on the ground by grabbing onto environmental objects for support).

Comorbid conditions associated with fear of falling appear to be similar to those responsible for falls, including visual impairment and gait and balance dysfunction. Cwikel et al. [14] found that, in those who fell, poor vision was more likely to cause them to restrict their activity and to be more cautious. In a study of older people who fell and were admitted to the hospital, Guimaraes and Isaacs [18] reported that the great majority of patients who expressed a fear of falling had an abnormal gait. In a comparison study of older persons with and without fear of falling, Tideiksaar [unpublished data] found that affected individuals often had disturbances in gait and balance when tested. Persons with fear of falling tend to display a slower walking pace, greater hesitancy and irregularity of steps, increased path deviation, and positive Romberg (increased sway) and pull test (impaired postural control after sternal nudge). Maki et al. [19] demonstrated that older persons with a fear of falling exhibited increased anteroposterior sway when blindfolded on measures of static balance. Fife and Baloh [20] studied a group of 26 patients older than 75 who complained of disequilibrium, with no apparent cause on clinical evaluation. Fear of falling was generally associated, though it was not formally assessed in the study. Seven patients had profound deficits on laboratory tests of vestibular function. The entire group showed increased sway and did not do as well on semiquantitative tests of gait and balance.

Whether gait and balance disorders are causes or effects of fear of falling remains speculative. Certainly cocontraction of postural muscles can influence the dynamics of postural control. In several studies of older persons with fear of falling and insecure gait, causative neurological abnormalities could not be defined [15, 21]. Laboratory evaluation of vestibular function may be useful in this context, as suggested by Fife and Baloh [20].

Clinical Presentation and Consequences

The spectrum and course of fear of falling is varied. It may start simply as an unpleasant feeling, the emotional aftermath of one or more recent falls or near-fall episodes. At this stage, individuals may feel that the consequences of the next fall may end either in psychological or in physical damage (i.e., embarrassment, injury, or functional dependency). As a result, these persons are more alert to potential hazards in their surrounding environment and perform activities of daily living cautiously. Within this context, however, fear of falling represents a normal or sensible reaction to possible danger and may protect persons from further falls.

However, fear of falling can progress beyond this point to become debilitating. Some persons develop a situational fear of falling: Fear is linked directly to a specific activity (i.e., walking outdoors, bathing, toileting, climbing stairs). Attempting the feared activity typically results in severe anxiety (i.e., heart palpitations, shortness of breath, feeling faint). Not surprisingly, such individuals lose confidence. They become uncertain as to whether they can perform the feared activity safely.

Anxiety also can lead to poor health and contribute to a worsening of comorbid medical conditions. Indirectly, anxiety may even predispose to further falls. Anxious persons experiencing periods of transient emotional stress or upheaval may be less alert to environmental hazards and less able to differentiate between safe and hazardous activities. If pharmacologic treatment is used to relieve a person's anxiety, any adverse drug effects may exacerbate the risk of falls. In an effort to reduce their anxiety and fear, anxious people commonly resort to avoidance behaviors. They circumvent those situations or activities associated with previous falls and risk of injuries or falls. For example, if a fall or near-fall occurred in the bathtub, the person may curtail (or abstain from) bathing altogether. Likewise, a fall that occurred outside the home may lead to decreased outdoor activities.

This condition can progress to a generalized or nonsituational fear of falling. Some individuals, for example, become so preoccupied with fall avoidance that they generalize their fear to all activities. At this stage, defensive adaptations become quite prominent in a patient's gait. Failure to secure a safe pattern of gait may further lead to multiple near-falls and falls, which heighten the element of fear and eventually lead to a curtailment of all physical activities.

Some persons develop a phobia or fear of falling that is excessive or unreasonable with respect to a particular situation. Several researchers have attempted to characterize this phobic reaction to fear of falling. Marks and Bebbington [22] described space phobia in a group of older women. The hallmark of this syndrome is an intense fear of falling associated with open space and the absence of visuospatial support in the environment. For example, sufferers may be unable to cross a room (except by going on their hands and knees) unless they can walk in close proximity to the wall. At least in the early stages, actual physical support is not needed, only visual evidence that such support is close by. When no visual support is available, patients experience an intense fear. For instance, one patient could dance on a crowded dance floor (visual support) but had to leave if the crowd left. Balaha et al. [21] used the term *ptophobia* to describe the phobic reaction to falls in a group of older persons. These patients exhibited a fear of sitting and standing without support. In some patients, walking was not feasible because of their intense fear of falling, whereas in others, maximal assistance in walking was required. Murphy and Isaacs [15] described the postfall syndrome in a group of hospitalized patients who expressed great fear of falling and were unable to walk unsupported after suffering a fall. In attempting to walk, many of these patients tended to grab and clutch onto environmental objects within their reach for physical support. Ptophobia commonly occurs in older persons who live alone and have poor balance and gait. This phobic reaction is triggered by a cluster of falls (although near-falls and isolated falls are not uncommon) and physical injury or prolonged postfall lie times [23].

Any prolonged restriction of activities that occurs as a result of fear of falling can lead to a loss of lower-extremity muscular strength and joint flexibility and to some loss of mobility. As a consequence, a number of morbid outcomes may occur. Persons may be fearful of performing activities by themselves and, eventually, become reluctant to attempt independent activities and may even become chair- or bedbound. Marks and Bebbington [22] found that several patients with space phobia progressed until confined to a wheelchair and were housebound. Subsequently, such persons become socially isolated and require assistance to accomplish everyday activities. Community-residing persons in this category are at risk for nursing home placement. Older hospital patients with fear of falling may delay or eventually refuse discharge to the community and, ultimately, may require nursing home placement. Of greater significance, fear of falling may be associated with increased mortality. Murphy and Isaacs [15] reported that in their patients with postfall syndrome, one-third died within 4 months of hospital admission, mainly due to bronchopneumonia, myocardial infarction, and pulmonary embolism [15].

Assessment

Whether older persons reside in community or institutional settings, a fall evaluation should always include an assessment of fear of falling. One method of accomplishing this is to simply ask patients, "Are you afraid of falling?" However, some older persons may deny the presence of fear in an effort to preserve their autonomy and to avoid creating an image of frailty [24]. As well, patients with cognitive impairment may not be able to express their fear.

An alternative method of determining the presence and extent of the phenomenon is to ask patients, "Has fear of falling made you avoid any activities?" Inquiring about whether patients have experienced a restriction of activities in association with recent near-falls and falls may be a better barometer of clinically significant fear of falling than asking patients directly if they are fearful. Most patients who have an aversion toward admitting that they are fearful will openly discuss their reluctance to pursue certain activities. As well, family members and other individuals, such as home attendants and institutional staff, can be asked whether the patient has avoided certain activities recently.

The falls efficacy scale (FES) (Fig. 18-2) was developed to measure fear of falling [25]. Self-efficacy refers to an individual's perception or self-confidence in performing an activity. The scale is based on the operational definition of fear as "low perceived self-confidence at avoiding falls during essential, relatively nonhazardous activities" [26]. Patients are asked to identify how confident they feel about performing each of the activities without falling. The total efficacy score represents the sum of scores on individual activity items. A high score represents higher efficacy or confidence, and a low score reflects lower confidence. Tideiksaar and Kay [23] developed another measure of this phenomenon, the fear-of-falling questionnaire (FOFQ) (Fig. 18-3). The FOFQ asks patients to indicate whether they avoid certain activities and situations, and to what degree. The greater the number of activities and situations shown to be avoided, the greater the fear of falling as a clinical problem. Both the FES and FOFQ are helpful in determining which activities or situations lead to either low confidence or fear of falling and are of benefit in developing treatment plans.

PSYCHOGENIC GAIT DISORDER

Functional disorders of gait are well described in the medical literature of the nineteenth century. Unexplained inability to use the legs in stance (astasia) and in walking (abasia) despite apparently normal strength was described by Jaccoud, Charcot, and Blocq, who coined the term *astasia-abasia* in 1888. While Charcot's case reports were young people, the disorder subsequently was observed to oc-

Instructions. Pose each question in the following manner: "How confident are you that you can [fill in activity] without falling?"

Activity	Rating
1. Take a bath or shower	1 2 3 4 5 6 7 8 9 10
2. Reach into cabinets or closets	1 2 3 4 5 6 7 8 9 10
3. Prepare meals not requiring heavy or hot objects	1 2 3 4 5 6 7 8 9 10
4. Walk around the house	1 2 3 4 5 6 7 8 9 10
5. Get in and out of bed	1 2 3 4 5 6 7 8 9 10
6. Answer the door or telephone	1 2 3 4 5 6 7 8 9 10
7. Get in and out of a chair	1 2 3 4 5 6 7 8 9 10
8. Get dressed and undressed	1 2 3 4 5 6 7 8 9 10
9. Do light housekeeping	1 2 3 4 5 6 7 8 9 10
10. Do simple shopping	1 2 3 4 5 6 7 8 9 10

Note: A rating of 1 denotes extreme confidence; a rising of 10 denotes no confidence.

Figure 18-2. Falls efficacy scale. Patients are asked to grade, on a scale of 1 to 10, their confidence level in performing certain tasks.

cur in all ages. Charcot characterized astasia-abasia as "a special variety of motor feebleness of the legs" confined to postural control and locomotion and emphasized its psychogenic nature, noting that in many cases "the condition develops suddenly after an emotion or traumatism" [27].

There was an explosion of interest in this phenomenon during World War I, when functional disorders were observed in the trenches of Europe. In a 1918 review on the psychoneuroses of war, Lhermitte and Roussy [28] described astasia-abasia as the most common form of conversion disorder to occur in combat. They described a similar disorder (paradoxical inability to use the legs in stance and gait, despite good function when tested in bed) related to extreme anxiety and phobia, which they termed *staso-basophobia*. They emphasized the difference

FEAR OF FALLING QUESTIONNAIRE

Name:____ Date:______________

Indicate the degree to which you avoid the following activities or situations because of fear or other unpleasant feelings (ie, embarrassment, anxiety).

1. Never avoid

2. Rarely avoid

3. Avoid most of the time

4. Always avoid

<table>
<tr><td>

ACTIVITIES:

☐ Walking alone outdoors

☐ Walking alone indoors

☐ Getting on/off the toilet

☐ Getting in/out the bathtub/shower

☐ Taking a bath/shower

☐ Getting in/out of chairs

☐ Getting on/off the bed

☐ Reaching up into closets/cabinets

☐ Bending down (cabinets, ground) to place/retrieve objects

☐ Climbing stairs/curbs

☐ Descending stairs/curbs

☐ Other activities (describe) __________

____

____

____

</td><td>

SITUATIONS:

☐ Living alone

☐ Housekeeping

☐ Shopping

☐ Using public transportation

☐ Visiting friends/family

☐ Visiting restaurants

☐ Attending movies, theater, concerts

☐ Other situations (describe)

____

____

____

____

____

</td></tr>
</table>

Figure 18-3. Fear-of-falling questionnaire.

between the hysterical and phobic forms of the disorder, though the manifestations are similar. Their manuscript also described *camptocormia* ("bent back") and other curious forms of gait disorder, such as walking "on a sticky surface" or progressing as if swimming through water. *Habit limping* is defined as an exaggerated postural abnormality that persists after the initial cause (often a minor injury to the lower limb) has long disappeared.

Recent reviews by Keane [30] and Lempert et al. [31] emphasize the continued occurrence of hysterical gait disorders in contemporary practice. Keane [30] notes that functional disorders account for roughly 3% of his patient population, though today more patients complain of fatigue and myalgia, and florid hysterical gaits are somewhat less common. Lempert et al. [31] prefer the term *psychogenic gait disorder*, which is value-neutral and encompasses a broader range of diagnoses beyond hysteria. Some such cases are related to depression, anxiety, and phobic disorders. An occasional patient with this presentation will have a factitious illness, such as Munchausen's syndrome or outright malingering.

Gait in Depression

Psychomotor retardation in a depressed patient can influence postural attitude and locomotion. Sloman et al. [29] studied 15 psychiatric inpatients, using frame-by-frame analysis of 16-mm film from a single stride. The depressed patients showed a lack of propulsion at the end of stance and a reduction in stride length compared to controls. This gives to the walking of depressed patients the appearance of lack of purpose. Cadence was not diminished, but velocity was reduced in proportion to stride. Presumably, the gait disturbance is reversible with treatment of the underlying depression, though follow-up studies are not available.

Anxiety and Phobia

Patients with anxiety disorders can develop an extreme and incapacitating timidity in their stance and gait. Typically, they complain of imbalance and fear of falling and manifest an inappropriately cautious gait. They may crouch slightly and abduct the arms, as if progressing across a slippery surface. This gait pattern is described by Lempert et al. [31] as "walking on ice." Sometimes such patients cling dramatically to walls or furniture and may not venture from the house. This state is a source of considerable disability (as described earlier under Fear of Falling).

Hysteria and Somatiform Disorders

Dramatic functional gait disorders have been observed on neurological wards since the nineteenth century. They are recognized by inconsistencies in neurological examination, phenomena that cannot be readily explained, and a negative evaluation for organic cause. The bias in medicine is to presume organic illness until normal neurological function has been demonstrated. There is an enormous diversity of these disorders, which can present at any age.

Keane [30] divided hysterical gait disorders into several broad categories. Of 60 patients in his series, 13 had hysterical hemiparesis, 10 exhibited paraparesis, and 24 patients had various ataxic gaits, characterized by dramatically exaggerated sway (without falling). Some patients exhibited the phenomenon of "tightrope balancing": maintenance of postural control on a narrow base with abduction of the arms. Of 60 patients, 9 were characterized as "tremblers," a condition that should not be confused with orthostatic tremor, a well-characterized organic disorder.

Lempert et al. [31] examined videotape from 37 inpatients with functional gait disorders, looking for clusters of features ("phenomenological clues") that would aid in recognition and diagnosis. They noted both dramatic moment-to-moment fluctuations in 19 of 37 patients and excessive hesitation (like slow motion or walking through a viscous fluid) in 19 of 37. Both Keane [30] and Lempert et al. [31] describe patients with buckling of the knees without falling. Uneconomical postures with wastage of muscular energy are depicted in Spillane's [32] atlas of classic neurological findings; Lempert et al. [31] had 11 such patients. A psychogenic Romberg test is characterized by buildup of sway, with a consistent tendency to fall toward the observer. Often this can be overcome by distraction, (examining the pupils while a patient stands quietly). These are the most common patterns, but there is a great diversity, and many unique styles are encountered. Keane [30] describes a patient who walked in a stiff-legged robotic fashion (like Frankenstein's monster). Such cases are seldom subtle and often are obvious to an experienced observer. In 73% of Lempert's patients, the pattern did not resemble neurological disease in any way.

A psychiatric history is often present in patients with conversion disorders. A psychiatric interview invariably provides data helpful in diagnosis [33]. The outlook generally is good for such patients, approximately half achieve a dramatic cure during initial evaluation and treatment.

TREATMENT

All these conditions should be viewed as reversible causes of gait failure in the elderly. Effective pharmacotherapy is available for anxiety disorders and depression. Benzodiazepines and sedating tricyclic drugs must be used with care in this age group, as such drugs can impair balance and increase the risk of falls [34]. Some forms of habituation therapy have been used with success in phobic patients. Graded exposure and physical therapy (e.g., gait and balance training, muscle strengthening exercises) appear to be successful in reducing mild cases of fear of falling [21, 35–37]. Graded exposure consists of asking the patient to participate in the feared activity or situation for increasing periods of time until their discomfort or fear is lessened or extinguished.

People who have gait disorders and for whom effective specific treatment is not available should be referred for physical therapy and gait training. Some patients with fear of falling benefit from the short-term use of a walker; the device provides both visual and physical support and proprioceptive feedback that improves balance. For those persons with increased postfall lie times, personal emergency alarm devices and training in how to get up from the floor by themselves are helpful. We employ a combination of supportive psychological therapy and gait-directed physical therapy for patients with hysterical gait disorders. Confrontation is avoided, though some patients benefit if a timetable is provided for the resolution of their symptoms. The approach is similar to the moral therapy employed near the turn of the century, providing encouragement and a milieu in which the patient can recover and save face.

Finally, a number of environmental interventions in the home and institutional setting can help to alleviate fear of falling and improve confidence: (1) Hazardous conditions that interfere with mobility and increase fall risk must be identified and eliminated. For example, a situational fear of falling related to walking on a stairway may be eliminated by altering the design of the steps to ensure proper and safe foot placement. (2) Mobility tasks should be simplified or maximized through the modification of furnishings or addition of durable medical equipment (e.g., grab-bars, toilet risers, bathrub benches).

REFERENCES

1. Rippeto RD. Social disabilities created by gait disturbances in the aged, *Geriatrics* 1967;22: 175–81.
2. Murray MP, Kory RC, Clarkson BH. Walking patterns in healthy old men, *J Gerontol* 1969;24:169–78.
3. Spielberg PI. Walking Patterns of Old People. In: Bernstein NA, ed. *Investigations on the Biodynamics of Walking, Running, and Jumping.* Moscow: Central Scientific Institute of Physical Culture, 1940.
4. Drillis R. The Influence of Aging on the Kinematics of Gait. In: *The Geriatric Amputee.* Washington, DC: National Academy of Science, 1961.
5. Craik R. Changes in Locomotion in the Aging Adult. In: Woollacott MH, Shumway-Cook A, eds. *Development of Posture and Gait Across the Life Span.* University of South Carolina Press, 1989.
6. Winter DA. *The Biomechanics and Motor Control of Human Gait: Normal, Elderly, and Pathological,* 2nd ed. Waterloo, Ontario: University of Waterloo Press, 1991.
7. Elble RJ, Hughes L, Higgens C. The syndrome of senile gait. *J Neurol* 1992;239;71–75.
8. Lundgren-Lindquist B, Aniansson jA, Rundgren A. Functional studies in 79-year-olds. *Scand J Rehabil Med* 1983;15:125–131.
9. Nutt JG, Marsden CD, Thompson MD. Human walking and higher-level gait disorders, particularly in the elderly. *Neurology* 1993;43:268–279.
10. Downton JH, Andrews K. Postural disturbance and psychological symptoms amongst elderly people living at home. *Int J Geriatr Psychiatry* 1990;5:93–98.
11. Walker JE, Howland J. Falls and fear of falling among elderly persons living in the community: Occupational therapy interventions. *Am J Occup Ther* 1991;45:119–122.
12. Tinetti ME, Speechley M, Ginter SF. Risk factors for falls among elderly persons living in the community. *N Engl J Med* 1988;319:1701–1707.

13. Baraff LJ, et al. Perceptions of emergency care by the elderly: Results of multicenter focus group interviews. *Ann Emerg Med* 1992;21:814–818.

14. Cwikel J, Fried AN, Galinisky D. Falls and psychosocial factors among community-dwelling elderly persons: A review and integration of findings from Israel. *Public Health Rev* 1989;17:39–50.

15. Murphy J, Isaacs B. The post-fall syndrome: A study of 36 elderly patients. *Gerontology* 1982;28:265–270.

16. Nevitt MC, et al. Risk factors for recurrent nonsyncopal falls. *JAMA* 1989;261:2663–2668.

17. Vellas B, et al. Prospective study of restriction of activity in older people after falls. *Age Ageing* 1987;16:189–193.

18. Guimaraes G, Isaacs B. Characteristics of the gait in old people who fall. *J Int Rehab Med* 1980;2:177–180.

19. Maki BE, Holliday PJ, Topper AK. Fear of falling and postural performance in the elderly. *J Gerontol* 1991;46:M123–131.

20. Fife TD, Baloh RW. Disequilibrium of unknown cause in older people. *Ann Neurol* 1993;34:694–702.

21. Bhala RP, O'Donnell J, Thoppil E. Phobic fear of falling and its clinical management. *Phys Ther* 1982;62:187–190.

22. Marks I, Bebbington P. Space phobia: Syndrome or agoraphobic variant? *Br Med J* 1976; 2:345–347.

23. Tideikasaar R, Kay AD. What causes falls? A logical diagnostic procedure. *Geriatrics* 1986;41:32–50.

24. Taylor SE, Brown JD. Illusion of well being: A social psychological perspective on mental health. *Psychol Bull* 1988;103:193–210.

25. Tinetti ME, Richman D, Powell L. Falls efficacy as a measure of fear of falling. *J Gerontol* 1990;45:P236–243.

26. Tinetti ME, Powell L. Fear of falling and low self-efficacy: A cause of dependency in the elderly persons. *J Gerontol* 1993;48:35–38.

27. Pasteur W. Thyssen on astasia abasia. *Brain* 1891;14:557–567.

28. Lhermitte JJ, Roussy G. *The Psychoneuroses of War.* (Trans. W Christophersen.) London: University of London Press, 1918.

29. Sloman L, et al. Gait patterns of depressed patients and normal subjects. *Am J Psychol* 1982;139:94–97.

30. Keane JR. Hysterical gait disorders. *Neurology* 1989;39:586–589.

31. Lempert T, Brandt T, Dieterich M, Huppert D. How to identify psychogenic disorders of stance and gait. *J Neurol* 1991;238:140–146.

32. Spillane JD. *An Atlas of Clinical Neurology.* London: Oxford University Press, 1968.

33. Lazare A. Conversion symptoms. *N Engl J Med* 1981:305:745–748.

34. Ray WA, et al. Psychotropic drug use and the risk of hip fracture, *N Engl J Med* 1987;316:363–369.

35. Discipio WJ, Feldman MC. Combined behavior therapy and physical therapy in treatment of a fear of walking. *J Behav Ther Exp Psychiatry* 1971;2:151–152.

36. Feldman MC, Discipio WJ. Integrating physical therapy with behavior therapy. *Phys Ther* 1972;52:1283–1285.

37. Watson JP, Gaind R, Marks IM. Prolonged exposure: A rapid treatment for phobias. *Br Med J* 1971;1:13–15.

19. Evaluating the Older Person Who Falls

Mary B. King

Falls are a common occurrence in the lives of older people; approximately 30% of community-dwelling older persons fall each year, and approximately half of these fall more than once [1, 2]. Though the majority of falls do not result in adverse health outcomes, a significant number of those who fall regularly suffer injury or restriction of activity. In addition, repeated falls may be a marker for disease or deteriorating physical function. In some cases, it is possible to identify a single etiology for the fall (e.g., syncope, onset of hemiparesis due to stroke, or overwhelming environmentally related accident). However, most falls do not have a clear cause; they result from the interaction of multiple factors. In this chapter, factors that contribute to falls and to injury due to falls are discussed, and evaluation of the older person who has fallen is reviewed.

CONSEQUENCES OF FALLING

The importance of falls lies in the adverse health outcomes associated with them, including injury, inability to get up from the floor, loss of function, and fear of falling. Minor injuries, such as bruises and abrasions, occur in approximately 30–55% of falls in men and women aged 65 and older living in the community [2–4]. Major injuries requiring hospitalization or immobilization occur in 2–10% of falls [1, 3, 5]. An additional 4–6% of falls result in fracture, one-fourth of these being hip fractures [1–3]. Complications from injurious falls are the leading cause of death due to injury in men and women older than age 65 [6].

Up to 50% of community-dwelling elderly persons who fall are unable to get up after falling [3, 7, 8]; however, most of these persons are not injured seriously [7]. In one study, inability to get up was associated with features suggestive of physical frailty: (1) age of 80 or older; (2) decreased strength in shoulders and knees; (3) poor balance; (4) arthritis; and (5) dependency in activities of daily living. When followed prospectively, these persons had further significant declines in ability to perform usual activities and showed a trend toward more frequent hospitalization or death [7].

Limitation of activity occurs in approximately 40% of those who fall, whether due to physical impairment from injury or to fear of future falls [3]. Falls and their sequelae were associated with 18% of restricted activity days, according to one national survey [9]. Approximately one-fifth of people who fell and were treated in an emergency room had persistent pain or limitation of activity when seen 7 months following their injury [8]. Older persons hospitalized for fall-related injuries are three times more likely to be discharged to a nursing home than are those hospitalized for non–trauma-related conditions [10].

Fear of falling is common in older people, regardless of whether an individual has fallen previously. Between 40% and 73% of elderly persons who have experienced a recent fall (and 20–46% of those who have not) acknowledge fear of falling [1, 2, 8, 11–13]. Thirty to fifty percent of older people who are fearful of falling eliminate social and physical activities because of that fear [1, 14].

FACTORS THAT CONTRIBUTE TO FALL RISK

Falls may be classified by contributing factors [15–20]. In nonsyncopal falls, the risk of falling is related to a number of factors (both short-term and long-term), intrinsic to the person who falls, and to extrinsic factors (including the activity that the person is pursuing at the time of the fall and existing environmental hazards). Stable intrinsic factors that increase the risk of falling are related to chronic disease or age-associated changes. Finding the predominant contributor to loss of postural control—decreased sensory input (e.g., poor vision, peripheral neuropathy), impaired central nervous system processing (e.g., dementia, Parkinson's disease), or motor response (e.g., muscle weakness, osteoarthritis)— is one way of categorizing the intrinsic factors involved in loss of balance [18]. Other intrinsic risk factors vary with time or may be present temporarily, such as acute illness or changes in medication [8, 15, 20]. Because of predisposing intrinsic factors, the person who falls is unable to produce an effective response to a postural challenge.

Extrinsic factors that challenge balance include environmental hazards, the physical demands of everyday activities and, in more frail individuals, movements such as turning, bending, and reaching. Most falls occur during routine activities at home, including walking or going up or down stairs [3]; only 2–5% of falls happen during hazardous activities, such as running or climbing ladders [3, 20]. Environmental hazards are involved in up to half of nonsyncopal falls [3]. Hazards include circumstances where sensory input is diminished (e.g., when there is poor lighting or excess glare or carpeting is thick). Other hazards involve challenges to the balance response by rapid displacement of the center of mass, such as a slip on a throw rug or waxed floor or a trip over an object, pavement crack, or electrical cord. Older persons who have decreased mobility or postural control may find routine movements used in daily activities (e.g., transferring from bed to chair, bending, turning, or reaching) sufficiently challenging to cause a fall [3].

Intrinsic and extrinsic factors are involved in the initiation of the fall event; other factors determine whether an injury will occur. These include area of impact during the fall, presence of protective responses to break the fall, natural padding of the body and hardness of the landing surface, and bone strength [21, 22]. Falls in which there is direct impact on the hip or wrist are more likely to result in fracture than those in which there is no direct impact [23–25]. Those who fall from less than body height or who are able to grab onto an object to decrease the energy of the fall are less likely to sustain a fracture than are those who fall from a greater height or have no protective responses [23–26]. Persons with a lower body mass index (BMI):

$$BMI = \frac{weight\ (kg)}{height\ (m)^2}$$

are at greater risk for hip fracture with a fall than those with a normal or increased BMI. Bone mineral density and other mechanical factors are important determinants of fracture risk. A decrease of one standard deviation of bone mineral density of the femoral neck increases the risk of hip fracture 2.7 times [24, 27]. The bending movement of the femoral neck becomes larger as its length increases, theoretically increasing the risk of fracture [28]. Hip axis length, the distance along the femoral neck axis from the greater trochanter to the inner pelvic brim, has been shown to be a predictor of both femoral neck fractures and trochanteric fractures in older women, independent of age and bone mineral density [27, 29].

EVALUATION OF THE OLDER PERSON WHO FALLS

Because the likelihood of a future fall is increased in persons who have fallen and because each fall carries approximately the same risk of injury [3], a careful evaluation of the person who fell is important. A description of the circumstances surrounding the fall will dictate the focus and extent of the evaluation. An active older person who has a single fall primarily because of an environmental hazard requires a less detailed assessment. Repeated falls and single falls at home during routine activity usually warrant a full evaluation. This evaluation should begin with a medical history and physical examination (supplemented by tests of physical performance) and should include an assessment of exposure to environmental hazards and a review of medications taken.

Circumstances

A history of the circumstances surrounding a fall may provide information about its cause and clues to important factors that increase risk of falling for the individual. It is necessary to establish whether or not the fall was due to a discrete neurological event or cardiovascular disorder. The person who fell should be questioned about loss of consciousness, which would suggest syncope. Affirmative answers to questions about dizziness, palpitations, or feeling faint at the time of the fall suggest postural hypotension or arrhythmia. Falls that occur after eating a meal are suggestive of postprandial hypotension. Sudden weakness is suggestive of a stroke. Acute illness, such as pneumonia, or flare-up of a chronic disease, such as congestive heart failure or arthritis, may contribute to the fall. A new medication or a change in dose of an old prescription may add to fall risk. Older people who have recently spent days in bed [4] or have been hospitalized

[30] are at higher risk of falling. The setting of the fall is one indicator of the functional reserve of the faller:

Did the fall take place at or away from home, indoors or outdoors?
Was an environmental hazard involved?
Was a displacing force involved, such as in a trip or slip, or was the person changing position, reaching, or turning?

Also of importance is an assessment of the consequences of the fall, as this will help guide treatment:

Is the person afraid of future falls, and are there activities that are no longer pursued because of this fear?
Did an injury occur with the fall, and has the person completely recovered function after the injury?

Once the circumstances and consequences of the fall are established, a medical evaluation can be tailored to the individual.

Falls that have a definite cause, including those occurring with syncope or overwhelming environmental hazard, usually do not warrant a full fall evaluation. If the circumstances of the fall indicate loss of consciousness, an evaluation of syncope should be undertaken. A decrease in cerebral perfusion gives rise to symptoms of presyncope or syncope; however, despite extensive evaluation, no etiology can be found for 30–50% of syncopal episodes [31, 32]. In other episodes of syncope, the etiology may be orthostatic or postprandial hypotension, medication effect, situational factors such as micturition, or a vasovagal response. Cardiac or pulmonary vascular disease may be a cause of syncope, due to obstruction of blood flow and decrease in cardiac output (e.g., aortic stenosis, pulmonary embolus). Cardiac tachyarrhythmias and bradyarrhythmias also may cause decreased cardiac output and syncope. Transient ischemic attacks and seizures are uncommon causes of syncope. The assessment of elderly persons with syncope has been reviewed recently [31, 32] and will not be addressed here. If a fall is due to an overwhelming hazard, such as being knocked down or slipping on an icy sidewalk, the evaluation should focus on consequences of the fall, including assessment of injury, decreased activity, and fear. If a fall occurs during an acute illness, such as pneumonia or exacerbation of congestive heart failure, the acute illness should be treated; a subsequent search for other risk factors for falls may be undertaken. Falls without a clear cause often have a multifactorial etiology and warrant a systematic evaluation as outlined in the following discussion and in Table 19-1. Appropriate laboratory testing will follow from abnormalities uncovered on history and physical examination.

Medical History and Physical Examination

For a fall evaluation, the medical history should include an assessment of usual activity and function, previous falls and fractures, and presence of chronic dis-

Table 19-1. Approach to the evaluation of the older person who falls

Circumstances of fall*

Loss of consciousness
Setting of fall (e.g., home, indoors, environmental hazard)
Activity at time of fall
Recent change in health
    Acute illness
    Change in activity level
    Recent hospitalization
    Medication change

History and physical examination

History
    Usual activity, functional independence
    Previous falls, fractures
    Chronic disease (e.g., diabetes mellitus, peripheral neuropathy, previous stroke, Parkinson's disease,
      osteoarthritis, joint replacement, dementia, depression)
Physical examination
    Cardiovascular (blood pressure lying, standing; heart arrhythmia, murmur)
    Neurological (vision, hearing; tremor; muscle tone, strength; sensory [vestibular, proprioceptive
      function]; cerebellar function; cognition, affect)
    Skeletal (joint swelling, deformity, kyphoscoliosis; range of motion, including neck, back; feet)
Factors that increase risk of injury
    Evaluate for osteoporosis, osteomalacia
    Height, weight (body-mass index)

Physical performance testing

Balance
Gait (including proper use of cane, walker)
Performance of daily activities

Review of medications

Prescription and over-the-counter medications
    Number of medications
    Change in dose
    Individual drugs

Home environment

Presence of environmental hazards
Need for assistive device, community services

* Syncope, overwhelming environmental hazard, acute illness warranting targeted evaluation; otherwise, comprehensive evaluation (see text).

ease. Because declining physical function and immobility often are associated with falls, a history concerning activities that the patient is and is not able to do should be obtained. The person who fell should be questioned about independence in activities of daily living (e.g., bathing, dressing, eating, transferring, toileting) [33], physical instrumental activities of daily living (e.g., transportation, shopping, cooking, housework, laundry) [34], and advanced activities (e.g., climbing stairs, walking a half-mile, and carrying groceries) [35, 36]. The use of an assistive device should be noted, as should whether it is fitted properly and used correctly. Older persons who have impaired mobility and whose daily activities are at the limits of their functional capabilities are at greater risk of falling than are those who are more cautious [37]. The availability of help or supervision for daily activities that cannot be performed independently should be ascertained.

Previous fractures may suggest the presence of osteoporosis or osteomalacia, which increase the risk of fracture with a future fall. Other chronic diseases may increase risk of falls both through the effects of the disease itself and by general reduction in mobility and activity. Diseases that have been associated with increased fall risk include diabetes mellitus, Parkinson's disease, previous stroke, osteoarthritis, dementia, and depression [1, 2, 38–41].

In the physical examination, special attention should be given to the cardiovascular, neurological, and skeletal systems. Cardiovascular assessment should include measurement of blood pressure and examination of the heart for murmur (particularly aortic stenosis) and arrhythmia. Dizziness or light-headedness due to reduced cerebral perfusion from cardiovascular disease without loss of consciousness may play a role in nonsyncopal falls. Postural hypotension, defined as a drop of 20 mm Hg or more in systolic pressure from the supine to the standing position, occurs in approximately 10–17% of older people living in the community [42, 43]. Orthostatic hypotension may be the result of underlying disease, such as peripheral autonomic dysfunction due to diabetic neuropathy or central nervous system autonomic dysfunction (e.g., Shy-Drager syndrome) or to medication effect (e.g., antihypertensives, tricyclic antidepressants) [44]. Most frequently, however, no underlying disease can be found [45].

A complete neurological examination will uncover the presence of chronic diseases and abnormalities resulting in decreased sensory input or impaired motor response to a postural challenge. Adequate sensory function, including vision, vestibular function, and proprioception, is necessary for postural control. Vision should be tested, as loss of visual acuity, contrast sensitivity, adaptation to the dark, peripheral vision, and accommodation may be due to age-related changes or to disease, and all may affect stability. Decreased vestibular system function may develop due to age-related change or disease and may affect spatial orientation. Proprioceptive loss can be detected by careful examination of the peripheral nerves and by testing neck range of motion while standing. Peripheral neuropathy due to diabetes, vitamin B_{12} deficiency, or other disease may be detected; damage to mechanoreceptors in the apophyseal joints of the cervical spine due to osteoarthritis or injury may result in unsteadiness on turning the head [20].

Any central nervous system process (e.g., Parkinson's disease, bilateral frontal-lobe dysfunction, previous stroke, and cerebellar disease) or peripheral neuromuscular disease (e.g., myopathy, spinal stenosis) may contribute to, or be the primary cause of, falling [45]. Muscle strength and tone, reflexes, coordination, and presence of tremor should be assessed. Observation of gait and turns provides important diagnostic information [45]. Gait apraxia, or a slow, sliding gait in which the person's feet seem adherent to the floor, is seen with bilateral frontal-lobe dysfunction. Patients with Parkinson's disease have difficulty with gait initiation and walk with small, shuffling steps, decreased arm swing, and anteroflexed posture. Ataxia and unsteady gait may be seen with cerebellar disorders or acute vestibular or brainstem lesions. Myopathy due to hypothyroidism or an inflammatory process results in bilateral proximal weakness and a characteristic waddling gait.

Mental status testing should be done to document the presence or absence of cognitive impairment, and mood, affect, and depressive symptoms should be assessed. Dementia increases the risk of falling, probably because of poor judgment exercised by persons with cognitive impairment. Dementia also may be a manifestation of a neurological disease that affects motor function, such as Parkinson's disease or multiple lacunar infarcts.

Skeletal abnormalities, such as joint instability, contractures, joint deformity and pain due to arthritis, or abnormal body alignment from severe kyphoscoliosis, may impair function and increase fall risk. A skeletal examination should include examination of range of motion, deformity, and evidence of active arthritis of the knees, hips, back, neck, and arms. Attention to the feet is important, as calluses, bunions, toe deformities, and ill-fitting shoes may cause pain and therefore instability [1, 19, 20]. The type of shoe worn by the patient should be assessed [46] (see Fig.11-11, 11-18, page 177).

Additional factors that affect risk of injury with a fall should be evaluated. Attention should be paid to nutritional status, with assessment of height and weight, as well as other nutritional factors when indicated. Osteoporosis is an important risk factor for fractures with falls, and if the history suggests its presence, further evaluation should be done.

Medications

A careful review of both prescription and over-the-counter medications should be made, as certain medications, recent changes in dose, and total number of prescriptions have been associated with increased fall risk [47, 48]. Specific medications, because they impair mental alertness, are implicated in falls; these include long-acting benzodiazepines, barbiturates, antidepressants, and neuroleptics [48–52]. The use of cyclic antidepressants [53, 54], long-acting benzodiazepines [53, 55], and neuroleptics [53] increase the risk of hip fracture with a fall. Antihypertensives may cause postural hypotension or fatigue, and diuretics may produce volume depletion or electrolyte imbalance [48]. Over-the-counter medications should not be overlooked, as many potentially cause drowsiness or postural hypotension.

Tests of Physical Performance

Whereas the presence of chronic disease is detected by physical examination, the role that deficits in balance, strength, and endurance play in restricting everyday activities is ascertained by tests of physical performance. Performance tests are attractive because they require little time or expertise, and loss of function that is

Table 19-2. Environmental safety around the home

Inside

Floors
  Remove throw rugs.
  Avoid wax or use nonskid wax.
  Remove clutter from traffic areas.
  Keep electrical and telephone cords near walls, out of walkways.
  Secure loose carpeting.
  Ensure that telephone can be reached from floor.
Lighting
  Adjust to decrease glare.
  Ensure adequate lighting exists from bedroom to bathroom at night.
  Ensure lights exist at top and bottom of stairways.
Stairways
  Ensure railings are secure and easily visible.
  Ensure stairs have nonskid surfaces.
Bathroom
  Install grab-bars in bath and next to toilet.
  Use rubber mat in bath or shower.
  Install raised toilet seat if needed.
Kitchen
  Keep food, dishes within easy reach.
  Do not use cupboards that are too high or too low.

Outside

Repair uneven pavement, cracked sidewalks.
Install railings for outdoor steps.
Use adequate lighting.
Keep shrubbery trimmed near walks.

otherwise inapparent may be observed directly [56]. There is no single measure or series of tests that has been used consistently to evaluate physical function. A battery of tests can be used, such as the Performance-Oriented Mobility Assessment [57] or the Balance Scale [58]. These batteries and other timed tests of lower-extremity function, such as gait velocity, the Get-Up-and-Go Test [59], and semitandem, tandem, and one-leg standing times [60], are quantitative measures that can be used for comparison at future examinations. Stair ascent and descent are important to observe, particularly if the older person must use stairs at home or in the community. The ability to get on and off the floor should be tested in frail older persons because of the potential of a long lie (i.e., an extended period waiting on the floor for assistance) with a fall.

Environmental Hazards

Because 75% of falls occur at home, it is important to assess aspects of the home environment that have the potential to challenge balance in an older person whose ability to maintain postural control may be compromised. A home assessment may be done through a home visit by medical personnel or by a checklist completed by the patient. The assessment should be followed by a discussion of ways to make the home safer. Both the existence of hazards in the home and the older person's frequency of exposure to these hazards should be determined. For example, a throw rug in a room that the older person never enters does not present a hazard; if a room can be well-lit by a lamp that is never turned on, a hazard exists. A summary of the most important environmental factors from several published lists is shown in Table 19-2 [19, 61].

SUMMARY

Falls occur frequently in older people and are an important cause of morbidity due to injury and restriction of activity. Prospective community studies have shown that the likelihood of a future nonsyncopal fall increases with the number of risk factors identified [1, 2]. A careful assessment should be done in an older person with impaired mobility or repetitive falling when the cause of the fall(s) is not readily apparent, in order to determine risk factors for falls and injury that can be modified or eliminated. Treatment of the person who fell then can be individualized, based on the findings of the fall assessment.

REFERENCES

1. Tinetti ME, Speechley M, Ginter SF. Risk factors for falls among elderly persons living in the community. *N Engl J Med* 1988;319(26):1701–1707.
2. Nevitt MC, Cummings SR, Kidd S, Black D. Risk factors for recurrent nonsyncopal falls. *JAMA* 1989;261(18):2663–2668.
3. Nevitt MC, Cummings SR, Hudes ES. Risk factors for injurious falls: A prospective study. *J Gerontol Med Sci* 1991;46(5):M164–170.
4. O'Loughlin JL, Robitaille Y, Boivin J, Suissa S. Incidence of and risk factors for falls and injurious falls among the community-dwelling elderly. *Am J Epidemiol* 1993;137:342–354.
5. Kellogg International Work Group on the Prevention of Falls in the Elderly. The prevention of falls in later life. *Dan Med Bull* 1987;34(Suppl 4):1–24.
6. Sattin RW. Falls among older persons: A public health perspective. *Annu Rev Public Health* 1992;13:489–508.
7. Tinetti ME, Liu W, Claus EB. Predictors and prognosis of inability to get up after falls among elderly persons. *JAMA* 1993;269:65–70.
8. Grisso JA, et al. The impact of falls in an inner-city elderly African-American population. *J Am Geriatr Soc* 1992;40:673–678.
9. Kosorok MR, et al. Restricted activity days among older adults. *Am J Public Health* 1992; 82:1263–1267.
10. Alexander BH, Rivara FP, Wolf ME. The cost and frequency of hospitalization for fall-related injuries in older adults. *Am J Public Health* 1992;82(7):1020–1023.
11. Walker JE, Howland J. Falls and fear of falling among elderly persons living in the community: Occupational therapy interventions. *Am J Occup Ther* 1991;45:119–122.
12. Maki BE, Holliday PJ, Topper AK. Fear of falling and postural performance in the elderly. *J Gerontol Med Sci* 1991;46(4):M123–131.

13. Tinetti ME, Mendes de Leon CF, Doucette JT, Baker DI. Fear of falling and fall-related efficacy in relationship to functioning among community-living elders. *J Gerontol Med Sci* 1994;49(3):M140–M147.

14. Downton JH, Andrews K. Postural disturbance and psychological symptoms amongst elderly people living at home. *Int J Geriatr Psychiatry* 1990;5:93–98.

15. Cummings RG, Kelsey JL, Nevitt MC. Methodologic issues in the study of frequent and recurrent health problems. *Ann Epidemiol* 1990;1:49–56.

16. Studenski S. A Model of Falls Risk for Clinical Research. In: Weinrach R, Hadley EC, Ory MG, eds. *Reducing Frailty and Falls in Older Persons.* Springfield, IL: Thomas, 1991. Pp 133–138.

17. Lach HW, et al. Falls in the elderly: Reliability of a classification system. *J Am Geriatr Soc* 1991;39:197–202.

18. Kiel DP. The evaluation of falls in the emergency department. *Clin Geriatr Med* 1993;9(3): 591–599.

19. Rubenstein LZ, et al. Falls and instability in the elderly. *J Am Geriatr Soc* 1988;36:266–278.

20. Tinetti ME, Speechley M. Prevention of falls among the elderly. *N Engl J Med* 1989; 320(16):1055–1059.

21. Cummings SR, Nevitt MC. A hypothesis: The causes of hip fractures. *J Gerontol Med Sci* 1989;44(4):M107–111.

22. Melton LJ, Riggs BL. Risk factors for injury after a fall. *Clin Geriatr Med* 1985;13(3):525–539.

23. Hayes WC, et al. Impact near the hip dominates fracture risk in elderly nursing home residents who fall. *Calcif Tissue Int* 1993;52:192–198.

24. Greenspan SL, et al. Fall severity and bone mineral density as risk factors for hip fracture in ambulatory elderly. *JAMA* 1994;271(2):128–133.

25. Nevitt MC, Cummings SR, Study of Osteoporotic Fractures Research Group. Type of fall and risk of hip and wrist fractures: the study of osteoporotic fractures. *J Am Geriatr Soc* 1993;41: 1226–1234.

26. Grisso JA, et al. Risk factors for falls as a cause of hip fracture in women. *N Engl J Med* 1991; 32(19):1326–1331.

27. Faulkner KG, et al. Simple measurement of femoral geometry predicts hip fracture: The Study of Osteoporotic Fractures. *J Bone Miner Res* 1993;8:1211–1217.

28. Nakamura T, et al. Do variations in hip geometry explain differences in hip fracture risk between Japanese and White Americans? *J Bone Miner Res* 1994;9:1071–1076.

29. Faulkner KG, McClung M, Cummings SR. Automated evaluation of hip axis length for predicting hip fracture. *J Bone Miner Res* 1994;9:1065–1070.

30. Mahoney J, Sager M, Dunham NC, Johnson J. Risk of falls after hospital discharge. *J Am Geriatr Soc* 1994;42:269–274.

31. Kapoor WN. Syncope in older persons. *J Am Geriatr Soc* 1994;42:426–436.

32. Lipsitz LA, Jonsson PV. Transient loss of consciousness. In: Katzman R, Rowe JW, eds. *Principles of Geriatric Neurology.* Philadelphia: Davis, 1992. Pp 300–313.

33. Branch LG, Katz S, Kniepman K, Papsidero JA. A prospective study of functional status among community elders. *Am J Public Health* 1984;74:266–268.

34. Lawton MP, Brody EM. Assessment of older people: Self-maintaining and instrumental activities of daily living. *Gerontologist* 1969;9:179–185.

35. Nagi S. An epidemiology of disability among adults in the United States. *Millbank Q* 1976; 54:439–468.

36. Rosow I, Breslau N. A Guttman health scale for the aged. *J Gerontol* 1966;21:556–559.

37. Studenski S, et al. Predicting falls: The role of mobility and nonphysical factors. *J Am Geriatr Soc* 1994;42:297–302.

38. Campbell AJ, Borrie MJ, Spears GF. Risk factors for falls in a community-based prospective study of people 70 years and older. *J Gerontol Med Sci* 1989;44(4):M112–117.

39. Morris JC, Rubin EH, Morris EJ, Mandel SA. Senile dementia of the Alzheimer's type: An important risk factor of serious falls. *J Gerontol Med Sci* 1987;42(4):412–417.

40. Buchner DM, Larson EB. Falls and fractures in patients with Alzheimer-type dementia. *JAMA* 1987;257(11):1492–1495.

41. Lipsitz LA, Jonsson PV, Kelley MM, Koestner JS. Causes and correlates of recurrent falls in ambulatory frail elderly. *J Gerontol Med Sci* 1991;46(4):M114–122.

42. Mader SL, Josephson KR, Rubenstein LZ. Low prevalence of postural hypotension among community-dwelling elderly. *JAMA* 1987;258:1511–1514.

43. Applegate WB, et al. Prevalence of postural hypotension at baseline in the Systolic Hypertension in the Elderly Program (SHEP) cohort. *J Am Geriatr Soc* 1991;39:1057–1064.

44. Onrot J, et al. Management of chronic orthostatic hypotension. *Am J Med* 1986;80:454–463.

45. Wolfson L. Falls and Gait. In: Katzman R, Rowe JW, eds. *Principles of Geriatric Neurology.* Philadelphia: Davis, 1992. Pp 281–299.

46. Dunne RG, et al. Elderly persons' attitudes towards footwear—a factor in preventing falls. *Public Health Rep* 1993;108(2):245–248.

47. Cumming RG, et al. Medications and multiple falls in elderly people: The St. Louis OASIS study. *Age Ageing* 1991;20:455–461.

48. Macdonald JB. The role of drugs in falls in the elderly. *Clin Geriatr Med* 1985;1:621–636.

49. Trewin VF, Lawrence CJ, Veitch GBA. An investigation of the association of benzodiazepines and other hypnotics with the incidence of falls in the elderly. *J Clin Pharm Ther* 1992;17: 129–133.

50. Sorock GS, Shimkin EE. Benzodiazepine sedatives and the risk of falling in a community-dwelling elderly cohort. *Arch Intern Med* 1988;148:2441–2444.

51. Spar JE, LaRue A, Hewes C, Fairbanks L. Multivariate prediction of falls in elderly inpatients. *Int J Geriatr Psychiatry* 1987;2:185–188.

52. Yip YB, Cumming RG. The association between medications and falls in Australian nursing-home residents. *Med J Aust* 1994;160:14–18.

53. Ray WA, et al. Psychotropic drug use and the risk of hip fracture. *N Engl J Med* 1987;316: 363–369.

54. Ray WA, Griffin MR, Malcolm E. Cyclic antidepressants and the risk of hip fracture. *Arch Intern Med* 1991;151:754–756.

55. Ray WA, Griffin MR, Downey W. Benzodiazepines of long and short elimination half-life and the risk of hip fracture. *JAMA* 1989;262:3303–3307.

56. Guralnik JM, Branch LG, Cummings SR, Curb JD. Physical performance measures in aging research. *J Gerontol Med Sci* 1989;44:M141–146.

57. Tinetti ME. Performance-oriented assessment of mobility problems in elderly patients. *J Am Geriatr Soc* 1986;34:119–126.

58. Berg K, Wood-Dauphinee S, Williams JI, Gayton D. Measuring balance in the elderly: Preliminary development of an instrument. *Physiother Can* 1989;41:304–311.

59. Mathias S, Nayak US, Isaacs B. Balance in elderly patients: The "get-up and go" test. *Arch Phys Med Rehabil* 1986;67:387–389.

60. Fornoff JER, et al. A cross-sectional validation study of the FICSIT common data base static balance measures [abstract]. *Gerontologist* 1993;33S:173.

61. Josephson KR, Fabacher DA, Rubenstein LZ. Home safety and fall prevention. *Clin Geriatr Med* 1991;7:707–731.

20. Interventions to Reduce the Multifactorial Risks for Falling

Laurence Z. Rubenstein and Karen R. Josephson

Though extremely common, falls are an exceedingly complex phenomenon in the elderly population and require a detailed evaluation and creative treatment strategies. As discussed in Chapter 2, the many risk factors for falls commonly interact and occur with varying prevalence among different subgroups of the aged population. Likewise, there is great variance in the prognostic significance of falls. A fall may be the first indicator of an acute problem (infection, postural hypotension, syncope), may indicate progression of a chronic disease (parkinsonism, dementia, diabetic neuropathy), or simply may be a marker for the onset of "normal" age-related changes in vision, gait, and strength.

No simple approach can be adequate for evaluating or treating falls. Diagnosis and preventive interventions must reflect the diverse nature of falling and must pay attention as well to maintaining optimal independence and quality of life without unduly restricting activity. Ideally, interventions directed to the underlying risk factors behind falls can and should improve quality of life even if they are not effective in reducing falls. (Causes and risk factors for falls are reviewed from an epidemiological perspective in Chapter 2.) This chapter discusses the principles of a multidimensional fall assessment from a geriatrician's perspective, along with the issues and research data related to developing successful fall interventions.

CAUSES OF FALLS

Determination of the major causes of falls has been attempted in numerous studies [1–12]. Though these studies have been useful, their data and conclusions have been limited by a lack of consistency in classifying falls. For example, a fall might be classified by a presenting symptom (e.g., dizziness, drop attack, slip, syncope), by a precipitating mechanism (e.g., postural hypotension, cardiac arrhythmia, environmental hazard), by categorical type (e.g., extrinsic versus intrinsic), or by underlying risk factors (e.g., antihypertensive medications, decreased vision, impaired gait). Other limiting factors include differences in study populations, variable patient recall, and lack of objective observer input. Probably the single major difficulty in classifying the causes of falls has been the fact that most falls have multifactorial causes (e.g., a trip over an electrical cord contributed to by both a gait disorder and poor vision). This complex relation-

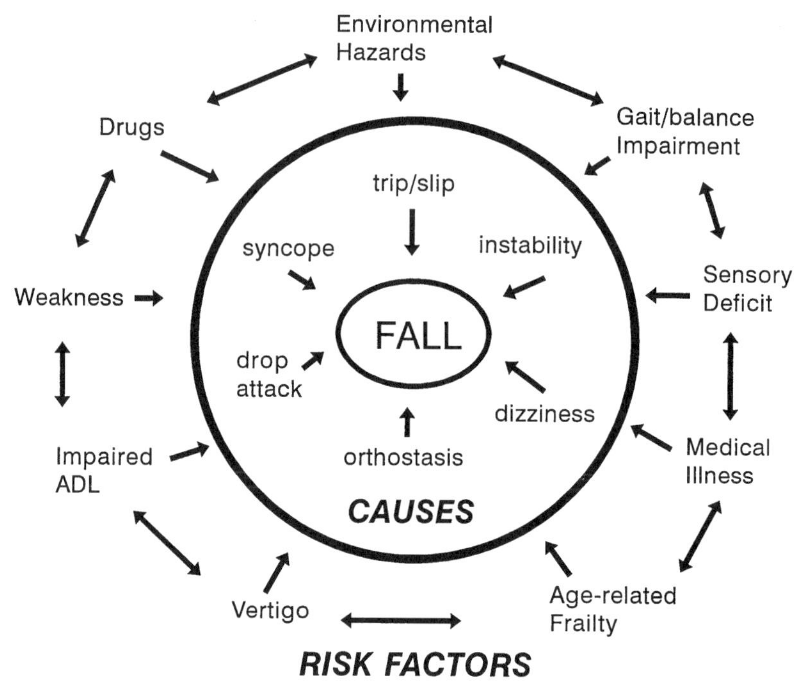

Figure 20-1. The multifactorial and interacting etiologies of falls. ADL = activities of daily living.

ship between risk factors, underlying causes, precipitating events, and falls is alluded to in Fig. 20-1. This multifactorial causality, which requires complex diagnostic and treatment strategies, is typical of geriatric syndromes generally and is part of what characterizes the approach of the geriatrician.

The major immediate causes of falls and their relative frequencies based on the major published literature are listed in Table 20-1. Not surprisingly, impairments of gait and balance are associated with the three most common causes of falls. Whereas so-called accidents or falls stemming from environmental hazards constitute the largest categorical cause of falls (accounting for 30–50% in most series), most falls in this category really stem from interactions between environmental hazards or hazardous activities (extrinsic factors) and increased individual susceptibility to hazards from accumulated effects of age and disease (intrinsic factors).

The broad category of gait and balance problems and weakness is the second most common cause for falls. As described in Chapters 5 and 6, gait and balance impairments can stem from age-related changes; specific dysfunctions of the nervous, muscular, skeletal, and circulatory systems; and from simple deconditioning following inactivity. Gait disorders affect 20–50% of the elderly population [13], and they are even more prevalent in persons who fall. Muscle weakness also is an extremely common finding among the aged population. Though there is general agreement that reduction in muscle strength accompanies the aging

Table 20-1. Causes of falls in elderly adults: Summary of twelve studies that carefully evaluated elderly persons after a fall and specified a most likely cause

Cause	Mean (%)[a]	Range (%)[b]
Accident or environment-related	31	1–53
Gait or balance disorders or weakness	17	4–39
Dizziness or vertigo	13	0–30
Drop attack	9	0–52
Confusion	5	0–14
Postural hypotension	3	0–24
Visual disorder	2	0–5
Syncope	0.3	0–3
Other specified causes[c]	15	2–39
Unknown	5	0–21

[a] Mean percent calculated from the 3,628 falls in the 12 studies.
[b] Ranges indicate the percentage reported in each of the 12 studies.
[c] This category includes arthritis, acute illness, drugs, alcohol, pain, epilepsy, and falling from bed.
SOURCE: Data from references [1–12].

process, much of it stems from disease and inactivity rather than from aging per se. Studies have reported the prevalence of grossly detectable lower-extremity weakness to range anywhere from 48% among community-dwelling older persons [14], to 57% among residents of an intermediate care facility [15], and more than 80% among nursing home residents [16]. Muscle weakness, especially of the quadriceps, plantar-flexors, and dorsiflexors, is a common cause of gait deviations in older persons.

Dizziness or vertigo syndromes constitute the third most common cause category for falling and may stem from very diverse etiologies, most of which can affect an individual's ability to maintain balance. True vertigo, a sensation of rotational movement, may indicate a disorder of the vestibular apparatus (e.g., benign positional vertigo, acute labyrinthitis, or Meniere's disease). Symptoms described as *imbalance on walking* often reflect a gait disorder. Many patients describe a vague light-headedness that may reflect cardiovascular problems, hyperventilation, orthostasis, drug side effect, anxiety, or depression.

Drop attacks, which appear as the fourth leading cause of falls, are defined as falls associated with sudden leg weakness but without loss of consciousness or dizziness. This syndrome has been attributed to transient vertebrobasilar insufficiency, although it probably is due to more diverse pathophysiological mechanisms, and many so-called drop attacks may be simply due to leg weakness or to a knee joint problem. Alternatively, lesions of brain structures involved in the maintenance of posture may predispose to sudden knee buckling. (Vascular causes of drop attacks are reviewed in Chapter 14.) Recent studies are reporting substantially fewer falls as drop attacks than did earlier studies, a finding probably related to better documentation and diagnostic precision; many current researchers believe that the 9% mean figure shown in Table 20-1 is much too high an estimate.

Other common causes of falls include confusion and cognitive impairment, orthostatic hypotension, and visual disorders. Important but less frequently cited causes of falls include syncope, arthritis, acute illnesses, disorders of the central nervous system, alcohol use, and drugs. Drugs frequently have side effects that result in impaired stability, gait, and mentation. Especially important are agents with sedative, antidepressant, and antihypertensive effects, particularly diuretics, vasodilators, and beta blockers [17, 18].

RISK FACTORS

Because a single specific cause for falling often cannot be identified and because falls are usually multifactorial in their origin, many epidemiological case-control studies have been performed in an attempt to identify specific risk factors that increase the likelihood of falling (see Chapter 2). The idea underlying these studies is that by identifying risk factors early, preventive strategies can be devised and instituted.

Though there are some differences in risk factors between community dwelling and institutionalized populations, many overlap. The most common single risk factors identified in 16 controlled studies [10, 11, 14–16, 18–28] are listed in Table 20-2, along with an approximate relative risk associated with each factor averaged over all studies that examined it. As can be seen, leg weakness increases risk of falling fivefold, whereas gait and balance impairments increase risk threefold. Limitation in mobility also has been identified as a separate risk factor, with a risk ratio of 2.5. Identifying risk factors for *injurious* falls is arguably more important than simply identifying risk factors for falls. These have been identified in six additional studies [11, 18, 29–32], and by and large the factors are the same as those for falls in general, with the addition of factors associated

Table 20-2. Important individual risk factors
for falls: Summary of sixteen controlled studies

Risk factor	Significant association/total[a]	Mean RR (OR)	Range
Weakness	11/11	4.9 (8)[b]	1.9–10.3
Balance deficit	9/9	3.2 (5)	1.6–5.4
Gait deficit	8/9	3.0 (5)	1.7–4.8
Visual deficit	5/9	2.8 (9)	1.1–7.4
Mobility limitation	9/9	2.5 (8)	1.0–5.3
Cognitive impairment	4/8	2.4 (5)	2.0–4.7
Impaired functional status	5/6	2.0 (4)	1.0–3.1
Postural hypotension	2/7	1.9 (5)	1.0–3.4

RR = relative risks (prospective studies); OR = odds ratios (retrospective studies).
[a] Number of studies with significant association/total number of studies examining each factor.
[b] Number in parentheses indicates the number of studies that reported relative risks or odds ratios.
SOURCE: Data from references [10, 11, 14–16, 18–28].

with osteoporosis, such as female gender and being underweight, and with use of physical restraints.

Perhaps as important as identifying individual risk factors is appreciating the interaction (and probable synergism) between multiple risk factors. Several studies have shown that the risk of falling increases dramatically as the number of risk factors increases [15, 16, 18]. In one study, the predicted 1-year risk of falling ranged from 12% for persons with none of three risk factors (i.e., hip weakness assessed manually, unstable balance, and taking four or more prescribed medications) to 100% for persons with all three risk factors [16].

In summary, studies clearly indicate a strong association between gait disorders, instability, and falls, and it is possible to identify persons at substantially increased risk of sustaining a fall or fall-related injury by detecting these and other risk factors.

MULTIDIMENSIONAL FALL ASSESSMENT

The goals of a multidimensional fall assessment are twofold: (1) to diagnose and treat patients after a fall and (2) to identify risk factors for future falls and implement appropriate interventions. The fall assessment should incorporate the basic principles of a comprehensive geriatric assessment—namely, a multidimensional assessment to quantify medical, psychosocial, and functional capabilities and problems so as to develop a comprehensive plan for therapy. The specific components of the fall assessment, however, may vary depending on the patient population being evaluated (e.g., community-dwelling versus nursing home residents).

For patients with a recent fall event, much of the focus of the fall assessment will be directed toward determining the etiology of the fall (already described in detail in Chapter 19). However, equal attention also should be paid to identifying risk factors that may predispose the patient to future falls or injuries. Most of these risk factors can be easily assessed in the physician's office by using basic examination techniques or standardized instruments (Table 20-3).

Components of the physical examination that are useful in identifying risk factors include postural blood pressure measurements, visual acuity testing, manual muscle testing of the lower extremities, neurological assessment, and a gait and balance assessment. In addition, a careful mental status examination using a standardized scale, such as the Folstein Mini–Mental State Examination [33] should be performed to screen for cognitive impairment.

A careful assessment of gait and balance is a particularly important component of the fall assessment, to detect abnormalities and to evaluate their impact on function. The complexity of this assessment can range from simple observation of a walking patient to computer analysis of motion and postural sway with video and forceplate equipment. For most clinical purposes, observational gait and balance analysis is sufficient, other more sophisticated testing methods usually being reserved for research purposes. Observational gait analysis generally consists

Table 20-3. Clinical approaches to specific causes
or common risk factors discovered in the fall assessment

Cause or risk factor	Evaluation	Therapeutic measure
Weakness	Review of medical problems and medications Complete neurological examination (quantifying severity; identifying central deficits, neuropathies, and myopathies) Physical therapy (PT) evaluation for therapeutic recommendations	Treatment of reversible causes Exercise regimen Prescribing appropriate assistive devices
Gait or balance deficit	Neurological examination (including gait analysis) PT evaluation for therapeutic recommendations Orthopedic, foot, and footwear evaluation	Treatment of reversible causes Gait or balance training Prescribe assistive device
Visual deficit	Vision examination	Corrective lenses, surgery, low-vision aids, and environmental adaptation
Environmental hazards	Environmental assessment (home visit or self-completed checklist)	Remove hazards Adaptive aids
Postural hypotension	Review of medical problems and medications (ruling out infection, dehydration, autonomic dysfunction, anemia, and drug effect)	Correct treatable problems (medication, dehydration, and infection) Teach adaptive behavior (slow rising, raised head of bed)
Confusion or delirium	Dementia or delirium evaluation (quantifying severity; identifying toxic or metabolic problem, ruling out structural lesion) Functional evaluation	Treat reversible problem Environmental safety adaptations
Syncope or arrhythmia	Full syncope evaluation (ruling out cardiac arrhythmia, valvular deficit, and metabolic abnormality)	Treat underlying problem
Dizziness or vertigo	Medical evaluation and medical review Neurological evaluation Vestibular evaluation	Treatment of underlying problem Prescribing exercises for benign postural vertigo, if appropriate

of observing, both from the side and from the back, a patient walking at a normal speed on a flat surface. Characteristics of gait to be noted include velocity and rhythm, stride length, double support time (the time spent with both feet on the floor), height of stepping, and degree of trunk sway. The fit and use of any assistive device and of footwear also are observed. Balance can be assessed by observing the patient attempting positions and position changes that stress stability (i.e., rising from a seated position, standing with eyes open and closed, tandem walk, neck flexion, turning in a circle, and sitting down). Simple scored screening scales for detecting and quantifying gait and balance problems have been developed [25, 34, 35]. The quantitative nature of these scales is useful for following progress over time.

In addition to identifying gait and balance deviations, it is important to assess functional mobility and physical activity. By determining the type of activities in which a patient actually engages, the clinician can make a more accurate appraisal of fall risk. Studies have suggested that patients who have fall risk factors and are physically active are at greater risk of falling than are similar patients who engage in little independent activity [28, 29]. For example, elderly men who were ambulatory with unstable gait had a fivefold increased risk of recurrent falls compared to men who were nonambulatory or ambulatory with stable gait [28]. Functionally independent nursing home patients with lower-extremity weakness also were found to be more likely to be injured from a fall than were dependent patients [29]. Optimally, it would be helpful to observe patients performing activities in their living environment, both to assess functional ability and to identify potential hazards. Though in the institutional setting this may be possible, among community-dwelling older adults the clinician must obtain this information by specific questioning. Numerous functional status scales have been developed for different populations of older adults [36–38]. The patient also should be questioned about more advanced physical activities, such as exercise, recreational activities, and work. Unfortunately, there are a lack of physical activity scales appropriate for testing sedentary or frail older adults. One scale that may be useful for less active populations quantifies kilocalorie expenditures on everyday tasks (cooking, housework, yardwork) [39] rather than looking solely at exercise activities.

Optimally, the multidimensional fall assessment will uncover direct or contributing causes amenable to medical therapy or other corrective interventions. Because of the multifactorial nature of falls, there is no standard approach to treatment or prevention. In cases in which the cause of a fall is due to an obvious acute problem, treatment may be relatively simple, direct, and effective (e.g., discontinuing medication that causes postural hypotension). However, patients with multiple risk factors often will require a combination of medical, rehabilitative, environmental, or behavioral intervention strategies (e.g., treating syncope, removing environmental hazards, prescribing a cane). Therapeutic measures that should be considered for the treatment of the most common risk factors for falls are listed in Table 20-3.

PREVENTION STRATEGIES

Prevention of falls and fall-related injuries has become an important goal of most geriatric outpatient and inpatient programs, with a recent heightened interest in finding effective strategies. Interventions have been developed and targeted to individual patients, caregivers, and the environment. Unfortunately, very few evaluative data exist, and most existing data are limited by small sample sizes, lack of control groups, or short follow-up periods. In 1990, the National Institute on Aging funded a series of eight innovative studies, the Frailty and Injuries: Cooperative Studies of Intervention Techniques (FICSIT) [40], for testing interventions to reduce fall-related injuries and frail health in older adults. Four of the studies have been published, and the results have added considerable new information to the literature on fall prevention. The types of preventive strategies described in the literature to date include postfall multidimensional assessment, risk factor identification and education programs, exercise and rehabilitation programs, nursing interventions, and protective devices. The design and outcomes of published intervention studies are presented in Table 20-4.

Multidimensional Postfall Assessment

The benefits of a multidimensional assessment have been reported by several study groups [9, 41, 42]. An outpatient falls clinic reported that among the first 36 patients evaluated, an average of three possible etiologies for falls or contributory factors were identified per patient, most of which were amenable to treatment. At 1-year follow-up, 78% of patients had reported no additional falls, and 17% had "fewer" falls. The calculated costs of the postfall clinic was $248 per patient [41]. In a randomized trial of a postfall assessment intervention [9], nursing home patients were assigned randomly within 7 days of a fall to receive either a comprehensive postfall assessment or usual care. The probable primary causes of the fall and secondary risk factors were identified for each intervention subject. Many remediable problems (e.g., weakness, environmental hazards, orthostatic hypotension, drug side effects, gait dysfunction) were detected, and many (mean, 2.8) specific treatment recommendations were given with good compliance (62% overall). At the end of a 2-year follow-up period, there were trends for intervention that showed subjects to have lower fall and death rates (9% fewer falls and 17% fewer deaths), but these did not reach statistical significance. Strikingly, the intervention group did experience significant reductions in hospitalizations (26%) and hospital days (52%) compared to controls. Both of these studies suggest that falls are markers of underlying disorders easily identifiable by a careful postfall assessment, which in turn can be treated with reduction in disability.

Risk Factor Identification and Education Interventions

There have been several published studies [43–46] describing results of intervention programs designed to identify and treat risk factors for falls or fractures prior to an actual fall. Each of these prevention programs targeted community-dwelling elders and provided a combination of intervention strategies to address physical risk factors (e.g., exercise, medication review, referrals to physicians), health behavior (e.g., group or individual education sessions), and environmental safety (e.g., home safety evaluations and assistance with home repairs). In a noncontrolled descriptive study, Tideiksaar [44] reported that 75% of patients who had multiple falls and participated in a fall prevention program had no further falls over a 2-year period. Reductions in fall rates also have been reported in two randomized controlled trials. In the first, Hornbrook et al. [46] found that a program that addressed home safety, exercise, and behavioral risks significantly decreased the odds of falling by 0.85, but there was only a nonsignificant trend for reductions in average number of falls and fall-related injuries.

Table 20-4. Intervention studies intending to prevent falls in elderly population

Reference	Population	Study design	Intervention	Outcome measures	Results	Effect on falls
Post-fall assessments						
Wolf-Klein et al. [41], New York	Community-dwelling Mean age = 78 N = 36	Descriptive 1-yr follow-up	Multidisciplinary falls clinic providing assessment and treatment (including home visits)	Fall rates	Majority of patients had 3–4 risk factors	78% had no falls, 17% fell less frequently, 5% no change
Rubenstein et al. [9], California	LTC residents Mean age = 79 N = 79;81	RCT 2-yr follow-up	Post-fall assessment (PE, labs, Holter monitor, environmental assessment) to detect causes, risk factors, and provide recommendations	Fall rates, hospital admits and days, mortality	2.1 active problems identified; 2.8 recommendations/subject; signficant reduction in hospital admits (26%) and days (52%); 17% reduction in mortality, nonsignificant	9% decrease, nonsignificant
Neufeld et al. [42], New York	LTC residents N = 24	Program description	Multidisciplinary falls consultation service to evaluate patients and provide recommendations	No evaluation conducted		
Risk factor identification and education						
Carpenter, Demopoulus [43], England	Community-dwelling Age ≥ 75 N = 272;267	RCT 3-yr follow-up	ADL questionnaire given by home visit volunteers Changes in ADL score led to referral to physician	Mortality, ADL scores, hospitals and nursing home admits, falls, use of community services	Reduction in long-term (> 6 months) nursing home admits	Controls had 47% increase in falls ($p < .001$), study group had no change

Tideiksaar [44], New York	Community-dwelling with multiple falls N = 28	Program description 2-yr follow-up	Community fall prevention program. Physician and patient education, evaluation and treatment of high-risk patients, referrals for home modifications	Fall rates		75% had no falls over 2 yr
Vetter et al. [45], Wales	Community-dwelling Age ≥ 70 N = 350; 324	RCT 4-yr follow-up	Home visit to assess fall and fracture risk and provide referrals, education, and exercise recommendations	Fall rates, fracture rates		More falls in study group at all levels of disability No difference in fracture rates
Hornbrook et al. [48], Oregon	HMO patients Age ≥ 65 At risk for falling N = 1323	RCT 2-yr follow-up	Behavioral program of walking, strength and balance training, home safety, mental imagery	Health status, functioning, falls, fall-related health care use and costs	Pending	No reduction in falls [61]
Tinetti et al. [47], Connecticut	Community-dwelling ≥ 70 years With 1 fall risk factor N = 301	RCT 1-yr follow-up	Multidisciplinary program to reduce risk factors. Behavioral and medication changes, education and exercise	Fall rates, injury rates, fear of falling	Intervention group had fewer risk factors and reduced fear of falling at 1 year follow-up	Significant reduction in falls and fall risk (approximately 30%)
Hornbrook et al. [46], Oregon	HMO Age ≥ 65 N = 1,611; 1,571	RCT 23-mo follow-up-	Home evaluation and recommendations, health behavior program, fall prevention exercises, assistance with home repairs	Fall rates, injury rates		Odds of falling significantly reduced No effect on number of falls or injuries
Reinsch et al. [55], California	Community-dwelling Mean age = 75 N = 230	RCT 1-yr follow-up	Exercise or cognitive behavioral programs: 3 times weekly for 12 mo	Falls, strength, balance, fear of falling, self-perceived health	No significant change in any measures	No reduction in falls

Table 20-4 (continued).

Reference	Population	Study design	Intervention	Outcome measures	Results	Effect on falls
Buchner et al. [56], Washington	Community-dwelling Ages 68–85 With leg weakness or gait deficit N = 100	RCT 3-mo follow-up	Strength training, endurance training, or combined: 3- or 6-mo interventions	Strength, aerobic capacity, gait, balance, falls, physical functioning	Pending	No reduction in falls [61]
Fiatarone et al. [60], Massachusetts	Nursing home Age ≥ 70 With previous fall or at ris] N = 100	RCT 6-mo follow-up	Resistance training or nutritional supplements: 3 times weekly for 10 weeks	Strength, mobility, nutritional status, muscle mass, falls	Exercise group showed significant improvement in muscle strength, gait velocity, physical activity, and muscle mass	No reduction in falls [61]
Wolf et al. [57], Georgia	Community-dwelling Age ≥ 70 N = 200	RCT 4-mo follow-up	Computerized balance training or Tai Chi training for 15 weeks	Grip strength, flexibility, blood pressure, functional status, falls, well-being	Reduced fear of falling in Tai Chi group and lower blood pressure	Subjects in Tai Chi group had 47.5% reduction in fall rate
Mulrow et al. [59], Texas	Nursing home residents Mean age = 80 N = 97;97	RCT 1-yr follow-up	Physical therapy (PT) 3 times weekly for 4 mo Control group received friendly visits	Physical function, ADL scores, self-perceived health status, falls	15.5% improvement in mobility scale for PT group, and reduced use of assistive devices at 4 mo	No reduction in falls
Wolfson et al. [58], Connecticut	Community-dwelling Age ≥ 75 N = 109	RCT 6-mo follow-up	Balance training or resistance training: 3 times weekly for 6 mo	Balance, gait, strength, fall rates	Balance training significantly improved balance measures; resistance training improved lower extremity strength	No reduction in falls [61]

Widder [68], Oregon	Hospital patients Age > 60 68 beds	Descriptive	Alarm device worn on leg that emits a sound when patient attempts to arise from bed	Falls	5-mo fall rates reduced by 45% on medicine and 33% on orthopedic wards
Dubner, Creech [69], United States	Psycho-geriatric unit patients	Descriptive	Monitoring for postural hypotension Infrared scanning system to detect patients arising from bed at night	Falls	Blood pressure monitoring did not reduce falls Scanning system reduced night falls significantly
Schmid [63], New York	Hospital patients	Descriptive 1-yr follow-up	Fall prevention program (fall risk assessment tool, alert signs, nursing evaluation of falls, safety vests, and bed alarms)	Falls	Average 20% reduction in monthly falls per patient day
Wallace et al. [72], Iowa	6 groups of older adults at high risk for falls or hip fracture	Descriptive	Protective hip pad worn during waking hours	Compliance rates, injury rates	Pending
Lauritzen et al. [71], Denmark	Nursing home patients 66% ≥ 80 years	RCT 11 mo	External hip protectors	Hip and nonhip fractures	Major reduction in hip fractures in study wards (relative risk 0.44). No hip fractures among study subjects who actually wore hip pads. No change in fall rates

LTC = long-term care facility; RCT = randomized controlled trial; PE = physical examination; admits = admissions; ADL = activities of daily living; HMO = health maintenance organization; PT = physical therapy.

In a study by Tinetti et al. [47], an in-home multifactorial intervention was used to modify known fall-risk factors. At 1 year follow-up, the risk of falling among intervention subjects was reduced by about 30% compared to the control group. Conversely, in a randomized trial of home visits to assess for fall risk, the experimental group actually sustained more falls than the control group over 4 years of follow-up, but there was no difference in fracture rates between the groups [45]. In another home visit trial, assessed subjects had no change in fall rates after 3 years of follow-up, whereas controls experienced a significant 47% increase [43]. The results are pending from an additional trial targeted to fall-prone individuals [48].

Exercise and Rehabilitation Interventions

There are numerous studies showing that specific risk factors in older adults, such as weakness [49–52] and instability [53, 54], can be reversed or improved following exercise or balance training. However, until recently these interventions have not been studied for their effectiveness in reducing falls, nor have they targeted fall-prone populations. Currently, there are six published studies—four among community-dwelling older adults [55–58] and two among nursing home patients [59, 60]—describing results of exercise interventions that included falls as an outcome measure. As shown in Table 20-4, five of the six studies reported improvements in strength or balance measures; however, only the Tai Chi intervention actually led to a significant reduction in falls [57]. These findings may stem from the dynamic interaction between exercise levels and falls: though exercise can lead to improved function and quality of life and to reductions in fall risk factors, it also increases the opportunity for falling. The relationship between short-term exercise and falls was further explored in a meta-analysis of seven of the FICSIT trials [61]. The combined analysis revealed that general exercise and balance training had a beneficial effect on fall incidence. However, because many different types of exercise were studied, it was impossible to determine which type was most effective.

Nursing Interventions

Nursing interventions probably are the most widely used fall prevention strategy in hospitals and nursing homes. Generally, these programs focus on identifying, at admission, those patients who are at high risk for falling and on instituting various kinds of precautions. To assist in identification of such high-risk patients, fall assessment tools have been developed and described in the literature [62, 63]. Using these tools, the nursing staff assesses such patient factors as mental status, history of falls, ambulation status, medications, physical status, continence, and sensory deficits. A patient's fall risk status is determined either by the number of risk factors present or by a summary score. Once a patient has been identified as being at high risk for falling, a nursing care plan usually is developed to include interventions aimed at injury prevention. Such interventions include (1) indicating on the medical chart and the patient's door that the patient is at high risk for falls; (2) moving high-risk patients to rooms that are close to the nursing station so as to increase observation; (3) periodic reassessment of patients following new episodes of illness or change in medication; (4) lowering side-rails and bed height for patients who climb out of bed; (5) increasing nurse-to-patient ratio; and (6) fall prevention education for patients and staff.

Few data have been published in support of the validity of assessment tools or of the effectiveness of these types of prevention programs. However, one non-controlled study [63] reported high reliability and validity of a scored fall assessment tool developed to identify hospitalized patients at high risk of falling. Implementation of this tool, along with standardized nursing care plans for high-risk patients and installation of new safety equipment (safety vests, bed alarm system) resulted in an average 20% decrease in falls over the first year of the program.

Fall Prevention Devices

Until recently, the most common "devices" used in nursing homes and hospitals to prevent falls were physical restraints, such as soft restraining vests and bedrails. In American nursing homes in the 1980s, the reported prevalence of restraint use ranged from 25–85% of residents [64]. Since new federal regulations went into effect in 1990 [65], there has been a major move away from the use of physical restraints, and research has shown that the adverse affects of physical restraints on functional status and quality of life outweigh any potential benefit in preventing falls. Specifically, there is evidence to suggest that physical restraints actually may contribute to falls [66], injuries [31], and death [67].

Technological devices that alert caregivers to patient movement or protect patients from fall injuries currently are being developed and marketed as possible alternatives to restraints. The most widely available devices are various alarm systems that are activated when patients try to get out of bed or ambulate unassisted. One such alarm system was pilot-tested both on an orthopedic and on a general medicine hospital ward. Preliminary 5-month data indicated that patient falls were decreased 33% and 45% on each ward, respectively [68]. An infrared scanning system, which activates a nursing station alarm when a patient sits up or gets out of bed, was found to reduce the incidence of nighttime falls from 2.8 to 1.0 falls per month when installed on a psychogeriatric unit [69]. Video-recording systems also are being used to acquire information about the circumstances and patterns of falls. This information then is used to devise specific interventions [70].

Injury prevention alternatives, such as protective hip pads, also are currently being tested [71, 72] but are not generally available. In one dramatic study from Denmark [71] protective hip pads were tested in a nursing home setting where hip fractures had been extremely common. In wards randomized to use the pads, hip fracture rates were markedly lower than in the comparison wards—almost a 60% reduction in risk. Even more striking was that no hip fracture occurred among patients actually wearing external hip pads.

CONSIDERATIONS IN DESIGNING FALL-PREVENTION STRATEGIES

From the foregoing discussion, it can be seen that fall prevention is a multifaceted endeavor. This stems from the multifactorial causes of falls, multiple contributing risk factors, issues of frailty and lack of responsiveness in many older persons to interventions, and the double-edged effect of many intervention strategies that may increase one fall risk factor while reducing another. An example has been given with regard to exercise and activity. Though activity is, and should be, encouraged as a positive goal leading to higher function and quality of life, activity also facilitates the opportunity for falling. Though the phenomenon is not well-studied, active individuals may have more falls, yet may have fewer falls per unit of activity. This theoretical relationship is indicated in Fig. 20-2. The interaction between falls, activity levels, frailty, and injury must be studied much more carefully.

Another issue has to do with the trade-off of targeting interventions only to those most likely to benefit. Though maximum impact per person enrolled certainly is higher with narrowly targeting interventions, the population served by the intervention may become overly small and possibly may have little overall effect on global fall rates.

Finally, there are subgroups of individuals with multiple or irreversible risk factors (e.g., blindness, progressive neurological diseases) for whom it will be ex-

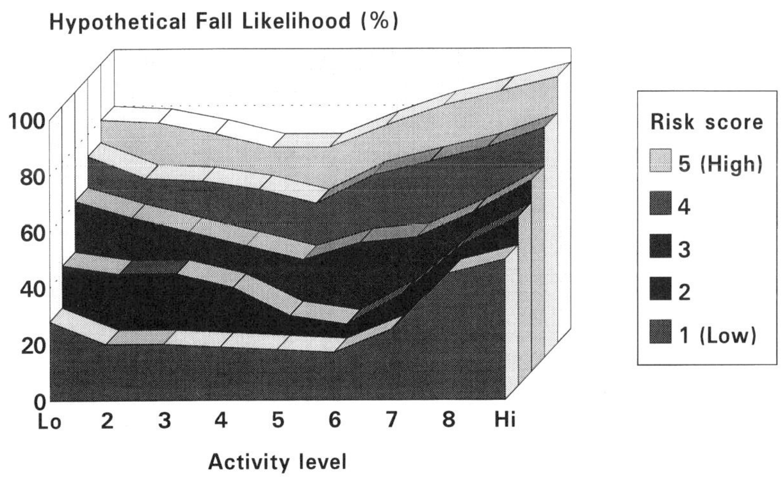

Figure 20-2. Fall likelihood: a function of risk and opportunity.

tremely difficult to devise effective interventions. For these individuals, the risks of falling must be weighed carefully against the risks of limiting activity.

In conclusion, a large proportion of falls and fall injuries in elderly people are due to gait and balance deficits, and many probably are preventable with careful medical and environmental evaluation and intervention. Therefore, regular screening for fall risk factors is prudent, and a vigorous diagnostic, therapeutic, and preventive approach clearly is appropriate in all older patients who fall and in those at high risk of falling.

REFERENCES

1. Sheldon JH. On the natural history of falls in old age. *Br Med J* 1960;2:1685–1690.
2. Clark ANG. Factors in fracture of the female femur. A clinical study of the environmental, physical, medical and preventative aspects of this injury. *Geront Clin* 1968;10:257–270.
3. Naylor R, Rosin AJ. Falling as a cause of admission to a geriatric unit. *Practitioner* 1970;205:327–331.
4. Lucht U. A prospective study of accidental falls and injuries at home among elderly people. *Acta Socio Med Scand* 1971;2:105–120.
5. Scott CJ. Accidents in hospital with special reference to old people. *Health Bull (Edinb)* 1976;34:330–335.
6. Exton-Smith AN. Functional Consequences of Aging: Clinical Manifestations. In: Exton-Smith AN, Grimley Evans J, eds. *Care of the Elderly: Meeting the Challenge of Dependency.* London: Academic, 1977. Pp 41–57.
7. Brocklehurst JC, et al. Fractures of the femur in old age: A two-centre study of associated clinical factors and the cause of the fall. *Age Ageing* 1978;7:2–15.
8. Morfitt JM. Falls in old people at home: Intrinsic versus environmental factors in causation. *Public Health* 1983;97:115–120.
9. Rubenstein LZ, et al. The value of assessing falls in an elderly population: A randomized clinical trial. *Ann Intern Med* 1990;113:308–316.
10. Lipsitz LA, et al. Causes and correlates of recurrent falls in ambulatory frail elderly. *J Gerontol* 1991;46:M114–122.
11. Svensson ML, et al. Accidents in the institutionalized elderly: A risk analysis. *Aging* 1991;3: 181–192.
12. Hale WA, Delaney MJ, McGaghie WC. Characteristics and predictors of falls in elderly patients. *J Fam Pract* 1992;34:577–581.
13. Sudarsky L. Geriatrics: Gait disorders in the elderly. *Curr Concepts Geriatr* 1990;322: 1441–1446.
14. Campbell AJ, Borrie MJ, Spears GF. Risk factors for falls in a community-based prospective study of people 70 years and older. *J Gerontol* 1989;44:M112–117.
15. Tinetti ME, Williams TF, Mayewski R. Fall risk index for elderly patients based on number of chronic disabilities. *Am J Med* 1986;80:429–434.
16. Robbins AS, et al. Predictors of falls among elderly people. Results of two population-based studies. *Arch Intern Med* 1989;149:1628–1633.
17. Granek E, Baker SP, Abbey H. Medications and diagnoses in relation to falls in a long-term care facility. *J Am Geriatr Soc* 1987;35:503–511.
18. Myers AH, et al. Risk factors associated with falls and injuries among elderly institutionalized persons. *Am J Epidemiol* 1991;133:1179–1190.
19. Whipple RH, Wolfson LI, Amerman PM. The relationship of knee and ankle weakness to falls in nursing home residents: An isokinetic study. *J Am Geriatr Soc* 1987;35:13–20.
20. Tinetti ME, Speechley M, Ginter SF. Risk factors for falls among elderly persons living in the community. *N Engl J Med* 1988;319:1701–1707.

21. Nevitt MC, et al. Risk factors for recurrent nonsyncopal falls. A prospective study. *JAMA* 1989;261:2663–2668.

22. Wickham C, et al. Muscle strength, activity, housing and the risk of falls in elderly people. *Age Ageing* 1989;18:47–51.

23. Gehlson GM, Whaley MH. Falls in the elderly: Part II, balance, strength, and flexibility. *Arch Phys Med Rehabil* 1990;71:735–738.

24. Jonsson PV, Lipsitz LA, Kelley M, Koestner J. Hypotensive responses to common daily activities in institutionalized elderly. A potential risk for recurrent falls. *Arch Intern Med* 1990;150:1518–1524.

25. Wolfson L, et al. Gait assessment in the elderly: A gait abnormality rating scale and its relation to falls. *J Gerontol* 1990;45:M12–19.

26. Mahoney J, et al. Risk of falls after hospital discharge. *J Am Geriatr Soc* 1994;42:269–274.

27. Maki BE, Holliday PJ, Topper AK. A prospective study of postural balance and risk of falling in an ambulatory and independent elderly population. *J Gerontol* 1994;49:M72–84.

28. Studenski S, et al. Predicting falls: The role of mobility and nonphysical factors. *J Am Geriatr Soc* 1994;42:297–302.

29. Tinetti ME. Factors associated with serious injury during falls by ambulatory nursing home residents. *J Am Geriatr Soc* 1987;35:644–648.

30. Grisso JA, et al. Risk factors for falls as a cause of hip fracture in women. *N Engl J Med* 1991;324:1326–1331.

31. Tinetti ME, Liu WL, Ginter SF. Mechanical restraint use and fall-related injuries among residents of skilled nursing facilities. *Ann Intern Med* 1992;116:369–374.

32. Mayo NE, Korner-Bitensky N, Levy AR. Risk factors for fractures due to falls. *Arch Phys Med Rehabil* 1993;74:917–921.

33. Folstein MF, Folstein SE, McHugh PR. "Mini-mental state." A practical method of grading the cognitive state of patients for the clinician. *J Psychiatr Res* 1975;12:189–198.

34. Tinetti ME. Performance-oriented assessment of mobility problems in elderly patients. *J Am Geriatr Soc* 1986;34:119–126.

35. Podsiadlo D, Richardson S. The timed "Up & Go": A test of basic functional mobility for frail elderly persons. *J Am Geriatr Soc* 1991;39:142–148.

36. Katz S, et al. Progress in the development of the index of ADL. *Gerontologist* 1970;10:20.

37. Lawton MP, Brody EM. Assessment of older people. Self-maintaining and instrumental activities of daily living. *Gerontologist* 1969;9:179–186.

38. Reuben DR, Siu AL. An objective measure of physical function of elderly outpatients. The physical performance test. *J Am Geriatr Soc* 1990;38:1105–1112.

39. DiPietro L, et al. A survey for assessing physical activity among older adults. *Med Sci Sports Exerc* 1993;25(5):628–642.

40. Ory MG, et al. Frailty and injuries in later life: The FICSIT trials. *J Am Geriatr Soc* 1993;41:283–296.

41. Wolf-Klein GP, et al. Prevention of falls in the elderly population. *Arch Phys Med Rehabil* 1988;69:689–691.

42. Neufeld RR, et al. A multidisciplinary falls consultation service in a nursing home. *Gerontologist* 1991;31:120–123.

43. Carpenter GI, Demopoulos GR. Screening the elderly in the community: Controlled trial of dependency surveillance using a questionnaire administered by volunteers. *Br Med J* 1990;300:1253–1256.

44. Tideiksaar R. Falls among the elderly: A community prevention program. *Am J Public Health* 1992;82:892–893.

45. Vetter J, Lewis PA, Ford D. Can health visitors prevent fractures in elderly people? *Br Med J* 1992;304:888–890.

46. Hornbrook MC, et al. Preventing falls among community-dwelling older persons: Results from a randomized trial. *Gerontologist* 1994;34:16–23.

47. Tinetti ME. A multifactorial intervention to reduce the risk of falling among elderly people living in the community. *N Engl J Med* 1994;331:821–827.

48. Hornbrook MC, Stevens VJ, Wingfield DJ. Seniors' program for injury control and education. *J Am Geriatr Soc* 1993;41:309–314.

49. Liemohn WP. Strength and aging: An exploratory study. *Int J Aging Hum Dev* 1975;6:347–357.

50. Aniansson A, Gustafsson E. Physical training in elderly men with special reference to quadriceps muscle strength and morphology. *Clin Physiol* 1981;1:87–98.

51. Frontera WR, et al. Strength conditioning in older men: Skeletal muscle hypertrophy and improved function. *J Appl Physiol* 1988;64:1038–1044.

52. Fiatarone MA, et al. High-intensity strength training in nonagenarians. *JAMA* 1990;263:3029.

53. Hopkins DR, et al. Effect of low-impact aerobic dance on the functional fitness of elderly women. *Gerontologist* 1990;30:189–192.

54. Roberts BL. Effects of walking on balance among elders. *Nurs Res* 1989;38:180–182.

55. Reinsch S, et al. Attempts to prevent falls and injury: A prospective community study. *Gerontologist* 1992;32(4):450–456.

56. Buchner DM, et al. The Seattle FICSIT/Move It study: The effect of exercise on gait and balance in older adults. *J Am Geriatr Soc* 1993;41:321–325.

57. Wolf SL, et al. Reducing frailty and falls in older persons: An investigation of Tai Chi and computerized balance training. *J Am Geriatr Soc* 1996;44:489–497.

58. Wolfson L, et al. Balance and strength training in older adults: Intervention gains and Tai Chi maintenance. *J Am Geriatr Soc* 1996;44:498–506.

59. Mulrow CD, et al. A randomized trial of physical rehabilitation for very frail nursing home residents. *JAMA* 1994;271(7):519–524.

60. Fiatarone MA, et al. Exercise training and nutritional supplementation for physical frailty in very elderly people. *N Engl J Med* 1994;330:1769–1775.

61. Province MA. The effects of exercise on falls in elderly patients: A preplanned meta-analysis of the FICSIT trials. *JAMA* 1995;273:1341–1347.

62. Berryman E, et al. Point by point: Predicting elders' falls. *Geriatr Nurs* (New York) 1989;10:199–201.

63. Schmid NA. Reducing patient falls: A research-based comprehensive fall prevention program. *Mil Med* 1990;155:202–207.

64. Schnelle JF, Simmons SF, Ory MG. Risk factors that predict staff failure to release nursing home residents from restraints. *Gerontologist* 1992;32:767–770.

65. Kapp MB. Nursing home restraints and legal liability. Merging the standard of care and industry practice. *J Legal Med* 1992;13:1–32.

66. Miller MB, Elliott DF. Accidents in Nursing Homes: Implications for Patients and Administrators. In: Miller MB, ed. *Current Issues in Clinical Geriatrics.* New York: Tiresias Press, 1979. Pp 97–137.

67. Miles SH, Irvine P. Deaths caused by physical restraints. *Gerontologist* 1992;32:762–766.

68. Widder B. A new device to decrease falls. *Geriatr Nurs* (New York) 1985;6:287–288.

69. Dubner NP, Creech R. Using infrared scanning to decrease nighttime falls on a psychogeriatric unit. *Hosp Common Psychiatry* 1988;39:79–81.

70. Cornell BR. Patterns of naturally occurring falls among frail nursing home residents. *Gerontologist* 1993;33:58.

71. Lauritzen JB, Petersen MM, Lund B. Effect of external hip protectors on hip fractures. *Lancet* 1993;341:11–13.

72. Wallace RB, et al. Iowa FICSIT Trial: The feasibility of elderly wearing a hip joint protective garment to reduce hip fractures. *J Am Geriatr Soc* 1993;41:338–340.

21. Physical Intervention for Elderly Patients with Gait Disorders

Margaret Schenkman and Cheryl Riegger-Krugh

Difficulties with walking are a key factor in loss of independence for older individuals [1–3]. These difficulties can result from a variety of sources: specific diseases or injuries, disuse or overuse, and nonspecific declines of physiological processing associated with aging. Disturbances of gait often present with similar characteristics [4, 5]. Gait slows with older age, and individuals become unsteady on their feet. Base of support tends to widen, step length shortens or becomes uneven, time spent in the double support phase of gait increases, and so on. Such individuals have particular difficulty in walking on uneven surfaces, in a crowd, or in the dark.

Treatment of gait disorders is designed to optimize gait, within the patient's inherent constraints and capabilities, for the purpose of improving function. The goal of intervention is not to achieve some "normal gait" as defined by biomechanical characteristics. Rather, the goal is to maximize the capacity for safe functional ambulation, including stability, speed and endurance, adaptability of speeds, adaptability in a variety of environments, energy efficiency, and appropriateness for the patient's lifestyle.

The first requirement of gait is safety. Improvements of speed of walking, body segment motions, and the like are of little value to a patient if the net result is an inherent instability that leaves the patient at risk for falls and injury. Second, the gait should be energy-efficient. To walk independently *without* a cane or walker may be of little value to a patient if the demands of the task are excessively energy-consuming as compared to walking with an assistive device. Third, the ability to walk quickly should be optimized but not at the risk of losing stability or endurance. Individuals will not be well served if they can achieve speed but cannot sustain a stable gait to cover needed distances. Fourth, adaptability to varying external conditions is desirable. To optimize function, patients should be able to walk in a variety of environments and on differing surfaces. They should be able to incorporate other activities while walking (e.g., carrying groceries). Patients are not well served if they are only safe, stable, and efficient when walking in a single environment and in a single direction. The extent to which variability is possible will determine the functionality of the patient's gait. Finally, gait should be appropriate to the patient's environment and lifestyle. The patient should be able to enter and leave a personal dwelling, to manage doors, and to negotiate stairs and curbs as the environment demands.

The similarity in presentation of gait disorders for different patients does not ensure a similarity of underlying causes for those gait disturbances. The similarity in goals of intervention does not indicate that the intervention should be the same. The clinician faces several challenges when initiating a physical intervention program. Specifically, the clinician must

1. Identify gait abnormalities.
2. Determine the causes of the patient's difficulty with gait.
3. Interpret the relationship between impairments and physical performance.
4. Set appropriate goals.
5. Choose an appropriate treatment strategy and techniques.

The decisions that the clinician makes regarding intervention should have a theoretical basis grounded in research. Unfortunately, there are few studies available that include investigating the rehabilitation of people with gait disturbances and delineating guidelines for rehabilitation [6, 7]. There is available, however, much conceptual information that serves as a theoretical basis for the approach to intervention outlined in this chapter, and this material functions as a framework that can be used to guide decisions.

A FRAMEWORK FOR MAKING CLINICAL DECISIONS REGARDING INTERVENTION

The goal of physical intervention is to optimize the patient's safe, functional, and efficient ambulation. A skilled clinician accomplishes this task by correctly interpreting the causes of dysfunction, setting priorities, and then choosing treatment strategies that are specific for the individual patient. No single set of physical intervention techniques can be used to correct gait deficiencies, even when patients have similar underlying pathological conditions or when their gait abnormalities appear similar. Physical intervention is most likely to be successful and efficient if the clinician has systematically analyzed the patient's deficits and has decided which problems to correct, which to compensate for, and which to prevent.

A patient often has myriad problems that could be evaluated and interpreted. Several authors have proposed strategies to organize information linking underlying difficulties within specific systems to the patient's overall function [8–13]. The systematic approach used in this chapter is based on conceptual work originally proposed by Nagi [9] and by the World Health Organization [10] and later adapted by The Committee Toward a National Agenda for the Prevention of Disabilities [11]. The practical use of this model for clinical decision-making purposes has been published elsewhere [8].

With this systematic approach, a clinician differentiates among functional limitations, physical performance of gait, underlying impairments, and underlying pathology. *Functional limitations* refer to those activities required in daily life that an individual cannot carry out successfully or efficiently (e.g., inability to enter or leave one's home independently). *Physical performance* refers to the manner in which activities are carried out. Physical performance of gait can be characterized through biomechanical characteristics and in terms of functional gait indicators.

Underlying impairments causing gait disturbances are deficits within systems (e.g. musculoskeletal deficits, such as weakness and contracture; neurological deficits, such as perceptual or coordination problems). Impairments are differentiated into direct effects, which occur as direct consequences of a disease process or injury (e.g., joint limitation with degenerative joint disease) and indirect effects, which occur as sequelae to the initial impairments (e.g., low endurance secondary to a sedentary lifestyle that results from pain) [8]. This differentiation helps the clinician determine those impairments that can potentially be corrected through physical techniques, those that are less likely to respond to physical intervention, and those that should be prevented (as will be illustrated throughout this chapter). *Underlying pathology* refers to interruption or interference of normal bodily processes. Pathology occurs at the level of cells and tissues and is one source of impairments.

Buchner et al. [13] identified three possible entrances to the cycle of pathology, impairments, functional limitations, and injury: (1) specific disease processes (e.g., osteoarthritis, cardiovascular disease, Parkinson's disease), (2) disuse (e.g., deconditioning due to a sedentary lifestyle), and (3) biological aging (e.g., slowing of nerve conduction velocities in the absence of specific disease). For some patients, the entrance to the cycle involving impairments, decline of physical performance, and functional limitations is a cumulative effect of many subtle changes rather than of a single event. Even when patients have specific disorders, such as a stroke or Parkinson's disease, they commonly have coexisting diseases, such as osteoarthritis, that compound their difficulties with gait.

The elements of the framework and decision-making process are outlined in Table 21-1; this framework is used throughout this chapter as an organizing principle. The clinician begins by identifying functional limitations based on an analysis of the physical performance of gait, including functional gait indicators and a biomechanical movement analysis (see Table 21-1). The next step is to determine underlying impairments and also to determine factors that modify a patient's response to impairments and functional limitations. Relevant modifiers include the patient's social support system, emotional state, premorbid lifestyle, and will to retain or achieve independence. Finally, the clinician interprets the observed impairments to identify the various entry points to the cycle of dysfunction (i.e., disease, injury, disuse, nonspecific aging, or some combination of these).

Because correction of a specific impairment may or may not lead to improved gait, the clinician must interpret the interrelationships between impairments, physical performance of gait, and functional limitations so as to direct treatment most efficiently. This interpretation includes (1) probable causes of underlying impairments; (2) consequences of impairments both with respect to the functional gait indicators and the biomechanical characteristics; (3) relative importance of the underlying impairments in producing the gait disturbance; and (4) expectation that specific underlying impairments can be corrected, compensated for, or prevented through physical techniques. Once this analysis is complete,

Table 21-1. Framework for decision making for
physical intervention of elderly patients with gait disorders

1. Identify functional limitations
2. Characterize physical performance of gait
    a. Functional gait indicators
        (1) Velocity
        (2) Endurance
        (3) Stability
        (4) Adaptability
        (5) Assistance
        (6) Safety
    b. Biomechanical analysis
        (1) Spatial characteristics
        (2) Temporal characteristics
        (3) Joint/segmental motion/alignment
        (4) Forces
3. Identify underlying impairments and modifiers related to gait and to the total
    physical assessment
    a. Impairments
        (1) Musculoskeletal
        (2) Neurological
        (3) Cardiovascular
    b. Modifiers
        (1) Mental status
        (2) Social support
        (3) Preexisting lifestyle
        (4) Preexisting medical conditions
4. Interpret the relationships between impairments and physical performance; identify
    the precipating causes of functional limitations; differentiate among direct, indirect,
    and composite effects of disease or injury
5. Determine problems to be treated
6. Set goals
7. Choose physical techniques for intervention

the clinician is ready to determine goals of intervention and to set the strategy
for physical intervention. This framework and systematic approach allows the
clinician to focus the evaluation process, to make logical decisions regarding intervention, and to make decisions regarding measurement of outcomes [8].

This process is illustrated by a frail elderly woman in early stages of Parkinson's disease, with mild osteoarthritic changes of the spine, moderate bilateral
osteoarthritis of the knees, and genu varum. This case example is used throughout the remainder of the chapter to illustrate decisions regarding the general approach to treatment and the actual techniques used:

Mrs. Warren past 76 years old, was 5 ft. 6 in., and weighed 110 pounds. She
was able to carry out basic activities of daily living independently, such as bathing
and dressing, but had neither the stability nor the endurance to cook, clean, or
manage the household independently. She tended to hold onto furniture when
she felt unsteady inside the house. She had had several near falls. Her 74-year-
old sister, with whom she lived, managed the household. On stairs, Mrs. Warren

Table 21-2. Framework for decision making: the characteristics of gait as illustrated by the evaluation of Mrs. Warren

1. Identify functional limitations
2. Characterize physical performance of gait
   a. Functional gait indicators
      (1) Velocity: 10 meters in 14 sec
      (2) Endurance: 846 feet in 6 min
      (3) Stability: adequate for household activities; assistance required to walk in the community
      (4) Adaptability
         Stairs: one step at a time
         Curbs: requires assistance
         Cannot carry items and walk at the same time
      (5) Assistance: sister's arm when in community
      (6) Safety: good judgment; appropriately conservative
   b. Biomechanical analysis
      (1) Spatial characteristics: short symmetrical step, narrow base of support
      (2) Temporal characteristics: slow velocity overall, symmetrical but slow knee motion
      (3) Joint/segmental motion/alignment: excessive subtalar eversion; continued trunk, hip, knee flexion throughout gait cycle; limited ankle dorsiflexion; upper body relatively immobile (no arm swing or pelvic rotation); genu varum
      (4) Forces: excessive force at heel strike
3. Identify underlying impairments and modifiers
4. Interpret relationships
5. Determine problems to be treated
6. Set goals
7. Choose physical techniques for intervention

held onto a railing and ascended or descended one step at a time. She had difficulty negotiating curbs. When Mrs. Warren walked outside the house, she held onto her sister's arm for stability. She tired easily and feared she would fall.

Identification of Gait Abnormalities

Before an intervention program can be established, the clinician must describe which aspects of gait dysfunction can and should be corrected. This requires accurate assessment of gait abnormalities. Disturbances or abnormalities of gait should be described from two perspectives: (1) functional gait indicators and (2) movement (biomechanical) analysis of the person's gait (Table 21-2). These descriptions of gait are the initial focus of assessing gait disturbances.

The term *functional gait indicators* identifies those attributes of gait that relate directly to functional use of gait at home or in the community. Functional gait indicators include speed (e.g., a person's ability to walk fast enough to cross a street before the light changes), endurance (e.g., walking far enough to accomplish grocery shopping or to go to the mailbox), balance control (e.g., whether assistance is required from devices or another person), adaptability (e.g., the ability to walk on different surfaces and terrain), and safety. Functional measures are available to capture speed of gait (e.g., the 10-meter walk test [14] and endurance (e.g., the

6-min. walk test) [15]. Stability and assistance requirements can be determined under increasingly difficult conditions (e.g., level surfaces, ramps, stairs).

In Mrs. Warren's case, three major areas of concern related to the functional use of gait. She had poor balance control and decreased endurance for walking, and she walked slowly and with effort. She had poor adaptability to changing surfaces, but (except for stairs and curbs) this was not a problem, because she limited her walking to the household and to level surfaces within the community.

Biomechanical characteristics of gait are identified and analyzed because they link functional gait problems to underlying causes and are used to determine appropriate physical intervention. The *biomechanical characteristics* of a person's gait include description of motion and alignment and of forces involved in producing movement [16]. We recommend both qualitative assessment (e.g., visual observation) and quantitative assessment (e.g., videotape, force platform, pressure platform analysis) of a person's gait, depending on what is appropriate and feasible. Each method of assessment of gait involves issues of convenience, time, equipment availability, patient fatigue, observation or technical skill, and so on, which have been addressed elsewhere [16, 17].

Difficulties during gait are localized to one or more of three basic tasks [16]: (1) weight acceptance, (2) single-limb support, and (3) (swing) limb advancement. For a more detailed analysis of gait, a number of formats may be followed. We recommend analyzing gait by observing or measuring gait parameters, including

1. Spatial or distance characteristics of foot-to-floor contact.
2. Temporal characteristics of gait.
3. Joint or segmental motions and alignments (e.g., individual joints and coordinated total body motions and alignment).
4. Internal and external forces.

Spatial characteristics of foot-to-floor contact are descriptors of how the foot contacts the floor. The important variables to note are step length, step width, angulation of the foot in relation to the path of progression (toe-out angle), and base of support (orientation of the feet on the floor and in reference to the body). Typical spatial characteristics noted in elderly people as compared to middle-aged adults are shortened step length, widened step width, increased toe-out angle, and increased base of support.

Temporal characteristics of gait encompass the gait velocity of the person, timing factors related to joint motions (e.g., faster subtalar eversion on one side) or to floor contact (e.g., longer stance time on one side), and symmetry of timing factors. Differences in temporal characteristics often noted in elderly people as compared to middle-aged adults include decreased velocity of gait, increased floor contact time overall and for each foot, and decreased velocity of joint motions. When specific pathology occurs, asymmetry within the gait pattern is often noted.

Joint or segmental motions and alignment include description of the motions and postures occurring at the joints, within the segments of the body, and for the total body and description of the symmetry of those motions. These motions and alignments are noted in a sequential manner from the ground up and include assessment of the toes, foot, ankle, knee, hip, pelvis, lumbar spine, thoracic spine, upper extremities, neck, and head. Compared to the gait of middle-aged adults, common findings in the gait of elderly people include decreased hip hyperextension, dorsiflexion, pelvic rotation, and arm swing. The end ranges of only four joint motions are required for normal gait: hip hyperextension, knee extension, ankle dorsiflexion, and great toe metatarsophalangeal hyperextension. Therefore, limited hip hyperextension would result in a gait disturbance, whereas limited knee flexion range may not. The sum of the timing and joint or segmental motion dictates the coordinated whole-body movement of gait.

The *forces* involved during gait include both external and internal forces. Relevant forces outside the body (external forces) include the effect of gravity on the person's posture, the magnitude and speed of contact of the foot on the ground, and the dampening (shock absorption) of the foot-to-ground contact forces. Significant forces inside the body (internal forces) include the force requirements from muscles, tendons, ligaments, bones, and fascia; the forces on the joints; and friction occurring between structures. Examples of forces relevant to elderly people would be excessive joint forces and pressures on the medial knee during walking for a person with a severe genu varum; the tendency for gravitational pull to increase the thoracic kyphosis of a person who already has an excessive thoracic kyphosis; or the potentially damaging effect of landing hard and fast on the heels, especially with a rigid foot structure or other deficit that makes shock absorption difficult [18] or for a person with bones weakened from osteoporosis. The forces of gait (and any movement pattern) are the most difficult of the four components to assess without sophisticated equipment.

The specifics of those concepts are illustrated by Mrs. Warren. The functional gait indicators and biomechanical characteristics of Mrs. Warren's gait are outlined in Table 21-2.

Interpretation of Underlying Causes of Gait Difficulties

Once the functional indicators of gait have been identified and the biomechanical analysis is complete, a clinician interprets the observed gait with respect to potential underlying causes of dysfunction (e.g., impairments). For example, a person may walk slowly (functional gait indicator) and take small steps (biomechanical characteristic) for many reasons. To interpret the causes, the clinician evaluates impairments in the different systems and decides whether specific impairments relate to the performance of gait and the extent to which the impairment can be improved with physical intervention.

Musculoskeletal, neurological, and cardiovascular impairments can influence gait directly and significantly (Table 21-3). Musculoskeletal impairments that can cause abnormal gait include alignment, posture, range of motion, muscle strength, and endurance. If any of these factors is not sufficient to support gait, an abnormality will occur in the phase of gait where that factor is required. For example, limited pelvic rotation, hip or knee extension, or ankle dorsiflexion

Table 21-3. Physical impairments that can influence gait

Musculoskeletal	Neurological	Cardiovascular
Posture	Sensory perception; sensory interpretation	Aerobic capacity
Joint structure	Motor planning*	Endurance
Joint alignment	Motor programming	Energy metabolism
Joint range of motion	Timing and coordination	Vascular integrity
Muscle length and flexibility	Sensory and motor integration	
Muscle strength and endurance	Pain	

* *Motor planning* refers to an action whose execution requires the sequential operation of a number of simple motor programs. Impaired motor planning is frequently observed in patients who have Parkinson's disease and is evidenced by the inability to carry out two actions simultaneously. The classic example is the patient who stands up to shake hands and either drops the oustretched hand or holds the hand outstretched while falling back onto the seat.
SOURCE: Adapted from TM Cutson. Assessment of motor planning deficits. *Top Geriatr Rehab* 1994; 10:56–69.

range of motion can each restrict step length (i.e., limb advancement) as can threatened balance control, knee pain, lack of cardiovascular endurance [19], and, therefore, speed of walking. Observed decreased step length would warrant investigation to determine which specific factors account for the decrease for a particular patient. Table 21-4 outlines musculoskeletal, neurological, and cardiovascular components of each of Mrs. Warren's three major areas of concern related to the functional use of gait.

The importance of each of the impairments as related to gait must be considered. Musculoskeletal problems may limit walking speed, endurance, and safety. Decreased ankle range of motion and strength most likely interfere with stability during gait and appear to be related to likelihood of falling [20, 21]. Loss of mobility of the lumbar and thoracic spine coupled with postural abnormalities set limits to the potential strategies for balance control [20] and is associated with performance of tasks such as reaching or turning 360 degrees while standing [22]. Weight bearing on malaligned joints may result in excessive joint contact pressures. Decreased hip hyperextension results in inability to stretch the hip flexors in terminal stance and, therefore, limits the rebound of the stretch that provides force for advancement of the swing limb.

The performance of gait also is determined by a person's neurological integrity and function, such as the capacity for motor control, as expressed through neuromuscular processing [3–5, 7, 23–25]. For example, loss of lower-extremity position sense may cause a person to reduce step length, to widen the base of support, and to be generally hesitant in walking, despite available range of motion. These gait abnormalities may be exaggerated when the person walks in the dark. Sensory losses may limit safety, speed, endurance, or adaptability. Impairments of motor planning may cause a person to have difficulty adjusting gait to changing circumstances and can lead to freezing during gait (as seen in Parkinson's disease). Impairments of timing and coordination (e.g., with cerebellar disease), can result in instability and incoordination. The combined abnormalities of timing, force production, and sensory processing (as occur with many strokes) may cause gait to become effortful, so that endurance and speed are compromised.

The performance of gait is dependent on an individual's physiological endurance for activity determined by cardiovascular condition. Impairments of the cardiovascular system frequently limit endurance or speed or gait-related activities (e.g., a person may no longer have the endurance to climb stairs).

The physical capacity for gait is tempered by modifying factors that include an individual's cognitive status, family and community support, and perhaps most important—the inherent motivation or will to succeed. Though a patient may have good musculoskeletal integrity, cardiovascular condition, and be without frank sensory motor deficits, without judgment and the ability to make appropriate decisions, such a patient would be unsafe alone and therefore extremely limited in functional capacity for gait. Alternatively, an individual might have severe musculoskeletal impairments, resulting in marked abnormalities of the physical performance of gait, and yet be functionally independent through determination to succeed. These concepts are illustrated by the impairments related to Mrs. Warren's gait (Table 21-5).

For the elderly patient, gait dysfunction often is a cumulative consequence of multiple underlying causes [4, 21]. Often, no single impairment on its own is severe enough to lead to gait disturbances, but the total multiple, subtle changes could cause functional limitations or disability. Several coordinated joint movement abilities, called *determinants of gait*, may allow the person to improve a gait disturbance. The determinants of gait include pelvic rotation, lateral tilt and lateral displacement of the pelvis, knee flexion in stance, and interrelated hip, knee, and ankle motion during walking. If the existing impairments are severe or numerous enough, the use of these determinants may not be adequate to normalize the person's gait.

Table 21-4. Example of impairments that affected Mrs. Warren's gait

Impairment	Musculoskeletal	Neurological	Cardiovascular
Poor balance control	Limited lower-extremity ROM Limited lumbopelvic ROM Excessive thoracic kyphosis	Retropulsion	
Decreased endurance for walking		Knee pain	Poor aerobic capacity
Slowness and effortful walking	Limited lower-extremity ROM	Bradykinesia; poor motor planning ability*	Poor aerobic capacity

ROM = range of motion.
* *Motor planning* refers to an action whose execution requires the sequential operation of a number of simple motor programs. Impaired motor planning is frequently observed in patients who have Parkinson's disease and is evidenced by the inability to carry out two actions simultaneously. The classic example is the patient who stands up to shake hands and either drops the outstretched hand or holds the hand outstretched while falling back onto the seat.
SOURCE: Adapted from TM Cutson. Assessment of motor planning deficits. *Top Geriatr Rehabil* 1994;10:56–69.

Table 21-5. Framework for decision making: impairments that affect gait as illustrated by the evaluation of Mrs. Warren

1. Identify functional limitations
2. Characterize physical performance of gait (see Table 21-2)
3. Identify underlying impairments and modifiers
   a. Impairments
      (1) *Musculoskeletal*
         Hip limited in all motions except flexion
         Knee limited for flexion and extension
         Ankle—limited dorsiflexion
         Excessive subtalar eversion
         Mild genu varum
         Mildly excessive thoracic kyphosis and loss of lumbar lordosis
         Pelvic mobility limited in all directions
      (2) *Neurological*
         Moderate rigidity
         Without tremor
         Retropulsion on postural pull test
         Mild motor planning deficits
      (3) *Cardiovascular*
         Generally deconditioned
   b. Modifiers
      (1) *Mental status*
         Folstein score* of 27
         Positive outlook
         No depression noted
      (2) *Social support*
         Strong family and community ties
      (3) *Preexisting lifestyle*
         Active and independent
      (4) *Preexisting medical conditions*
         None
4. Interpret relationships
5. Determine problems to be treated
6. Set goals
7. Choose physical techniques for intervention

* See MF Folstein, SE Folstein, PR McHugh. "Mini-mental state": A practical method for grading the cognitive state of patients for the clinician. *J Psychiatr Res* 1975;12:189–198.

The clinician's task in linking impairments to physical gait performance parameters is to make judgments regarding (1) the relative impact of the different impairments on the patient's gait, (2) the extent to which treating these deficits will improve gait, (3) whether deficits should be corrected by physical intervention or by compensation, and (4) impairments that are potential precursors to future problems and should be prevented.

The interpretation of the four major areas of concern related to Mrs. Warren's physical gait performance illustrates this process (i.e., poor balance control, decreased endurance for walking, slow and effortful walking, and landing hard and fast on her heels). The clinician interpreted each of these problems with respect to musculoskeletal, neurological, and cardiovascular causes (see

Table 12-4). In addition, the clinician developed hypotheses regarding which aspect of the dysfunction were direct effects of the underlying pathological processes, which were indirect effects, and which had multiple underlying causes. For example, cardiovascular deconditioning could result from this woman's sedentary lifestyle alone but probably is compounded by Parkinson's disease and by the knee pain that she experiences with activity. Limited knee range of motion and articular changes can be direct effects of the arthritic condition but also can occur as an indirect effect of the Parkinson's disease, compounding the loss of range. Excessive thoracic kyphosis tends to increase with increasing age [22, 26] but also can occur as an indirect effect of the bradykinesia and rigidity of Parkinson's disease [27].

On the basis of these analyses, the clinician can hypothesize which problems are likely to be corrected through physical techniques, which should be prevented, and to what extent compensatory strategies might be needed. In Mrs. Warren's case, limited range of motion and cardiovascular endurance can be corrected or at least improved. As range of motion increases, stability, speed, and endurance for walking also may improve. Similarly, if cardiovascular endurance increases, speed and endurance for walking may improve. In contrast, poor postural control that occurs as a direct effect of Parkinson's disease will not respond appreciably to physical intervention. Mrs. Warren should be encouraged to use a cane (rather than her sister) to **compensate** for those aspects of poor balance control that cannot be corrected with physical intervention. This will increase her independence and allow her to have a more normal gait pattern.

The clinician also predicts, and attempts to **prevent**, the indirect effects of disease that are likely to occur in the future. For example, loss of neck, trunk, and extremity range of motion commonly occurs as an indirect effect of Parkinson's disease, as does altered posture (excessive thoracic kyphosis and flexed postures of the extremities) [27, 28]. These impairments may further compromise balance control, aerobic capacity, and therefore stability and speed of gait. The pain and restricted motion occurring with arthritis of the knees may result in a more sedentary life, which leads to decreased cardiovascular endurance. Prevention or correction of indirect as well as direct effects of disease can break the spiraling cycle of disease/pathology/impairments/functional limitation. In the example given, increases in thoracic kyphosis and knee malalignment should be **prevented,** along with pneumonia, a common problem for elderly individuals who have Parkinson's disease.

Finally, the clinician assesses the modifying factors that either facilitate or limit functional performance. Mrs. Warren was motivated and had a good family and social support system. Her sister was willing and able to take her to the clinic for physical intervention, and Mrs. Warren was able to continue exercises on her own after the intervention program was completed. An exercise program might not have been appropriate had she been poorly motivated and unable to take responsibility for her intervention. There is little point in correcting impairments if the patient will not take responsibility for her intervention. There is little point in correcting impairments if the patient will not take responsibility to retain the gains achieved. Most patients will not have access to continuous assistance from a skilled clinician in order to retain the gains.

In summary, it is important to be methodical in interpreting the causes of a person's gait dysfunction. An effective system assists a clinician in interpreting causes of dysfunction and allows for differentiation between those impairments that can be corrected by physical intervention and those that cannot. When the underlying dysfunction can be corrected, the clinician should select the most appropriate approaches. When the underlying dysfunction cannot be corrected, the system guides the clinician's determination of appropriate ways for an individual to compensate for the disorder. Future problems should be anticipated and prevented.

PRACTICAL CONSIDERATIONS IN SETTING GOALS FOR TREATMENT

Before initiating an intervention program, the clinician should decide on the goals of intervention, with respect to both the person's gait and the underlying impairments. Specifically, a decision should be made as to the extent to which the functional limitations will be treated and whether underlying impairments will be corrected, compensated for, or prevented. Based on these decisions, the clinician sets goals that serve to structure the actual treatment program. There are no absolute guidelines regarding the most appropriate choice of intervention; rather, the intervention is developed from scientific rationale. General considerations that should shape the goals of intervention are outlined here.

The goals must be consistent with the patient's own goals, with his or her lifestyle and expectations, and with the total medical picture. There is little point to a goal of maintaining an aerobic walking program unless an individual understands the relevance of the program and has a commitment to its goals. A goal of being able to walk three miles daily may not be realistic if the patient has not been a community ambulator for the past 15 years. Even if it is mechanically feasible for a person to walk independently, setting independent ambulation as a goal is contraindicated if the person's judgment is so severely impaired that falls and injuries are likely.

The goal of treatment is to improve gait for functional use; hence, the overall goals of treatment should be functionally relevant. The clinician must decide which functional characteristics of gait are problematic for each patient. Does the patient need to walk faster? Should endurance increase? Is safety an issue? Does the patient require greater adaptability before gait is functional? The goal of treatment is not always to correct a problem but may be to prevent further injury or dysfunction. For example, abnormal forces occurring during gait can be a precipitant of serious long-term wear and tear on joints. Landing hard and fast on the heels during weight acceptance (especially with inadequate knee flexion for shock absorption) can result in excessive forces on the knee and ultimately can lead to osteoarthritis [18].

The clinician always must balance that which *could* be changed with that which

Table 21-6. Framework for decision making:
goals and treatment as illustrated by Mrs. Warren

1. Identify functional limitations
   Cannot cook or carry out heavy housework
   Tendency to fall entering tub
   Cannot walk safely in the community
2. Characterize physical performance of gait (see Table 21-2)
3. Identify underlying impairments and modifiers (see Tables 21-4, 21-5)
4. Interpret relationships
5. Determine problems to be treated
6. Set goals
   Increase aerobic capacity without mechanical damage
   Normalize thoracolumbopelvic mobility
   Normalize hip, knee, and ankle range
   Improve balance control and posture
   Improve ability to gauge activity to protect joint (of knee and spine)
   Improve movement stategies for sit to stand and gait
7. Choose physical techniques for intervention
   Aquatics for aerobic condition, strength, and flexibility (substitutions: biking
      [reclining] for aerobic conditioning; nonaquatic lower-extremity stretching and
      strengthening)
   Cushioned and supportive shoe wear
   Assistive device: straight cane
   Movement reeducation: land softly to protect joints; sitting to standing; gait
   Practice in a variety of environments to enhance functionality

---

should be changed. Goals for correction of gait deficits must be realistic in context of the patient's total circumstances. This requires interpretation of the gait deficits in the context of all comorbidities as well as the patient's lifestyle and goals.

The requirements for optimal movement performance depend on the specific nature of a task. For example, gait requires full extension of the knee but only approximately 50 to 70 degrees of flexion [29] whereas going from sitting to standing normally requires both full extension of the knee and at least 95 to 100 degrees of flexion, depending on the height of the seat. Similarly, loss of subtalar motion may not interfere with walking on level surfaces but may lead to inability to compensate for uneven terrain and may, therefore, contribute to a patient's tendency to fall when walking outside. Strengthening, increasing range of motion, and improving balance control can be appropriate goals for selected patients.

In Mrs. Warren's case, both safety and endurance limited function (Table 21-6). She tired easily, was afraid of falling, and used her sister's arm for stability in the community. Goals related to the functional aspects of gait included safe, independent ambulation within the house; safe ambulation with an appropriate assistive device when accompanied by another person outside the house; and adequate speed and endurance to walk distances that would allow her to accomplish desired community activities. Target speed was 10 meters in 8 seconds; target distance was 1,100 feet in 6 minutes.

Analysis of Mrs. Warren's gait impairments (and modifying factors previously described) guided the clinician's decisions regarding how to improve the functional indicators of gait. Though there were no specific goals to correct these biomechanical characteristics of gait, they should improve as underlying impairments are corrected. The one exception was the problem of landing hard and fast on the heels. The clinician specifically identified correction of this gait characteristic as a goal because it was evident even with visual observation of Mrs. Warren's gait and was judged to be potentially damaging.

The impairments that appeared most relevant were knee pain, limited joint motion, and cardiovascular condition (see Table 21-4). Rigidity was judged to contribute to the limited joint range of motion and to postural abnormalities. Bradykinesia and motor planning deficits were only minimally present at the time of this evaluation, although they may worsen as the Parkinson's disease progresses. Malalignment of the knees was long-standing and did not respond to such physical intervention as orthotics in the shoes. The excessive subtalar eversion was a necessary compensation to let the medial heel reach the ground. The goal with respect to knee pain was to help Mrs. Warren to determine realistic boundaries for physical activity that would allow her to accomplish her social and household activities without unduly exacerbating the arthritic condition of her knees. Mrs. Warren was advised regarding joint protection to prevent or lessen further degenerative changes. Joint protection included use of one or two canes, movement reeducation to ensure landing more softly, and cushioned and supportive shoes.

The impairments that specifically contributed to Mrs. Warren's slowness of gait included decreased hip and knee extension, decreased lumbopelvofemoral mobility, poor movement coordination, and knee pain (see Table 21-4). Increased range of motion for both the lower extremities and the thoracolumbopelvic area might reduce the mechanical stress to the knees and improve speed of walking. Movement reeducation was necessary for Mrs. Warren to maximize use of newly gained mobility. Goals included increasing knee and hip extension range of motion, ankle dorsiflexion and lumbopelvofemoral motion in all planes, improving coordinated functional movement for gait, and improving aerobic capacity.

The impairments that appeared most relevant to Mrs. Warren's poor balance control were a primary deficit of postural control due to Parkinson's disease and loss of mobility throughout the spine and lower extremities. Difficulty with motor planning was very mild and judged to be noncontributory. Retropulsion (uncontrolled stepping or falling backwards when pulled backwards from the waist) occurs as a direct effect of the Parkinson's disease and does not appear to be corrected through physical intervention. The other contributors to loss of balance control could, however, be treated. Goals included increased mobility of the lumbar spine in all directions, increased range of motion of the lower extremity (including hip and knee extension), hip rotation, and ankle dorsiflexion.

In summary, many elderly individuals have a host of impairments that could be treated physically. Judgment is essential as the clinician decides which ones to attempt to correct. The clinician must prioritize to correct those impairments that most limit the functional characteristics of gait and must know which impairments are most likely to respond to physical intervention. For example, restrictions of muscle length and loss of strength should respond to physical intervention, even among the elderly [30–33]. The clinician must:

1. Recognize fixed deformities unlikely to respond to physical intervention (e.g., long-standing excessive kyphosis or malalignment of the knees secondary to osteoarthritis).
2. Know whether the impairment limits function now or is likely to in the future.
3. Decide whether modifying factors (the patient's motivation, cognitive ability, and judgment) contraindicate correction of certain impairments.
4. Consider the patient's ability and willingness to take responsibility for the physical intervention program.
5. Not spend valuable time correcting musculoskeletal impairments if the patient will resume a sedentary lifestyle posttherapy and the return of impairments is likely.
6. Focus on correcting underlying impairments that are clearly identified if gait is the only or main movement problem. The interpretation of direct, indirect, and composite effects of pathology and interpretation of their ramifications for performance of gait can assist the clinician in deciding which impairments are of high priority and should be corrected.

CHOOSING THE APPROPRIATE TREATMENT APPROACH

Once the goals of intervention have been established, the clinician must decide on a treatment strategy. Decisions must be made with respect both to the techniques that will be used and to delivery of the treatment program. A variety of techniques are used routinely in clinical settings for correcting impairments and improving functional use of gait [7, 34–36]. There are few comparisons of the efficacy of one approach to another. The clinician, therefore, depends on analysis of the underlying deficits (coupled with personal or others' experience) when deciding which techniques to use with a particular patient. Techniques should be based on the patient's specific impairments, the severity of the impairments that limit gait, and other limiting factors (e.g., cancer and resulting impairments unrelated to gait that alter the patient's potential to regain optimal gait). The patient's specific abilities and limitations and preferred learning style also are important determinants of the clinician's choice of intervention. General considerations that help to determine specific treatment techniques are discussed here, using treatment of Mrs. Warren to illustrate which decisions were made and why.

Mrs. Warren's difficulties with gait were interpreted within a broader functional context. She was an independent ambulator in that she could walk without assistance. However, Mrs. Warren was having increasing difficulty moving from a sitting to a standing position independently. She had a tendency to fall back onto the seat before achieving the erect standing posture. A person who cannot

Table 21-7. Outline of the physical intervention program for Mrs. Warren (treatment related to endurance, flexibility, balance control, posture, strengthening, and function)

Goal 1: Increase aerobic capacity without damaging joint mechanics
    Aquatics program: 2–3 times per week, gradually increasing from 10 min to 30–40 min
    Walking forward, backward, sideways with the incorporation of upper-body motion, eventually while holding empty closed plastic milk or water jugs
    Reclining bike as an alternative
    Outcome measures: time of continued activity, heart rate, perceived exertion

Goal 2: Normalize flexibility of thoracic and lumbar spine, pelvis, hips, knees, and ankles[a]
    Axial mobility exercises [38] from stages I, II, III
    Aquatics exercises used for lower-limb flexibility
    Wall stretches for ankle flexibility
    Outcome measures: thoracic and lumbar mobility measured by kyphometer and BROM, respectively.[b] Hip, knee, and ankle range of motion measured by goniometer

Goal 3: Improve balance control[a]
    Axial mobility exercises [38], stage V
    Balance activities involving self-initiated perturbations in sitting and standing
    Structured walking on uneven surfaces
    Outcome measures: functional reach

Goal 4: Normalize posture[a]
    Visualization exercises for improved posture (e.g., visualizing raising the sternum toward the ceiling
    Outcome measures: thoracolumbar posture by kyphometer, overall posture[b] visual inspection

Goal 5: Strengthen back extensors and lower-limb muscles (especially antigravity lower-limb muscles)[a]
    Back extensors by walking backward during aquatics (emphasized over walking forward)
    Lower-limb muscles by walking in all directions during aquatics
    Antigravity lower-limb muscles by stationary bike
    Outcome measures: dynamometry for lower-limb muscles

Goal 6: Improve ability to gauge physical activity while conserving energy and protecting joints[a]
    Movement re-education strategies, emphasizing landing softly on the heels while walking and generally moving with smooth flowing motions
    Cushioned shoe inserts, especially on the heels
    Training in the safe use of an assistive device for gait
    Training in the efficient and effective use of movement strategies, such as backlying to stand
    Training in the safe modification of velocity changes during gait
    Axial mobility exercise [38], stage V
    Outcome measures: distance walked in 6 min; time to walk 10 m at self-selected and maximal safe speed; ability to use a cane safely in various environments; loading rate at initial contact of gait as measured on a force plate

[a] Treatment related to goals 2–6: Two to three sessions per week for 40 minutes for 1 month for training; supervision and progression tapered to one session weekly, then monthly for 4 months.
[b] See, for example, M Schenkman et al. Relationships between mobility of axial structure and physical performance. *Phys Ther* 1996; 76:276–285.

transfer independently cannot be functionally independent, regardless of ability to "walk." Intervention for Mrs. Warren's gait difficulties necessarily included intervention for her difficulties moving from a sitting to a standing position.

Treatment included a combination of techniques for specific impairments and a functional approach (Table 21-7). On initial evaluation the clinician had identified significant weakness of the quadriceps muscles. Observation of Mrs. Warren's transfer performance indicated that her alignment was poor and that she did not have range of motion of the lumbopelvofemoral area adequate to maintain an appropriate posture of the upper body while executing the task. Furthermore, her balance control was compromised, and she had knee pain at the initiation of standing. All these difficulties contributed to compromised transfer ability and were interpreted as limiting factors for Mrs. Warren's gait. Treatment began with correction of specific impairments and with her transfer performance.

Treatment of Specific Impairments

A host of approaches could be used to treat impairments of range of motion, alignment, strength, balance control, and pain. For example, range of motion can be corrected either by stretching or relaxation techniques or by movement re-education [35, 37–39]. In Mrs. Warren's case, the relaxation approach [38], rather than forceful stretching, was chosen for improving range of motion of axial structures (cervical, thoracic, and lumber spine), the shoulder complex (connecting scapula to thorax and to humerus), and for muscles that connect the pelvis and lower extremities. (See Appendix A for a summary of this treatment approach.) This choice was made because it has been suggested that postural deformity associated with Parkinson's disease is a result of rigidity coupled with bradykinesia. To counteract the effects of rigidity, a relaxation approach to exercise has been suggested for persons with Parkinson's disease [27]. Furthermore, the clinician wanted to avoid stressful activities that could exacerbate Mrs. Warren's underlying osteoarthritis of the spine. Relaxation techniques have the added benefit of reducing any existing discomfort or pain. In contrast, range of motion of the distal extremities (e.g., ankle and foot or elbow and wrist) was achieved most easily by using stretching, with the understanding that flexibility gains must be gradual and take longer with elderly people [40]. This part of the program was incorporated with pool exercises (as described below) in light of the osteoarthritic condition of Mrs. Warren's knees. Regardless of whether a stretching or relaxation-based approach is used, the clinician must decide whether to use passive techniques (applied by the therapist), active techniques (applied by the patient), or both. In Mrs. Warren's case, all range-of-motion exercises were performed actively by the patient, who was highly motivated and had good cognitive ability to correctly monitor her performance of the exercises.

With respect to muscle strengthening, decisions must be made regarding the speed at which strengthening will occur (slow or fast), where in the joint range to strengthen, and whether to strengthen in an open or closed kinetic chain [41]. Both concentric and eccentric strengthening are advised because muscles contract in both modes during transfers and gait. *Concentric strengthening* refers to strengthening while the muscle is shortening under a load (e.g., the quadriceps muscle acts to extend the knee, in sitting to standing, against gravity). *Eccentric strengthening* refers to strengthening as the muscle lengthens under a load (e.g., the quadriceps muscle acts to control the return of the extended knee to the flexed position when returning to sitting). Training in one mode does not ensure strengthening in the alternate mode. Strengthening should occur at differing speeds, and those speeds should be functionally relevant. Patients should be able to generate appropriate force in muscles at variable speeds so as to function under a diversity of environmental conditions. Specific choices will be dictated by the functional tasks for which strengthening is indicated.

Mrs. Warren had compromised quadriceps strength. She had difficulty standing from the seated position, controlling standing-to-sitting performance, and with quick contractions of the quadriceps muscles during gait. For transferring in and out of chairs, improving strength at lower speeds and in both concentric and eccentric contractions was a goal. To improve strength and timing for walking, a strengthening program was implemented using faster speeds of muscle contraction and emphasizing appropriate timing of muscle contractions and strength.

Aerobic conditioning can be achieved by using any activity that increases heart rate to within the patient's aerobic conditioning range. This can be accomplished through a walking program, arm ergometry, bicycling, or pool therapy. The choice of technique will be dictated by the patient's overall status and by convenience. A walking program was contraindicated for Mrs. Warren because she had significant knee joint malalignment. Knee pain secondary to the malalignment was exacerbated by walking distances, and there was a potential to worsen the joint deformity with the repetitive stresses of gait. Arm ergometry, stationary biking, or aquatic therapy were appropriate for her safe aerobic conditioning. For patients who do not have access to a pool or a stationary bike, a restorator might be appropriate, or an individualized exercise program, such as the stretch-and-strengthen program of Watson [37], may be used.

Approaches to management of pain include methods of pain alleviation and compensation for underlying conditions that produce the pain. For example, ultrasound, heat or cold, and analgesics may be used to alleviate pain. Stretching of soft tissue, strengthening of appropriate muscles, and muscle reeducation may contribute to alleviation of underlying causes of pain [42]. Orthotics were not helpful in this case. Cushioned and supportive shoe wear did help, as did learning to land more softly on the foot when walking. Mrs. Warren also was advised to avoid prolonged knee flexion in sitting.

The clinician should treat as many impairments as possible with one set of exercises. In Mrs. Warren's case, the weakness, decreased cardiovascular conditioning, losses of range of motion, and pain were effectively treated together by using an aquatics program. The patient's cardiovascular deconditioning could be improved while she strengthened her lower extremities and improved joint flexibility. Joints were protected from excessive pressure by having her exercise in water.

Posture and joint alignment should be optimized when stretching or strengthening muscles to ensure that the intended result will be achieved. The alignment of Mrs. Warren's axial structures was not optimum for either gait or transfers. She had excessive thoracic kyphosis and loss of lumbar lordosis. In addition, she had limited lumbar and thoracic range of motion in all planes (rotation and lumbar lateral flexion were particularly compromised). She learned a series of exercises to increase range of motion of the axial structures and to correct her postural alignment. Improvement in alignment and range of motion simultaneously improved endurance and control of the back extensor muscles and general postural control during movement. (Trunk mobility, endurance, and balance control are all prerequisites to effective gait). The specific series of exercises used for this purpose has been described elsewhere [38] and key exercises are presented in Appendix A, page 415.

Treatment in the Context of Function

Exercises used should be relevant to the intended function. Mrs. Warren's posture, alignment, and range of motion precluded ability to perform tasks appropriately in a functional context. The program focused initially on correction of those underlying impairments and included exercises illustrated in Appendix A (see Figs. A-1, A-2, A-3, pages 419–422). As Mrs. Warren's mobility, posture, and endurance improved, exercises were practiced in the context of functional tasks (e.g., reaching for objects, bending over to tie her shoes).

Correction of the underlying axial impairments does not translate necessarily and directly into improved transfer ability. Mrs. Warren tended to come from sitting to standing from an excessively kyphotic posture, with her pelvis posteriorly tilted (which makes this a very difficult task). As she gained increased mobility and control of lumbopelvofemoral mobility, movement reeducation for this functional task was initiated and included exercises illustrated in Appendix A (see Figs. A-4, A-5, pages 424, 425). Emphasis was on a more erect posture, improved lumbar lordosis prior to initiation of the activity, and on retaining the extended posture of the spine throughout the sitting-to-standing activity. Practiced with good posture and control, this activity was used to increase the strength and endurance of the trunk and lower-extremity muscles and to develop adequate balance control during the self-initiated perturbation imposed by moving from the stable position of sitting to the inherently less stable posture of standing. This progression of exercises illustrates a systematic combination of activities designed to correct several specific impairments, physical performance, and finally performance of functional activities.

Correction of underlying impairments does not ensure optimal gait. Normal gait requires appropriate coordination of motion of the different body segments [29]. Mrs. Warren tended to keep her thorax flexed relative to the pelvis in stance and in walking. She never achieved full extension of the hips in gait and had limited trunk and pelvic rotation. These movement patterns contributed to her poor balance control and resulted in small step lengths. Movement reeducation was required for each element of gait to optimize her movement performance; see, for example, Fig. A-6 in Appendix A, page 427 [38]. Movement reeducation also was necessary for disrupted motor planning due to Parkinson's disease and for alteration of motor performance related to the osteoarthritis.

Movement reeducation in the clinical setting is of little value if it does not translate into more efficient and effective walking in functional contexts. Each situation relevant to the individual patient is evaluated and, when necessary, the clinician and patient together determine the barriers to functional gait performance and establish strategies to eliminate those barriers. For example, sitting-to-standing activity was practiced from a variety of chairs, so that Mrs. Warren would regain the ability to control this activity from the different seat heights and surfaces (e.g., soft versus hard) in her home and be able to get up from the seated position with and without arm rests. Similarly, individuals must be able to vary speed of walking from slow speeds used to accomplish household activities to the fast speeds used for distance walking and aerobic conditioning. One patient may have difficulty walking rapidly enough to cross a busy street in the neighborhood. Another may have difficulty with the slower gait used in dressing, cooking, and house cleaning, due to poor balance control. Exercises can be implemented for these different causes of difficulty with functional gait. Mrs. Warren needed to walk in a variety of environments (e.g., home, clinic, across streets, and in busy shopping malls). She was advised to use one or two canes to improve stability outside the house. (If one cane was used because one knee was especially painful, the cane was held in the hand opposite the more painful knee). She needed practice to use the cane effectively going up and down stairs and ramps and in and out of doorways. In contrast, she had little need to walk on a variety of surfaces (e.g., grass, gravel, uneven terrain). These situations were not emphasized in her treatment program.

The Use of Feedback

Another consideration is how much and what kind of feedback the clinician should use. To what extent should the clinician instruct verbally, demonstrate visually, or use hands to correct the patient's performance? There are several issues to take into consideration when making this decision. Ultimately, the patient must be able to carry out the program independently if it is to have lasting benefit. Knowledge of performance (i.e., how the task was carried out) and knowledge of results (i.e., whether it was accomplished successfully, regardless of the specific elements) both play roles during motor learning [43, 44].

Sometimes underlying deficits are too severe for the patient to correct them initially without assistance. For example, Mrs. Warren was able to carry out the lower-extremity stretching and strengthening program and the cardiovascular conditioning independently after the clinician described the exercises to her. On the other hand, she needed guidance from the clinician's hands initially as she began the exercises to improve axial mobility and movement reeducation for transfers and gait. As she gained an appreciation of the appropriate way to coordinate movement of the axial structures in these tasks, she was able to perform these exercises with less guidance—first with verbal instructions and finally independently.

In summary, the patient must understand the task before it can be practiced effectively and independently. The amount of guidance needed will depend on the degree of limitation and on the patient's capacity for independent learning. By its very nature, movement reeducation is likely to require some form of specific guidance from the clinician, whether in the form of verbal, visual, or hands-on instruction.

The Effect of Variability

In general, learning is made more functional with variability of practice [43, 44]. The need for variability must be balanced against the patient's capacity for learning and the patient's needs. For patients who have learning difficulties (whether due to cognitive deficits or as a result of their specific injury), excessive variability in practice initiated too early in the program can lead to confusion rather than to effective learning. In general, the clinician can start the program with limited variability and build in variability of practice depending on the patient's response. For example, initially, Mrs. Warren practiced transferring into and out of a chair without varying either the chair height or the instructions, until she was able to correctly coordinate the movements of the trunk, pelvic complex, and extremities for efficient transfer. As she gained the ability to accomplish the task under one set of circumstances, the chair was varied, the order of the exercise was varied, and so forth. This progression from simple to more complex was important for Mrs. Warren, who had some difficulty with movement reeducation stemming from subtle motor planning deficits associated with Parkinson's disease.

Ending Treatment

The end point of any intervention is determined by the patient's independence from the program and achievement of the goals. The time required for a patient to achieve independence depends on the severity of dysfunction and on motivation and capability for motor learning. Mrs. Warren was able to become independent in the pool program almost immediately, with the clinician progressing the exercises as appropriate. She needed more guidance with the motor reeducation part of the program for the reasons previously described.

When change no longer occurs, treatment should be terminated. As with all other decisions that the clinician must make, there are no hard and fast rules regarding the appropriate length of guidance during the exercise program. For some patients, a few sessions with a treating clinician can translate into significant and necessary functional gains or in prevention of potentially damaging impairments. For other patients, the directed exercise program might require weeks, months, or even a year for completion. For patients with chronic progressive conditions, such as Parkinson's disease and osteoarthritis, the exercise program may continue indefinitely. In these cases, the patient should become independent in carrying out the program as part of the daily routine and may see the clinician on a periodic basis for modifications to the program as the disease progresses.

Functional change is the essential determinant of appropriate duration of intervention. The clinician must clearly delineate the functional gains that are sought, both for the short and long term of the completed program, and must then be able to document that relevant changes are occurring consistently (even if slowly) over the course of treatment. Even slow change is valuable if the change leads to maintained independence or significantly lessens the amount of assistance that a patient requires.

Measuring Outcomes

Both the clinical and research communities should document outcomes of interventions. This chapter illustrates interrelationships in the pathway to disability that can focus decisions regarding the choice of outcome measures to use during physical intervention. The complexity of the interrelationship of impairments and the choice of appropriate functional outcome measures for gait increase with multiple pathologies. Though much *can* be measured, it is necessary to decide what *should* be measured in a given context.

Schenkman [8] has outlined a general strategy for deciding what should be measured, both to interpret underlying causes of dysfunction and to measure change. There are several considerations that relate specifically to gait in the measurement of functional outcomes:

1. Measures of functional gait performance should be linked to measures of relevant impairments (identified as underlying causes of dysfunction).
2. Physical performance measures of gait must be interpreted in the context of the normal or abnormal biomechanics associated with the person's gait.
3. Interpretation of functional gait performance should be made in the context of norms for different groups distinguished by age, physical activity level of the individuals (at the time and perhaps over the lifetime) and pathology.

Increasingly it is evident that improvements of underlying impairments must be linked to functional outcomes to assess the true success of interventions. Recent investigations have begun to assess underlying impairments and functional gait indicators. For example, Minor et al. [45] investigated three programs (pool, walking, and range of motion) for persons with rheumatoid arthritis and osteoarthritis in weight-bearing joints. They demonstrated a significantly different and decreased timed walk for the pool and walking subjects but not for the range-of-motion subjects. Fisher et al. [46, 47] used a 16-week individualized program for subjects with osteoarthritic knees and included isotonic and isometric strengthening, range of motion, functional training, and patient education. Their results demonstrated a significantly decreased 50-foot walk time (mean decrease, 12%). Kovar et al. [48] studied osteoarthritic knee patients and compared an 8-week program of supervised fitness walking and patient education to standard routine medical care. They reported a significant increase in distance walked in 6 minutes for the experimental group but not for the control group (mean increase, 18%). Judge et al. [49] demonstrated significant increases in both lower extremity muscle strength and gait velocity following a 12-week resistance and balance training program compared with flexibility exercises performed in a chair. Lord et al. [50] demonstrated improvements in five lower limb muscle groups as well as walking speed, cadence, stride length, and stride time for exercises compared with control subjects following a 22-week exercise program.

In the literature, there are only a few reports of physical intervention of Parkinson's disease [51–55]. Not all included objective measures of gait. A 13-week exercise program including walking, marching to music, and exercise designed to improve general flexibility resulted in significant improvement in step length and average walking speed [51]. A 12-week study comparing two different exercise programs demonstrated improvements in a gait index (sec/30-foot walk × the number of steps) for both exercise approaches [52]. In contrast, investigation of an intervention program by Pedersen et al. [53] revealed decreased maximum velocity and stride length. Most recently, Schenkman et al. [55] demonstrated significant improvements in axial mobility, with clear-cut gains in standing, functional reach, and supine-to-stand time following a 12-week axial mobility program for participants in the early and mid-stages of Parkinson's disease.

When appropriate, physical performance measures of gait should be linked to the normality or abnormality of the **biomechanics** of gait used to attain the desired functional outcome [56, 57]. In general, such data are not yet available in the literature. Numerous investigators [45–48, 58–62] have studied the benefits of a walking program for people with lower-limb joint degeneration (osteoarthrosis) and have reported improvements in such **functional indicators** as aerobic capacity, distance walked in 6 minutes, and measures from the Arthritis Impact Measurement Scales [63] (e.g., decreased depression, anxiety, and pain; increased physical activity tolerance and desire; increased knee strength and flexibility). The hazards of physical activity are well recognized, and people with this pathology historically have been advised to rest and unburden their joints without being given an option of wise physical activity. Normal physiological loading, such as occurs during walking, may damage an arthritic joint further in a person with skeletal malalignment or damaging joint mechanics [18, 64]. Yet none of the aforementioned investigations of exercise benefits for persons with arthritis reported on joint alignment for individual subjects. Also, they did not include the effect of the intervention on the joint malalignment (or vice versa) or the advisability of the specific intervention based on the patient's particular joint alignment.

A few investigators have studied the biomechanics of gait in those with Parkinson's disease [65–67]; none of the available intervention studies have reported on the benefits of intervention with respect to these findings. Similarly,

Morey et al. [68] recently reported on the impact of two years of supervised fitness program (including 30 minutes of walking) for community-dwelling veterans without regard to specific underlying pathology. These investigators demonstrated significant improvements of physical performance related to cardiovascular function and flexibility but did not include specific measures of gait.

Outcome measures for gait should be interpreted on the basis of appropriate norms. Norms for physical measures of gait performance should be distinguished by age and physical activity levels of subjects and by any chronic pathology in the subject population. Murray [69, 70] reported that a number of gait variables in subjects aged 20 to 87 changed at different age intervals (e.g., some at 65, some at 70). Riegger-Krugh and Parker [71] compared healthy people with approximately the same physical activity status during the main occupation of their lifetime and in their current spare time. These investigations revealed significant differences for subjects ages 50 to 60 compared with those 70 to 80 in walking speed at self-selected velocity and maximal speed and time to cross a street. In contrast, Gabell and Nayak [72] grouped all subjects older than mid-60s together and reported fewer differences in gait with age. Recently, Morris et al. [73] published data comparing temporal spatial measures of community-dwelling subjects with and without Parkinson's disease. Their data demonstrate substantial declines in walking speed, cadence, and stride length for those with Parkinson's disease. In general, norms by physical activity level and for selected chronic conditions are not yet available and will be required for adequate interpretation of functional gait measures in a variety of clinical situations.

To date, most investigations reporting gait-related outcomes following physical intervention have been restricted to persons with specific types of injury or pathology (e.g., arthritic conditions [45–48]. Frequently, an older individual with gait dysfunction has multiple underlying impairments stemming from a variety of pathologies, coupled with disuse or misuse syndromes. The complexity of the interrelationship of impairments, the choice of intervention, and the choice of appropriate functional outcome measures is therefore intensified. In Table 21-7 we illustrate measures, combining both functional indicators of gait and biomechanical measures, that were chosen to document change during physical intervention for Mrs. Warren.

SUMMARY

There are no hard and fast rules for physical management of gait disorders of elderly persons. A treatment program should be guided by the specific impairments related to physical performance or movement, the patient's total situation, and personal goals and lifestyle. Intervention is most effective when the approach to treatment is based on a systematic interpretation of underlying impairments and consequences. There are strategies for making decisions and for specific treatment approaches, illustrated by Mrs. Warren, a woman who has early-stage Parkinson's disease and significant osteoarthritic changes in her knees. These concepts illustrate the decisions that are made in physical management of gait for any elderly individual.

REFERENCES

1. Friedman PJ. Gait recovery after hemiplegic stroke. *Int Disabil Stud* 1990;12:119–122.
2. Sauvage LR, et al. A clinical trial of strengthening and aerobic exercise to improve gait and balance in elderly male nursing home residents. *Am J Phys Med Rehab* 1992;71:333–342.
3. Alexander, NB. Gait disorders in older adults. *J Am Geriatric Soc* 1995;43:1198–1206.
4. Sudarsky L, Ronthal M. Gait Disorders in the Elderly: Assessing the Risk for Falls. In: Vellas B, et al., eds. *Falls, Balance and Gait Disorders in the Elderly*. Paris: Elsevier Press, 1992. Pp 117–127.
5. Nutt JG. Gait Disorders. In: Jankovic J, Tolosa E, eds. *Parkinson's Disease and Movement Disorders*, 2nd ed. Baltimore: Williams & Wilkins, 1993. Pp 433–441.
6. Oatis C. Perspectives on the Evaluation and Treatment of Gait Disorders. In: Montgomery PC, Connolly BH, eds. *Motor Control and Physical Therapy*. Hixon, TN: Chattanooga Group, Inc., 1991. Pp 141–155
7. Sullivan PE. Ambulation: An Integrated Framework to Achieve a Functional Outcome. In: Guccione A, ed. *Geriatric Physical Therapy*. St Louis: Mosby, 1993. Pp 253–268.
8. Schenkman M. Evaluation and measurement considerations for physical rehabilitation of patients who have neurological deficits. *Top Geriatr Rehabil* 1994;10:1–21.
9. Nagi SZ. Some Conceptual Issues in Disability and Rehabilitation. In: Sussman MB, ed. *Sociology and Rehabilitation*. Washington DC: American Sociological Association, 1965. Pp 100–113.
10. Wood PHN. The language of disablement: A glossary relating to disease and its consequences. *Int Rehabil Med* 1980;2:86–92.
11. Pope AM, Tarlov AR, eds. *Disability in America. Toward a National Agenda for Prevention*. Washington, DC: National Academy Press, 1991. Pp 5–15.
12. Verbrugge LM, Jette AM. The disablement process. *Soc Sci Med* 1994;38:1–14.
13. Buchner DM, Cress ME, Wagner EH, de Lateur BJ. The Role of Exercise in Fall Prevention: Developing Targeting Criteria for Exercise Programs. In: Vellas B, et al. eds. *Falls, Balance and Gait Disorders in the Elderly*. Paris: Elsevier, 1992. Pp 55–67.
14. Schenkman M, et al. Reliability of physical performance measures for patients with Parkinson's disease. *Phys Ther* (in press).
15. Guyatt GH, Sullivan MJ, Thompson PJ. The 6 minute walk: A new measure of exercise capacity in patients with chronic heart failure. *Can Med Assoc J* 1985;32:919–923.
16. Perry J. *Gait Analysis: Normal and Pathological Function*. Thorofare, NJ: Slack, Inc., 1992.
17. Smidt G, ed. *Gait in Rehabilitation*. New York: Churchill Livingstone, 1990.
18. Radin EL, Yang KN, Riegger-Krush CL, et al. Relationship between lower limb dynamics and knee joint pain. *J Orthop Res* 1991;9:398–405.
19. Perry J. Kinesiology of lower-extremity bracing. *Clin Orthop* 1974;102:18–31.
20. Schenkman M. Neuromuscular and Musculoskeletal Factors in Balance Control. In: Duncan PW, ed. *Balance. Proceedings of the APTA Forum*. Alexandria, VA: American Physical Therapy Association, 1990. Pp 29–42.
21. Duncan PW. How do physiological components of balance affect mobility in elderly men? *Arch Phys Med Rehabil* 1993;74:1343–1349.
22. Schenkman M, et al. The relationship between axial mobility and physical performance. *Phys Ther* 1996;76:276–285.
23. Messert B, Neal HB. Syndrome of progressive spastic ataxia and apraxia associated with occult hydrocephalus. *Neurology* 1966;16:440–452.
24. Masdeu JC, Gorelick PB. Thalamic astasia: Inability to stand after unilateral thalamic lesions. *Ann Neurol* 1988;23:596–603.

25. Meyers JS, Barron DW. Apraxia of gait: A clinico-physiological study. *Brain* 1960;83:261–284.

26. Lewis CB. Musculoskeletal Changes with Age: Clinical Implications. In: *Aging: The Health Care Challenge*, 2nd ed. Philadelphia: Davis, 1990. Pp 135–161.

27. Schenkman M. Physical Therapy Intervention for the Ambulatory Patient. In: Turnbull G, ed. *Physical Therapy Management of Parkinson's Disease.* New York: Churchill Livingstone, 1992. Pp 137–192.

28. Schenkman M, Morey M, Cutson Tm, Kuchibhatla M. Axial mobility, axial configuration, and physical performance of community dwellers with and without Parkinson's disease. Presented at the Annual Meeting of the American Physical Therapy Association, Minneapolis, MN. June 1996.

29. Inman VT, Ralston HJ, Todd F. *Human Walking.* Baltimore: Williams & Wilkins, 1981.

30. Fiatarone M, Marks E, Ryan N, et al. High-intensity strength training in nonagenarians— Effects of skeletal muscle. *JAMA* 1990;263:3029–3034.

31. Brown M, Rose S. The effects of aging and exercise on skeletal muscle; clinical considerations. *Top Geriatr Rehabil* 1985;1:20–30.

32. Goldberg AP, Hagberg JM. Physical Exercise in the Elderly. In: Schneider EL, Rowe JW, eds. *The Handbook of the Biology of Ageing*, 3rd ed. San Diego: Academic 1990. Pp 407–428.

33. Lord SR, Ward JA, Williams P, Strudnick M. The effect of a 12 month exercise trial on balance, strengths, and falls in older women: A randomized controlled trial. *J Am Geriatr Soc* 1995;43:1198–1206.

34. Shepherd R, Sidney K. Exercise and aging. *Exerc Sports Sci Rev*, 1978;6:1–57.

35. Voss DE, Ionta M, Myers BJ. *Proprioceptive Neuromuscular Facilitation*, 3rd ed. Philadelphia: Harper & Row, 1985.

36. Bobath B. *Adult Hemiplegia: Evaluation and Treatment*, 2nd ed. London: Heinemann, 1978.

37. Watson M. Stretching and Strengthening Videotape and Manual. MHW Tapes, 3213 Carroll Woods, Chapel Hill, NC.

38. Schenkman M, et al. *Axial Mobility Exercise Program. An Exercise Program to Improve Functional Ability.* Durham, NC: Claude D. Pepper Older Americans Independence Center, Duke University, 1993.

39. Feldenkrais M. *Awareness Through Movement.* New York: Harper & Row, 1977.

40. Lewis CB, Knortz K. *Orthopedic Assessment and Treatment of the Geriatric Patient.* St. Louis: Mosby, 1993.

41. Judge JO. Resistance training. *Top Geriatr Rehabil* 1993;8:38–50.

42. Neuman D. Arthrokinesiologic Considerations in the Aged Adult. In: Guccione A, ed. *Geriatric Physical Therapy.* St. Louis: Mosby, 1993. Pp 47–70.

43. Schmidt RA. Motor Learning Principles for Physical Therapy. In: Lister MJ, ed. *Contemporary Management of Motor Control Problems. Proceedings of the II Step Conference.* Alexandria, VA: Foundation for Physical Therapy, 1991. Pp 49–66.

44. Shumway-Cook AS, Woollacott M. *Motor Control. Theory and Practical Application.* Baltimore: Williams & Wilkins, 1995.

45. Minor MA, et al. Efficacy of physical conditioning exercise in patients with rheumatoid arthritis and osteoarthritis. *Arthritis Rheum* 1989;32:1396–1403.

46. Fisher NM, et al. Quantitative effects of physical therapy on muscular and functional performance in subjects with osteoarthritis of the knees. *Arch Phys Med Rehabil* 1993;74:840–847.

47. Fisher NM, Perdergast DR, Gresham GE, Calkins E. Muscle rehabilitation: Its effect on muscular and functional performance of patients with knee osteoarthritis. *Arch Phys Med Rehabil* 1991;72:367–374.

48. Kovar PA, et al. Supervised fitness walking in patients with osteoarthritis of the knee. *Ann Intern Med* 1992;116:529–534.

49. Judge JO, Underwood M, Gennos T. Exercises to improve gait velocity in older persons. *Arch Phys Med Rehabil* 1993;74:400–406.

50. Lord SR, et al. The effect of exercise on gait patterns in older women: A randomized controlled trial. *J Gerontol Med Sci* 1996;51A:M64–M70.

51. Szeleky BC, et al. Adjunctive treatment in Parkinson's disease: Physical therapy and comprehensive group therapy. *Rehabil Lit* 1982;43:72–76.

52. Palmer SS, et al. Exercise therapy for Parkinson's disease. *Arch Phys Med Rehabil* 1986;67: 741–745.

53. Pedersen SW, Oberg B, Insulander A, Vretman M. Group training in parkinsonism: Quantitative measurements of treatment. *Scand J Rehabil Med* 1990;22:207–211.

54. Comella CL, Stebbins GT, Brown-Toms N, Goetz CG. Physical therapy and Parkinson's disease: A controlled clinical trial. *Neurology* 1994;44:376–378.

55. Schenkman M, et al. Physical intervention and Parkinson's disease. Presented at the Annual Meeting of the Gerontological Society of America, Washington, DC. November 1996.

56. Panush RS, Lane NE. Exercise and the Musculosketal System. In: Panush RS, Lane NE, eds. *Baillière's Clinical Rheumatology: Exercise and Rheumaic Disease* (vol 8). Philadelphia: Saunders, 1994. Pp 79–102.

57. Ytterberg SR, Mahowal MC, Krug HE. Exercise for Arthritis. In: Panush RS, Lane NE, eds. *Baillière's Clinical Rheumatology: Exercise and Rheumatic Disease* (vol 8). Philadelphia: Saunders, 1994. Pp 161–189.

58. Beals CA, et al. Measurement of exercise tolerance in patients with rheumatoid arthritis and osteoarthritis. *J Rheum* 1985;12:458–461.

59. Ekblom B, et al. Effect of short-term physical training on patients with rheumatoid arthritis. *Scand J Rheumatol* 1975;4:87–91.

60. Ekdahl C, Broman G. Muscle strength, endurance, and aerobic capacity in rheumatoid arthritis: A comparative study with healthy subjects. *Ann Rheum Dis* 1992;51:35–40.

61. Minor MA. Physical activity and management of arthritis. *Ann Behav Med* 1991;13:117–124.

62. Minor MA, et al. Exercise tolerance and disease related measures in patients with rheumatoid arthritis and osteoarthritis. *J Rheum* 1988;15:905–911.

63. Hughes SL, et al. Reliability and validity of The Arthritis Impact Measurement Scales for elderly respondents. *Arthritis Rheum* 1991;34:856–865.

64. Radin EL, et al. Mechanical determinants of osteoarthrosis. *Semin Arthritis Rheum* 1991; 21(suppl 2):12–21.

65. Ueno E, Yanagisawa N, Takami M. Gait disorders in parkinsonism. A study with floor reaction forces and EMG. *Adv Neurol* 1993;60:414–41.

66. Morris ME, Iansek R, Matyas TA, Summers JJ. The pathogenesis of gait hypokinesia in Parkinson's disease. *Brain* 1994;117:1169–1181.

67. Morris ME, Iansek R, Matyas TA, Summers JJ. Ability to modulate walking cadence remains intact in Parkinson's disease. *J Neurol Neurosurg Psychiatr* 1994;57:1532–1534.

68. Morey MC, et al. Two-year trends in physical performance following supervised exercise among community-dwelling older veterans. *J Am Geriatr Soc* 1991;39:986–992.

69. Murray MP, Kory RC, Clarkson BH. Walking patterns in healthy old men. *J Gerontol* 1969;24:169–178.

70. Murray MP, Kory RC, Sepic SB. Walking patterns of normal women. *Arch Phys Med Rehabil* 1970;51:637–650.

71. Riegger-Krugh C, Parker D. Some normative data on knee strength, flexibility, and timed functional tasks in healthy women aged 50–60 and 70–80. *J Aging Phys Act* 1993;1:108–109.

72. Gabell A, Nayak USL. The effect of age on the variability in gait. *J Gerontol* 1984;39:662–666.

73. Morris ME, Matyas TA, Iansek R, Summers JJ. Temporal stability of gait in Parkinson's disease. *Phys Ther* 1996;76:763–777.

22. Improving Balance in Older Adults: Identifying the Significant Training Stimuli

Robert H. Whipple

Deterioration of balance is a well-documented hallmark of the aging process [1, 2]. Poor balance is initially detectable in the sixth decade of life but then accelerates so that it becomes the rule rather than the exception by one's late eighties [3, 4]. It is unclear, however, to what degree balance can be restituted in fully functioning older adults who are free from disease that could affect balance directly (e.g., neurological diagnoses, severe musculoskeletal and cardiovascular problems).

A number of reviews of balance in the elderly [5–7] have described it as a highly complex set of overlapping sensorimotor, musculoskeletal, psychoemotional, and perceptual functions. Compounding this complexity are diverse additional factors such as age, gender, unmanifest disease, learning, activity level, genetic endowment, socioeconomic status, risk-taking behavior, and fitness.

Because balance is an ill-defined and nonunitary entity, it is not surprising that endeavors to improve it have met with mixed success. Although some laudable efforts have been made to place balance in the elderly within a cohesive theoretical framework [6, 8–11], there have been few attempts to improve balance in older adults with theory-based intervention strategies. This lack is frequently reflected in the geriatric balance training literature in a medley of nonspecific interventions characterized by conventional calisthenic (coordination) exercises, which often include aerobic or muscle-strengthening components. Additionally, guidelines for the establishment of effective balance enhancement techniques often are difficult to derive from the balance-training literature because of imprecision in sample selection, the absence of validated yardsticks for the measurement of balance, and the lack of true controls in experimental design.

In this chapter an attempt will be made to operationalize the many physical circumstances that challenge balance in the course of daily life and to group them according to shared functional demands. The geriatric balance-training literature will be reviewed and used as a basis for examining study features, interventions, and balance outcome measures. Each study is profiled on the basis of (1) the number and degree of balance challenges that the intervention provided and (2) the type and variety of tests of balance that were used as outcome measures. From this information, the training and testing features of interventions in which training resulted in improved balance will be characterized.

Finally, a few potentially fruitful areas for new interventions are examined. These areas include the roles played by multisensory interaction, body awareness, eye-head control, vestibular and proprioceptive input, and spatial orientation. One model for a theoretically driven intervention is presented, based on the Farmington-FICSIT (Frailty and Injuries: Cooperative Studies of Intervention Techniques) study. Tai Chi is discussed as an example of an approach that systematically uses many of the aforementioned training features.

PHYSICAL CHALLENGES TO BALANCE

An examination of the balance assessment literature reveals the use of a wide variety of methods for the creation of a *balance-challenging condition*, here defined as a circumstance whereby a force tends to move the vertical projection of the body's center of mass away from its neutral position over its base of support. These challenges span a spectrum ranging from daily activities, such as walking and picking up an object from the floor, to attempts to replicate forces acting on the body through the use of force platforms or the manipulation of sensory inputs. The wide diversity of possible challenges to balance were arranged into three naturalistic balance-challenge domains (BCDs) encompassing a total of 13 categories and numerous subcategories:

1. Predictable challenges occurring during bipedal activities (Table 22-1; seven categories).
2. Postural transitions during ground-level activities (lying-to-standing; Fig. 22-1; one category).
3. Environmentally induced (extrinsic) destabilizations while erect (Table 22-2; five categories).

The designation *category* reflects a dimension of challenges to balance derived from the intervention components described below in the balance-training literature. Numerous subcategories of these conditions were created on the basis of the author's subjective impression of the prevalence of certain functional movements in daily life and on the nature of challenges to balance encountered in the balance and functional test literature [12–14]. The choices of subcategories are necessarily arbitrary at this stage and are meant merely to serve as guidelines. It should be noted that a balance-challenge subcategory often can be viewed as both a training stimulus and as an outcome measure.

Although balancing activities are clearly dependent on the proper functioning of intricate higher-order neural mechanisms [8], all balancing tasks vary in degree of difficulty (e.g., a moderate lean versus a maximal reach) and hence require different intensities of movement control. Motor complexity aside, the intensity of response to a balance challenge can be grossly viewed in terms of (1) amplitude, (2) speed, (3) imposed resistance, and (4) duration of required movement. These features are inextricably associated with muscle strength, joint flexibility, and endurance. Insofar as great demands can be made on head and eye control during many movements, vestibulo-ocular processing can be considered as yet another feature of the intensity sphere. Age-related decrements in these

Table 22-1. Common challenges to erect balance in the absence of external provocations or tripping*

Destabilizing conditions	Real-life activities
1. Decreased bipedal base	
Normal-width foot separation	
Symmetrical weight on heels	Leaning or reaching backward
Symmetrical weight on balls of feet	Leaning or reaching forward
Assymmetrical weight between feet	Leaning or reaching in oblique directions
Narrowed stance	
Feet close together (Romberg)	Narrowed floor space (or diminished ROM)
Tandem, semitandem	Narrowed floor space (or diminished ROM)
Feet crossed	Dictated by available floor space
2. One-legged stance	Put on pants; leaning to side
3. Limits of stability	
(Maintenance of center of force on perimeter of base of support)	Extreme reaching (e.g., painting, dusting)
4. Ambulatory conditions	
Normal walk	
Forward, usual speed, > 1 m/sec	Conventional walking
Backward	Dancing, IADLs
Maximum speed walk	Hurrying, exercising
Running or jogging	Hurrying, exercising
Side-stepping	Dancing; navigation at home, crowds
Stepping over	Obstacles in path
Narrowed (tandem) walk	
Forward (heel-to-toe-like)	Limited floor space; diminished abduction ROM
Backward (toe-to-heel-like)	Limited floor space; diminished abduction ROM
Slow-as-possible walk	In dark or on uncertain floor conditions
Using reduced area of foot	
Walk on toes	Hiking, dancing, uncertain floor conditions
Walk on heels	Backward loss of balance, dancing, pain under forefoot
5. Turning	
Segmental rotations (head, torso, pelvis)	Twists in daily activities
Pivots/spins of whole body	Fast turns without stepping
Step-pivots, > 180 degrees	Turns with steps, reverse direction of walk
6. Upper-extremity movements	
Casual movements	Unstressed daily activities
Fast	Reactive or catching movements
With loads	Lift bags, place objects
7. Vertical body movements	
Nonstepping	
Tranfers	Sit-to-stand
Jumps, hops	Emergency movements, exercise
Other	Stoop, squat, bend, pick up
While stepping	Stairs, curbs, stools

IADL = instrumental activities of daily living; ROM = range of motion.

* While weight bearing on feet on a flat horizontal surface that is at least equal to the weight-bearing surface of the foot (feet).

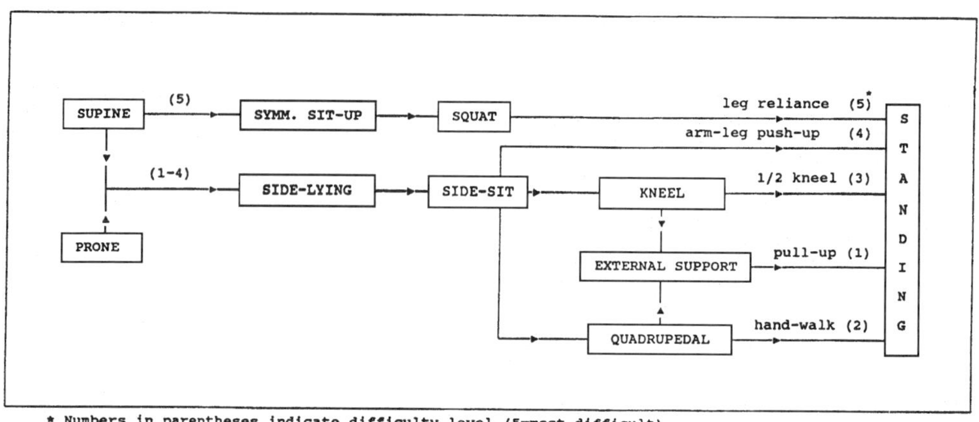

Figure 22-1. Ground-level transfers to stand. Numbers in parentheses indicate difficulty level (*1* = least difficult, *5* = most difficult).

intensity cofactors of movement are universally acknowledged and are associated with falls and loss of mobility and function [15–18].

Predictable Challenges to Balance During Bipedal Activities

The first domain of challenges to balance (see Table 22-1) consists of predictable destabilizing situations that can occur during unassisted and unprovoked weight bearing on the lower extremities. Most routine bipedal activities thus can be encompassed within the seven categories of challenges to balance listed in Table 22-1. Poor performance in most of these areas, which are closely linked to function, has often been associated with either falls or abnormal measures of balance [17, 19, 20].

As indicated earlier, the intensity cofactors can be closely associated with any of the balance activities. For example, lower-extremity strength is necessarily involved with larger-amplitude vertical movements of the center of gravity, whereas high-speed locomotion, turning, and vertical activities together will make greater demands on vestibulo-ocular processing. Controlling limits of stability during maximal leaning will tax ankle flexibility and strength, which are often reduced in aging [18, 21], whereas prolonged one-legged standing may rely on strong hip musculature [22] to stabilize the pelvis [23].

Ground-Level Functional Balance

The standing-to-floor movement (and its reverse) represents a high order of balance challenge (see Fig. 22-1), under which most easier transfer activities can be subsumed (e.g., rolling, coming to sit). It demands considerable flexibility, lower- and upper-extremity strength, and multisegmental interactions. The functional importance of this ground-level activity in aging has been deemphasized in the literature, perhaps because of the lifelong bias for chair use in industrialized so-

Table 22-2. Unexpected or unusual external challenges to balance

Destabilizing conditions	Real-life activities
1. Surface instabilities	
Horizontal plane	
Translations	Buses, trains, boats, escalators, moving walkways
Slippery or loose surfaces	Ice, loose rugs, gravel (stance-phase challenges)
Saggital and frontal plane (tilts)	
Inclines (static)	Ramps, sloping terrain
Evoked sudden tilts	Vehicles, small boats, planes
Compliant (yielding) tilts	Foam, floor-rug transitions, sand
Sway-referenced tilts	Posturography platforms
Vertical dimension	
Surface movement under both feet	Boats, elevators, escalators, buses
Surface movement under one foot	Boat-dock, floor-elevator
Surface height differential	Potholes, rugged terrain, missteps
Compliant surfaces	Rugs, sand, foam, mud, sneakers, snow
2. Body perturbations	
Sudden pushes and pulls	Crowds, pets, team sports
Gradual onset	Pets
Sudden cessation	Object (pet) giving way while leaning against it
3. Reduced surface area	
Reduced anteroposterior dimension	Stand/walk on short object or terrain
Reduced mediolateral dimension	Stand/walk on narrow beam, plank, irregular terrain
4. Obstacle contact-ambulation	
Trips and stumbles	Edges of rug, cracks, cords, clutter
Anticipated resistances	
At lower-extremity level	Walk in snow, water, leaves
At body level	Push-pull doors, pets, mowers, vacuum
5. Aberrant visual input	
Reduced or absent input	Moving in darkness
Distorted or confusing input	In moving vehicles, ships

cieties. However, long lies after falls (i.e., long periods of waiting for assistance) and fear both of falling and arising are issues that relate to the perception of balance self-efficacy and ultimately bear on an individual's sense of demoralization and quality of life [24, 25].

Although not usually considered a daily activity in Western cultures, transferring to and from supine lying on the ground is among the most difficult functions for older adults. Few attempts have been made to typify this complex righting activity [26], but it is clear that aging and frailty result in the adoption of compromised performance strategies. Figure 22-1 traces the course of five different pathways that can be taken by a person when progressing from ground supine lying to erect standing. Each entails diverse mixes of bipedal, tripedal, and quadrupedal balancing efforts and is numbered in ascending order of difficulty. Path 5, the most difficult, requires enough balance, flexibility, and mass extensor strength to quickly and symmetrically bring the individual forward from a full squat to standing [26]. Path 1, the easiest, involves kneeling, followed by arm assistance against a piece of furniture to attain the erect posture.

Unexpected or Unusual External Challenges to Balance

Many of the less common (and for that reason, unexpected) causes of falls are hazardous environmental conditions, such as slips, trips, and pushes [20]. Five categories of external destabilization have been formulated (see Table 22-2), along with examples of the natural circumstances in which they occur:

1. Instabilities of the support surface;
2. Forces acting on the body;
3. Reduced areas of support;
4. Obstacles during ambulation;
5. Reduced or distorted visual input;

As in the case of unprovoked balance tasks (see Table 22-1), in Table 22-2 there is much overlapping of categories, the examples provided are not meant to be exhaustive, and less common athletic activities (skateboarding, judo) are not included.

These challenges to balance occur within the contexts of high velocities and hazardous terrain and are, therefore, more likely to result in more severe injuries [27]. Highly varied, unexpected, and fast onsets of destabilizing forces also demand faster neuromuscular responses. Ironically, people with higher mobility levels are placed at greater risk for falls because of their greater exposure to such environmental destabilizers, particularly if their balance and judgment are marginal [28]. Theoretically then, any balance-training paradigm that aimed to lower the risk from environmental injury without restricting mobility would, of necessity, have to offer the opportunity for the repeated and systematic practice of balancing acts that were reasonable facsimiles of real-world hazards.

STUDIES OF BALANCE TRAINING IN OLDER ADULTS

Tables 22-3 and 22–4 summarize the salient features of 25 "balance-training" studies [29–53] performed with older adults. Improving balance appeared not to be the primary objective in 13 (52%) of the 25 studies. However, if a study showed at least one quantifiable balance outcome measure other than (or in addition to) gait, it was considered a balance intervention.

Tables 22-3 and 22-4, which differentiate nonrandomized control (see Table 22-3) from randomized control trials (see Table 22-4), portray the studies in terms of number, subject population (fraility and gender), age, exercise frequency, intervention components, balance outcome measures, and effect of the intervention. In considering the conclusions reached by each study, tempered by the author's subjective assessment of the presence of analytical flaws, it appears that 10 (40%) of the studies [29, 30, 33, 35, 39, 42, 50–53] resulted in no sig-

Table 22-3. Description of intervention, balance measures, and outcome results of training studies with older adults: nonrandomized control trials

Study	No. and group	Study population	Age	Exercise frequency	Intervention description	Balance outcomes	Significant change[a]
Barry et al. [29]	8 Exp 5 Cnt	Community	71	13 wk, 3×/wk, 40 min	Bicycle ergometer (10–15 min submaximum; 6–10 min near maximum at ≥ 130 beats/min)	Toe stand (eo/ec) 1-legged stand (2-inch beam)	No No
Bassett et al. [30]	16 Exp	Community	74	10 wk, 3×/wk, 30 min	"Nonstrenuous" stretching and exercises for quad strength and balance and hip-shoulder-knee flexibility; with music and dowels	1-legged stand	No
Binder et al. [31]	8 Exp	Community (frail)	79	8 wk, 3×/wk	"Moderate intensity," focused on LE strengthening, flexibility, "increased speed"; seated, standing, and on mats	Romberg, tandem, semitandem gait velocity, sit-stand	Yes Yes
Brown and Holloszy [32]	62 Exp 13 Cnt	Community	65	13 wk, 5×/wk, 60 min	48 "Low-intensity" strengthening and flexibility exercises using body and limb weight; 1-legged stand, heel-toe walk, rock on heel and toes	1-legged stand (eo) 1-legged stand (ec)	Yes (women) No
Clark et al. [33]	10 Ext 13 Cnt	Psychiatric patients	69	12 wk, 5×/wk, 60 min	Light rhythmical activities, including stretching, postural exercises, modified weight and circuit training, and dancing	Bilateral toe stand 1-legged stand 1-legged stand (2-inch beam)	No No No
Fiatarone et al. [34]	10 Exp	Nursing home	90	8 wk, 3×/wk, 30 min	PRE of quadriceps, 2 sets at 80% of one-repetition maximum	Tandem gait Usual gait	Yes No
Gutman et al. [35]	19 Exp1 13 Exp2	Congregate living	72	6 wk, 3×/wk, 60 min	Feldenkrais group exercised on mat (low effort/flexibility plus body awareness); Exp2 = walk, run in place, bend, walk straight line	Walk on balance beams	No
Lord and Castell [36]	40 Exp 40 Cnt	Community	62	10 wk, 2×/wk, 60 min	Walking; flexibility and modified aerobics; specific graded strengthening of LEs using body weight; balance exercises	Sway (ec) Sway (ec + foam) Sway (ec + foam)	Yes Yes Yes
Rikli et al. [37]	21 Exp 13 Cnt	Congregate living	70	3 years 3×/wk, 1 hr	Aerobics (60–70% maximum heart rate); standing and floor exercises for balance, strength, coordination; static stretch (flexibility)	1-legged stand	Yes

Table 22-3 (continued).

Study	No. and group	Study population	Age	Exercise frequency	Intervention description	Balance outcomes	Significant change[a]
Roberts [38]	27 Exp 25 Cnt	Community	72	6 wk, 3×/wk, 30 min	Walking (60–70% maximum heart rate)	Sum of 8 stances (eo/ec)[a]	Yes
Sauvage et al. [39]	8 Exp 6 Cnt	Nursing home (men)	73	12 wk, 3×/wk, 45–75 min	Bicycle ergometer; PRE using weights to hip (abduction, adduction, flexion, extension), knee (extension), and ankle (plantar flexion)	Normal AP sway Tinetti ("balance") Gait velocity	No No Yes
Stones and Kozma [40]	80 Exp 87 Cnt	Community	63	1 yr, 2×/wk, 45 min	30-min endurance, 15-min flexibility exercises	1-legged stand[b]	Yes
Vanfraechem and Van-fraechem [41]	10 Exp1 10 Exp2	Congregate living (women)	75	8 wk, 2×/wk, 60 min	"Physical training activities adapted . . . to age"; (Exp1 group were sedentary, Exp2 group had been exercising for years)	1-legged stand, ec	Yes

AP = anteroposterior; Cnt = control group; ec = eyes closed; eo = eyes open; Exp = experimental group; LE = lower-extremity; PRE = progressive-resistance exercise.
[a] Weight on balls of feet; 1-legged stand (on floor and 3-inch beam).
[b] Free foot against calf.

Table 22-4. Description of intervention, balance measures, and outcome results of training studies with older adults: randomized control trials

Study	No. and group	Study population	Age	Exercise frequency	Intervention description	Balance outcomes	Significant change[a]
Crilly et al. [42]	25 Exp 25 Cnt	Congregate or nursing home (women)	82	12 wk, 3×/wk, 35 min	Unspecified 1- and 2-legged balance, co-ordination, breathing, flexibility, antigravity-trunk-ankle strength, relaxation	Sway (eo/ec)	No
Era [43]	13 Exp1	Community (men)	76	8 wk, 2×/wk, 60 min	Exp1: isometric and dynamic strengthening of limbs and trunk	Sway eo	Yes Exp1
	11Exp2 18 Cnt				Exp2: "traditional" weight-bearing, rhythmical, and flexibility	Sway ec Tandem stand	Yes Exp2 Yes Exp1
Fansler et al. [44]	12 Exp1 12 Exp2 12 Cnt	Congregate living (women)	79	3 days 5 min/day	Exp1: 3× 1-legged stand after relaxation tape Exp2: 3× 1-legged stand after relaxation and ideokinetic facilitation tape (mental practice)	1-legged stand	Yes
Hopkins et al. [45]	35 Exp 30 Cnt	Community (women)	65	12 wk, 3×/wk, 50 min	20-min aerobics to music (stretching, walking, progressive dance movements); 30-min warm-up and cool-down; 100–120 heart rate	1-legged stand	Yes
Hu and Wooll-acott [46]	12 Exp 12 Cnt	Community	75	2 wk, 10×, 40 min	Ten 10-sec trials in each of the 8 combinations of standing with eyes open and closed, on firm or foam surface, head neutral or extended	1-legged stand DP	Yes Yes
Johanssen and Jarnlo [47]	18 Exp 16 Cnt	Community (women)	70	5 wk, 2×/wk, 60 min	Walk and dance steps to music, different directions and speeds often combined with arm-neck-trunk movement; sit-stand	1-legged stand Maximum walk speed	Yes Yes
Judge et al. [48]	12 Exp1 9 Exp2	Community (women)	68	26 wk, 3×/wk, 60 min	Exp1: 20-min walk (70% of maximum HR); PRE knee extension, leg press; low weight hip abduction/extension; bridge, lunge, pelvic tilt, lie-to-stand; static stretch; balancing (slow weight shifts, forward and backward steps, pivots). Exp2: same stretch and balance exercises (30 min/wk)	1-legged stand Semi-1-legged stand	No Yes

Table 22-4 (continued).

Study	No. and group	Study population	Age	Exercise frequency	Intervention description	Balance outcomes	Significant change[a]
Ledin et al. [49]	15 Exp 14 Cnt	Community	73	9 wk, 2×/wk, 45 min	Jog, jump, walk on toes or heels, sudden turns, walk sideways, backward, sit-to-stand, 1-legged stand (eo/ec), head movement during visual fixation, playing ball, trampoline	1-legged stand plus head shake Walk-turn time DP[a]; 1-legged stand (eo)	Yes Yes No
Lichtepstein et al. [50]	24 Exp 26 Cnt	Community women living alone	77	16 wk, 3×/wk, 60 min	Stretching, static balance, tandem walk, walking on line, performing maneuvers in response to color signals, walking	1-legged stand, eo/ec Normal AP sway	No No
McMurdo and Burnett [51]	44 Exp 43 Cnt	Community	65	32 wk, 2×/wk, 45 min	30-min exercise to music (contained elements of endurance, low resistance strengthening and suppleness); 15-min warm-up	Normal AP sway	No
Reinsch et al. [52]	123 Exp 101 Cnt	Community	74	52 wk, 3×/wk, 60 min	Specified number of stand-ups from a chair and step-ups to a 6-inch stool; warm-up and cool-down stretching and movement to music	1-legged stand, ec 10 sit-stand	No No
Topp et al. [55]	25 Exp 30 Cnt	Community	71	12 wk, 3×/wk, 60 min	Resistance exercise for UE and LEs using surgical tubing of progressively increasing thickness (2 out of 3 sessions unsupervised at home)	Backward tandem walk 1-legged stand, ec[b]	No No

AP = anteroposterior; CNT = control group; DP = dynamic platform; ec = eyes closed; eo = eyes open; Exp = experimental group; LE = lower extremity; PRE = progressive-resistance exercise; UE = upper extremity.
[a] Not significant after Bonferroni correction.
[b] Free foot against calf.

nificant improvement in one or more balance outcome measures. Randomized control trials were equally represented within the improvement versus nonimprovement categories.

By dichotomizing the studies into those with and without positive balance outcomes and by using the operationally defined BCD scheme (discussed in Predictable Challenges to Balance During Bipedal Activities), we can address the following issues:

1. Do the balance test outcome measures used in the interventions reflect the full range of BCD categories?
2. How well do current approaches to balance training reflect the BCDs?
3. What aspects of testing, training, research design, and subject characteristics differed between studies with significant (versus nonsignificant) balance outcomes?

Representation of the Balance-Challenge Categories Within the Tests of Balance Used in 25 Interventions

The second column of Table 22-5 shows the percentage of times that a specific balance test was included as an outcome measure. The one-legged stance time was by far the most frequently used test (in 68% of the studies) and occurred almost three times more often than did the next two most frequently used tests. Fifteen of the 17 studies using one-legged stance employed the traditional eyes-open condition, whereas six used eyes closed, and four used both.

There was no consistent use of any other test. Decreased bipedal base and standing sway were each employed in six (24%) studies, whereas tandem walks occurred in four. The categories of surface instability, vertical body movements, and turns received only token representation. No category appeared consistently superior to another with respect to how often it was used to detect a significant outcome (see Table 22-5, column 3).

Tests representing dynamic movement patterns (vertical body movements, turns, ambulatory conditions, upper-extremity movements, and forces acting on the body) rarely appeared, and the measurement of anteroposterior limits of stability, obstacle contact during ambulation (see Table 22-2), and ground-level activities (see Fig. 22-1) were absent. Standing or walking on reduced areas of support (narrow beam walk or one-leg stand on narrow beam) appeared in 16% of studies. Reduced visual input (eyes closed) occurred in 40% of the studies but usually in the context of one-legged standing or normal sway. Although 11 of the 13 major categories of challenge to balance were represented among the 25 studies, the average number of categories per study was only 2.0 ± 1.1. Just three of the investigations [38, 47, 49] employed as many as four BCD categories, and only one [39] incorporated eight (in the form of Tinetti's performance-oriented mobility assessment) [14].

Table 22-5. Usage frequency of balance tests in intervention studies

Categories and individual tests	Percentage and number of studies using test	Percentage and number studies with a positive outcome
One-legged stand	**68 (17)**	**65 (11/17)**
With eyes open	60 (15)	53 (8/15)
With eyes closed	24 (6)	50 (3/6)
On narrow beam	8 (2)	50 (1/2)
With head shake	4 (1)	100 (1/1)
Reduced bipedal base of support	**24 (6)**	**67 (4/6)**
Balls of feet (eyes open)	12 (3)	33 (1/3)
Balls of feet (eyes closed)	8 (2)	50 (1/2)
Tandem (eyes open)	8 (2)	50 (1/2)
Romberg (eyes open)	8 (2)	33 (1/3)
$^1/_2$ Tandem (eyes open)	4 (1)	100 (1/1)
Romberg (eyes closed)	4 (1)	0 (0/1)
1-legged stand plus toe-touch	4 (1)	100 (1/1)
Standing sway (normal stance)	**24 (6)**	**33 (2/6)**
With eyes open	24 (6)	17 (1/6)
With eyes closed	12 (3)	67 (2/3)
Tandem (-like) walks	**16 (4)**	**25 (1/4)**
Narrow beam walk	8 (2)	0 (0/2)
Forward tandem	4 (1)	100 (1/1)
Backward tandem	4 (1)	0 (0/1)
Unstable surface	**12 (3)**	**67 (2/3)**
Sway-referenced tilts	8 (2)	50 (1/2)
Foam	4 (1)	100 (1/1)
Vertical COG control	**12 (3)**	**33 (1/3)**
Sit-to-stand	8 (2)	50 (1/2)
Tinetti	4 (1)	0 (0/1)
Horizontal body or head movement	**2 (3)**	**67 (2/3)**
Walk with fast turns	8 (2)	50 (1/2)
1-legged stand or head shake	4 (1)	100 (1/1)

COG = center of gravity.

Representation of the Balance-Challenge Categories Within the Balance-Training Protocols of 25 Interventions

Only 6 of the 13 BCD (see Tables 22-1 and 22-2) categories occurred in 50% or more of the intervention (Table 22-6, column 3). They were ambulation, decreased base, one-legged stance, turning, and upper extremity and vertical movements. Training by means of aberrant visual input, surface instabilities, ground activities, and limits of stability occurred rarely (8–12%). Totally absent were the external destabilization categories of body perturbations, reduced surface areas, and obstacle contact.

Table 22-6. Usage rank and frequency of balance-challenge categories in 25 studies of balance training in older adults

Balance categories	Rank and percentage of studies using a balance test	Rank and percentage of studies using a balance intervention
One-legged stance	1 (72)	4 ($\approx$50)[a]
Absent or altered vision	2 (44)	5 (12)
Decreased bipedal base	3 (28)	4 ($\approx$50)[a]
Tandem walk[b]	4 (20)	7 (4)[c]
Reduced surface area	5 (16)	8 (0)
Vertical center of gravity	5 (16)	2 (72)
Unstable support surface	6 (12)	6 (8)
Upper-extremity movements	7 (4)[d]	2 (72)
Turns	7 (4)[d]	3 (64)
Fast gait[b]	7 (4)	1 (76)
Body perturbations	7 (4)[d]	8 (0)
Limits of stability (backward)	7 (4)[d]	6 (8)
Unexpected obstacles	8 (0)	8 (0)
On-ground activities	8 (0)	5 (12)

[a] Approximation.
[b] Components of ambulation category.
[c] Presence of category not clear.
[d] Included in Tinetti's performance-oriented mobility assessment (POMA).

Comparisons of Balance Test Characteristics Between Studies With and Without Successful Balance-Training Outcomes

Studies with negative outcomes tended to show less diversity in their use of different balance tests ($\overline{X}$ = 1.6 versus 2.2, $p < .09$). Forty percent of the studies with unsuccessful outcomes included tests of unstressed (eyes-open sway) balance, and in 50% of these, eyes-open sway was the only test modality employed. Only one of the positive outcome trials included eyes-open sway as a test. This suggests that a possible reason for a negative response to training could be the use of insufficiently challenging tests.

The one-legged stance test was used 65% and 50% of the time, respectively, in studies with significant versus nonsignificant outcomes (NS, X^2). Moreover, in the latter group, one-legged stance was never tested with eyes closed. Furthermore, a lack of control over the design details of this balance test might also have adversely influenced study outcome.

Although one-legged standing was the most frequently used of the outcome measures, it is a complex activity with many degrees of freedom of movement, which in turn could be easily affected by inconsistencies in test procedure. Leg dominance, footwear (shoes, sneakers, unshod), practice trials, scoring manner (e.g., best versus average of trials), support surface quality (carpeting, wood), arm placement, and raised foot posture (suspended versus closed-loop contact with calf) are examples of features that must be controlled to maximize reproducibility. However, an average of only 2.75 (range, 0–6) of the 7 considerations mentioned above were accounted for in the 16 studies using the one-legged stance test on a normal surface. Interestingly, in the 11 studies with successful outcomes, a mean of 3.18 of the control features were specified, whereas in the 5 with nonsuccessful outcomes, only 1.1 items were stipulated ($p < .05$, t test). It is not surprising, then, that oversights in the one-legged stance test protocol might account for failure to detect a training effect.

Comparisons of Intervention Characteristics Between Studies With and Without Successful Balance-Training Outcomes

In order to characterize the balance-stimulating elements within an intervention, the training procedures of each study were expressed in terms of the 13 BCD categories, as well as 3 "other" training modes encountered in the literature: vestibulo-ocular, Tai Chi Chuan, mental imagery (Tables 22-7 and 22-8). Scores of 0 to 3 (0 = absent, 1 = minimal, 2 = moderate, 3 = abundant) were used to rate the degree to which a category was represented in an intervention based on the authors' descriptions of their procedures. A total balance score also was derived from the sum of 15 balance-training classifications (see Tables 22-7, 22-8; 12 BCD* + "other").

Scoring was difficult and often subjective, as most studies provided only abbreviated descriptions of the training procedures and frequently used terms such as "coordination," "traditional," "flexibility," "dance-like," and "postural" to portray what probably were groups of highly specific movements. For example, turn and upper-extremity components had to be inferred from "dance-like" movements, whereas vertical movements were assumed to be present in abundance during what was described as aerobics, but minimally during walking. It is likely that many movements subsumed under designations such as "strengthening" and "flexibility" may unintentionally have been richly endowed with balance components and hence were lost to analysis. If not controlled for, the natural tendency for overlapping and sharing of features under the labels balance, strengthening, and endurance training also confounds our ability to attribute the outcomes of interventions to specific training paradigms.

The endurance and strength classifications were assessed in order to gain insights into the possible roles played by intensity factors such as aerobic training and resistance exercise, and a frailty rating also was derived (see Tables 22-7 and 22-8). The frailty level of a study sample was estimated by assigning values of

---

* Decreased bipedal base and one-legged stance were combined into the single base of support category because of the frequent difficulty in discerning these categories from the intervention descriptions.

Table 22-7. Scoring of components of training and related factors in 10 studies with nonsignificant improvements in balance outcomes

Study	A M B	B O S	L O S	T U R	U E	V E R	G G R	S I N	B O D	R S A	O B S	V I S	V O C	T C	I M G	TOT	E N D	V E S	S T R	F R A
RC trials																				
Crilly et al. [42]	1	1	0	1	1	1	0	0	0	0	0	0	0	0	0	5	1	1	0	0
Lichtenstein et al. [50]	2	2	0	0	1	1	0	0	0	0	0	0	0	0	0	6	1	1	0	1
McMurdo and Burnett [51]	1	1	0	1	1	1	0	0	0	0	0	0	0	0	0	5	2	1	0	2
Reinsch et al. [52]	1	1	0	1	1	2	0	0	0	0	0	0	0	0	0	6	2	1	0	1
Topper et al. [20]	0	0	0	0	3	0	0	0	0	0	0	0	0	0	0	3	1	2	3	2
Non-RC trials																				
Barry et al. [29]	0	0	0	0	0	0	0	0	0	0	0	0	0	0	0	0	3	0	0	2
Bassett et al. [30]	1	1	0	1	1	1	0	0	0	0	0	0	0	0	0	5	1	0	0	2
Clark et al. [33]	1	1	0	1	1	1	0	0	0	0	0	0	0	0	0	5	1	1	0	1
Gutman et al. [35] (Exp1)	0	0	0	0	1	1	0	0	0	0	0	2	2	0	2	8	0	1	0	1
(Exp2)	2	2	0	0	0	1	0	0	0	0	0	0	0	0	0	5	1	1	0	1
Sauvage et al. [39]	0	0	0	0	0	0	0	0	0	0	0	0	0	0	0	0	2	0	3	0

RC = randomized control; AMB = ambulatory conditions; BOS = base of support; LOS = limits of stability; TUR = turns;
UE = upper extremity; VER = vertical movement of center of gravity; G, GR = ground; SIN = surface instabilities; BOD = body
 perturbations; RSA = reduced surface area; OBS = obstacle contact; VIS = aberrant visual input; VOC = vestibulo-ocular; TOT = total.
END = endurance; FRA = frailty; IMG = imagery; STR = strength; TC = Tai Chi; VES = vestibular.
NOTE: Base of support (BOS) is a combination of diminished base and one-legged stance (see text); 0 = absent; 1 = minimal;
2 = moderate; 3 = abundant.

Table 22-8. Scoring of components of training and related factors in 15 studies with significant improvements in balance outcomes

	Functional challenges to balance								Provoked				Other training				Miscellaneous factors			
	Voluntary						G													
Study	AMB	BOS	LOS	TUR	UE	VER	GR	SIN	BOD	RSA	OBS	VIS	VOC	TC	IMG	TOT	END	VES	STR	FRA
RC trials																				
Era [43] (Exp1)	0	1	0	1	1	1	0	0	0	0	0	0	0	0	0	4	2	1	3	3
(Exp2)	1	1	0	1	1	1	0	0	0	0	0	0	0	0	0	5	1	1	0	3
Fansler et al. [44]	0	0	0	0	0	0	0	0	0	0	0	0	0	0	3	3	0	0	0	2
Hopkins et al. [45]	2	1	0	2	1	2	0	0	0	0	0	0	1	0	0	9	3	3	0	2
Hu and Woollacott [46]	0	0	2	0	0	0	0	3	0	0	0	2	0	0	0	7	0	1	0	2
Johanssen and Jarnlo [47]	2	1	0	2	1	2	0	0	0	0	0	0	0	0	0	8	2	3	0	2
Judge et al. [48]	2	1	0	1	0	1	2	0	0	0	0	0	0	2	0	9	3	1	2	3
Ledin et al. [49]	3	3	0	3	2	3	0	2	0	0	0	2	0	0	0	18	3	3	0	3
Non-RC trials																				
Binder et al. [31]	1	1	0	1	1	2	2	0	0	0	0	0	0	0	0	8	2	2	0	1
Brown and Holloszy [32]	1	1	2	2	2	2	2	0	0	0	0	0	0	0	0	12	2	1	0	2
Fiatarone et al. [34]	0	0	0	0	0	0	0	0	0	0	0	0	0	0	0	5	2	0	2	0
Lord and Castell [36]	2	2	0	2	1	2	0	0	0	0	0	0	0	0	0	9	2	2	0	3
Rikli and Edwards [37]	1	2	0	2	1	2	0	0	0	0	0	0	0	0	0	8	2	2	0	1
Roberts [38]	2	0	0	0	0	0	0	0	0	0	0	0	0	0	0	2	2	1	0	2
Stones and Kozma [40]	2	1	0	1	1	1	0	0	0	0	0	0	0	0	0	6	3	1	0	2
Vanfraechem and Vanfraechem [41]	1	1	0	1	1	1	0	0	0	0	0	0	0	0	0	5	1	1	0	1

RC = randomized control; AMB = ambulatory conditions; BOS = base of support; LOS = limits of stability; TUR = turns; UE = upper extremity; VER = vertical movement of center of gravity; G, GR = ground; SIN = surface instabilities; BOD = body perturbations; RSA = reduced surface area; OBS = obstacle contact; VIS = aberrant visual input; VOC = vestibuloocular; TC = Tai Chi; IMG = imagery; TOT = total; END = endurance; VES = vestibular; STR = strength; FRA = frailty.

NOTE: Base of support (BOS) is a combination of diminished base and one-legged stance (see text); 0 = absent; 1 = minimal; 2 = moderate; 3 = abundant.

0, 1, 2, or 3, respectively, to nursing home residents, community dwellers with obvious deficits, "normal" community dwellers, and "fit" community dwellers. Vestibular contribution was considered as a separate factor for analysis and is a composite approximation of activities in the vertical, turning, and surface instabilities categories. Running and aerobic activities also were considered examples of the vestibular factor.

The total (Table 22-9) balance training score (derived from summing the 12 functional challenges to balance plus the 3 "other training" categories from Tables 22-7 and 22-8) was significantly greater in the 15 studies with positive balance outcomes ($\overline{X}$ = 7.6 versus 4.15, $p < .01$). This implies that a greater "dosage" of balance-enhancing features may have been partially responsible for the successful outcomes in this subgroup of studies. Diversity alone did not appear to account for the difference. If a 1 was awarded to an intervention each time a balance category was represented and the sums were compared, no significant difference emerged between study groups (see Table 22-9).

A number of other balance-related elements were selected for comparison from Tables 22-7 and 22-8 and are summarized in Table 22-9. Age and training duration (number of weeks of intervention plus number of minutes per session* were similar for both negative and positive outcomes. The base of support (a composite of the one-legged stance and decreased bipedal base categories of Table 22-3), and upper-extremity movement categories did not differ. However, there were trends showing vertical movements ($p < .1$), ambulation ($p < .08$), and endurance exercise ($p < .07$) to be higher in the successful outcome interventions. The turns category and vestibular factor were significantly greater in the studies with positive outcomes ($p < .01$ and $p < .025$, respectively).

A glance at the training variables that were more strongly represented in the successful outcome studies suggests certain common underlying qualities in these interventions. Activities in which the above-listed movement factors occur appear to share elements of (1) high body or head velocity, which frequently requires fast interactive movements of body segments and eyes in a horizontal plane; (2) larger-amplitude vertical movements of the center of gravity, which requires task-associated thigh and hip strength; and (3) endurance activities during full-body weight bearing. The acronym *5V* describes the essence of these movement features: *velocity, vestibular, vision, vertical,* and *vigor.*

An unexpected finding was the significantly frailer status of subject samples in the nonsuccessful studies ($p < .025$). Previous work in fitness training [54] indicated that frailer subjects might show greater early training effects. Hence, it was expected that studies with positive outcomes would have had a frailer sample makeup. It is certainly possible that our basis for designating frailty is flawed or (given the relatively small number of 10 negative-outcome studies) that this was

---

* $\leq$ 30 min = 1, ~ 30–45 min = 2, > 45 min = 3; < 10 weeks = 1, $\geq$ 10 weeks = 2. The number of weeks of intervention were given weights of 1 (< 10 weeks) and 2 ($\geq$ 10 weeks). Number of minutes per session were weighted as 1 ($\leq$ 30 min), 2 (> 30–45 min), or 3 (> 45 min).

Table 22-9. Comparison of balance variables (means) between studies with successful and unsuccessful balance outcomes

Variable	Nonsignificant-outcome balance studies (N = 10)	Significant balance outcome studies (N = 15)
Total balance-training score	4.14	7.6[a]
Training diversity	3.3	4.2
Age	72.8	72.1
Frailty	1.2	1.9[b]
Training duration	4.3	3.7
Vertical	0.8	1.3[c]
Ambulation	0.8	1.3[c]
Endurance	1.5	2.0[c]
Turns	0.5	1.3[a]
Vestibular	0.7	1.5[b]

[a] $p < .01$.
[b] $p < .025$.
[c] $p < .1$

a chance finding. On the other hand, the significant underrepresentation of most of the key BCD training categories and intensity factors (see Table 22-9, total) within the unsuccessful-outcome studies may indicate either a deliberate or an inadvertent lowering of the exercise dosage for subjects who might have been viewed as intolerant of a more intensive intervention. Yet another explanation might be that, although frailer individuals may respond more readily to endurance and strengthening programs, improvements in balance may be more recalcitrant to change.

An examination of the studies for other features reveals possible additional reasons for negative outcomes. In keeping with the 5V thesis, which presupposes training during weight bearing, 4 of the 10 negative-outcome studies were carried out during non–weight bearing [29, 35, 39, 53]. Although two positive-outcome interventions were also non–weight bearing, they were atypical and highly focused forms of training. Fansler et al. [44] employed 5 minutes of daily body imagery over a brief (3-day) period, whereas Fiatarone et al. [34] used intensive quadriceps strengthening in the very frailest sample (90-year-old nursing home residents) of the studies analyzed.

A disproportionate number of negative-outcome studies (70%) consisted of extremely low-intensity interventions [29, 30, 33, 35, 42, 51, 52]. Only two of the positive-outcome studies could be categorized as low-intensity [44, 46]; however, both involved very specific and concentrated training efforts. A total of 9 of the 10 unsuccessful trials could be classified as either low-intensity [29, 30, 33, 35, 42, 51, 52], non–weight-bearing [29, 35, 39, 53], or both [29, 35].

DISCUSSION

Limitations of Balance Tests and Interventions in Reflecting Challenges to Balance Found in Daily Life

Testing

Of the 13 major BCDs, (see Tables 22-1, 22-2), only one-legged standing was used consistently in testing. Tests of decreased bipedal base of support occurred infrequently, whereas four other areas (turns, vertical body movements, surface instabilities, and tandem walks) had only token representation. Of the more than 50 subcategories of balance challenge listed in Tables 22-1 and 22-2, only 15 appeared in test form, and 53% of the latter were concentrated within only 2 of the 13 major categories (one-legged stance and decreased bipedal base).

In addition to the underrepresentation of commonplace balance challenges within testing, there is also a lack of concordance between the kinds of balance tasks encountered in testing and the forms of balance training used during the 25 interventions (see Table 22-9). For example, one-legged stance, aberrant visual input, and decreased bipedal base are the most frequently used categories of balance testing. In contrast, ambulation, vertical body movements, upper-extremity movements, and turns occur most often as training components. Clearly, there are likely to be many varieties of improvements in balance that go undetected, either because of an inappropriate mesh of test and training categories or because of the near absence of variety in test categories. This may in part account for negative outcomes in many (40%) of the studies.

Training

Six of the categories in the domain of predictable challenges to balance (see Table 22-1; ambulation, one-legged stance, decreased bipedal base, upper-extremity movements, turning, and vertical body movements) occurred with regularity in the interventions (all six components appeared in 53% of the studies). Conspicuously absent or underrepresented (≤ 12% of studies) were the domains of ground activities (see Fig. 22-1), unexpected destabilizations (see Table 22-2), and limits of stability (see Table 22-1).

Frequency of falling increases in older adults [19, 20, 27] during hazardous circumstances, and often it is the unpredictable nature of the balancing demands that constitutes the hazard (poor lighting, irregular surface, slip, push, over-leaning, fast turns). Data from Topper et al. [20] indicated that 60% of falls were associated with external perturbations of the surface or body. It is ironic, then, that opportunities for practice in the domain of unpredictable balance challenges are lacking in most intervention studies.

If one assumes that (1) balance has multiple dimensions and (2) any balancing skill is to some degree a byproduct of exposure to the circumstances that stimulate the use of that skill, it follows that in order to enhance a given balance skill, training must be carried out in a context-specific manner. Although recent neurophysiological findings indicate that there is an inherent adaptive plasticity to many sensorimotor processes [9, 55, 56], recurring exposure to specific postural and balancing demands is likely to be necessary for the acquisition of skill.

Barring changes in habit or lifestyle, if an individual's customary activity pattern leads to a frequent exposure to certain categories of balance challenge (e.g., gardening, narrow stairs, crowds), it would be desirable to attempt to replicate as many as possible of the key features of these events during training. After a person is "innoculated" with a program that includes unpredictable balance challenges in the safety of an intensive one-on-one training program, it is conceivable that the enhancement of a balance skill might be carried over into the posttraining period. After cessation of formal training, occasional "booster shots" with the same (or a similar) balance challenge may result in the maintenance of the original skill. This might be especially true if training resulted in a higher level of functioning, along with lifestyle modifications that included balance-enriched elements (e.g., walking on sand, practicing Tai Chi, ballroom dancing, aquatic activities, riding).

Criteria for Effective Balance Training in Older Adults

As a group, the studies with successful outcomes appeared to take a more intensive approach to training. Propulsive movements, in both horizontal and vertical planes, and activities involving endurance and quick turns seemed to predominate. Some task-specific contexts that were encountered in these studies and incorporated many of these dynamic features were (1) ambulation, (2) jogging, (3) aerobic dancing, (4) sit-stand and ground-stand movements, and (5) "calisthenics."

Some calisthenic programs undoubtedly contained such dynamic features, but the extent usually was difficult to infer from the abbreviated descriptions. It is likely that many calisthenic or coordination exercises may have only accidentally contained dynamic balance-stimulating elements. Future studies should consider choosing or assembling movement patterns with the intent of including specific "dosages" of 5V components.

Higher-velocity movements and turns place great demands on vestibulo-ocular processing and head control, and the successful execution of such motions of necessity must be mediated by high-speed and high-intensity contractions of the lower extremity musculature, particularly of the proximal groups (quadriceps, hip extensors).

Balancing on one leg and in narrowed stances occurred with approximately equal frequency in both classes of studies, although this often had to be inferred from the abbreviated descriptions of procedures. These abilities frequently improved with training, which bodes well for the prospects of falls prevention. It is interesting and auspicious to note that the capacity to stand on one leg appeared to improve in a universal manner in response to many different forms of training. For example, Hu and Woollacott [46] observed significant increases in one-legged standing time in response to multisensory training on an unstable surface, whereas Fansler et al. [44] reported improvements resulting from body awareness and mental imagery practice. Wolfson et al. [22] have also reported improvement in single stance time in both balance- and strength-trained older subjects.

NEW DIRECTIONS AND RECOMMENDATIONS.

The foregoing trends from the intervention literature do not do justice to some emerging strategies for balance retraining in the elderly. The multisensory-interaction [46] and mental imagery [44] approaches already have been mentioned. In a study with healthy elderly by Wolfson et al. [22], balance was effectively trained through the use of a wide representation of BCD categories: (1) unstable (foam) surfaces, (2) narrowed base in stance, (3) one-legged stance, (4) video feedback of the standing center of pressure, (5) training at the limits of stability, (6) manual delivery of body perturbations, (7) various forms of nonendurance ambulation, and (8) visual occlusion. The categories were combined whenever possible in order to maximize the challenge level (e.g., walking backward on foam with eyes closed, or tandem standing on foam with eyes closed while receiving manual perturbations).

Balance training in a diversity of categories led to improvement in multiple-outcome measures (dynamic platform balance, one-legged stance time, and a limits of stability test), lending support to the thesis that balance enhancement may indeed be task-specific to some degree. It is interesting to note that there was no significant increase in lower-extremity strength. This may have been a consequence of the lack of representation of challenging vertical movements of the center of gravity.

Recently, vestibulo-ocular exercises have been effectively used to ameliorate balance in individuals with vestibular hypofunction or with benign positional nystagmus [57]. When used for these clinical conditions, such tactics may spur the development of compensatory capacities within the CNS [55]. Moreover, many ostensibly disease-free elderly with balance problems may be suffering from occult neurological dysfunctions that are directly or indirectly associated with vestibulo-ocular processing [58]. In such cases, vestibulo-ocular approaches may hold promise as well.

Much progress is being made in the area of spatial perception, a function that declines steeply with age [59, 60]. As in the case of vestibular compensation, there may be a potential for plasticity within the neural networks that process spatial relationships between body segments and of the body in space [61]. Improvements in spatial orientation may result from prolonged task-specific training. Schaie and Willis [62] have found that a brief period (five 1-hour sessions) of cognitive spatial retraining (mental rotation of figures) in 64- to 95-year-olds resulted in a significant reversal of decline in this function.

Tai Chi Chuan is a movement technique that directs attention to spatial intersegmental associations and to body orientation in space. Guidelines are provided for changing the habitual alignments between body segments and for developing new spatial frames of reference for posture and movement. Body imagery and awareness procedures are used to enhance the perceptions of verticality, weight distribution, and pelvic alignment. In two recent studies [63, 64], Tai Chi training resulted in significant improvements in balance [22] and reduction of falls [65] in older adults.

Work by Roll et al. [66] and Vallar et al. [67] indicate that increased levels of Ia and vestibular sensory inputs, respectively, can affect short-term spatial perception. Sustained vestibular stimulation, lateral head-eye movements, and visual imagery are all known to affect the metabolic activity of brain regions associated with spatial processing [68–70]. Repeated exposure to kinesthetic matching tasks in the elderly [71] has resulted in enhanced foot position perception. Tai Chi, mental imagery, and related approaches that involve attention to multiple sensory inputs (both real and imagined) may represent reasonable tools for creating long-term change.

CONCLUSIONS

Although there are an infinite number of biomechanical contexts that challenge balance, an attempt has been made to operationalize them into categories and subcategories. A healthy nervous system has been shown to be able to adapt its sensorimotor response patterns to many contexts after repeated exposure [72–74]. Future success in enhancing the balance of older adults may depend on training designs that incorporate (1) sustained (and safe) exposure to a wide variety of functional balance-challenging contexts, (2) opportunities for multimodal sensory processing, and (3) focused attention on real or imagined spatial references.

REFERENCES

1. Overstall PW, Exton-Smith AN, Imms FJ, Johnson AC. Falls in the elderly related to postural imbalance. *Br J Med* 1977;1:261–264.
2. Wolfson LI, Katzman R. The Neurologic Consultation at Age 80. In: Katzman R, Terry R, eds. *The Neurology of Aging*. Philadelphia: Davis, 1983. Pp 75–88.
3. Panzer V, Kaye J, Edner A, Holme L. Standing Postural Control in the Elderly and Very Elderly. In: Woollacott M, Horak F, eds. *Posture and Gait: Control Mechanisms*. Eugene, OR: University of Oregon, 1992. Pp 220–223.
4. Wolfson L, et al. A dynamic posturography study of balance in healthy elderly. *Neurology* 1992;42:2069–2075.
5. Alexander NB. Postural control in older adults. *J Am Geriatr Soc* 1994;42:93–108.
6. Horak FB, Shupert CL, Mirka A. Components of postural dyscontrol in the elderly: A review. *Neurobiol Aging* 1989;10:727–738.
7. Stelmach GE, et al. Age-related decline in postural control mechanisms. *Int J Aging Hum Dev* 1989;29:205–223.
8. Dietz V. Human neuronal control of automatic functional movements: Interaction between central programs and afferent input. *Physiol Rev* 1992;72:33–69.

9. Keshner EA. Controlling stability of a complex movement system. *Phys Ther* 1990;70:844–854.

10. Nashner LM, McCollum G. The organization of human postural movements: A formal basis and experimental synthesis. *Behav Brain Sci* 1985;8:135–172.

11. Woollacott MH, Shumway-Cook A, Nashner LM. Aging and posture control: Changes in sensory organization and muscular coordination. *Int J Aging Hum Dev* 1986;23:97–114.

12. Berg K, Wood-Dauphinee S, Williams JI, Gayton D. Measuring balance in the elderly: Preliminary development of an instrument. *Physiother Can* 1989;41:304–311.

13. Reuben DB, Siu AL. An objective measure of physical function of elderly outpatients: The physical performance test. *J Am Geriatr Soc* 1990;38:1105–1112.

14. Tinetti ME. Performance-oriented assessment of mobility problems in elderly patients. *J Am Geriatr Soc* 1986;34:119–126.

15. Buchner DM, Wagner EH. Preventing frail health. *Clin Geriatr Med* 1992;8:1–17.

16. Hinchcliffe R. *Hearing and Balance in the Elderly.* Edinburgh: Churchill Livingstone, 1983.

17. Tinetti ME, Williams TF, Mayewski R. Fall risk index for elderly patients based on number of chronic disabilities. *Am J Med* 1986;80:429–434.

18. Whipple R, Wolfson L, Amerman P. The relationship of knee and ankle weakness to falls in nursing home residents: An isokinetic study. *J Am Geriatr Soc* 1987;35:13–20.

19. Nevitt MC, Cummings SR, Hudes ES. Risk factors for injurious falls: A prospective study. *J Gerontol* 1991;46:M164–170.

20. Topper AK, Maki BE, Holloday PJ. Are activity-based assessments of balance and gait in the elderly predictive of risk of falling and/or type of fall? *J Am Geriat Soc* 1993;41:479–487.

21. Vandervoort AA, McComas AJ. Contractile changes in opposing muscles of the human ankle joint with aging. *J Appl Physiol* 1986;61:361–367.

22. Wolfson L, et al. Balance and strength training in older adults: Intervention gains and Tai Chi maintenance. *J Am Geriatr soc* 1996;44:498–506.

23. Mouchnino L, Aurenty R, Massion J, Pedotti A. Coordination between equilibrium and head-trunk orientation during leg movement: A new strategy built up by training. *J Neurophysiol* 1992;67:1587–1598.

24. Tinetti ME, Liu WL, Claus E. Predictors and prognosis of inability to get up after falls among elderly persons. *JAMA* 1993;269:65–70.

25. Tinetti, Richman D, Powell L. Falls efficacy as a measure of fear of falling. *J Gerontol* 1990;45:P239–243.

26. VanSant AF. Life-span development in functional tasks. *Phys Ther* 1990;70:788–798.

27. Speechley M, Tinetti M. Falls and injuries in frail and vigorous community elderly persons. *J Am Geriatr Soc* 1991;39:46–52.

28. Arfken CL, Birge SJ, Miller JP. Maladaptive behavior: A risk factor for falls resulting from slips and trips. *J Am Geriat Soc* 1991;39:A39.

29. Barry AJ, Steinmetz JR, Page HF, Rodahl K. The effects of physical conditioning on older individuals: II. Motor performance and cognitive function. *J Gerontal* 1967;21:192–199.

30. Bassett C, McClamrock E, Schmelzer M. A 10-week exercise program for senior citizens. *Geriatr Nurs* 1982;3:103–105.

31. Binder EF, Brown MB, Birge SJ. Effects of moderate intensity exercise program at reducing risk factors for falls in frail older adults. *J Am Geriat Soc* 1991;39:A50.

32. Brown M, Holloszy JO. Effects of a low intensity exercise program on selected physical performance characteristics of 60- to 71-year-olds. *Aging* 1991;3:129–139.

33. Clark BA, Wade MG, Massey BH, Van Dyke R. Response of institutionalized geriatric mental patients to a twelve-week program of regular physical activity. *J Gerontol* 1975;30:565–573.

34. Fiatarone MA, et al. High-intensity strength training in nonagenarians. *JAMA* 1990;263:3029–3034.

35. Gutman GM, Herbert CP, Brown SR. Feldenkrais versus conventional exercises for the elderly. *J Gerontol* 1977;32:562–572.

36. Lord SR, Castell S. Physical activity program for older persons: Effect on balance, strength, neuromuscular control, and reaction time. *Arch Phys Med Rehabil* 1994;75:648–652.

37.   Rikli RE, Edwards DJ. Effects of a three-year exercise program on motor function and cognitive processing speed in older women. *Res Q Exerc Sport* 1991;62:61–67.

38.   Roberts BL. Effects of walking on balance among elders. *Nurs Res* 1989;38:180–182.

39.   Sauvage LR, et al. A clinical trial of strengthening and aerobic exercise to improve gait and balance in elderly male nursing home residents. *Am J Phys Med* 1992;71:333–342.

40.   Stones MJ, Kozma A. Balance and age in the sighted and blind. *Arch Phys Med Rehabil* 1987;68:85–89.

41.   Vanfraechem J, Vanfraechem R. Studies of the effect of a short training period on aged subjects. *J Sports Med* 1977;17:373–380.

42.   Crilly RG, et al. Effect of exercise on postural sway in the elderly. *Gerontology* 1989;35:137–143.

43.   Era P. Posture control in the elderly. *Int J Technol Aging* 1988;1:166–179.

44.   Fansler CL, Poff CL, Shepard KF. Effects of mental practice on balance in elderly women. *Phys Ther* 1985;65:1332–1338.

45.   Hopkins DR, Murrah B, Hoeger WWK, Rhodes RC. Effect of low-impact aerobic dance on the functional fitness of elderly women. *Gerontologist* 1990;30:189–192.

46.   Hu MH, Woollacott MH. Multisensory training of standing balance in older adults: I. Postural stability and one-leg stance balance. *J Gerontol* 1994;49:M52–M61.

47.   Johansson G, Jarnlo G. Balance training in 70-year-old women. *Physiother Theory Pract* 1991;7:121–125.

48.   Judge JO, Lindsey C, Underwood M, Winsemius D. Balance improvements in older women: Effects of exercise training. *Phys Ther* 1993;73:254–262.

49.   Ledin T, et al. Effects of balance training in elderly evaluated by clinical tests and dynamic posturography. *J Vestib Res* 1991;1:129–138.

50.   Lichtenstein MJ, Shields SL, Shiavi RG, Burger MC. Exercise and balance in aged women: A pilot controlled clinical trial. *Arch Phys Med Rehabil* 1989;70:138–143.

51.   McMurdo MET, Burnett L. Randomised controlled trial of exercise in the elderly. *Gerontology* 1992;38:292–298.

52.   Reinsch S, MacRae P, Lachenbruch PA, Tobis JS. Attempts to prevent falls and injury: A prospective community study. *Gerontologist* 1992;32:450–456.

53.   Topp R, et al. The effect of a 12-week dynamic resistance strength training program on gait velocity and balance of older adults. *Gerontologist* 1993;33:501–506.

54.   Buchner DM, deLateur BJ. The importance of skeletal muscle strength to physical function in older adults. *Ann Behav Med* 1991;13:91–98.

55.   Llinas R, Walton K. Vestibular Compensation: A Distributed Property of the Central Nervous System. In: Asanyma H, Wilson VT, eds. *Integration in the Nervous System*. Tokyo: Igaku-Shoin, 1979. Pp 145–166.

56.   Moore SP, Rushmer DS, Windus SL, Nashner LM. Human automatic postural responses: Responses to horizontal perturbations of stance in multiple directions. *Exp Brain Res* 1988;73:648–658.

57.   Herdman SJ. *Vestibular Rehabilitation*. Philadelphia: Davis, 1994.

58.   Yamasoda T, et al. Ischemic brain lesions in aged patients. *Acta Otolaryngol Head Neck Surg* 1993;119:1346–1350.

59.   Howieson DB, et al. Neurologic function in the optimally healthy oldest old: Neuropsychological evaluation. *Neurology* 1993;43:1882–1886.

60.   Schaie KW. The course of adult intellectual development. *Am Psychol* 1994;49:304–313.

61.   Llinas RR. The intrinsic electrophysiological properties of mammalian neurons: Insights into central nervous system function. *Science* 1988;242:1654–1664.

62.   Schaie KW, Willis SL. Can decline in adult intellectual functioning be reversed? *Dev Psych* 1986;22:223–232.

63.   Wolfson L, et al. Training balance and strength in the elderly to improve function. *J Am Geriat Soc* 1993;41:341–343.

64.   Wolf S, Kutner N, Green R, McNeely E. Reducing frailty in elders: Two exercise interventions at Emory University and Wesley Woods Geriatric Center. *J Am Geriat Soc* 1993;41:329–332.

65. Wolf S, et al. Reducing frailty and falls in older persons: An investigation of Tai Chi and computerized balance training. *J Am Geriatr Soc* 1996;44:489–497.

66. Roll JP, Hay L, Quoniam C, Roll R. Muscle Proprioception: A Powerful Sensory Input for Postural Adaptation in Man. In: Vellas B, et al., eds. *Falls, Balance and Gait Disorders in the Elderly.* Paris: Elsevier, 1992. Pp 161–182.

67. Vallar G, Bottini G, Rusconi ML, Sterzi R. Exploring somatosensory hemineglect by vestibular stimulation. *Brain* 1993;116:71–86.

68. Brandt Th, Dieterich M, Danek A. Vestibular cortex lesions affect the perception of verticality. *Ann Neurol* 1994;35:403–412.

69. Gross Y, Franko R, Lewin I. Effects of voluntary eye movements on hemispheric activity and choice of cognitive mode. *Neuropsychologia* 1978;16:653–657.

70. Roland PE, Gulyas B. Visual imagery and visual representation. *Trends Neurosci* 1994;17: 281–287.

71. Meeuwsen HJ, Sawicki TM, Stelmach GE. Improved foot position sense as a result of repetitions in older adults. *J Gerontol* 1993;48:137–141.

72. Horak FB, Nashner LM. Central programming of postural movements: Adaptation to altered support-surface configurations. *J Neurophysiol* 1986;55:1369–1381.

73. Macpherson JM, Horak FB, Dunbar DC, Dow RS. Stance dependence of automatic postural adjustments in humans. *Exp Brain Res* 1989;78:557–566.

74. Nashner LM. Organization of Human Postural Movements During Standing and Walking. In: Grillner S, et al., eds. *Neurobiology of Posture and Locomotion.* London: Macmillan, 1986. Pp 637–648.

23. Resistance Training

James O. Judge

Resistance training holds great promise to prevent or reverse many age-associated losses of function, including gait. Studies that have demonstrated impressive muscle strength gains have been widely reported. This chapter reviews the theoretical reasons for an association between muscle strength and gait and the relationship between muscle strength and gait found in cross-sectional studies. Finally, the limited experience of resistance interventions on gait are discussed.

AGE-ASSOCIATED CHANGES IN GAIT

Usual and maximal gait velocity is maintained until the seventh decade and thereafter declines at a rate of 12–16% per decade for usual gait and approximately 20% for maximal gait [1–3]. A shortened step length is responsible for most of the decline in gait velocity [1, 2, 4, 5]; cadence (steps/min^{-1}) usually is maintained [1, 2, 4]. A shorter step length is associated with decreased pelvic rotation and decreased hip flexion and extension [2, 4]. Stance time (proportion of gait cycle with the foot on the ground) increases in men from 0.59 in 20-year-olds to 0.63 in 70-year-olds, resulting in substantial increases in double-stance time (proportion of time when both feet are on the ground) in the same groups: from 18% to 26%, respectively [6].

The pattern of an increase in double-stance time and a shortened step may be an appropriate response to declines in balance or may be primarily due to lack of muscle power. In older persons, limited range of motion rarely impacts gait.

THEORETICAL RELATIONSHIP BETWEEN MUSCLE STRENGTH AND GAIT

Muscle forces are required to accelerate and decelerate the limbs and torso and, thus, are an absolute requirement for upright stance and walking. Maximal muscle force is a powerful predictor of performance in a short burst of work (50-m dash or 30-sec maximal bicycle work) but may be less important in sustained submaximal activities such as walking. Figure 23-1 describes the gait kinematics during usual gait of young and older subjects. Figure 23-2 is the surface electromyography (EMG) recordings of leg muscles during several gait cycles. These figures highlight one major point: Joint moments, joint power, and muscle activity are developed in bursts—each muscle group is quiet during a large proportion of the gait cycle. The hip generates substantial power in extension in

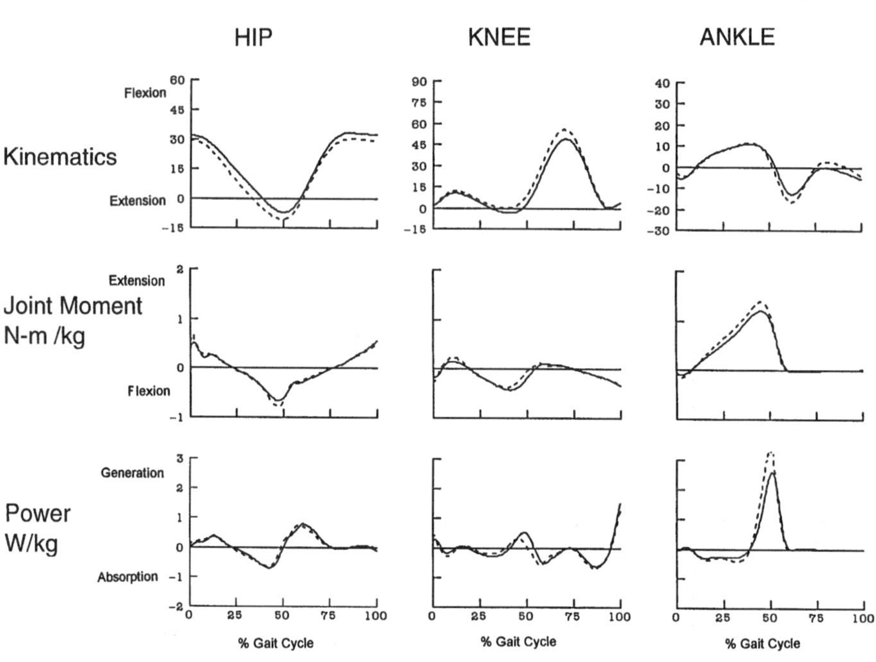

Figure 23-1. Gait kinematics of young and older subjects. The ordinate is a complete gait cycle (GC), or stride, where 0% represents initial foot contact, and 100% initial foot contact of the next stride. The stance phase is from 0 to 60% GC in the younger subjects and 0 to 63% in the older subjects. The top row represents the joint angle (kinematics of the three joints) during one complete gait cycle. The middle row represents the joint moment, or torque. The bottom row represents joint power generated or absorbed at the joint. The dotted line is the mean for younger subjects; the solid line is the mean for older subjects. (From Judge JO, Davis RB, Ounpuu S. Step length reductions in advanced age: The role of ankle and hip kinetics. *J Gerontol Med Sci* 1996.

early stance and power in flexion during late stance. The ankle develops substantial power in late stance, which is termed the "push-off" phase of gait [7]. The "off" time during the gait cycle is important to prevent muscle fatigue during repetitive motions, such as walking. The integrated surface EMG activity of leg muscles is similar in younger and older women in usual gait [6].

If muscle power were the primary determinant (or limiting factor) of usual gait, the joint-power tracings in Figure 23-1 suggest that hip flexion and ankle plantar flexion would be the joint movements where muscle weakness could limit velocity. If muscle power were the primary determinant of usual gait velocity, it would be very difficult to increase step length or gait velocity. However, people of all ages can walk faster than usual when instructed, by increasing step length and cadence. Usual gait velocity is approximately 72–75% of maximal gait velocity. When instructed, persons of all ages can increase gait velocity by approximately 30%, with a combination of increasing step length by 20–22% and cadence by 12% [8–10]. Does the muscle force developed during the bursts of activity in gait approach the maximum possible force? Unfortunately, there are

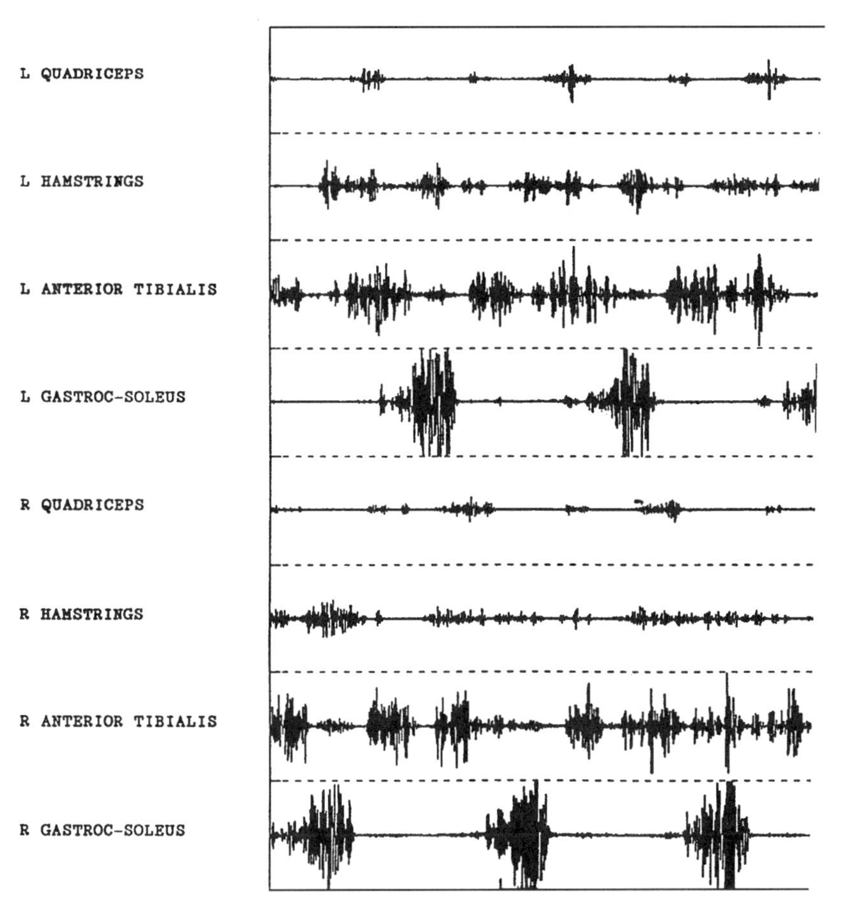

Figure 23-2. Surface electromyography of several gait cycles at usual pace.

no studies of gait kinetics at varying velocity in older persons to determine whether hip extension power or ankle plantar flexor power is a limiting factor in step length [11]. In addition, pelvic motion in the transverse plane (forward rotation of the pelvis on the femur in the direction of travel), which requires power developed by the internal rotators of the hip and power absorbed by the deceleration of the swing leg, also contributes to step length. The kinetics of pelvic motion have not been determined.

The moment and power tracings at the knee in Figure 23-1 might imply that control of the knee may not be important, as the power developed at the knee is small relative to the hip and ankle joints. However, control of the knee is probably very important. Knee flexion during early stance, termed the *loading response*, absorbs power generated by the opposite leg and contributes to step length and gait efficiency [12]. The peak knee flexion occurs during the initial portion of the single-stance phase of gait. Control of the knee during single stance may be challenging for persons with weakness in the quadriceps and hamstrings. (Fig. 23-2 demonstrates cocontraction of the hamstring and quadriceps during the loading response and coactivation of the gastrocnemius and tibialis anterior.) Cocontraction of agonist and antagonist increases the stiffness and control of the joint. In addition, the thigh muscles act to transmit plantar flexor moment to accelerate the body and to generate hip extensor moment [13]. Preliminary work in our laboratory suggests that healthy older subjects do not increase ankle plantar flexor moment or power when walking at maximum speed compared to their preferred speed. In contrast, hip flexion and hip extension moment and power increased at maximum speed [11]. This indirect data supports the hypothesis that ankle plantar flexion strength may be responsible for the decline in gait velocity and step length with usual aging.

Extensive data show that there are limits to maximum walking cadence. Usual and maximum cadence is related inversely to leg length and inertial mass of the leg by scaling laws [14]; that is, short persons will have a higher cadence and shorter step length. The combination of effects results in velocity, which is only slightly affected by differences in height. However, step length must be corrected for leg length (or height) in comparative studies of young and older persons because of the cohort effect on height (young persons are taller and have longer legs).

PHYSICAL ACTIVITY AND FUNCTIONAL LOSS

Several epidemiological studies have demonstrated that physical activity reduces the risk of functional dependence after correcting for comorbidity. Some studies have followed persons long enough to suggest that physical activity may be the most important preventive intervention to reduce future dependence.

Almost one-half of the older population engages in no regular physical activity [15]. In prospective studies, lack of usual physical activity is an independent risk factor for all-cause and cardiovascular mortality [16–18] and functional dependence [19, 20]. After correcting for comorbid conditions, physical inactivity (never walking a mile, no regular exercise) increased the risk of future functional loss by 50% [20]; another large 4-year prospective study found that frequent activity (walking, gardening, vigorous exercise)—not exercise—reduced the risk of mobility loss in women by 40%, after correcting for comorbidity [21]. Declines in functional status are related closely to chronic disease burden [19, 22], but physical activity may delay disability by delaying the onset of chronic disease and by maintaining endurance and body composition (muscle mass, percentage body fat, and bone mineral density [23].

PHYSICAL ACTIVITY AND GAIT SPEED

One study of women over age 65 compared the role of physical activity (three levels: sedentary, active, and regular exercisers) and age on gait. The exercise group walked faster at usual and maximal pace than did sedentary women (1.57 m/sec^{-1} compared to 1.29 m/sec^{-1}) but were 10 years younger (71 compared to 81 years) [10]. After correcting for age, the level of physical activity did not predict gait velocity or step length. Though these data suggest that physical activity may not be important, these statistical findings may be due to the limitations in characterizing physical activity.

PHYSICAL ACTIVITY, MUSCLE MASS, AND MUSCLE FORCE

Muscle mass is lost at a rate of 0.5% to 1.0% annually in women and men past 60 [24, 25], and muscle strength loss varies from 20–40% from the third to the eighth decades [26–28] and may be even greater in the eighth decade [29]. Weakness is due to loss of muscle mass and contractility (force/cm^2 of muscle cross section) [30–32]. Vigorous physical activity is associated with maintaining muscle strength, mass, and contractility [33, 34]. Thus, muscle strength measurements are dependent on *both* muscle mass and physical activity.

MUSCLE STRENGTH AND GAIT

Muscle strength is associated with gait velocity and step length in older persons [3, 35–37]. Both knee extension strength and ankle plantar flexion strength predict step length and gait velocity. Figures 23-3 and 23-4 illustrate the bivariate relationships between ankle plantar strength and gait velocity in relatively healthy volunteers over age 75. Knee extension strength also was associated with gait velocity in healthy women [3] and in nursing home residents over 90 years of age [36]. In middle-aged subjects with polio, knee extensor strength and ankle plantar flexor strength were associated with step length, but ankle plantar flexor strength was the only independent predictor in multivariate analysis.

Ankle plantar flexor strength also predicts gait velocity in older persons [37]. In a study comparing healthy adults, who were age-matched with diabetic patients with peripheral neuropathy, ankle plantar flexor strength predicted ankle plantar flexor power and moment in late stance, whereas disease status and gait velocity did not [39]. Though this evidence is not conclusive, it suggests that gastrocnemius-soleus strength may be a prime determinant of gait velocity in older persons. However, the contribution of proximal strength to gait velocity still may be important.

RESISTANCE TRAINING

Strength Response of Older Persons

Numerous manuscripts have demonstrated impressive strength gains in studies of older persons from the seventh through tenth decades of life. Heavy, progressive resistance training programs are superior to low-intensity training in achiev-

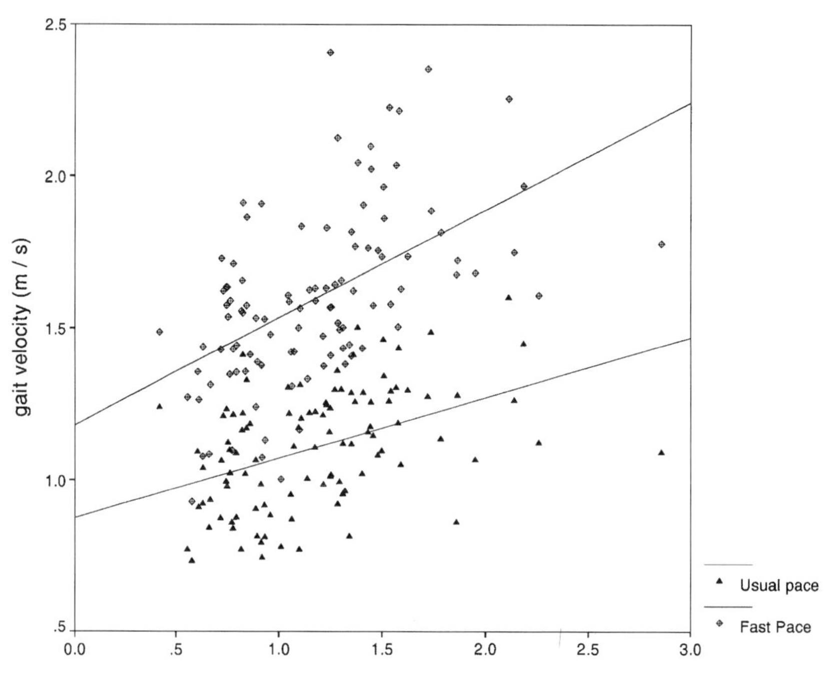

Figure 23-3. Gait velocity at usual and at fast pace is related to isokinetic knee extensor strength, corrected for body mass (peak moment at 60 degrees/sec^{-1}). N = 110, subjects are age 75 or older. The relationship between strength and gait velocity was stronger for fast pace (r^2 0.18 for usual pace, r^2 = 0.28 for fast pace).

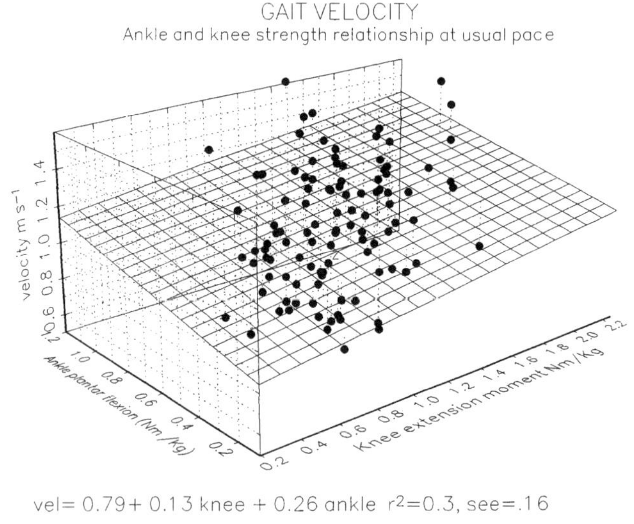

Figure 23-4. Association between ankle plantar flexion strength (isokinetic joint moment at 30 degrees/sec^{-1}) and usual gait velocity in healthy older subjects over 75 years of age.

ing strength gains in a short time (3 months or less) [40, 41]. The strength gains, whether measured in maximum weight lifted on the machine used in training or isokinetic moment exerted at the joint axis, are much larger than increases in muscle mass or muscle cross-sectional area.

The increase in muscle strength with training is dependent on (1) the intensity of training, (2) the strength measure used as outcome, and (3) how hard the exerciser works. There is a consensus that rapid increases in strength (over 3 months or less) are achieved by training multiple sets at a resistance that is a high proportion of the maximum lift. Resistance (weights, air, or hydraulic) is increased frequently to maintain the same relative intensity of exercise as strength improves. Resistance is set at between 70% and 80% of the maximum lift, and the greatest strength improvements have been seen in studies that trained at a resistance of 80% of the maximum lift [30, 41]. There are no studies of older subjects using higher than 80% resistance for training. As the blood pressure response is much greater when resistance settings exceed 80% of the maximum lift, the resistance used in training should not exceed that level. Because of demonstrated efficacy and safety in patients with stable and controlled coronary artery disease, resistance training is now a component of many cardiac rehabilitation programs [42].

Limitations

Short-term resistance training increases muscle contractility, but the effects on muscle hypertrophy are small [41, 43]. Resistance training results are most impressive when the outcome is how much one can lift on the training machine (at the velocity used in training). The gains are much smaller when the outcome is strength on another machine or strength at a different velocity of contraction [44]. Two recent studies illustrate this point. We trained ankle dorsiflexion in a sitting position. Though the maximum lift performed on the training machine increased 58–73% ($p < .001$), improvements in isokinetic strength (measured in a supine position with the knee extended) were much smaller (25%, $p > .05$) [45]. Nursing home residents trained in an intense (80% of maximum lift resistance) 10-week program. Leg muscles were trained in isolated motions (knee extension), and some subjects trained in multiple-joint motions resistance exercises (leg press). Strength gains were greatest in the isolated knee extension measure, which increased between 156% and 215%. Another measure of combined leg power—stair-climbing power—increased from 23% to 38%. As stair climbing was not trained in the program, stair-climbing power improvements can be considered a "generalizable" improvement in muscle power that is directly relevant to function. Large increases in leg strength in nursing home patients resulted in clinically meaningful improvements in stair climbing, but the improvement in a functional activity was much smaller than the improvement in isolated knee extension strength.

The specificity of resistance training suggests that to improve performance of real-world tasks—such as stair climbing, rising from a chair, or walking up a hill—

resistance training should include multijoint exercises similar to the speed and pattern of muscle contraction of such tasks. A 12-week pilot trial trained older persons in movements important to function, using resistance supplied by body weight, sandbags, and weight vests. Multijoint movements were trained, specifically, combined hip and knee extension and plantar flexion were performed on a step-up bench [46]. Plantar flexion was trained in a standing position. Resistance was increased by adding weights to a weight vest and by increasing the step height. Muscle contractility was not measured. However, subjects performed a series of functional tasks (picking objects off the floor, placing objects on a shelf, climbing stairs) faster after training, compared to the control group (physical performance test) [47].

EXERCISE INTERVENTIONS: EFFECT ON GAIT

If the relationship between leg strength and gait velocity found in cross-sectional studies represents a causal relationship, interventions to increase muscle strength should increase gait velocity and step length. The data from intervention trials is mixed.

Resistance Training and Gait Outcomes

Seven trials of resistance training in the elderly have reported gait outcomes. Two studies of nursing home residents showed similar positive results. The Boston Frailty and Injuries: Cooperative Studies of Intervention Techniques (FICSIT) study enrolled 100 nursing home residents who had a baseline gait velocity of 0.46 m/sec^{-1} and who were randomized either to a control group or to resistance training. Subjects also were randomized to a nutritional supplement or placebo supplement, which had no effect on performance. After 10 weeks of high-intensity resistance training, usual gait velocity increased 0.05 m/sec^{-1} (a 12% improvement), whereas the control group members did not improve their velocity. Subjects trained in knee and hip extension, and some residents trained on a sitting leg press (which involves simultaneous hip and knee extension and ankle plantar flexion). The maximum lift increased 5 kg, and hip extension increases averaged 7 kg, which represented more than doubling of knee extension strength.

A second small nursing home study using elastic bands for resistance noted a similar increase in gait velocity (0.06 m/sec^{-1} from 0.44 ± 0.05 m/sec^{-1} to 0.50 ± 0.05 m/sec^{-1}, $p = .01$), and an increase of 7 cm in step length (from 55 ± 6 cm to 66 ± 6 cm, $p = .003$).

A resistance training program using elastic bands and enrolling community-dwelling subjects did not improve gait velocity. Gait velocity declined in the resistance-trained group (from 1.24 to 1.19 m/sec^{-1} treatment effect, $p = .01$), whereas the gait velocity of the control group increased from 1.12 to 1.15 m/sec^{-1} velocities [48].

Combined Resistance-Walking Programs

A combined modified resistance-walking program increased 6-minute walk distance 9% (from 337 to 367 m, $p < .05$, paired t-test) and increased maximum gait velocity 9%, (from 1.19 m/sec^{-1} to 1.28 m/sec^{-1}, $p < .05$ compared to control group), with a trend to increase usual velocity (6% improvement, $p = .2$ compared to control group) [45].

A combined walking and low-resistance training program did not improve gait velocity in subjects with a baseline velocity of 1.13 m/sec^{-1} [49]. A second study by the same researchers compared sequential training and resistance training for 3 months followed by endurance exercises for 12 months (a combination of walking, uphill treadmill walking, bicycling, and jogging) at 75–85% of maximum heart rate [50]. The results are striking: The 3-month program of resistance training increased plantar flexor strength between 17% and 23%, and knee extension between 7% and 12%. Gait velocity did not change (1.09 m/sec^{-1}). The 12-month endurance program increased gait velocity 8% (1.09 to 1.17 m/sec^{-1}), maintained but did not increase quadriceps strength, and increased isometric plantar flexor strength significantly compared to strength following resistance training (68 Nm to 79 Nm). Isokinetic strength measures at 60 degrees and 120 degrees/sec^{-1} were unchanged. The authors imply that isometric measures are appropriate for a measure of gait because the greatest ankle extensor moment occurs when the ankle is not moving. The ankle tracings in Figure 23-1 and the electromyogram (EMG) tracings in Figure 23-2 support this argument; the greatest ankle moment and muscle activation occurs just as plantar flexion is initiated, and the greatest ankle plantar flexor power occurs immediately thereafter. To simplify the kinetics, it means that the ankle plantar flexor velocity and range of motion (the slope of the kinematic tracing) is dependent on the forces and power generated at the initiation of plantar flexion.

Two important observations can be inferred from this study. First, high levels of physical activity can maintain or increase strength gains achieved from resistance training. Second, the performance gains are training-specific; for example, walking training will improve walking more than resistance training.

Combined Resistance and Balance Training

A combined resistance-training and balance-training protocol increased usual gait velocity 8% (from 1.04 m/sec^{-1} to 1.12 m/sec^{-1}) in a small study in life-care community residents. In this study, baseline gait velocity was 1.04 m/sec^{-1}. Maximum gait velocity also improved in the trained group, compared to the control group [9]. In contrast, another study by our lab, which enrolled community-dwelling subjects free of significant neurological or cardiovascular diseases, found no increase in gait velocity after 13 weeks of either resistance training, balance training, or combined resistance and balance training. Baseline gait velocity was higher in the community-dwelling subjects (1.10 m/sec^{-1}) [45].

Resistance Training in Arthritis

Several researchers have demonstrated that strength gains in knee extension can be achieved in persons with knee arthritis. A large prospective trial of resistance training in knee arthritis is in progress and should provide definitive findings and suggestions for training in this group of older persons. Two interventions have improved gait velocity with resistance training. Resistance training lasting 3 months improved gait velocity approximately 6% in older subjects who had knee arthritis with a baseline gait velocity of 1.45 m/sec^{-1}, determined from a 50-foot walk test [51]. A combined resistance and walking program improved 6-minute walk distance 18% (from 381 to 451 m, $p < .001$) in subjects with knee arthritis and yielded a baseline gait velocity of 1.03 m/sec^{-1} (based on 6-minute walk distance) [52].

Figure 23-5 plots the change in gait velocity in the isolated resistance interventions previously cited, compared with the mean baseline gait velocity of the subjects. There is not sufficient data to draw firm conclusions on the effects of resistance training and gait velocity. However, Figure 23-5 illustrates that the studies enrolling slow walkers noted substantial improvements in gait velocity with resistance training, whereas the three studies that had negative results (no improvement in gait velocity) enrolled subjects with relatively high gait veloci-

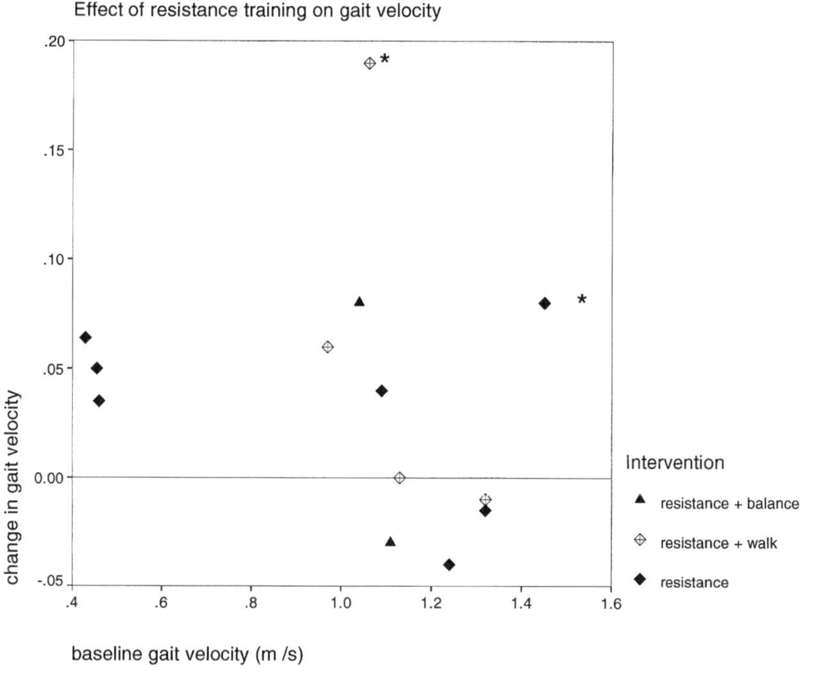

Figure 23-5. Results of resistance training on gait velocity. Cited references are for resistance, resistance-balance, and resistance and walking programs. The asterisks (*) represent two interventions in subjects with knee arthritis.

ties. In two nursing home studies [41, 53], subjects were still walking very slowly after resistance training (i.e., resistance training improved but did not correct the gait deficits found in these nursing home residents).

CONCLUSION AND CLINICAL RECOMMENDATIONS

The overall effect of resistance training programs on gait velocity is modest, and the improvement in gait velocity is greater in studies that enrolled persons with very low baseline gait velocity. That suggests that resistance training in persons with slow gait can improve gait velocity. The improvements are statistically significant and are likely to be clinically meaningful, but training does not achieve normal gait velocity. There is little evidence that short-term resistance training can reverse much of the age-associated decline in gait velocity in relatively healthy older persons living in the community. This suggests that improving muscle strength using resistance training is not sufficient to correct age-associated changes in gait. Resistance training may be necessary, but short-term training is not sufficient to correct age-associated declines in gait velocity. There is no evidence of a positive interaction between resistance and balance training.

In contrast, substantial prospective data suggest that physical activity preserves independent function, after correcting for associated comorbid conditions. However, there are no long-term data to determine whether long-term physical activity will maintain gait velocity.

In older persons with no complaints and with clinically normal gait, a high level of physical activity is recommended. The activity should be enjoyable and designed to preserve endurance and muscle strength. Walking programs probably are the most easily started and maintained and should be recommended to nearly all sedentary but able older persons. A high level of physical activity probably is the best way to maintain gait function and muscle strength.

In older persons with slow or impaired gait, resistance training is indicated to increase muscle contractility (strength). Resistance training alone may have a modest effect on gait velocity. It is likely that a combined resistance and walking training (sequential or simultaneous) will be the most effective method to improve gait. Resistance training may be a critical component to gait retraining, but it will not achieve good results in isolation.

REFERENCES

1. Hinman JE, et al. Age-related changes in speed of walking. *Med Sci Sports Exerc* 1988; 20:161–166.
2. Murray PM, Kory RC, Clarkson BH. Walking patterns in healthy old men. *J Gerontol* 1969;24:169–78.
3. Aniansson A, Rundgren A, Sperling L. Evaluation of functional capacity in activities of daily living in 70-year-old men and women. *Scand J Rehabil Med* 1980;12:145–54.

4. Hageman PA, Blanke DJ. Comparison of gait of young women and elderly women. *Phys Ther* 1986;66:1383–1387.

5. Crowinshield RD, Brand RA, Johnston RC. The effects of walking velocity and age on hip kinematics and kinetics. *Clin Orthop* 1978;132:140–144.

6. Finley FR, Cody KA, Finizie RV. Locomotion patterns in elderly women. *Arch Phys Med Rehabil* 1969;50:140–146.

7. Davis R, et al. A gait analysis data collection and reduction technique. *Hum Mov Sci* 1991;10:575–589.

8. Larish DD, Martin PE, Mungiole M. Characteristic patterns of gait in the healthy old. *Ann NY Acad Sci* 1988;515:28–31.

9. Judge JO, Underwood M, Gennosa T. Exercise to improve gait velocity in older persons. *Arch Phys Med Rehabil* 1993;74:400–406.

10. Leiper CI, Craik RL. Relationships between physical activity and temporal-distance characteristics of walking in elderly women. *Phys Ther* 1991;71:791–803.

11. Judge JO, Davis RB, Ounpuu S. Step length reductions in advanced age: The role of ankle and hip kinetics. *J Gerontol Med Sci* 1996 (in press).

12. Dec JB, et al. *J Bone Joint Surg* 1953;35:543–558.

13. Zajac FE. Muscle coordination of movement: A perspective. *J Biomech* 1993;26(suppl): 109–124.

14. Holt K, Hamil J, Andres R. Predicting the minimal energy costs of human walking. *Med Sci Sports Exerc* 1991;23:491–498.

15. Wagner EH, et al. Effects of physical activity on health status in older adults I: Observational studies. *Annu Rev Publ Health* 1992;13:451–468.

16. Paffenbarger, RS, Jr, et al. Physical activity, all-cause mortality, and longevity of college alumni. *N Engl J Med* 1986;314:605–613.

17. Blair SN, Kohl HW, Paffenbarger RS, et al. Physical fitness and all-cause mortality. *JAMA* 1989;262:2395–2401.

18. Rakowski W, Mor V. The association of physical activity with mortality among older adults in the longitudinal study of aging (1984–1988). *J Gerontol Med Sci* 1992;47:M122–129.

19. Jette AM, Branch LG, Berlin J. Musculoskeletal impairments and physical disablement among the aged. *J Gerontol Med Sci* 1990;45:M203–208.

20. Mor V, Murphy J, Masterson-Allen S, et al. Risk of functional decline among well elders. *J Clin Epidemiol* 1989;42:895–904.

21. LaCroix AZ, et al. Maintaining mobility in late life: II. Smoking, alcohol consumption, physical activity, and body mass index. *Am J Epidemiol* 1993;137:858–869.

22. Badley EM, Wagstaff S, Wood PHN. Measures of functional ability (disability) in arthritis in relation to impairment of range of joint movement. *Ann Rheum Dis* 1989;43:563–569.

23. Kohrt WM, Obert KA, Holloszy JO. Exercise training improves fat distribution patterns in 60 to 70-year-old men and women. *J Gerontol* 1992;47:M99–M105.

24. Aloia JF, et al. Relationship of menopause to skeletal and muscle mass. *Am J Clin Nutr* 1991;53:1378–1383.

25. Flynn MA, et al. Total body potassium in aging humans: A longitudinal study. *Am J Clin Nutr* 1989;50:713–717.

26. Larsson L. Aging in Mammalian Skeletal Muscles. In: Mortimer JA, Pirazzolo FJ, Maletta GJ, eds. *The Aging Motor System.* New York: Praeger, 1982. Pp 60–96.

27. Murray PM, et al. Age-related changes in knee muscle strength in normal women. *J Gerontol* 1985;40:275–280.

28. Stalberg E, et al. The quadriceps femoris muscle in 20 to 70-year-old subjects: Relationship between knee extension torque, electrophysiologic parameters and muscle fiber characteristics. *Muscle Nerve* 1989;12:382–389.

29. Aniansson A, Grimby G, Hedbert M. Compensatory muscle fiber hypertrophy in elderly men. *J Appl Physiol* 1992;73:812–816.

30. Frontera WR, et al. A cross-sectional study of muscle strength and mass in 45- to 78-yr-old men and women. *J Appl Physiol* 1991;71:644–650.

31. Kallman DA, Plato CC, Tobin JD. The role of muscle loss in the age-related decline of grip strength: Cross-sectional and longitudinal perspectives. *J Gerontol* 1990;45:M82.

32. Overend TJ, et al. Knee extensor and knee flexor strength: Cross-sectional area ratios in young and elderly men. *J Gerontol* 1992;47:M204–210.

33. Sipila S, et al. Muscle strength in male athletes aged 70–81 years and a population sample. *Eur J Appl Physiol* 1991;63:399–403.

34. Klitgaard H, et al. Functional, morphology and protein expression of ageing skeletal muscle: A cross-sectional study of elderly men with different training backgrounds. *Acta Physiol Scand* 1990;140:41–54.

35. Ito H, et al. Age related changes in the walking cycle during fastest walking in healthy male subjects. *Nippon Ronen Igakkai Zasshi* 1989;26(4):347–352.

36. Fiatarone MA, et al. High intensity strength training in nonagenarians: Effects on skeletal muscle. *JAMA* 1990;263:3029–3034.

37. Bassey EJ, Bendal MJ, Pearson M. Muscle strength in the triceps surae and objectively measured customary walking activity in men and women over 65 years of age. *Clin Sci* 1988;74:85–89.

38. Judge JO, Smyers D, Wolfson L. Muscle strength predicts gait measures in older adults [abstract]. *J Am Geriatr Soc* 1992;40:SA27.

39. Mueller MJ, et al. Difference in the gait characteristics of patients with diabetes and peripheral neuropathy compared with age matched controls. *Phys Ther* 1994;74:299–313.

40. Fleck SJ, Kraemer WJ. *Designing Resistance Training Programs*. Champaign, IL: Human Kinetics Books, 1987.

41. Fiatarone MA, et al. Exercise training and nutritional supplementation for physical frailty in very elderly people. *N Engl J Med* 1994;330:1769–1775.

42. Verril D, et al. Resistive exercise training in cardiac patients: Recommendations. *Sports Med* 1992;3:171–193.

43. Frontera WR, et al. Strength conditioning in older men: Skeletal muscle hypertrophy and improved function. *J Appl Physiol* 1988;64:1038–1044.

44. Fleg JL, Lakatta EG. Role of muscle loss in the age-associated reduction in VO_2 max. *J Appl Physiol* 1988;65:1147–1151.

45. Judge JO, Whipple RH, Wolfson LI. Effects of resistive and balance exercises on isokinetic strength in older persons. *J Am Geriatr Soc* 1994;42:937–946.

46. Judge JO, Schechtman K, Cress E: The relationship between physical performance measures and independence in Instrumental Activities of Daily Living. *J Am Geriatr Soc* 1996;44 (in press).

47. Reuben DB, Siu AL. An objective measure of physical function of elderly outpatients. *J Am Geriatr Soc* 1990;38:1105–1112.

48. Topp R, Mikesky A, Wigglesworth J. The effect of a 12-week dynamic resistance strength training program on gait velocity and balance of older adults. *Gerontologist* 1993;33:501–506.

49. Brown M, Holloszy JO. Effects of a low intensity exercise program on selected physical performance characteristics of 60- to 71-year olds. *Age Ageing* 1991;3:129–139.

50. Brown M, Holloszy JO. Effects of walking, jogging and cycling on strength, flexibility, speed and balance in 60- to 72-year olds. *Aging Clin Exp Res* 1993;5:427–434.

51. Fisher NM, Gresham G, Pendergast DR. Effects of a quantitative progressive rehabilitation program applied unilaterally to the osteoarthritic knee. *Arch Phys Med Rehabil* 1993;74:1319–1326.

52. Kovar PA, et al. Supervised fitness walking in patients with osteoarthritis of the knee. *Ann Intern Med* 1993;116:529–534.

53. Sauvage LR Jr, et al. A clinical trial of strengthening and aerobic exercise to improve gait and balance in elderly male nursing home residents. *Am J Phys Med Rehabil* 1992;71:33–42.

24. Environmental Factors in the Prevention of Falls

Rein Tideiksaar

Falls are among the most common problems faced by older persons. Approximately 30% to 50% of persons aged 65 and older residing in the community and institutional setting (i.e., acute care hospital, nursing home) will fall each year [1, 2]. Of these individuals, up to one-half will fall repeatedly [1].

The causes and risk factors associated with falls in older persons are multiple. Typically, they involve an interaction between intrinsic or host-related factors (e.g., acute and chronic medical conditions, medication effects) and extrinsic or environmental factors (e.g., environmental hazards and obstacles). This chapter reviews the extrinsic causes of falls, discusses the clinical approach governing assessment of the designed environment, and outlines environmental strategies aimed at reducing fall-risk.

EXTRINSIC FACTORS

Physical Environment

Although some community-based studies have found that older persons experience a high proportion of falls outdoors [3, 4], most studies have shown that the overwhelming majority of falls experienced by older individuals occur indoors and at home [5–8]. Furthermore, the risk of suffering a fall at home increases with advancing age [3]. Most falls at home take place in the bedroom, bathroom, living room, kitchen, and on stairways [9–13]. There are several possible explanations for these findings. It may be that older persons, particularly those at fall-risk, spend more time at home and, as a consequence, are exposed to domestic environmental hazards for greater periods of time. Also, persons may be less cautious or careless around the familiar surroundings of the home. It is also possible that the home environment is unsafe.

In acute-care hospitals and nursing homes, most falls by older patients occur in the bedroom and bathroom [14, 15]. Again, this may reflect the time spent by patients in these locations, that the bed and bathroom are unsafe, or that these older patients are unfamiliar with new environmental surroundings.

In any case, the environment has been implicated as a contributing factor in one-third to one-half of all falls occurring in homes and institutions [1, 2, 5, 11, 16, 17]. Most of these falls occur during the performance of common, activities of daily living wherein a person's center of gravity is displaced beyond the base of support and, as a result, balance stability is threatened. Activities that threaten stability include (1) transferring from low or elevated bed heights or climbing over side rails; (2) getting up from or sitting down on unstable, low-seated, and armless chairs and on low toilet seats that lack grab bar support; (3) walking in poorly illuminated areas; (4) tripping over low-lying objects (objects resting outside one's field of vision), or tripping on such floor coverings as door thresholds, thick pile carpets, and unsecured carpet or rug edges; (5) slipping on highly polished or wet ground surfaces, such as kitchen, bathroom, and bathtub or shower floors and on sliding rugs; (6) climbing and descending steps and stairways with faulty handrail support, poor illumination, and unsafe coverings on tread surfaces; and (7) reaching up (on tiptoes or step stools and chairs) and bending down to place or retrieve objects from high or low kitchen or closet shelves [18, 19]. This list is by no means exhaustive, but it does reflect the variety of environmental factors that have been implicated.

Though no one would argue with the assertion that environmental factors probably contribute to falls in older persons, the true extent of this contribution and the precise etiology of falling is currently unknown. There are several reasons that account for the lack of knowledge. First and foremost, most studies are not designed to allow for the evaluation of environmental hazards as risk factors. More specifically, they lack standard definitions of the word "hazard"; validated and reliable instruments to assess environmental hazards are not employed; and comparison control groups that assess the risk of exposure to environmental hazards are not included [20, 21]. The few available prospective studies that have examined the risk of falls due to environmental hazards in the home are inconclusive [5, 8].

Second, the majority of falls (in both homes and institutions) are not observed events. As a result, the causative role of environmental factors typically is obtained either from self-report or from researchers who list what they consider to be hazardous conditions present at the time of the fall [20]. This can lead to either an overrepresentation or an underrepresentation of environmental factors, depending on the subject's recall of hazardous conditions and his or her willingness to identify features of the environment as being hazardous [21]; the researcher's self-created definition of what constitutes a hazardous condition also plays an important role. Often older persons, their family members, and health care providers blame the environment—understandably, but mistakenly.

Last, most studies do not categorize falls according to whether they are exclusively due to an environmental factor or to a combination of both extrinsic and host-related factors that lead to fall-risk [2].

Though Speechley and Tinetti [22] found that (in contrast to frail individuals) healthy, active older persons do experience falls because of environmental hazards, the chance of the surrounding environment contributing to falls is greatest in those persons with underlying mobility problems [23]. In this scenario, an environmental hazard, such as a low toilet seat or elevated bed height (both easily negotiated by a healthy person), can become a major obstacle for someone with neuromuscular impairment. In other words, the less mobile the individual, the greater the impact of environmental factors on the person.

Devices

Assistive devices (e.g., canes, walkers, wheelchairs) used to support mobility have been found to contribute to the problem of falls [14]. Canes and walkers can lead to unsafe mobility if their size is inappropriate (i.e., too high or low in height), if they are used improperly, or if they are in a poor state of repair (e.g., worn rubber tips, structural deterioration). Wheelchairs contribute to falls when older persons use improper transfer techniques (e.g., not locking wheel brakes or clearing the footplates with lower extremities) or when the wheelchair is in poor repair (e.g., faulty locking mechanisms).

Physical restraints, used in hospitals and nursing homes to reduce the risk of falls, often fail to achieve their intended purpose and have been found to increase the likelihood of falls [24, 25]. Presumably, the immediate cause of restraint-induced falls is improper application or patient removal. The contribution of restraints to falls becomes even more plausible, however, when the deconditioning, muscle wasting, and exacerbation of underlying gait and balance abnormalities they can cause are considered [26]. In addition, side-rails employed to guard against bed falls can lead to falls and increase the risk of physical injury [27, 28]. Patients agile enough may climb over the top of these rails when exiting from bed and catch their limbs in the rails, falling as a result. Further, bed rail–related falls may lead to injuries (e.g., fractures, head trauma) brought on by the distance of falling (from the top of an elevated rail to the floor) and the impact against a hard floor surface. Durable medical equipment (e.g., toilet risers, bathtub seats or benches, grab bars,) can lead to falls as well, particularly if they do not support the mobility requirements of older persons or if they are in disrepair.

Footwear

Although footwear is not typically considered a part of the environment, footwear interfaces directly with host-related factors (e.g., decreased step height) and ground conditions (e.g., slippery and irregular floor surfaces) and, therefore, should be included when considering fall risk. Improper footwear can alter an individual's gait and balance. High-heeled shoes can cause instability [29]; specifically, they narrow the standing and walking base of support, decrease stride length, and cause a person to assume a forward-leaning posture. Poorly fitting shoes (particularly when loose) can also alter gait patterns. For example, in an effort to keep loose shoes from falling off, people often assume a shuffling gait that can cause tripping. Wearing leather- and plastic-soled shoes or wearing socks without shoes promotes slipping. Rubber crepe soles, promoted for their slip-resistant qualities, may stick to linoleum and carpeted floor surfaces. As a result, in those persons with decreased foot-ground clearance, slip-resistant soles can cause halting gait, ending in balance loss and falls. Thick-soled footwear (e.g., running shoes, tennis sneakers) may decrease proprioceptive feedback gained from the foot striking the ground and may contribute to balance loss [30].

Situational Circumstances

Length of Stay

In institutions, older patients fall most often during the first week of admission [31, 32]. Various explanations have been offered for this phenomenon, including (1) the presence of acute diseases (e.g., altered homeostasis) and chronic neuromuscular diseases (e.g., altered mobility) or (2) unfamiliarity with the surrounding environment. In hospitals, the former is more likely. In nursing homes (where residents are generally medically stable but have a high prevalence of chronic disease), a poor fit between the person's mobility capacity and the surrounding environment is a more plausible causative factor. In acute-care hospitals, increased length of patient stay is correlated with increased falls [33], an incidence presumably due to a greater chance of iatrogenic factors that contribute to fall-risk.

Time of Fall

In the home, most falls occur during daylight hours [11, 13]. Falls during these periods probably are related to getting out of bed and using the bathroom. Some researchers have found that falls occur more often during weekends than on weekdays [11]. One explanation for this may be that persons spend more time at home during weekends, hence are exposed to domestic environmental hazards for longer periods. In hospitals and nursing homes, falls are more likely to occur at night and during certain daytime hours (6 AM to 10 AM, 4 PM to 8 PM) that are associated with increased bed- and bathroom-related activities [34]. Falls generally are distributed evenly over the days of the week.

Caregiving Patterns

Institutional staffing patterns and the number of nurses and aides available also may influence fall occurrence. Most studies have found an inverse relationship between falls and the number of available staff [35] (i.e., increased fall rates with decreased staff and decreased falls with increased staff) [36, 37]. However, sometimes this relationship is reversed; that is, falls increase with increased staff [38]. The reasons for this anomaly are not entirely clear and may not relate to the number of staff present or to nurse-staff ratios, but rather to the availability of nurses and to their attitudes toward fall prevention (i.e., assessing for fall-risk and assisting mobility-dependent patients with activities) [39]. Also, the location of a patient's bedroom in relation to the nursing station may play a contributing role. For example, if the patient's bedroom is located a long distance from the nursing station, this distance may prohibit the nurse from making multiple visits to the bedroom to assist the patient. In the community, there is a probable connection between falls and the number and availability of caregivers (e.g., family members, attendants), although this relationship has not been examined.

THE ENVIRONMENTAL ASSESSMENT

Although there are no definitive studies that demonstrate the advantages of environmental modifications in reducing the risk of falls, a few recent studies have shown promising results [40–42]. This suggests that attention to the identification and correction of environmental fall hazards in both homes and institutions may help to reduce fall-risk.

Safety Checklists

Safety checklists commonly are used both to identify and correct environmental hazards in homes and institutions. There are several safety checklists available for health professionals and lay persons [17, 43–45]. Table 24-1 summarizes the most common hazards and suggested modifications from several of these safety checklists. In the community, safety checklists frequently are used when a home visit is not possible. Home safety checklists often are distributed to those older persons at fall-risk, those who have experienced falls in the home, and (if available) their family members. Through a program of patient education, individuals are instructed on how to recognize and eliminate environmental hazards found in the home. During subsequent office or clinic visits, discovered hazards and proposed modifications can be reviewed.

In hospitals and nursing homes, safety checklists are frequently employed by nursing and physical or occupational therapy staff for guidance on the correction of environmental hazards in the institution. In addition, home safety checklists are sometimes provided to patients and family members prior to the patient's discharge to the home.

Safety checklists can be valuable; however, there are a number of problems associated with their use. In general, definitions of what constitutes a hazard are rarely clear. For example, low illumination and thick carpets may interfere with safe ambulation, but it is unclear how poor lighting must be or how thick carpets must be before they become hazards [21]. Such ambiguity can lead to problems with suggested modifications. For the same example, how much additional lighting should be provided, or how thin should replacement carpeting be? To add to the confusion, some checklists include suggestions such as, provide "chairs and beds of proper height," "sufficient lighting," and "secure handrails"—suggestions that are much too vague and inexplicit to be of any real use.

Another problem with safety checklists is that a hazardous condition (e.g., a low toilet seat) may be unsafe for some persons but not for others; many hazards are patient specific. As a result, the proposed modification or elimination of a hazard (e.g., a low toilet seat) may be beneficial for some persons but not for others. In fact, any attempted modification in such an instance (e.g., providing a

Table 24-1. Environmental hazards and modifications

	Hazard	Modification
Pathways	Low-profile furnishings obstructing walking paths	Arrange furnishings so that pathways are clear; avoid cluttered pathways
Illumination	Low lighting	Provide increased lighting in all areas (100-watt bulbs, fluorescent lights, night lights)
	Excessively bright lighting	Use rheostatic and three-way light switches to adjust lighting levels
	Lighting glare	Use frosted bulbs or translucent shades to reduce glare
	Decreased access	Provide nightlight and sound-activated lighting sources
Floor surfaces	Worn carpet and rug edges	Repair or replacement
	Sliding rugs	Replace, or apply slip-resistant backing
	Upended carpet edge	Tack or tape down
Chairs	Unstable; tippable	Replace with stable seating
	Lack of armrests	Provide chairs equipped with armrest that extend to seat edge
Beds	Low bed height	Replace, or use thick mattress to increase height; height-adjustable beds
	Elevated bed	Replace, or use thin mattress to decrease height; height-adjustable beds
Stairway	Lack of handrail	Install handrails on both sides of stairway
	Slippery steps	Apply nonslip adhesive strips to steps
	Inadequate lighting	Provide adequate lighting at top and bottom steps
Bathroom	Slippery tub surface	Apply nonslip strips or rubber bathmat; install grab bars
	Toilet seat too low	Install grab rails, or use toilet riser

raised toilet seat) may potentially create a hazard where there formerly was none, thus increasing the risk of falls for some people. Similarly, maintaining clear circulation pathways (e.g., removing furnishings from narrow passageways) may provide safe ambulation for most persons, but for some individuals (those with balance instability), furnishings placed along pathways can be grasped to provide ambulation support. Ironically, strict adherence to recommended modifications of environmental hazards, without considering individual mobility patterns or the need for specific environmental modification, can be dangerous for persons residing in the community or an institution, ultimately increasing the risk of falls.

Performance-Oriented Environmental Assessments

Given the limitations and potential dangers associated with safety checklists, the assessment and modification of environmental hazards must be based on an older person's mobility status and, in those persons with falls, the precipitating circumstances. To obtain this information, older persons can be asked directly about their mobility (e.g., their capacity to transfer from beds, chairs, toilets; and their ability to get into or out of bathtubs or showers, to climb and descend stairways, etc.). Similar details can be obtained from family members (spouses, adult children), if available.

Persons who have experienced recent falls should be questioned about (1) the surrounding circumstances, (2) the specific location or area in which the fall occurred, (3) the activity being performed at the time (e.g., transferring from the bed, descending stairs), and (4) the immediate condition of the environment (e.g., wet floor, unstable chair). This is helpful in detecting environmental problems that may be contributing to decreased mobility and fall-risk. However, if taken alone, the information will fail to clarify the specific contribution of environmental factors. Often, any conclusions formed about the role of environmental factors in causing mobility problems or heightening fall-risk are left to individual or family interpretations, which may or may not always be an accurate reflection of the situation. Consequently, the most accurate way to assess the true extent and role of environmental factors contributing to dysmobility and the risk of further falls is to observe the person's mobility performance within his or her living environment.

Several instruments (the *Get-up-and-go-test* and the *Performance-oriented Assessment of Mobility*) can be used to assess an older person's mobility [46, 47]. The basic components of these mobility instruments consist of asking an older person to perform a number of gait and balance maneuvers and observing the manner in which each task is accomplished. We have adapted performance-oriented mobility screen from the aforementioned instruments in Fig. 24-1. Any observed abnormality signifies altered mobility, which helps to localize possible organ system involvement and provides clues to contributing environmental problems (Table 24-2).

These mobility instruments, however, have limitations. For example, any mobility assessment performed outside the patient's living environment (e.g., in a private office or outpatient clinic) typically will fail to elicit specific information about the person's mobility status with respect to conditions in the usual environment. Also, a test of mobility performance in an outpatient setting may be influenced by several environmental conditions (e.g., type of floor surface, carpet versus linoleum, the amount of lighting, and the design of chairs used to evaluate transfers), which may not reflect the conditions present in the patient's living environment. For example, it is not unusual for persons to perform poorly in the clinic but better at home, and vice versa. Therefore, mobility assessment is best accomplished in the person's living environment (the home or an institution). This will allow for the evaluation of environmental conditions and hazards that interfere with mobility and for the design of intervention strategies.

In the home, mobility assessment is accomplished by observing the person transferring from chairs, beds, and toilets; getting in and out of bathtubs; walking and turning about in different rooms and areas; climbing and descending stairs; and reaching up and bending over to place and retrieve objects from shelves. Also, the person's mobility can be examined with respect to the type and

PERFORMANCE ORIENTED MOBILITY SCREEN (POMS)

Instructions: Ask the patient to perform the following maneuvers. For each maneuver, indicate whether the patient's performance is normal or abnormal.

ASK PATIENT TO:	OBSERVATION			
	NORMAL		ABNORMAL	
Sit down in chair (select a chair with armrests approximately 16–17 inches in seat height)	☐ Able to sit down in one smooth, controlled movement without using armrests		☐ Sitting is not a smooth movement; falls into chair or needs armrests to guide	
Rise up from chair	☐ Able to get up in one smooth movement without using armrests		☐ Uses armrests and/or moves forward in chair to propel self up; requires several attempts to get up	
Stand (approximately 30 seconds) after rising from chair	☐ Steady, able to stand without support		☐ Unsteady, loses balance	
Stand with eyes *closed* (approximately 15 seconds)	☐ Steady, able to stand without support		☐ Unsteady, loses balance	
Stand with eyes *open*; nudge on sternum with light pressure 3 times	☐ Steady, needs to move feet, but able to withstand pressure and maintain balance		☐ Unsteady, begins to fall	
Walk in a straight line (approximately 15 feet) at "usual" pace, then back again	☐ Gait is continuous without hesitation; walks in a straight line and feet clear		☐ Gait is non-continuous with deviation from straight path; feet scrape or shuffle on floor	
	☐ WITH AID	☐ WITHOUT AID	☐ WITH AID	☐ WITHOUT AID
Walk a distance of 5 feet and turn around	☐ No staggering; steps are smooth and continuous		☐ Staggering; steps are unsteady and discontinuous	
	☐ WITH AID	☐ WITHOUT AID	☐ WITH AID	☐ WITHOUT AID

Note: If the patient uses a walk aid such as a cane or walker, the walking maneuvers are tested separately, with and without the aid. Indicate type of aid used:

☐ Cane   ☐ Walker   ☐ Other   ☐ None

Figure 24-1. Performance-oriented mobility screen.

Table 24-2. Differential diagnoses of abnormal mobility maneuvers

Impaired maneuver	Organ systems	Environmental factors
Chair transfer	Parkinsonism Arthritis Deconditioning	Poor chair design (possibly faulty bed, toilet, and bathtub design)
Standing balance	Postural hypotension Vestibular dysfunction	
Romberg	Proprioceptive dysfunction	Poor illumination Overly absorptive footwear or carpeting
Sternal nudge	Parkinsonism Normal-pressure hydrocephalus	May require assistive device for balance support
Walking and turning	Gait disorders (parkinsonism, hemiparesis, or foot problem) Sensory dysfunction	Improper footwear Improper size or use of ambulation devices Hazardous ground surfaces (wet, irregular)

conditions of floor surfaces, lighting, footwear, and the use of any assistive devices, and durable medical equipment can be examined. At the same time, the individual's motivation to perform tasks and his or her cognitive ability (e.g., judgment and comprehension) to perform each task in a safe manner can be assessed. The presence of any and all hazardous environmental conditions should be noted. After these factors are identified, recommendations for environmental interventions must be made. (See Environmental Strategies to Reduce Fall Risk). In hospitals and nursing homes, the assessment process is similar. However, the scope of the mobility evaluation (those activities and environmental features assessed) in institutions is different from the home evaluation and is primarily limited to those activities and environmental locations available to patients and residents.

It is important to remember that mobility (both in the home and in the institution) is not a static but a dynamic process, that is subject to change (i.e., to decline or improve based on the stability or instability of an individual's medication and medical and mobility status. Likewise, environmental conditions are subject to change. Depending on the person's mobility status, safe environmental conditions may become hazardous, and vice versa. Subsequently, mobility and environmental assessments should be completed on a regular basis or whenever the person experiences a change in health or environmental conditions.

Currently, researchers are developing instruments for clinicians so that specific hazardous environmental conditions in homes and institutions can be assessed. We have developed the Performance-Oriented Environmental Mobility Screen (POEMS) that assesses several mobility domains in relation to the person's hospital or nursing home environment (see Appendix B). Presently, the

POEMS is being designed for use in the home to include the addition of steps and stairways, bathtubs and showers, doorways, living rooms, dining rooms, kitchens, and immediate outdoor areas. Chandler and Duncan [48] have developed an instrument that allows the clinician to assess performance-based environmental risk in the home. Rodriguez et al. [21] have developed a home environment assessment instrument that uses both direct observation of the home and patient interviews.

ENVIRONMENTAL STRATEGIES TO REDUCE FALL-RISK

The design of environmental strategies intended to support safe mobility and reduce fall-risk consists of three general approaches. The goal of the first approach is to eliminate those environmental conditions that interfere with mobility. This task is accomplished by modifying or altering hazardous features of the existing physical environment and by using durable medical equipment to simplify and maximize mobility tasks. The second approach strives to maintain safe mobility through use of appropriate ambulation devices and footwear. The third approach attempts to reduce the risk of injurious falls (i.e., hip fractures, prolonged postfall lie times) through the use of hip pads and personal emergency response systems. The last approach emphasizes individual compliance with the recommended interventions. In most cases, a management approach will include features from each of the approaches described previously. Although there is little direct evidence of the effectiveness of these approaches, these recommendations make intuitive sense and should be attempted.

Physical Environment

Circulation Pathways

The paths through hallways, doorways—indeed, all floor space—should permit safe ambulation. The arrangement of furnishings (e.g., chairs, tables, beds) should allow an individual sufficient space for walking and turning around without bumping into objects. Clear walking space is especially important for those persons dependent on assistive ambulation devices (e.g., canes, walkers) and wheelchairs. Furnishings should be arranged so that they do not protrude into natural walkways. In particular, low-profile furniture that may fall outside the field of vision (e.g., coffee tables, small step-stools, chair legs) and might cause trips should be relocated. Also, the path from the bed to the bathroom should be clear and well illuminated (particularly at night), as older persons commonly get up during the night to urinate. Nightlights can be used to provide sufficient lighting; however, for some patients with Alzheimer's disease, such lights may be dangerous, as they tend to cast shadows and images that may cause hallucinations and paranoia.

Some older persons with balance loss and fear of falling feel safer ambulating if they are able to hold onto furnishings every few feet for guidance, balance support and, if a stumble occurs, recovery. Preferable to wide-open spaces in these instances are pieces of furniture (e.g., sturdy, high-backed chairs; tables; dressers) that can be used to accommodate individuals who prefer to walk while holding onto one object as they move toward the next. This strategy is also useful if furniture placement or lack of ambulation space prohibits the use of walkers.

Lighting
The proper amount of illumination in the environment is dependent on the person's needs. As a general rule, older people require two or three times more light than younger persons to facilitate vision and compensate for the functional visual changes that accompany the aging process. However, note that this is a generalization; there are instances when lower levels of lighting may be more appropriate. For example, persons who have cataracts and glaucoma and tend to be sensitive to bright lights would do better with lower lighting. Under ideal circumstances, the individual should be able to regulate and maintain levels of illumination appropriate for his or her own safe mobility. Rheostatic light switches allow the individual (or staff members in an institutional setting) to regulate illumination levels as desired. However, such individual control of lighting may not always be feasible, especially in persons who are cognitively impaired. As a consequence, the best method of determining lighting needs is to observe individual ambulation in the environment and to adjust lighting levels accordingly.

Lighting levels can be increased by using 100-watt bulbs, employing light-colored wall coverings (to increase the reflective quality of light), replacing incandescent lights with fluorescent lightning, and providing extra lighting sources, such as night lights that turn on automatically when lighting levels are low. A red bulb is suggested for night lights, because it reduces the time required for dark adaptation. Any sudden increase or decrease in lighting levels (moving from dark to bright areas and vice versa) should be avoided, as the ability to adapt to changes in illumination declines with age. Rheostatic and three-way light switches vary the amount of light available and control the distribution of lighting and can be used to avoid sudden and pronounced shifts in illumination typical of toggle light switches. Also, lighting sources (e.g., switchplates, lamps) should be easily accessible, particularly in high fall-risk locations (i.e., top and bottom of stairways, bedrooms, bathrooms) and during situations likely to cause falls (getting out of bed at night). The use of a "clapper light" (a device that turns on lights automatically in response to clapping the hands) is a viable alternative.

Glare from sunlight shining through windows or from unshielded light bulbs reflecting on polished floor surfaces may impair vision and should be avoided. Direct window glare can be eliminated with sheer shades or tinted glass. Light bulb glare is reduced with frosted bulbs or translucent lighting shades. Floor glare can be controlled with carpets or low-luster polishes that diffuse light.

Floor Surfaces
Patterned carpets, rugs, and tiled floors (checkered or floral designs) should be avoided. These coverings tend to interfere with depth perception and balance

stability. Floor coverings should be solid colors. Sliding throw rugs should be replaced; or, as an alternative, nonslip backing (double-sided adhesive tape, matting) can be placed under the rug to prevent sliding. Linoleum and wooden floors are made slip-resistant by applying nonskid finishes. Bathroom tiles can be rendered slip-resistant by applying nonskid adhesive strips or decorative decals on the floor next to the toilet, sink, and bathtub (areas prone to wetness).

Low-density indoor-outdoor carpeting on bathroom floors has similar benefits. (Deep-pile carpet can cause halting gait and become a tripping hazard for persons with decreased foot-ground clearance. Also, the force required to propel rolling walkers and wheelchairs increases on thick carpets.) Low-pile carpets offer several advantages. They decrease the risk of slips, because friction between footwear and carpet surface is great (even if footwear is slip-resistant). Also, low-density carpets that provide cushioning help to reduce the impact of a fall and minimize the risk of injury. Carpet edges prone to buckling or curling should be tacked or taped down.

Beds

Elevated and low bed heights and soft mattresses contribute to balance loss and fall-risk. Bed height is appropriate when a person is able to sit on the edge of the mattress with the knees flexed at 90 degrees and both feet planted on the floor. At home, elevated bed heights can be reduced by replacing thick mattresses with something thinner and, conversely, low bed heights can be raised with mattresses that are thicker. All mattresses should be firm enough to support sitting and transfer balance. In institutions, height adjustable "hi-low" beds can be used to maintain proper bed heights. Side rails that extend one-half the length of the bed can be used as assistive transfer devices for persons with poor balance. The floor surface along the length of the bed should be slip-resistant to support safe transfers. If floor surfaces are slippery, have the person wear traction-soled socks or slippers. Beds that slide away during transfers can be placed against the wall for support (if feasible).

Persons who have poor mobility and altered cognition and get out of bed by themselves are at great risk for falls. One way to resolve this problem without the use of physical restraints is to place either a bed alarm underneath the patient's bedding or mattress (in a hospital or nursing home) or an electronic alarm mat on the floor next to the bed (in the home). Both are pressure-sensitive devices that activate a warning alarm when patients are transferring out of bed. A number of studies have found bed alarm systems to be effective in preventing bed falls [49, 50] as they alert staff and family that a patient who should not be attempting to leave his or her bed unassisted (or independently) is doing so and, consequently, prompts the assistance the patient needs.

Seating

The seating height of chairs (the distance from the floor to the front edge of the seat) is critical for effective transfers [51]. Low seats require greater knee flexion and muscle strength to initiate and support both rising and sitting. Conversely, it is much easier to transfer on and off seats that are higher, as less joint flexion and muscle strength are required. Seat height is appropriate when it allows the patient to sit with both feet firmly planted on the floor with the knees flexed at 90 degrees. To support seated transfers, all chairs used by older persons should be equipped with armrests. Armrests provide leverage during rising and gradual deceleration when sitting. Armrests usually can compensate for low seat heights. Armrests located approximately 7 inches above the seat and extending slightly beyond the front seat edge provide maximum support. A cushion can be added to increase the height of low-seated chairs. The cushion's thickness is determined by how much height is needed to accomplish independent transfers.

Bathroom

Armrest toilet grab bars compensate for low toilet heights. These devices are adjustable in height and width and offer better support and leverage than do conventional wall-mounted grab bars. Towel bars used for balance support should be replaced with wall-mounted grab bars. The grab bars should be round (for easy hand grasp), slip-resistant, color contrasted with the wall for visibility, and securely fixed to the studs of the wall for adequate support. To guard against hand slippage, nonslip adhesive strips can be placed on the top of sink edges if these surfaces are used for balance support. A rubber mat or nonslip adhesive strips applied to the bathtub and shower floor surface provide stable footing. Wall-mounted grab bars in the bathtub and shower provide support during transfers and bathing. Their location is determined by where persons customarily place their hands during tub or shower transfers. In institutions, a grab bar that extends completely around the perimeter of shower stalls is preferable. In the home, a grab bar that attaches onto the edge of the bath rim can be used for further transfer support. For those persons with balance loss, the use of bathtub chairs or benches and extended shower hoses can serve as alternatives and ensure safe bathing.

Stairs

The negotiation of stairs requires both visual feedback (to detect and judge the position of steps) and kinesthetic input (to ensure adequate foot placement). To ensure the safety of these passages, certain conditions must be met. All stairways should be equipped with handrails for support. The rails should be round and slip-resistant (for secure hand grasp) and color-contrasted for visibility. Step surfaces should be in good repair and slip-resistant. Geometric or floral trend designs should be avoided, as these patterns can disguise step edges and cause foot misplacements. Contrasting colored nonslip adhesive strips placed along step edges eliminate slipping and aid visibility. Adequate stairway illumination, especially at the top and bottom steps, is important to safeguard initial stairway approach. Light sources should be positioned to eliminate glare and shadow, which may obstruct the view of steps.

Storage Areas

Closet and kitchen shelves that are too high or too low may contribute to balance loss and falls when persons reach up or bend down beyond their safe capacity to retrieve and place objects. To remedy this problem, frequently used items should be placed on shelves that lie between a person's eye and hip level. A hand-held reaching device can be employed as an alternative.

Ambulation Devices

Assistive ambulation devices (e.g., canes and walkers) are designed to improve gait and balance; they provide a greater base of support, reduce the load on weight-bearing joints (e.g., hips and knees), and supply proprioceptive feedback through the handle. Also, such ambulation devices (particularly walkers) may help reduce the fear of falling, as they provide the person with a visual presence of physical support and instill a sense of confidence during walking.

To ensure that ambulation devices achieve these goals, they should be "prescribed" individually to correct specific gait and balance problems and should be tailored to fit both the person (properly sized) and the living environment (e.g., the space requirements or limitations). Also, persons who require an ambulation device must be instructed on the proper use of the device (e.g., walking on level ground and steps; transferring activities). This is best accomplished by referring patients to a physiatrist or physical therapist. Also, canes and walkers should be checked by clinicians on a regular basis for defects (e.g., worn rubber tips, structural weakness, loose wheels, etc.), and should be replaced when necessary. Patients should be asked to perform walking and transferring maneuvers with the cane or walker, observed to determine whether it is being done properly, and examined to see that the device meets their mobility needs.

Footwear

All footwear (e.g., shoes, slippers) worn by patients should fit properly and have slip-resistant soles. If foot problems such as hammer toes, bunions, calluses, or nail disorders prohibit the wearing of properly sized shoes, the patient should be referred for podiatric care. For optimal balance stability, shoes with thin, hard soles are preferable to those with thick, absorbent soles that detract from proprioceptive feedback [30]. Shoes and slippers with rubber or crepe soles provide adequate slip-resistance on linoleum floor surfaces. Socks with nonskid sole tread are a good choice, especially for persons who frequently get up at night (i.e., those with nocturia). However, for some patients with poor step height (i.e., inability to pick up the feet adequately from the floor), slip-resistant soles may stick to floor surfaces. For these patients, footwear with leather soles that promote gliding on linoleum and carpeted floors may be a better choice. High-heeled shoes should be avoided in favor of flat heels. If patients insist on wearing high-heeled shoes out of vanity or because they must (a lifelong wearing of high heels leads to shortening of the achilles tendon and thus necessitates their use), shoes with flared-wedge heels are recommended as they provide a better base of support.

Injury Prevention Devices

Several factors are associated with the risk of hip fractures following a fall: decreased bone strength, loss of normal protective postural responses, and the type of surface struck (hard versus absorptive) [52]. However, one of the principal determinants of injury is the reduction of soft tissue or fat covering the hip (poor energy absorption and distribution) [53]. As a result, external hip pads (consisting of two shock-absorbent pads inserted in a wraparound pelvic garment worn under outer clothing and over underwear) may be useful to guard against hip fractures. They are designed to act as shock absorbers and to divert the direct impact of a fall away from the bone. The efficacy of hip pads in protecting against hip fractures was demonstrated by Laurtzen et al. [54] in the nursing home setting. However, because only 24% of the nursing home residents who received hip pads wore them regularly, noncompliance may be a problem. Conversely, we found that hip pads were well-accepted by a group of community-residing older females at risk for hip fracture and fear of injury [55]. Thus, the use of hip pads may be beneficial in reducing hip fractures when other measures fail to prevent falls.

Some studies suggest that falls with prolonged lie times are associated with increased morbidity, particularly fear of falling [13, 56]. For persons who are at risk for long lies (e.g., those who live alone, are at fall-risk, and have difficulty getting up from the floor unassisted), a personal emergency response system (PERS) may be beneficial. Such devices are worn by the patient as a neck pendant and are designed to summon assistance in the event of a fall that results in a long lie. Compliance with PERS is greatest in those persons with a positive fall history [57].

Compliance

A final item to consider, particularly in the community-residing population, is whether the suggested environmental modifications will be accepted by the older person. At issue is whether the individual will change the environment. For example, older persons may not alter the environment if they do not perceive themselves as being at fall-risk or if they do not think that the environment is hazardous. In general, compliance with environmental modifications improves with an individual's perception of risk. Those most likely to comply with recommendations to change their environment are older persons at risk for falls and injury (those with gait and balance impairments and older women with low bone density) and those who have experienced a clustering of recent falls at home, particularly in association with untoward consequences (e.g., fear of falling, prolonged postfall lie times, and restricted mobility).

Also, a host of other factors influence compliance, some of which include

(1) the availability and cost of modifications and (2) the capability of individuals or availability of family members and others to institute the required modifications. In addition, the elimination of certain hazardous items, such as a sliding carpet, may be difficult if it is expensive or if it is an heirloom. In general, compliance is enhanced if the following criteria are met:

1. The patient understands the reason for the environmental change.
2. The modification improves mobility (gait and balance).
3. The modification is aesthetically appealing.
4. The modification is affordable, easily obtained, and simple to implement [57].

REFERENCES

1. Tinetti ME, Speechley M. Prevention of falls among the elderly. *N Engl J Med* 1989;320:1055–1059.
2. Rubenstein, LZ, et al. Falls and instability in the elderly. *J Am Geriatr Soc* 1988;36:266–278.
3. Blake AJ, et al. Falls by elderly people at home: Prevalence and associated factors. *Age Ageing* 1988;17:365–372.
4. Reinsch S, Tobis JS. Intervention Strategies to Optimize Health Behaviors and Environment: A Cognitive-Behavior Approach. In: Weindruch R, Hadley EC, Ory MG, eds. *Reducing Frailty and Falls in Older Persons.* Springfield, IL: Thomas, 1991. Pp 293–306.
5. Tinetti ME, Speechley M, Ginter SF. Risk factors for falls among elderly persons living in the community. *N Engl J Med* 1988;319:1701–1707.
6. Hale WA, Delaney MJ, McGagie WC. Characteristics and predictors of falls in elderly patients. *J Fam Pract* 1992;34:577–581.
7. Shepherd J, et al. Patients presenting to family physicians after a fall: A report from the ambulatory sentinel practice network. *J Fam Pract* 1992;35:43–47.
8. Nevitt MC, et al. Risk factors for recurrent nonsyncopal falls. *JAMA* 1989;261:2663–2668.
9. Campbell AJ, et al. Circumstances and consequences of falls experienced by a community population 70 years and over during a prospective study. *Age Ageing* 1990;19:136–141.
10. DeVito CA, et al. Fall injuries among the elderly: Community-based surveillance. *J Am Geriatr Soc* 1988;36:1029–1035.
11. Lucht U. A prospective study of accidental falls and resulting injuries in the home among elderly people. *Acta Socio-Medica Scand* 1971;3:105–120.
12. Schelp L, Svanstrom L. One year incidence of home accidents in a rural Swedish community. *Scand J Soc Med* 1986;14:75–82.
13. Wild D, Nayak US, Isaacs B. How dangerous are falls in old people at home? *Br Med J* 1981;282:266–268.
14. Berry G, Fischer RH, Lang S. Detrimental incidents, including falls, in an elderly institutional population. *J Am Geriatr Soc* 1981;29:322–324.
15. Dimant J. Accidents in the skilled nursing facility. *NY State J Med* 1985;85:202–205.
16. Waller JA. Falls among the elderly—Human and environmental factors. *Accid Anal Prev* 1978;10:21–23.
17. Kellogg International Work Group on the Prevention of Falls by the Elderly. The prevention of falls in later life. *Dan Med Bull* 1987;34:1–24.
18. Tideiksaar R. *Falling in Old Age: Its Prevention and Treatment.* New York: Springer, 1989. Pp 49–51.
19. Tideiksaar R. *Falls in Older Persons: Prevention and Management in Hospitals and Nursing Homes.* Boulder, CO: Tactilitics, 1993. Pp 33–34.

20. Sattin RW. Falls among older persons: A public health perspective. *Annu Rev Public Health* 1992;13:489–508.

21. Rodriguez JG, et al. Developing an Environmental Hazards Assessment Instrument for Falls Among the Edlerly. In: Weindruch R, Hadley EC, Ory MG, eds. *Reducing Frailty and Falls in Older Persons.* Springfield, IL: Thomas, 1991. Pp 263–276.

22. Speechly M, Tinetti M. Falls and injuries in frail and vigorous community elderly persons. *J Am Geriatr Soc* 1991;39:46–52.

23. Houge CC. A Person-Environment Model for Understanding Fall Risk. In: Weindruch R, Hadley EC, Ory MG, eds. *Reducing Frailty and Falls in Older Persons.* Springfield, IL: Thomas, 1991. Pp 96–105.

24. Tinetti ME, Wen-Liang L, Ginter SF. Mechanical restraint use and fall-related injuries among residents of skilled nursing facilities. *Ann Intern Med* 1992;116:369–374.

25. Evans LK, Strumpf NE. Tying down the elderly: A review of the literature on physical restraint. *J Am Geriatr Soc* 1989;37:65–74.

26. Marks W. Physical restraints in the practice of medicine: current concepts. *Arch Intern Med* 1992;152:2203–2206.

27. Morse JM, et al. A retrospective analysis of falls. *Can J Public Health* 1985;76:116–118.

28. Rubenstein HS, et al. Standards of medical care based on consensus rather than evidence: The case of routine bedrail use for the elderly. *Law Med Health Care* 1983;11:27–276.

29. Gabell A, Simons MA, Nayak US. Falls in the elderly: Predisposing causes. *Ergonomics* 1985;28:965–975.

30. Robbins S, Gouw GJ, McClaran J. Shoe sole thickness and hardness influence balance in older men. *J Am Geriatr Soc* 1992;40:1089–1094.

31. Coyle N. A problem-focused approach to nursing audit: Patient falls. *Cancer Nurs* 1979; 2:389–391.

32. Tinker GM. Accidents in a geriatric department. *Age Ageing* 1979;8:196–198.

33. Catchen H. Repeaters: Inpatient accidents among hospitalized elderly. *Gerontologist* 1983; 23:273–276.

34. Heslin K, et al. Managing Falls: Identifying Population-Specific Risk Factors and Prevention Strategies. In: Funk SG, Tornquist EM, Champagne MT, et al., eds. *Key Aspects of Elder Care.* New York: Springer, 1992. Pp 70–88.

35. Elliott DF. Accidents in nursing homes: Implications for Patients and Administrators. In: Miller M, ed. *Current Issues in Clinical Geriatrics.* New York: Tiresias, 1979. Pp 97–137.

36. Kalchthaler T, Bascon RA, Quintos V. Falls in the institutionalized elderly. *J Am Geriatr Soc* 1978;26:424–428.

37. Clark G. A study of falls among elderly hospitalized patients. *Aust J Adv Nurs* 1985;2:34–44.

38. Sehested P, Severin-Nielsen T. Falls by hospitalized elderly patients: Causes, prevention. *Geriatrics* 1977;4:101–108.

39. Harris PB. Organizational and staff attitudinal determinants of falls in nursing home residents. *Med Care* 1989;27:737–749.

40. Tideiksaar R. The Biomedical and Environmental Characteristics of Slips, Stumbles, and Falls in the Elderly. In: Gray BE, ed. *Slips, Stumbles, and Falls: Pedestrian Footwear and Surfaces.* Philadelphia: American Society for Testing and Materials, 1990. Pp 17–27.

41. Wolf-Klein GP, et al. Prevention of falls in the elderly population. *Arch Phys Med Rehabil* 1988;69:689–691.

42. Tideiksaar R. Falls among the elderly: A community prevention program. *Am J Public Health* 1992;82:892–893.

43. Tideiksaar R. Preventing falls: Home hazard checklist to help older patients protect themselves. *Geriatrics* 1986;41:26–28.

44. *Home Safety Checklist for Older Consumers.* Washington, DC: United States Consumer Product Safety Commission, 1985.

45. Dalziel WB, Kelley FA, Cherkin A. *80 Do's and Don'ts for Your Safety: A Practical Guide for Eldercare.* Sepulveda, CA: Geriatric Research Education and Clinical Center, 1985.

46. Mathias S, Nayak US, Isaacs B. Balance in the elderly: The "get-up and go" test. *Arch Phys Med Rehabil* 1986;67:387–389.

47. Tinetti ME. Performance-oriented assessment of mobility problems in elderly patients. *J Am Geriatr Soc* 1986;34:119–126.

48. Chandler JM, Duncan PW. Balance and Falls in the Elderly: Issues in Evaluation and Treatment. In: Guccione AA, ed. *Geriatric Physical Therapy.* St. Louis: Mosby, 1993. Pp 237–251.

49. Tideiksaar R, Feiner CF, Maby J. Falls prevention: The efficacy of a bed alarm system in an acute care setting. *Mt Sinai J Med* 1998;60:522–527.

50. Tideiksaar R, Osterweil D. Prevention of bed falls: The Sepulveda GRECC method. *Geriatr Med Today* 1989;8:70–78.

51. Weiner DK, et al. When older adults face the chair-rise challenge. *J Am Geriatr Soc* 1993;41:6–10.

52. Cummings SR, Nevitt MC. A hypothesis: The cause of hip fractures. *J Gerontol* 1989; 44:M107–111.

53. Lutz JC, Hayes WC. The use of quantitative computed tomography to estimate the risk of fracture of the hip from falls. *J Bone Joint Surg* 1990;72A:689–700.

54. Laurtzen JB, Peterson MM, Lind B. Effect of external hip protectors on hip fractures. *Lancet* 1993;341:11–13.

55. Tideiksaar R. The compliance of older persons with external hip protectors: A device to prevent hip fractures. Proceedings of the Thirteenth Annual Southern Biomedical Engineering Conference, Washington, DC, April 16–17, 1994.

56. Gryfe CI, Amies A, Ashley MJ. A longitudinal study of falls in an elderly population. I: Incidence and morbidity. *Age Ageing* 1977;6:201–210.

57. Levine D, Tideiksaar R. Personal emergency response systems: Factors associated with use among older persons. *Mt Sinai J Med* 1995;62:293–297.

58. Tideiksaar R. Environment adaptations to preserve balance and prevent falls. *Top Geriatr Rehabil* 1990;5:78–84.

Appendices

A. The Axial Mobility Exercise Program

Margaret Schenkman

This program was developed at Duke University Medical Center as part of the work of the Claude D. Pepper Older Americans Independence Center. A therapist's manual, and videotapes available through the center, describes the exercises in detail and the philosophy on which they were based. Appendix A includes an introduction to the program,* a brief summary of the exercises, and several examples of exercises.*

INTRODUCTION

This exercise program is designed to improve mobility, function, and postural alignment. It is intended to increase axial and extremity range of motion through the relaxation of synergistic muscles and the lengthening of soft-tissue structures. As this occurs, postural alignment improves, and the ability to use muscle groups with appropriate mechanical advantage is enhanced. This increased capacity allows decreased effort and increased efficiency of movement so that optimal movement patterns can be achieved. A main objective is to integrate isolated and coordinated movement into daily activities.

The exercises are based on several principles.

1. These exercises are not designed to increase strength or mobility beyond normal levels but to enhance participation of appropriate synergistic muscles. Participation of muscles that are overactive should be decreased, and participation of muscles that are not active enough should be increased.

2. Individuals can increase range of motion and ability to coordinate movement through exercises that emphasize relaxation as opposed to effort.

The participant should be as relaxed as possible prior to initiating these exercises. Gentle diaphragmatic breathing promotes relaxation of musculature throughout the body so as to achieve optimal relaxation prior to initiating exercises.

Muscle groups can be relaxed through deep breathing at the point in the range of motion in which they first become tight. Deep breathing can be used at this point to increase range of motion through relaxation.

3. The axial structures form the base from which extremity and whole-body motions occur.

---

* From M. Schenkman, J. Keysor, J. Chandler, K. C. Laub, H. MacAller. *The Axial Mobility Exercise Program: An Exercise Program to Improve Functional Ability. Therapist's Manual* (2nd ed). Durham, NC: Claude D. Pepper Older American's Independence Center at Duke University, 1994.

The exercises are organized in such a way that relaxation and mobility of axial segments always precede mobility of limb segments. This proximal-to-distal progression is designed to ensure the optimum participation of all body segments during functional movement.

4. Isolated efficient movement of the axial skeleton can be learned best in supported positions so that the participant can focus attention on a minimum number of body segments.

5. The exercises become increasingly complex as the participant's proficiency increases.

Complexity is achieved by increasing the number of segments that are moved coordinately (e.g., upper extremities and lower extremities together in supine position; alternating between symmetrical and asymmetrical movement patterns).

Complexity also is achieved by decreasing the support structures (e.g., progressing from supine to sitting to standing). As the support surface is decreased, there are increased demands for balance control, and it is necessary for more body segments to participate in the desired movement.

6. Each stage of the exercise program builds on previous stages. The participant should always begin the program with the early stage exercises in order to enhance relaxation and to retain optimal range of motion. As the participant progresses through the stages, s/he may use the more complex coordinated exercises in each previous stage. The instructor may emphasize specific exercises according to the participant's individual needs.

7. The goal is for the participant to become independent in these exercises.

The program should be simple so that the participants will be able to follow the exercises and remain compliant.

The instructor should use a variety of handling techniques as needed to guide the desired movements and facilitate the participant's ability to learn the correct movement patterns. As the participant learns the appropriate execution of the exercises, the instructor should diminish the use of handling techniques and verbal cues until the participant is entirely independent.

Functional mobility training and the home program are integral components of the exercise program.

These activities are designed to complement each exercise stage in several ways:

1. Assisting the participant to become independent in the execution of the program.
2. Assisting the participant to incorporate isolated coordinated movement into relevant functional activities of daily life.

To achieve the goals of this exercise program, both therapist and participant should observe several principles:

1. The exercises are to be performed slowly, in a relaxed and precise manner.

a. *The participant should be conscious of achieving the desired movements with minimal effort.* The effort used should be just enough to perform the movement so that substitution by accessory muscles is minimized. Initially, neither the number of repetitions nor completion of a movement is important.

b. *Breathing is used to enhance relaxation.* Breathing can be used to enhance total body relaxation prior to initiating exercise. Breathing also can be used at the end of the range of available motion to promote relaxation of specific muscle groups and to increase range of specific body segments.

c. *Positioning is essential to optimum relaxation.* Throughout the program, the participant must be optimally positioned with pillows or bolsters to provide support and to encourage relaxation. The instructor will modify the positioning as needed. In all cases, the goal is to achieve alignment as close to neutral as possible.

   Neutral alignment. In standing, ideal plumb line alignment runs through the external auditory meatus, the glenohumeral joint, posterior to the greater trochanter, anterior to the center of the knee joint, and anterior to the lateral maleolus. Alignment in the supine position is similar. In sitting, the upper body is aligned as described above, and the lower body is positioned with the feet flat on the supporting surface, with 90-degree angles at the hips, knees, and ankles. In the prone position, the spine should be as close as possible to the described position for standing, using pillows and towel rolls as needed. The shoulders are positioned in abduction with the elbows flexed.

d. *Segments that are not participating in the desired motion must remain relaxed.* For example, the shoulder complex should stay relaxed during sitting exercises to increase thoracic and lumbar rotation.

2. The instructor modifies the exercises as needed based on the participant's orthopedic, muscular, or neurologic impairments.

   These exercises can be used appropriately with almost all people. Precautions and appropriate modifications should always be considered when working with participants who have diagnoses and conditions including but not limited to:

   a. Osteoarthritis.

   b. Osteoporosis.

   c. Spinal fusions.

   d. History of low-back pain.

   e. Other painful conditions of the spine and extremities.

   f. Severe cardiovascular disease.

   Modifications include but are not limited to the following:

   a. Limiting movement to a pain-free range of motion.

   b. Modifying positions to minimize pain (e.g., using pillows for comfortable positioning).

    c. Avoiding positions and movements that could cause fracture in an osteoporetic participant (e.g., consulting with attending physician as necessary).

    d. Monitoring cardiovascular status in positions and during activities that could unduly stress the cardiovascular system (e.g., quadruped, prone, sit-to-stand).

    e. Deleting exercises if they are inappropriate (e.g., quadruped for individuals who have severe thoracic kyphosis).

3. The instructor modifies the progression of the exercises as needed. If a participant does not make gains in a particular stage, it may be necessary to move to the next stage while continuing to work on the earlier stage. The instructor should not feel that the participant must completely master all aspects of a particular stage before advancing.

4. Each participant should perform daily the exercises specified by the instructor in an individual *home exercise program*. The beginning of each session should consist of fundamental exercises from stages I, II, and III (see Summary of Exercises), to promote relaxation and preparation for more advanced exercises. The majority of time spent should be on the exercise of each specific stage and on specific impairments of the participant. All of the exercises, including functional mobility, should carryover and be incorporated into daily functional activity and mobility.

Summary of Exercises

Stage I. Relaxing while increasing range of motion in the supine position

Goals:

1. Relaxing the trunk, hip, shoulder, and neck regions.
2. Increasing range of motion while retaining relaxation.
3. Retaining the relaxation of antagonist and accessory muscles while moving.

EXERCISE	PURPOSE
Deep breathing	Learn the use of breathing to promote relaxation
Double hip rotation (see Fig. A-1)	Relax axial musculature for optimal elongation of lower-trunk muscles
Single hip rotation	Relax the hip abductors and adductors and rotator muscles for their optimal elongation and for appreciation of isolated movement
Shoulder rotation	Relax the shoulder complex and upper-trunk musculature for isolated internal and external glenohumeral motion
Neck rotation	Relax cervical musculature to improve range of motion and head position

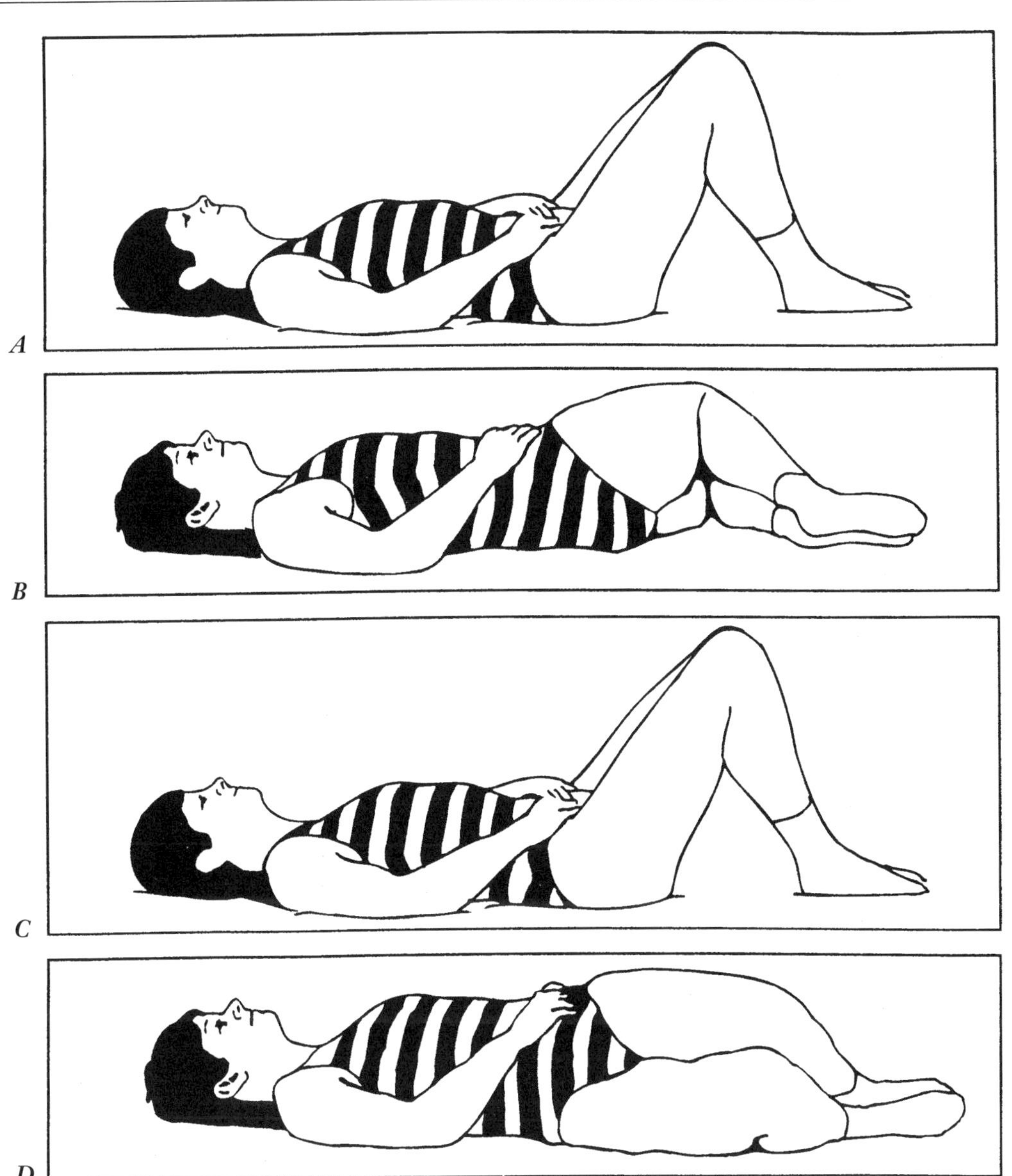

Figure A-1. (*A-D*) Trunk: Double hip rotation. *Purpose: Relax axial musculature for optimal elongation.* Participant flexes hips and knees (hook lying position) and, keeping knees together, moves them side to side to achieve lower-trunk rotation and elongation. The motion should be gentle to achieve relaxation of the axial structures, and the instructor should be able to feel a reduction in the participant's total body tension. The low back should not lift from the mat more than a few inches.

Coordinated neck, shoulder, and hip motion	Develop smooth coordinated motion of multiple segments

Stage II. Segmental motion of the spine and upper quadrant, with emphasis on the thorax

Goals:

1. Isolating thoracic movement on a stable pelvis.
2. Isolating scapular movement on the thorax.
3. Coordinating movement of the glenohumeral, scapular, and thoracic regions on a stable pelvis.

EXERCISE	PURPOSE
Thorax	Increase thoracic rotation
Scapula on thorax	Isolate scapular and glenohumeral motion without thoracic motion; optimize orientation of the scapula and movement of the scapulothoracic joint
Scapula and thorax on a stable pelvis (see Fig. A-2)	Coordinate glenohumeral and thoracic motion

Stage III. Segmental motion of the spine and isolated motion of the lower extremities on a stable pelvis (prone)

Goals:

1. Assuming symmetrical prone position.
2. Increasing thoracic and lumbar extension.
3. Isolating internal and external rotation of the lower extremities on the pelvis.
4. Increasing hip internal and external rotation range of motion.

EXERCISE	PURPOSE
"Wiggle" (see Fig. A-3)	Promote relaxation of the spine and the pelvofemoral area in preparation for extension exercises
Prone on elbows	Increase flexion and extension of the thoracic and lumbar spine
Internal and external hip rotation	Relax the internal and external hip rotators and increase their range of motion

Stage IV: Segmental motion of the spine and pelvis (quadruped)

Goals:

1. Increasing mobility in the lumbar, thoracic, and cervical regions.
2. Isolating motion throughout the spine.
3. Coordinating dynamic movement of the shoulders, hips, and spine.

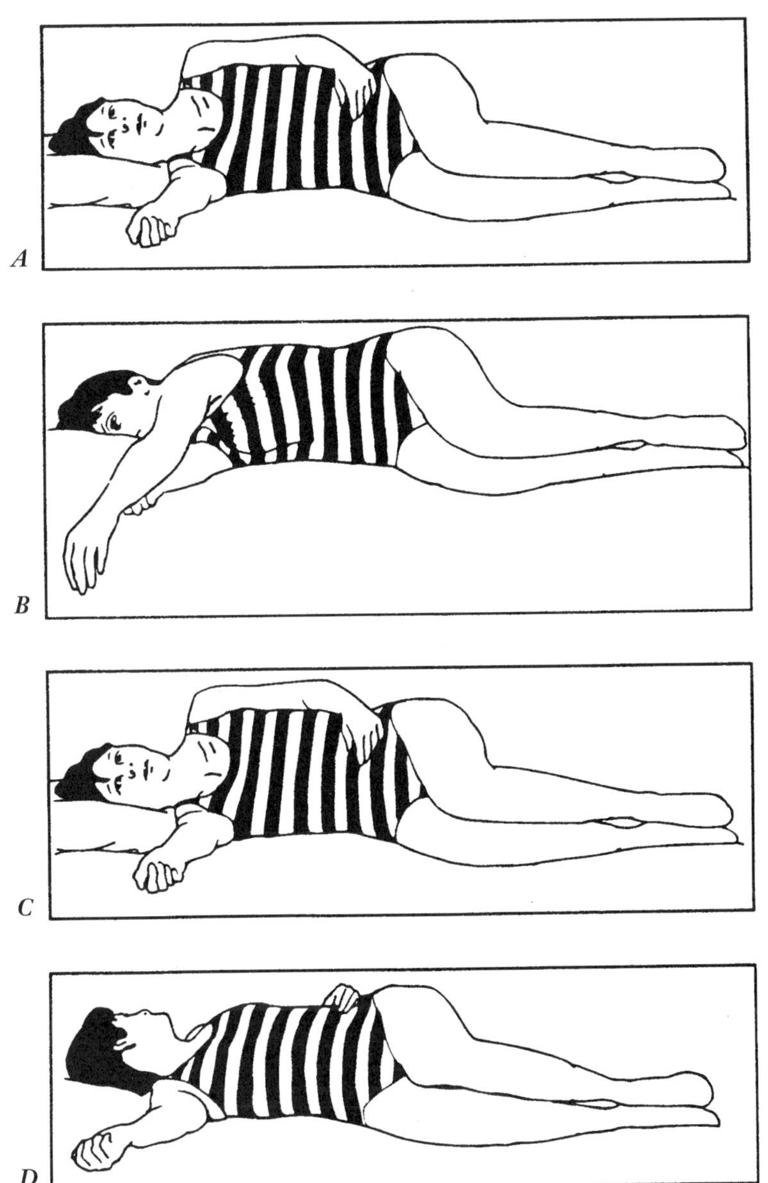

Figure A-2. (*A-D*) Scapula and thorax on a stable pelvis. *Purpose: Coordinate glenohumeral and thoracic motion.* The participant reaches forward and backward with the humerus in the sagittal plane of the body. The movement should include thoracic rotation with respect to the fixed pelvis. The motion of the thorax and upper extremity should be smooth and coordinated while the pelvis remains relatively fixed. As the participant gains scapulothoracic motion, s/he may reach in various planes as long as the upper extremity remains relaxed and abduction of the extremity is avoided.

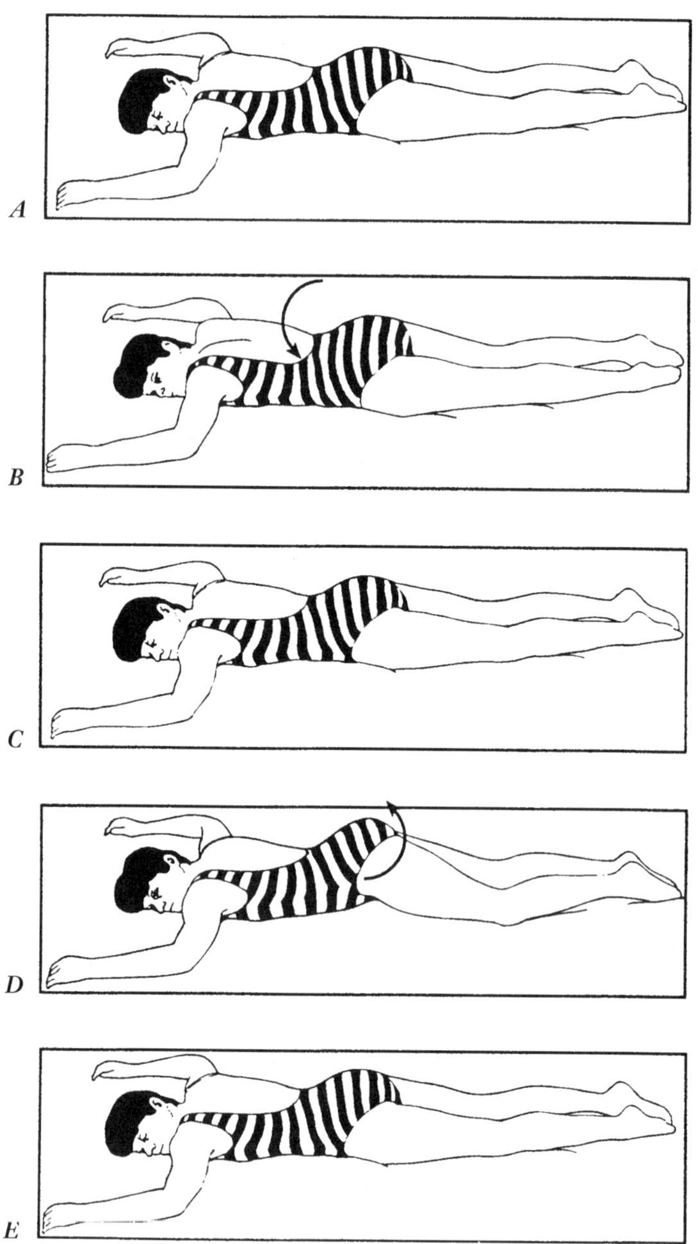

Figure A-3. (*A-E*) "Wiggle." *Purpose: Promote relaxation of the spine and pelvofemoral area in preparation for extension exercises.* The participant gently "wiggles" the pelvis rhythmically and in a relaxed manner to the right and left to achieve movement and relaxation of the lower back and axial structures. The emphasis of this motion is on rotation of the lumbar and low thoracic region.

EXERCISE	PURPOSE
Cat, camel	Increase range of motion and control of extension and flexion of the entire spine
Isolated flexion and extension of the lumbar region	Isolate motion of the lumbar spine and of the thoracic spine
Forward and backward rock (sagittal plane)	Stretch the soft-tissue structures of the low back, pelvis, hip, and shoulder complex; increase coordinated movement in less supported positions
Forward and backward rock (diagonal plane)	Stretch the lateral soft-tissue structures of the thorax, pelvis, hip, and shoulder complex; increase coordinated movement in less supported positions

Stage V. Segmental motion of the spine and pelvis (sitting)

Goals:

1. Assuming an erect sitting posture with neutral alignment.
2. Increasing lumbar flexion and extension in the unsupported position.
3. Isolating and coordinating lumbopelvic motion in unsupported sitting.

EXERCISE	PURPOSE
Isolated anterior/ posterior pelvic tilt (see Fig. A-4) Trunk flexion over stable base	Increase lumbopelvic motion; stabilize the thorax in an upright position while moving the pelvis Increase hip extensor muscle length; develop the ability to maintain neutral trunk alignment while moving the trunk in relation to the hips
Diagonal trunk flexion over a stable pelvis (see Fig. A-5)	Increase hip abduction and adduction and extensor range of motion; increase the ability to coordinate complex lumbopelvic motion; increase balance control through small displacements of the trunk
Lateral tilt of the trunk and pelvis	Isolate lumbar lateral flexion in sitting
Pelvic clock	Isolate pelvic movement in all planes in sitting
Chin tuck motion	Improve head and neck alignment and mobility

Stage VI. Coordinated trunk and upper-extremity movement in an unsupported position (sitting)

Goals:

1. Coordinating movement of bilateral upper extremities and trunk.
2. Maintaining an erect posture and initiating weight shift from the pelvis as the movement is performed.

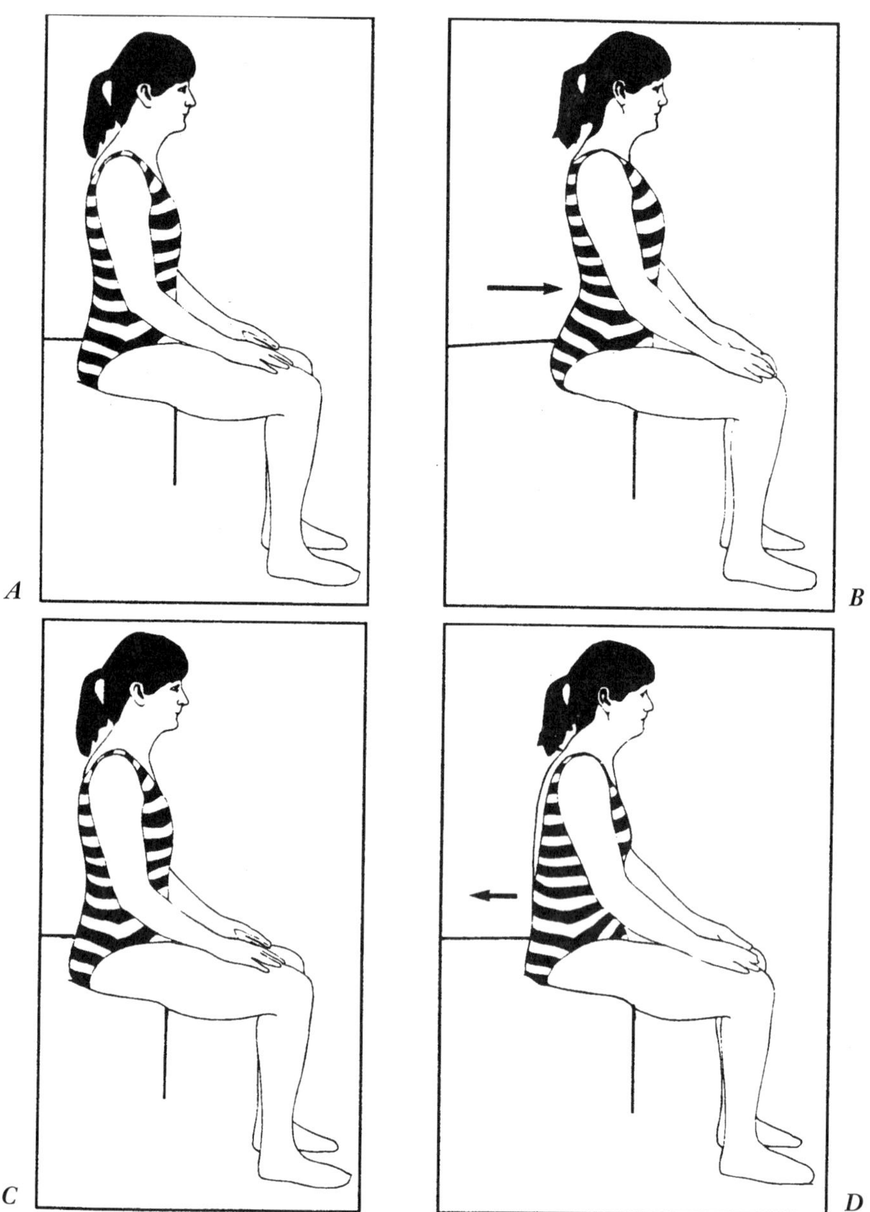

Figure A-4. (*A-D*) Isolated anterior/posterior (A/P) pelvic tilt. *Purpose: Increase lumbopelvic motion; stabilize the thorax in an upright position while moving the pelvis.* The participant will perform an A/P pelvic tilt, with the emphasis on isolated pelvic movement. The shoulders should be held relatively stationary over the greater trochanters while the pelvis is rotated forward and backward. Verbal and tactile cues may be indicated until the concept is understood. It is frequently helpful for the instructor to place his/her hands over the lateral aspects of the pelvis and/or on the lumbar spine. One technique that may help the participant to recognize motion in the lumbar region, is to have her/him assume a slouched position, and then to sit erect with emphasis on slight lumbar extension.

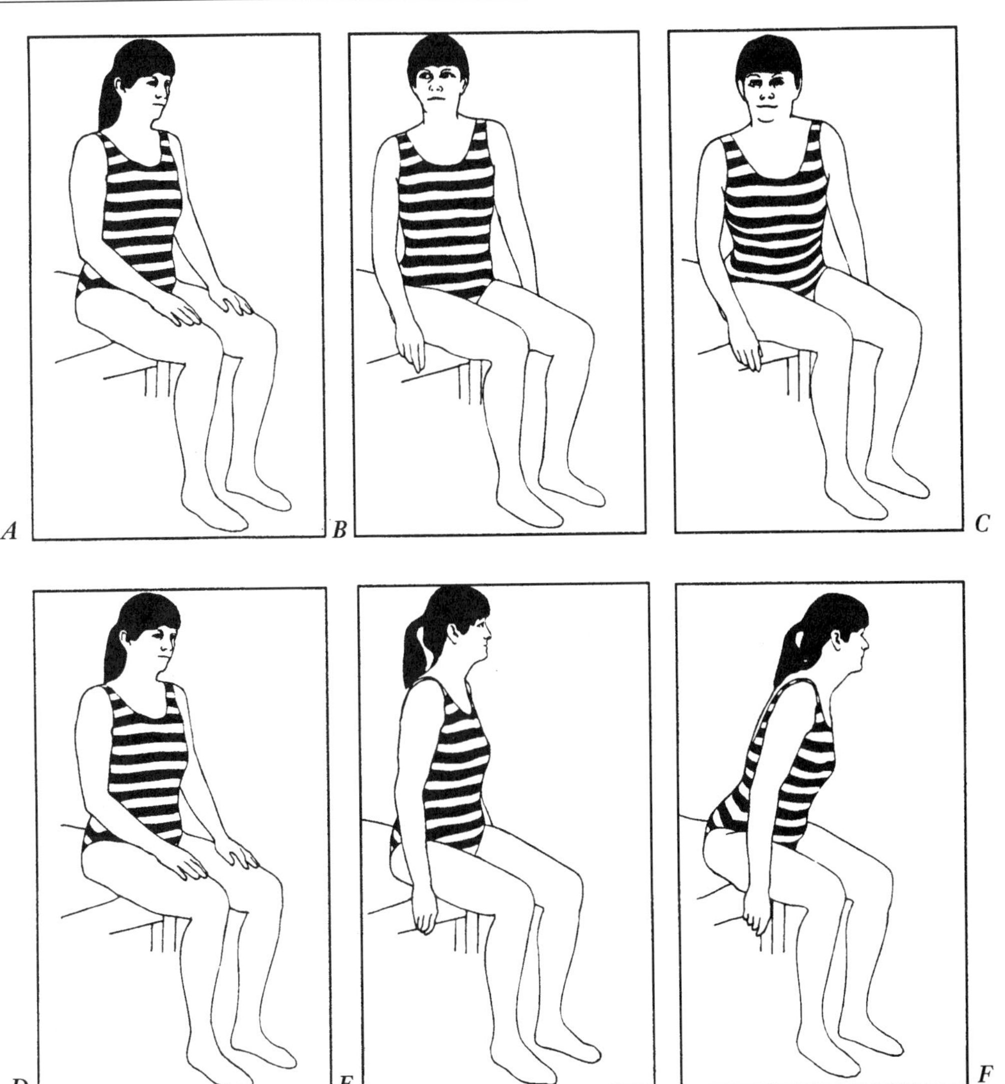

Figure A-5. (*A-F*) Diagonal trunk flexion over a stable pelvis. *Purpose: Increase hip abduction/adduction and extensor range of motion; increase the ability to coordinate complex lumbopelvic motion; increase balance control through small displacements of the trunk.* The participant rotates the pelvis and entire trunk to the right, and allows his/her weight shift to the right buttock. S/he flexes the trunk forward over the right femur in a diagonal plane. The thorax is stabilized. Repeat the movement to the left.

EXERCISE	PURPOSE
Trunk rotation	Develop range of motion of trunk rotator musculature and control of movement in the transverse plane
Trunk extension from a flexed position	Achieve segmental extension
Trunk flexion and extension in the diagonal plane	Achieve coordinated trunk extension, rotation, and weight shift

Stage VII. Axial mobility in standing

Goals:

1. Using the axial and segmental motion gained from the previous stages for co-ordinated dynamic movement in standing.
2. Performing isolated and coordinated motions at all spinal segments and regions.

EXERCISE	PURPOSE
Lateral trunk flexion	Lengthen soft tissues of the lateral trunk
Relaxed trunk and lower-extremity rotation	Achieve relaxed rotation in standing
Isolated lower-trunk rotation	Learn to rotate the lower trunk and pelvis relative to a stable upper trunk
Isolated upper-trunk rotation	Achieve upper-trunk rotation relative to a fixed pelvis and lower extremities
Lateral pelvic tilt in standing	Learn to initiate lateral weight shift at the pelvis
Forward and backward weight shifts (see Fig. A-6)	Use the pelvis to initiate and control weight shift in functional planes
Dynamic activities	Incorporate the segmental movement gained in the previous exercises into dynamic movement

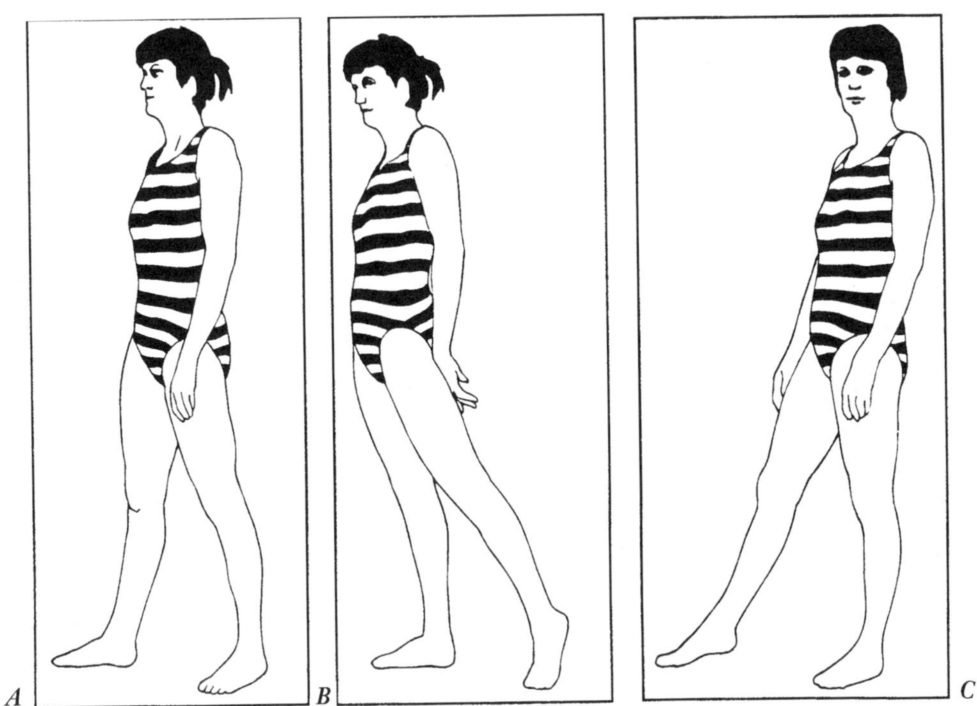

Figure A-6 A-C. Forward and backward weight shifts. *Purpose: To use the pelvis to initiate and control weight-shifts in functional planes.* The participant stands with one foot in front of the other, as if taking a step. S/he then shifts weight from one extremity to the other, initiating movement from the pelvis. The knees should remain relatively straight. As weight is shifted anteriorly over the foward foot, the heel of the posterior foot is allowed to rise. As the weight is transferred back to the posterior foot, the toe of the forward foot is allowed to rise. The participant should feel the weight shift from the heel to

B. Performance-Oriented Environmental Mobility Screen

Rein Tideiksaar

Instructions: Ask the patient or resident to perform the indicated maneuvers. If the individual uses ambulation device (e.g., cane, walker), each maneuver is tested with the device as appropriate. For each maneuver, indicate whether the person's performance is independent or impaired.

Maneuver	Observation	
	✓ Independent	✓ Impaired
Sit down and rise up from chairs(s)	☐ Chair transfer is smooth, controlled movement (sits down and rises from chair in one attempt: does not use armrests; chair does not tip or slide away)	☐ Chair transfer is not smooth movement (requires several attempts to sit or rise; falls onto seat; uses armrest or seat edge to guide transfers: chair tips or slides away)
	☐ Sitting balance is stable (does not use armrest support to maintain balance)	☐ Sitting balance is unstable (stables down from seat or uses armrest support to maintain balance)
	☐ Seated, both feet rest flat on ground	☐ Seated, feet do not rest on ground
		☐ Unable to perform maneuver
Device used to perform maneuver ☐ Yes ☐ No	☐ Device appropriate for space (able to transfer with device)	☐ Device not appropriate for space (unable to transfer with device)
	☐ Device used correctly for transfers	☐ Device used incorrectly for transfers
Stand in place (for approximately 15 seconds) with arms by side and eyes open	☐ Steady; able to stand without balance loss	☐ Unsteady; unable to maintain standing balance
	☐ Does not use chair or other furnishing to maintain balance	☐ Uses chair or other furnishings to maintain balance
	☐ Does not use device to maintain balance	☐ Uses device to maintain balance
		☐ Unable to perform maneuver

Maneuver	Observation	
	✓ Independent	✓ Impaired
Standing in place with both eyes closed (for approximately 15 seconds)	☐ Steady; able to stand without balance loss ☐ Does not use chair or other furnishing to maintain balance	☐ Unsteady; unable to maintain standing balance ☐ Uses chair or other furnishing to maintain balance ☐ Unable to perform maneuver
Stand in place (both eyes open); nudge person's sternum lightly three times	☐ Steady; able to withstand pressure without balance loss ☐ Does not use chair or other furnishing to maintain balance	☐ Unsteady; unable to withstand pressure and maintain balance ☐ Uses chair or other furnishing to maintain balance ☐ Unable to perform maneuver
From standing position, bend down and pick up object from ground	☐ Steady; able to bend down and rise up without balance loss ☐ Does not use furnishings to maintain balance ☐ Does not use device to maintain balance	☐ Unsteady; unable to bend down and rise up and maintain balance ☐ Uses furnishings to maintain balance ☐ Uses device to maintain balance ☐ Unable to perform maneuver
Transfer onto and up from bed	☐ Bed transfer is smooth, controlled movement (sits on and rises from bed in one attempt) ☐ Feet do not slide away on ground during transfers ☐ Bed does not slide away during transfers ☐ Sitting balance is stable (does not use arm support to maintain balance) ☐ Able to lie down (in supine position) and rise in one smooth, controlled movement	☐ Bed transfer is not smooth (requires several attempts to sit or rise; falls onto mattress; uses mattress edge to guide transfers) ☐ Feet slide away on ground during transfers ☐ Bed slides away during transfers ☐ Sitting balance is unstable (uses arm support to maintain balance) ☐ Unable to lie down (in supine position) or rise in one smooth, controlled movement ☐ Unable to perform unassisted transfers

Device used to perform maneuver ☐ Yes ☐ No	☐ Device appropriate for space (able to transfer with device) ☐ Device used correctly for transfers	☐ Device not appropriate for space (unable to transfer with device) ☐ Device used incorrectly for transfers
Walk and turn in bedroom and bathroom	☐ Gait is continuous, without hesitation ☐ Gait is straight, without deviation from path ☐ Both feet clear ground surface ☐ Turns are smooth, continuous, without balance loss ☐ Does not use wall, furnishings, sink, or towel bar for balance support	☐ Gait is noncontinuous, with hesitation ☐ Gait deviates from straight path ☐ One or both feet scrape ground surface ☐ Turns are discontinuous, with balance loss ☐ Uses wall, furnishings, sink, or towel bar for balance support ☐ Unable to perform maneuver
Device used to perform maneuver ☐ Yes ☐ No	☐ Device appropriate for space (able to walk without environmental interference) ☐ Device used correctly for walking and turning	☐ Device not appropriate for space (unable to walk due to environmental interference) ☐ Device used incorrectly for walking and turning
Sit on and rise from toilet	☐ Toilet transfer is smooth, controlled movement (sits down and rises from toilet in one attempt; does not use grab bars, seat, or sink edge for support; feet do not slide away on ground) ☐ Seated, both feet rest flat on ground	☐ Toilet transfer is not smooth movement (requires several attempts to sit or rise; falls onto toilet seat; uses grab bars, seat, or sink edge for support; feet slide away on ground) ☐ Seated, feet do not fest flat on ground

Subject Index

A

Acaudate posture, 60
Achilles tendon
    corticosteroid injection of, 179
    immobilization of, 178
    irritation of, 176
    rupture of, 176, 192
    tendinitis of, 181
Adaptation
    balance improved by, 84
    context-dependent, 71–73
    defined, 84
    reflex-dependent, 71–73
Akinesia, 216
Alcoholic consumption
    spinocerebellar anterior lobe atrophy, 266
Amyloid angiopathy, 236
Ankle
    flexion strength, 386
    immobilization of, 168, 179–180, 192
    pressures on, 162
    strategy. *See* Ankle strategy
Ankle disorders, 159–193
    arthritis causing, 177
    causes of, 165–167
    defined, 165
    etiology of, 173–190
    evaluation and treatment of, 190–193
    iatrogenic causes of, 190
    inflammation causing, 180
    rheumatoid arthritis causing, 182
    sports injuries causing, 188
    trauma causing, 173–177
Ankle joint
    anatomy of, 159–160
    arthritis in, 177
    stiffness in, 168
Ankle sprain, 175
Ankle strategy, 39, 109, 265
Ankle-foot orthosis (AFO), 168
Ankylosis, 168–169
    spondylitis, 182
    subtalar, 170
Anxiety, 292
Aphasia, evidence of, 247
Apraxia, 216

Arteriosclerosis, 221
Arthritis
    foot and ankle, 177–179
    gait disorders compared, 148
    resistance training, 390
Arthritis Impact Measurement Scales, 349
Astasia-abasia. *See also* Subcortical disequilibrium
    history of, 2, 141, 289
    symptoms of, 153
Automatic postural movements
    coordination of, 43–44
    electromyelography caused by, 42
Axial mobility
    exercise program for, 415–426
    improvement in PD patients, 349

B

Balance. *See also* Posture
    anticipatory postural reflexes, 137
    assessing, traditional approaches to, 107–
        108
    base of support. *See* Base of support
    bipedal activities, 358
    center of gravity. *See* Center of gravity
    clinical assessment of, 111–119
    clinical management of, 50
    defined, 37–38, 108
    external challenges to, 359–360
    ground-level functional, 358
    hearing loss affecting, 80
    hip strategy. *See* Hip strategy
    impairment. *See* Balance impairment
    improving. *See* Balance training
    laboratory measures of, 23
    limits of stability. *See* Limits of stability
    morphology, role of, 82
    movement strategies, 39–41
    moving platforms perturbing. *See* Moving
        platforms
    multidisciplinary approach to, 3–4
    muscle activation. *See* Muscle response
    muscle coordination, 109–111
    overview of, 1–10
    physical challenges to, 356–360
    physiology of, 4–5, 37

Balance (*contd.*)
  postural movement control. *See* Postural
    movement control
  prevalence of, 2–3
  proactive control of, 110–111
  protective reactions, 137
  reaction time affecting, 81
  reactive control of, 109–110
  reactive postural reflexes, 137
  reflexes evaluating, 108
  repetitive motor tasks improving, 84
  rescue reactions, 137
  research methods for study of, 108–110
  sensory components of, 45–49, 79–81, 111
  single stance. *See* Single stance
  somatosensory input, 46, 48, 100
  stabilometry measuring, 107
  subsystem evaluation of, 113
  surface conditions affecting, 118
  sway. *See* Sway
  systems approach to, 37–50, 108, 119
  vestibular input, 46
  visual input, 46
Balance impairment
  disease-related, 88
  functional and therapeutic implications of,
    87–89
  men and women compared, 86–88
  muscle mass, loss of, 81
  nursing home patients, 88
  old and young compared, 86
  pain sensitivity, loss of, 79–80
  sensorimotor processing, 81–84
  thermal sensitivity loss, 79–80
  visual input. *See* Visual impairment
Balance tests, 113–114, 138, 365–372
  comparisons of, 367–368
  lifting and pushing tasks, 111
  limitations of, 113, 373–374
  toes-up and toes-down rotation, 84
  turns, negotiating, 138
  types of, 124, 366
  usage of, 366
  vestibular impairment. *See* Vestibular
    impairment
  vibratory sensitivity, loss of, 80
Balance training, 355–376
  criteria for, 374
  resistance training, 389
  studies of, 360–374
  test for. *See* Balance tests
Basal ganglia disease, 138
Basal ganglia lesions, 225

Base of support
  defined, 38
  functional, 85
  narrowed, 85–86
  sitting, 95
Binswanger's disease, 151, 222
Bipedal locomotion. *See also* Walking
  neurophysiology of, 73–76
  requirements for, 73
Body alignment, evaluation of, 116
Bone cysts, 184
Bone mineral density, loss of, 27
Bradykinesia, 340, 343
Brain. *See also* specific regions of
  compartmental models of, 59
  movement controlled by, 58
  posture controlled by, 58
  vascular supply to. *See* Cerebrovascular
    diseases
Brain stem
  cell loss in, 99
  dorsal tegmental field (DTF). *See* Dorsal
    tegmental field (DTF)
  ischemia. *See* Cerebrovascular diseases
  mesencephalic locomotor region. *See*
    Mesencephalic locomotor region (MLR)
  spinal cord functioning together with, 57
  stimulation of. *See* Brain stem stimulation
  subthalamic locomotor region. *See*
    Subthalamic locomotor region (SLR)
  transection of. *See* Brain stem transection
  ventral tegmental field (VTF). *See* Ventral
    tegmental field (VTF)
Brain stem stimulation
  decerebration, 62–68
  intact central nervous system, 68–71
Brain stem transection, 58
  rigidity caused by, 62

C
Canes
  falls caused by, 397, 408
  use of, 337, 346
Capsular lesions, 225
Cardiovascular impairments, 334
Cataracts, 79
Caudate nuclei ablation, 60
Cautious gait
  psychological state, 153, 283–285
    clinical presentation, 285
    factors underlying, 285
    treatment of, 293

Center of gravity (COG)
  defined, 38
  parkinsonism, 210
  senses measuring, 45
  shifts in, 137
  sway angle, 39
Center of mass (COM)
  force plates measuring, 132
  gait initiation, 94
  measuring, 116
  posterior displacement of, 100
Center of pressure (COP)
  defined, 107
  force plates measuring, 132
  gait initiation, 94
  posterior displacement of, 100
  stability gauged by, 107–108
Central nervous system ablation, 58
Cerebellar ataxia
  gait affected by, 140, 151
  sensory ataxia compared, 1–2, 143
  white-matter disease compared, 235
Cerebellar hemorrhages, 230–232
Cerebellar impairment, 266–270
  EMG responses indicating, 267
  gait disturbances in, 269
Cerebellum
  anterior lobe atrophy, 266, 268
  anterior vermis lesions in, 151
  cell loss in, 99
  diseases of, 268
  flocculonodular lobe disorders, 151
  infarcts of, 151
  olivopontocerebellar atrophy in, 151
  rhythmic signals reaching, 67
  role in locomotion, 62–63
  spinocerebellar lesions, 266, 269
  spinocerebellar loop, 63
  vestibulocerebellar lesions, 151, 266, 2
    69
Cerebral blood flow (rCBF) reduction,
    249
Cerebral cortex
  cell loss in, 99
  loss of. *See* Decerebration
  role in locomotion, 55–76
  SLR lesions of, 61
  spinal pathways to, 55–57
Cerebrospinal fluid (CSF)
  absorption, 256
  drainage of, 247–248
  infusion tests, 250
  pressure monitoring, 249

Cerebrovascular disorders, 221–250
  classification of, 222
  history of, 221
Cervical spondylosis
  defined, 148, 197
Cervical spondylotic myelopathy, 197–208
  cervical decompression, 205
  defined, 197
  diagnosis of, 200–201
  history of, 197
  imaging of, 200
  motor findings of, 199
  pathophysiology of, 197–198
  physical therapy for, 204
  posterior decompression, 205
  reflex changes, 199
  sensory changes, 199
  surgery for, 204–207
  symptoms of, 198
  tests to confirm, 200
  treatment of, 201–207, 211–212
  x-rays, 200
Chair, rising from, 95, 138, 346
Charcot's arthropathy, 182, 184
Choreic gait, 140
Cisplatin neurotoxicity, 274
Cisternography, 249
Clinical Test for Sensory Interaction in Balance
    (CTSIB), 117
Computer tomography, 154
Contact, postural reactions to, 75
Corticobasal ganglionic degeneration (CBGD),
    215

D
Decerebration
  acute, 63–68
  gait pattern, changes in, 67–68, 72
  locomotor phase control system, 63, 66–67
  locomotor rhythm-releasing system,
    64–65
  postural tonus-regulating system, 65–66
Decorticate posture, 59–60
Dementia
  NPH, 245
  Parkinson's Disease, 215
  white matter changes with, 233
Depression, 292
Diabetes
  autonomic neuropathy of, 182–183
  foot disorders caused by, 172
Diffuse Levy-Body disease (DLBD), 215

Dopamine loss
  agonists as treatment for, 211
  balance affected by, 82
  percentage of age-related, 99
Dorsal root ganglion cells
  degeneration of, 275
  toxins attacking, 273
Dorsal tegmented field (DTF)
  hindlimbs controlled by, 65
  stimulation of, 65, 68–71
Dorsolateral systems ablation, 57–58
Drop attacks
  falls caused by, 311
  symptoms of, 237–239
Dynamics, 131–132
Dystonic gait, 140

E
Electromyography, 42
Electromyography
  motion analysis, 126
    gait cycles, 383
    leg muscles, 381
    muscles activated by, 109
    repeatability of, 132
En bloc turning, 210
Encephalopathy, 152
Environmental hazards causing falls, 97, 304
  assessments of, 400
  bathroom, 407
  beds, 406
  circulatory pathways, 404
  floor surfaces, 405
  lighting, 405
  modifications of, 400
  removal of, 30, 395–398
  seating, 406
  stairs, 407
  storage areas, 408
  strategies to reduce, 404–410
Equilibrium, 136–137
Exercise. *See also* Strength training
  axial mobility. *See* Axial mobility
  choosing appropriate, 345
  falls reduced by, 30, 321
  gait, effect on, 388
  oseoarthritis, 348
  Parkinson's disease, 349
  performance-oriented environmental
    mobility, 429–431
  rheumatoid arthritis, 348
  stretching and relaxing compared, 343

F
Fall prevention, 315–324
  caregiving patterns, 398
  compliance with, 409
  devices for, 322
  education interventions for, 316
  environmental factors in, 395–410
  environmental hazards. *See* Environmental
    hazards causing falls
  exercise reducing, 321
  hearing and, 80
  hospital patients, 31, 321, 395
  length of stay, 398
  medical history, 300–303
  nursing home patients, 321, 395
  physical exam, 300–303
  risk factor identification, 316
  safety checklists, 399–400
  strategies for, 323
  studies for, 29–31
  studies of, 316–322
  time of fall, 398
  visual input, 79
Fall-related deaths
  age and, 14
  gender and, 14
  prevalence of, 297
  race and, 14
Fall-related injuries. *See also* Balance
    impairment; Fractures
  as cause of death. *See* Fall-related deaths
  mechanics of, 28
  prevalence of, 297
  risk factors for
    falls compared, 27–29
    intrinsic, 20–22
    methodological issues of, 20
    multifactorial etiology of, 19
  types of, 17
Falls
  affective disorders as risk factor for, 23
  age-related diseases causing, 88
  backward, 100, 280
  causes of, 108, 119, 300, 309–312
  circumstances of, 299
  clinical tests as predictors of, 23
  cognitive impairment as risk factor for, 23
  consequences of, 297, 316
  costs of, 18
  death caused by. *See* Fall-related deaths
  defined, 13
  devices contributing to, 397
  disability resulting from, 18

environmental hazards causing. *See*
    Environmental hazards causing
    falls
etiology of, 310
evaluation of, 299–305, 313–315
fear of. *See* Fear of falling
footwear contributing to, 397, 408
fractures affected by mechanics of, 28
frequency of, 15–16
hospital patients suffering. *See* Hospital
    patients
injuries from. *See* Fall-related injuries
mechanics of, 28
medications causing, 24, 303
men and women compared, 15
muscle weakness causing, 23
nursing home patients suffering. *See* Nursing
    home patients
overview of, 13
parkinsonism, 210
prevalence of, 395
prevention of. *See* Fall prevention
psychological results of, 18
risk factors for, 19–29, 124, 298, 312
    activity-related, 25–27
    behavioral, 25–27
    environmental, 25–27
    injurious falls compared, 27–29
    intrinsic, 20–22
    methodological issues of, 20
    multifactorial etiology of, 19
    self-reported, 20
sitting to standing position causing, 95
slow reaction time causing, 23
sway as predictors of, 24
sway velocity and, 107
vision impairment causing, 21
Falls efficacy scale (FES), 289
Fear of falling, 140, 153
    assessment of, 289–291
    clinical presentation, 287
    consequences of, 288
    defined, 286
    prevalence of, 285
    treatment of, 293
    underlying factors, 286
Festination, 210
Fibrosis, 182
Foot
    anatomy of, 159–164
    biomechanics of, 159–164
    bones and joints of, 161
    COM on, 132
    COP on, 132
    hindfoot, 159
    immobilization of, 172, 179–180,
        192
    midfoot, 160
    plantar fascia, 160, 162
    pressures on, 162, 164
    standing vs. normal gait, 162
    tibialis anterior, 160, 162
    vibration sensation loss in, 100
Foot disorders, 159–193. *See also* specific
    diseases, e.g. Tendinitis
    anklosing spondylitis causing, 182
    arthritis causing, 177
    causes of, 165–167
    congenital deformities, 184
    contusions causing, 176
    defined, 165
    diabetic, 172
    etiology of, 173–190
    evaluation and treatment of, 190–193
    forefoot, 171
    fractures causing. *See* Fractures
    heel pad, 172
    iatrogenic causes of, 190
    inflammation causing, 180
    metatarsophalangeal joint, 181
    midfoot, 171
    neuropathy causing, 182–184
    psoriatic arthritis causing, 182
    rheumatoid arthritis causing, 182
    sports injuries causing, 188
    subtalar and transverse tarsal joints, 169–
        170
    trauma causing, 173–177
Footwear contributing to falls, 397, 408
Force plates, 126, 132
Fractures. *See also* type of fracture
    ankle, 174–177
    bone mineral density, loss of, 27
    calcaneus, 176
    detecting, 191
    fibular, 176
    foot, 174–177
    impact needed for, 27
    mechanics of falls affecting, 28
    tibia-fibula, 174
    women with, 17
Freezing, 138, 143, 210
Frontal gait, 144, 150
Functional reach
    decline of, 85
    test for, 112–113

G

Gait. *See also* Balance; Posture; Stride;
　　Walking
　biomechanics of, 332, 349
　clinical analysis of, 123–133
　COM. *See* Center of mass (COM)
　COP. *See* Center of pressure (COP)
　defined, 125
　diseases affecting, 98–99
　drunken, 63
　dynamics of. *See* Dynamics
　external and internal forces affecting, 333
　functional indicators of, 331, 349
　initiation, 93–95, 137
　kinematics of. *See* Kinematics
　laboratory analysis of. *See* Motion analysis
　　laboratories
　muscle strength and, 381–384
　normal aging, 93–101
　old and young compared, 164
　parkinsonian gait. *See* Parkinsonian gait
　performance indicating, 124
　physiology of, 4–5
　requirements for, 327–328
　spatial characteristics of, 332
　temporal characteristics of, 332
　video recording of, 124–125
Gait cycle, 96, 162
Gait disorder treatments, 327–350
　axial mobility improving after, 349
　choosing appropriate, 341–350
　clinical decision-making for, 328–338
　ending, 347
　exercise. *See* Exercise
　feedback from clinician, 346
　functional tasks, related to, 345–346
　goals of, 327, 338–341
　independence, increasing patient, 337, 346
　lifestyle of patient, 336
　medical conditions of patient, 336
　mental status of patient, 336
　outcomes, measuring, 348
　outline for physical program for, 342
　pain management, 344
　social support of patient, 336
　stretching and relaxing compared, 343
　systematic approach to, 328
Gait disorders. *See also* specific types
　arthritis compared, 148
　brain-imaging studies of, 154
　causes of, 333
　cerebellar ataxic. *See* Cerebellar ataxia
　classification of, 139–145, 148
　death caused by, 3
　defined, 135
　depression causing, 153
　diseases related to, 139
　etiology of, 148–149
　evaluation of, 153–155, 331
　frontal disequilibrium, 143–144
　heterogeneity of, 147–148
　historical aspects of, 1–2
　hospital patients with, 147
　initiation failure, 143
　multidisciplinary approach to, 3–4
　myelopathy. *See* Myelopathy
　neurophysiology of, 154
　nosology of, 135–145
　nursing home patients with, 147
　overview of, 1–10
　paraplegic, 140
　parkinsonism. *See* Parkinson's disease
　peripheral factors in, 279–281
　physical intervention for. *See* Gait disorder
　　treatments
　prevalence of, 2–3, 147, 310
　prioritizing, 340
　psychogenic. *See* Psychogenic gait disorders
　sensory impairment causing. *See* Sensory
　　impairment
　somatosensory impairment causing. *See*
　　Somatosensory impairment
　subcortical disequilibrium, 140–143
　terms used to describe, 142
　treatment of. *See* Gait disorder treatments
　trepidant abasia, 143
　vestibular impairment causing. *See*
　　Vestibular impairment
　without identifiable cause, 153
Gait rehabilitation, 155
Gait tests, 113–114, 138. *See also*
　　Electromyography; Force plates;
　　Kinematics; Kinetics
　digital computers, 125
　laboratories for, 155
　repeatability of, 132
　turns, negotiating, 138
　types of, 124
Gait velocity
　muscle strength and, 386
　resistance training, 382, 391
　stride and cadence determining, 96
Ganglion cysts, 184
Ganglionopathy, 273–274
Get-Up-and-Go Test, 112, 124
Glaucoma, 79

Gout, 182
Guillain-Barré syndrome (GBS), 278

H
Hallux rigidus, 177–178
Hallux valgus, 183, 185–187
    weight shift caused by, 172
Hammertoes, 187–189
Hearing loss affecting balance, 80
Heel spurs, 181
Hemiplegic gait, 140
Hemorrhages
    cerebellar, 230–232
    mesencephalic region, 227
    symptoms of, 268
Hindlimbs
    MLR-induced rhythmical oscillation of,
        65
    stimulation of DTF and VTF areas affecting,
        65
Hip fractures
    annual occurrence of, 3
    death caused by, 15
    mechanics of falls affecting, 28
    obesity protecting against, 28
    prevention of, 322, 409
Hip rotation, 419
Hip strategy, 110
Hospital patients
    fall prevention, 321, 395
    falls, rate of, 16
    falls, risk of, 397
    gait disorders in, 147
Hydrocephalus, 144, 150
    aphasia, evidence of, 247
    brain imaging, 248
    congenital, 247, 256
    predicting surgical outcome for, 246
    rCBF reduction, 249
    risk factors for, 256
    shunt surgery. *See* Shunt surgery
    systemic hypertension, 255
Hypertension
    cerebellar hemorrhage, 231
    hydrocephalus, 255
    posterior tibial tendon rupture caused by,
        179
    prevalence of, 235
    treatment of, 236–237
Hypokinesia
    locomotor ataxia compared, 138
Hysteria, 292–293

J
Joint
    alignment, 332, 344
    deformity, 166

K
Kinematics, 127–130
    accelerometers, 129
    computer-controlled precision cameras,
        129
    errors in, 130
    goniometers, 129
    old and young compared, 98, 382
    repeatability of, 132
    rotation, measurement of, 128
Knees
    extension of, 339, 385
    flexion of, 383
    joint malalignment, 344

L
Labyrinthine function, postural reactions to,
        75
Learning
    difficulties, 347
    postural adjustments improved by, 84
    variability, need for, 347
Leukoaraiosis, 235
Lhermitte's sign, 276
Ligament sprains, 175
Limbs, stimulation of, 65
Limits of stability
    defined, 38–39
    FBOS measuring, 85
Locomotion
    afferent and sensory pathways compared, 74
    automatic and volitional control compared,
        58–62
    bipedal. *See* Bipedal locomotion
    central rhythm generator, 75
    cortical control of. *See* Cerebral cortex
    defined, 137
    pontine-induced changes in. *See* Pontine
        locomotor region
    proprioceptive information. *See*
        Proprioception
    pyramidal tract ablation affecting. *See*
        Pyramidal tracts
    somatic sensation, 74
    spinal cord, role in. *See* Spinal cord
    stimulus site-specific changes in, 69–70

Locomotion (*contd.*)
ventromedial system ablation affecting. *See* Ventromedial systems
volitional and automatic control compared, 58–62
Locomotor ataxia
hypokinesia compared, 138
Locomotor preparation, 62
Long-loop reflexes, 83–84, 235

M
Macular degeneration, 79
Magnetic resonance imaging, 154
Mallet toes, 188
Marche à petits pas. See Short steps
Medications
falls caused by, 24, 303
percentage of prescribed, 30
Mesencephalic locomotor region (MLR)
decerebration, 62–64
GABA antagonists injected into, 62
hemorrhage in, 227
intact central nervous system, 68–71
pontine locomotor region. *See* Pontine locomotor region
stimulation of, 63–65
Mobility Skills Protocol, 113
Motor analysis laboratories, 125, 133, 155
Motor blocks, 210
Motor planning, 334
Moving platforms
EMG responses elicited by, 261–262
muscle coordination, 109
proprioceptive input, 264
sensory input, 264
Muscle mass loss
age-related, 164
balance impaired by, 81
prevalence of, 385
Muscle response
electromyography, 109
old and young compared, 85
vestibular impairment, 265
Muscle spindle syndromes, 277–279
Muscle strengthening, 343
Muscle weakness
age-related, 164
ankle disorders caused by, 168
falls caused by, 23, 310
foot disorders caused by, 166
gait impaired by, 99
gait velocity, 381–385

nutritional inadequacy causing, 30
reversing, 387
Musculoskeletal impairments, 140, 333
Musculoskeletal stiffness, 99
Myelopathy, 148

N
Nerve fibers, loss of, 280
Neurological impairments, 334
Neuropathy
ataxic, 273–276
carcinomatous sensory, 273–274
chronic ataxic sensory, 275
foot disorders caused by, 182–184
idiopathic acute sensory, 275
nitrous oxide-related, 275
peripheral, 152
pyridoxine-related, 275
Nudge Test, 116, 138
Nursing home patients
ambulation, loss of, 3
balance impairment in, 88
fall prevention, 321, 395
falls, rate of, 16
falls, risk of, 397
gait disorders in, 147
morbidity of, 3
resistance training, 388
Nutritional inadequacy, 30

O
Obesity, posterior tibial tendon rupture caused by, 179
Obstacles, negotiating. *See* Environmental hazards causing falls
Olivopontocerebellar atrophies (OPCA), 213
Orthostatic tremor, 216
Osteoarthritis, exercise program for, 348

P
Pain management, 344
Pantalar arthrodesis, 170
Parkinson's Disease
biomechanics of gait, 349
case example of, 330
clinical features of, 209
dementia, 215
drug-induced, 149
exercise program for, 349
falls caused by, 210

gait. *See* Parkinsonian gait
history of, 2
motor blocks, 209
postural adjustment in, 337
prevalence of, 149, 209
retropulsion, 340
rigidity in, 343
standing, preparation for, 94
Parkinsonian gait, 99
disequilibrium, 142
secondary causes of, 214
Pedunculopontine nucleus, 227
Pelvis rotation, 420–422
Pernicious anemia, 276
Perturbations
response to, 83–84, 109, 116
Phobia, 292
Plantar fascia, 172, 181
Plantar fibroma, 184
Pontine locomotor region, 64, 70–71
Pontomesencephalic gait failure, 226
Posterior tibial tendon
rupture, 179
tendinitis of, 181
Postural adjustments
learning improving, 84
old and young compared, 83–84
Parkinson's disease, 337
vestibular impairment, 263
Postural movement control. *See also* Balance;
     Gait
automatic, Automatic postural movements
motor aspects of, 115–117
physiology of, 41–44
sensory aspects of, 45–49, 117–119
voluntary. *See* Voluntary postural movements
Posture. *See also* Balance
cerebellar influences on, 266
COM. *See* Center of mass (COM)
COP. *See* Center of pressure (COP)
labyrinthine function, 75
orientation, 108
proprioception, 75
righting reactions, 136
stimulus site-specific changes in, 69–70
stooped, 99
supporting reactions, 136
tactile input, 75
thalamic. *See* Thalamic movement
visual input affecting, 75
Posturography, 264. *See also* Moving platforms
Presbyopia, 79
Progressive supranuclear palsy (PSP), 213

Proprioception
defined, 74
postural reactions to, 75
Romberg's test for, 138
Proprioceptive impairment, 273–281
Psoriatic arthritis, 182
Psychogenic gait disorders, 153, 289–292
treatment of, 293
Purkinje cells
atrophy of, 99
discharge frequency of, 66
Pyramidal tracts
ablation of, 57–58
ischemia, 238
neurons, discharge patterns of, 60

R
Range of motion
stretching and relaxing compared, 343
Reaction time
changes in, 81
falls caused by slow, 23
Reiter's syndrome, 182
Resistance training
arthritis, 390
balance training, 389
functional loss, 384
gait speed, 384
gait velocity, 382, 391
high intensity, 30
limitations of, 387
nursing home patients, 388
outcomes, 388
walking programs for, 389
Reticulospinal cells
axon collaterals, branching patterns of, 57
hindlimbs activating, 67
neuron discharge of, 65
Rheumatism, 182
Rheumatoid arthritis
ankle disorders caused by, 182
exercise program for, 348
Rigidity
brain stem transection causing, 62
Parkinson's Disease, 343
Romberg's Test, 138, 267
exaggerated sway, 153

S
Safety checklists for fall prevention, 399–400
Scarpa's ganglion nerve cell loss, 100

Senile gait, 216, 284
Sensory ataxia
    cerebellar ataxia compared, 1–2, 143
Sensory impairment
    isolating conditions of, 47, 152
    peripheral, 140
Sensory organization
    defined, 46
    under changing conditions, 48
    with known diseases, 48–49
Sensory Organization Test, 111
Short steps, 2, 144, 210
Shuffling, prevalence of, 2–3
Shunt surgery
    checking shunt function, 253
    complications in, 251–252
    improvement after, 253–255
    patient selection for, 246, 251
    purpose of, 252
Single stance
    ability to maintain, 85
    time measuring, 87
Sitting, 94–96
    base of support for, 95
Sjögren's disease, 274
Somatosensory impairment
    isolating conditions of, 48
    Romberg's test for, 152
Space phobia, 288
Spastic paraparesis, 199
Spinal cord. *See also* specific diseases of
    brain stem functioning together with, 57
    dorsolateral systems. *See* Dorsolateral
        systems
    pyramidal tracts. *See* Pyramidal tracts
    role in locomotion, 55–76
    subcortical pathways, 56
Spinal stepping generator, 75
Spinocerebellar lesions, 266, 269
Sports injuries
    ankle disorders caused by, 188
Stability, limits of. *See* Limits of stability
Stairs, descending, 97
Standing, 94–96
    foam, 118
    Parkinson's disease affecting, 94
    requirements of, 138
    sitting to, 95, 138, 346
Start-hesitation, 93–95, 137, 210
Stasobasophobia, 141
Stepping
    coordinating mechanism for, 74
    disrupted, 138

forward, 93
    newborns, in, 74
    Purkinje cell discharge, 66
    short. *See* Short steps
    step length defined, 162
    strategy, 110
Strength training, 30
Striatonigral degeration (SND), 213
Stride
    defined, 96
    length defined, 162
    performance indicated by, 124
    reduction in, 97
Stroke
    alcohol consumption as risk factor for,
        232
    cerebrovascular disease causing, 221
    ischemic, 268
    lacunar, 231
    postural control affected by, 151
    presentation of, 232
    smoking as risk factor for, 232
Subcortical disequilibrium, 141, 223
Substantia nigra (SN), GABA antagonists
        injected into, 62
Subthalamic locomotor region (SLR)
        stimulation
    decerebration, 61
    intact central nervous system, 68–71
Sway
    backward, 162, 280
    center of gravity determined by, 39
    control of, 136
    falls predicted by, 24
    forward, 162
    measurement of, 82–83, 107
    Romberg's test for. *See* Romberg's
        Test
    tactile-proprioceptive input, 82–83
    visual input affecting, 82–83
    voluntary, 85
Sway Direction Histogram (SDH), 267

T

Tai chi chuan, 375
Tardive dyskinesia, 149
Tendinitis, treatment of, 181
Thalamic astasia, 223–224
Thalamic movement, 60
Thermal sensitivity, loss of
    balance impaired by, 79–80
Timed Up-and-Go Test, 112

Tinetti's Balance and Mobility Scale, 113
    as predictor of falling, 124
Toes
    deformities of, 167, 185–188
Toes-up and toes-down rotation, 84, 262
Turns
    en bloc, 210
    negotiating, 138

V
Vascular diseases, 151
Ventral muscles, contraction of, 93, 95
Ventral tegmented field (VTF)
    hindlimbs controlled by, 65
    stimulation of
        intact central nervous system, 68–71
Ventromedial systems
    ablation of, 56
    dorsolateral systems compared, 57
Vertebrobasilar ischemia, 237
Vertigo, falls caused by, 311
Vestibular hair cell loss, 100
Vestibular impairment
    gait disturbances caused by, 265
    moving platforms. *See* Moving platforms
    muscle response to, 265
    old and young compared, 263
    physiology of, 261
    postural adjustment, 263
    prevalence of, 152
    sensory input, 263
    stance, 263
Vestibular vascular diseases, 229–230
Vestibulocerebellar lesions, 151, 266, 269
Vestibulospinal cell activation, 67–68
Vibratory sensitivity, 80
Video recording of walking, 124–125

Visual impairment
    balance affected by, 79, 100. *See also* eye-
        related diseases, e.g. Glaucoma
    falls caused by, 21
    postural reactions to, 75
    sway affected by, 82–83
Vitamin B12 deficiency, 276
Voluntary postural movements, 44

W
Walking
    biomechanics of, 49
    cadence, 384
    mechanical aids for, 147
    normal, 135–138
    old and young compared, 97, 350
    phases of, 96
    requirements for, 136
    stepping and balance movements in, 49
    straight line heel-to-toe, 138
    toe-floor clearance during, 97
    velocity. *See* Gait velocity
    video recording of, 124–125
Walking velocity. *See* Gait velocity
Wallenberg's syndrome, 229–230
Wheelchairs contributing to falls, 397,
        408
White-matter disease
    cerebellar ataxia compared, 235
    clinical correlates of, 233
    hypertension as risk factor for, 236
    neuroimaging findings, 232
    pathology of, 235
    prevalence of, 233
    risk factors for, 235
    treatment of, 236
Wrist fractures, obesity protecting against, 28